Practical Trends in Anesthesia and Intensive Care 2026

Davide Chiumello • Andrea De Gasperi
Editors

Practical Trends in Anesthesia and Intensive Care 2026

Springer

Editors
Davide Chiumello
Department of Anesthesia and
Intensive Care
ASST Santi Paolo e Carlo, San Paolo
University Hospital
Milan, Italy

Department of Health Sciences
University of Milan
Milan, Italy

Coordinated Research Center
on Respiratory Failure
University of Milan
Milan, Italy

Andrea De Gasperi
Former Director AR2
Ospedale Niguarda Ca' Granda
Milano, Italy

ISBN 978-3-032-25720-8 ISBN 978-3-032-25721-5 (eBook)
https://doi.org/10.1007/978-3-032-25721-5

The original submitted manuscript has been translated into English. The translation was done using artificial intelligence. A subsequent revision was performed by the author(s) to further refine the work and to ensure that the translation is appropriate concerning content and scientific correctness. It may, however, read stylistically different from a conventional translation.

This Springer imprint is published by the registered company Springer Nature Switzerland AG
The registered company address is: Gewerbestrasse 11, 6330 Cham, Switzerland

Foreword

I feel honored to write the foreword for the *Practical Trends in Anesthesia and Intensive Care 2026*. Anesthesia and intensive care are the essential pillars of modern medicine. Together, they make complex and high-risk surgeries feasible, ensuring patient safety and improving survival in life-threatening conditions. Advances in technology, newer drugs, advanced monitoring techniques, and evidence-based protocols have reshaped clinical care and the scope of our services. These advances help reduce complications, shorten recovery time and hospital stay, thereby optimizing healthcare resources.

Being one of the fastest-evolving fields in medicine, rapid updating of knowledge and skills in anesthesia and intensive care is paramount to ensure patient safety and improve outcomes. The Editors have carefully selected the most relevant perioperative and intensive care issues to be addressed, ranging from advances in airway management to cardiorespiratory monitoring of ARDS, including human factor considerations.

The authors of the chapters have done stupendous work in maintaining a fine balance between foundational principles and the latest developments in the field. Importantly, the book provides evidence-based guidance while acknowledging areas of ongoing uncertainty, encouraging the readers to think critically and even challenge dogma. With the synthesis of the updated evidence and practical guidance, the book stands as both a reference and a reflection of the evolving nature of anesthesia and intensive care medicine, making the principles outlined practical, adaptable, and globally relevant.

I congratulate the Editorial team and the authors for putting together this excellent resource. May this book inspire continued excellence in clinical care and research to those entrusted with our care at the most critical moments.

Sheila Nainan Myatra
Department of Anaesthesiology Critical Care and Pain
Tata Memorial Hospital
Mumbai, India

Preface

Keeping pace with the rapidly evolving clinical and technological landscape of modern medicine represents one of the most demanding challenges for clinicians. Physicians involved in anesthesia, perioperative care, and intensive care medicine are required to engage in continuous professional development, integrating into everyday practice advances in basic sciences, surgical frontiers, emerging technologies—including advanced monitoring systems and ventilation modalities—and innovations in pharmacological therapy. These developments, whether or not perceived by the busy practitioner, increasingly shape clinical decision-making, with the ultimate aim of improving patient outcomes and quality of care. The management of complex perioperative patients, critical conditions in emergency and intensive care settings, difficult decisions driven by surgical innovation, and the ethical challenges arising from new medical frontiers are now integral components of anesthesiology and critical care practice. The topics selected for this 2026 edition of *Practical Trends* reflect these evolving needs and include technical innovations, novel monitoring strategies and future perspectives, practical clinical challenges in general and locoregional anesthesia, and updated approaches to cardiac arrest and resuscitation. With this volume, we hope to contribute to continuing medical education in anesthesia and intensive care medicine by providing clinically relevant, evidence-based, and up-to-date insights for practitioners. As nicely emphasized by Prof. Sheila N. Myatra in her Foreword to this book, scientific progress and technological innovation must always remain aligned with patient safety, dignity, and respect. While the challenge for every physician is to continuously advance medical care, the core of the mission is to preserve empathy and an indispensable human touch with patients and their families.

Finally we wish to honor the memory of two outstanding figures, Professor Luciano Gattinoni and Professor Biagio Allaria—brilliant "doctors" who profoundly renewed the care of the critically ill patients. They encouraged physicians to delve deeper into every clinical case, never to accept the first explanation uncritically, and always to look beyond the obvious. Through their intellectual curiosity and scientific activity, they inspired and nurtured generations of clinicians to combine a physiological approach, a clinical rigor, and the enthusiastic passion for teaching. We are grateful for the privilege of having worked with these two *Maestri*.

Milano, Italy — Davide Chiumello
Milano, Italy — Andrea De Gasperi

Contents

Part I

Anesthesia

Hypotension in Anesthesia and in the Critically Ill Patient: Mechanisms and Prevention

1

Marta Iaconi, Laura Cascarano, Dojna Stavri, Maria Vittoria Antonica, and Luigi Tritapepe

1.1 Introduction

Worldwide, more than 300 million patients undergo non-cardiac surgery each year [1]. Postoperative mortality is a public health issue, with rates ranging from 1% to 4% [2, 3]. High-risk patients are more likely to experience perioperative complications and death. Furthermore, patients who have experienced and survived postoperative complications have a shorter life expectancy compared to those without complications [3]. Reducing postoperative complications decreases mortality. Some risk factors are non-modifiable, including those related to the patient or the surgery itself, while others, such as perioperative hypotension, are modifiable risk factors [4]. Perioperative hypotension appears to be strongly associated with a higher incidence of death, myocardial injury, and acute kidney injury (AKI) [2, 5–8].

Perioperative hemodynamic monitoring aims to detect physiological alterations and achieve therapeutic targets that may improve outcomes. Heart rate (HR) and blood pressure (BP) alone are insufficient for this purpose. More advanced and comprehensive monitoring, which measures cardiac output (CO), volume status, and tissue perfusion, assists clinicians in identifying the causes of perioperative hypotension and treating it with fluids and vasoactive drugs. This targeted approach is known as goal-directed therapy (GDT). However, an Italian survey revealed that GDT protocols are implemented by only 29.1% of anesthesiologists [7].

M. Iaconi · L. Cascarano · M. V. Antonica · L. Tritapepe (✉)
Department of Anesthesia and Intensive Care, San Camillo-Forlanini, Rome, Italy
e-mail: miaconi@scamilloforlanini.rm.it; lcascarano@scamilloforlanini.rm.it; mantonica@scamilloforlanini.rm.it; luigi.tritapepe@uniroma1.it

D. Stavri
Residency Program in Anesthesia and Intensive Care, Tor Vergata University, Rome, Italy
e-mail: dstavri@scamilloforlanini.rm.it

D. Chiumello, A. De Gasperi (eds.), *Practical Trends in Anesthesia and Intensive Care 2026*, https://doi.org/10.1007/978-3-032-25721-5_1

1.2 Definition of Hypotension

Blood pressure management is a cornerstone of perioperative anesthetic care, yet the definition of hypotension remains debated [9]. Numerous studies support the need for perioperative blood pressure regulation, but there are no universally accepted blood pressure thresholds to define hypotension. Hypotension is usually defined using absolute or relative thresholds for various blood pressure components and may also include the duration of exposure. Most commonly, hypotension is defined by changes in systolic arterial pressure (SAP), mean arterial pressure (MAP), or a combination of both. Many studies report a MAP <60 mmHg and/or a SAP <90 mmHg as the absolute numerical threshold for defining hypotension. Other studies have used a relative threshold, most often showing a percentage decrease (from 10% to 60%) from baseline MAP or SAP [10]. The incidence of intraoperative hypotension can vary between 5% and 99%, depending on the definition used [2, 11]. For example, a hypotension intraoperative, defined as a MAP <65 mmHg, occurs in 65% of surgeries, while considering a 20% reduction in MAP from baseline, it occurs in 94% of cases [5]. A MAP <65 mmHg is often used to define intraoperative hypotension and as a threshold value for intervention, since MAP values <60–70 mmHg are associated with a higher incidence of myocardial injury, AKI, and death in adults undergoing non-cardiac surgery. However, a single threshold value cannot define intraoperative hypotension without overlooking individual variations in blood pressure; in such cases, the true incidence of this problem may be underestimated, exposing patients to serious risks. Other, more sophisticated definitions take into account the duration of exposure, such as cumulative minutes with MAP <65 mmHg, or the duration and severity of exposure, such as the area under a threshold value, measured in mmHg x minute, which is not immediately applicable [2].

1.3 A Bit of Physiology

Blood pressure (BP) is the product of cardiac output (CO) and systemic vascular resistance (SVR) (Fig. 1.1). Systolic arterial pressure (SAP), mean arterial pressure (MAP), and diastolic arterial pressure (DAP) are its components and represent different phases of the cardiac cycle, with ventricular contraction during systole and relaxation during diastole [3]. SAP is the highest pressure measured in the arterial vessels and is generated by left ventricular contraction. It depends on stroke volume (SV), heart rate (HR), SVR, and the compliance of the aorta and large arteries near the heart. The lowest pressure recorded in the arterial tree is the DAP. DAP is influenced by SVR, vascular compliance, the duration of diastole, and the length of the cardiac cycle. MAP is the average arterial pressure during a cardiac cycle [10]. CO

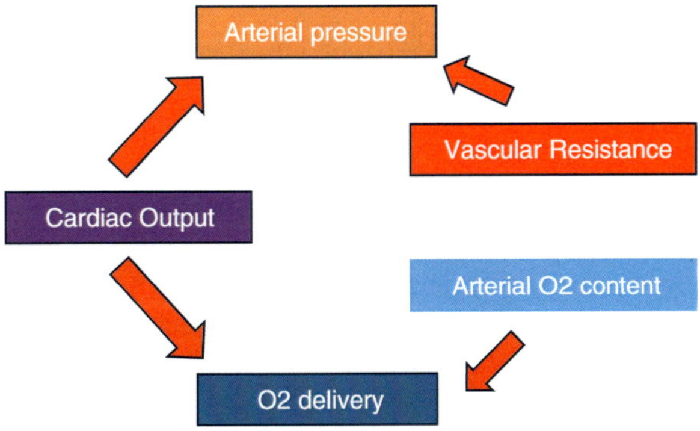

Fig. 1.1 Relationship between cardiac output, hypotension, and tissue hypoxia

assesses cardiac function and is a determinant of oxygen delivery (DO_2) together with arterial oxygen content, as shown by the following formula[1]:

$$DO_2 = CO \times CaO_2$$

$$CaO_2 = (SaO_2 \times Hb \times 1.36) + 0.02 \times PaO_2$$

BP is directly proportional to CO; during hypotensive episodes, tissues will receive a reduced supply of oxygen. The reduction in microcirculatory flow, due to reflex vasoconstriction, may be associated with an increased incidence of postoperative complications. In patients undergoing high-risk surgical procedures, fluids and inotropes may act on the microvascular flow, improving organ perfusion.

At any given SV, the arterial system (resistance, compliance, specific impedance, arterial wave reflection) determines BP by modulating pressure-volume relationships. BP changes according to variations in SV, the arterial system, or both. The cardiovascular system meets the metabolic demands of the body by decreasing or increasing the supply of oxygen and nutrients. Cardiac function, arterial and venous tone, and the metabolic needs of the body interact with each other. During the perioperative period, tissue oxygen demand increases to cope with the increased workload imposed on the body. If the patient is unable to increase cardiac output, tissues do not receive the required oxygen supply, resulting in dysfunction and tissue hypoxia. This creates an oxygen debt that leads to increased postoperative complications and mortality [3, 5, 10].

The Frank-Starling law describes how the heart is able to accommodate incoming blood and then eject it. An increase in preload increases the distensibility of cardiac myocytes, lengthening the sarcomere and enhancing contractile force, resulting in a greater volume of blood ejected. The venous system serves as a blood reservoir that can be directed to the heart according to the body's needs, as the majority of blood volume, about 70% of the total, is contained within it. Under steady-state conditions, CO and venous return are identical. Venous return and

[1] SaO_2 arterial oxygen saturation, 1.36 oxygen-carrying capacity of Hb, Hb hemoglobin, 0.03 oxygen solubility coefficient, PaO_2 arterial partial pressure of oxygen.

changes in venous tone support CO. We can deduce that any changes in venous return and venous tone will affect the left ventricular CO and thus systemic hemodynamics.

1.4 Anesthesia and Hypotension

During surgical procedures, various factors act on the venous system, leading to a reduction in CO and BP. General anesthesia causes: myocardial depression, reduced vascular tone in both arteries and veins, decreased CO, and hypotension. The use of intermittent positive pressure ventilation reduces venous return and increases right ventricular (RV) afterload, decreasing CO and BP. The opposite occurs during expiration. The magnitude of this variation is proportional to the degree of preload dependence of the patient. If the heart is operating on the flat portion of the Frank-Starling curve (Fig. 1.2), the pulse pressure variation (PPV) and stroke volume variation (SVV) volume (SVV) are low, whereas if the heart is operating on the ascending portion of the Frank-Starling curve, PPV and SVV increase [3, 7].

Pulsatile arterial flow, resulting from the intermittent nature of cardiac output, is modulated by the vascular tone of resistance arterioles to maintain arterial pressure (AP) at levels suitable for the capillary lumen. Precapillary arterioles, through vasoconstriction, regulate capillary blood flow and organ perfusion. When pressure values decrease, the tone of arterioles and capillaries diminishes to increase blood flow reaching the organ. The mediators of these mechanisms are induced by tissue hypoxia and produced at the endothelial level. Tissue ischemia, regardless of AP, reduces arteriolar tone in the affected tissues. The body centrally controls AP and autoregulates organ blood flow according to specific metabolic demands. An increase in oxygen demand is associated with heightened sympathetic tone, which directs blood flow from less active tissues (skin and muscles) to more vital organs (heart, kidneys, and brain). Increased venous tone enhances venous return. The result is a rise in AP. When AP remains above a certain threshold, these mechanisms

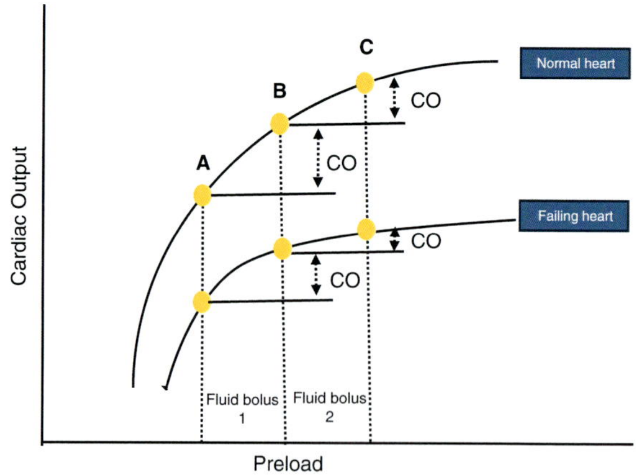

Fig. 1.2 Frank-Starling curve, fluid responsiveness

are preserved, ensuring adequate organ blood flow; when AP falls below this threshold, autoregulation is lost. At this point, blood flow to various organs becomes dependent on perfusion pressure, as there is widespread peripheral vasodilation in an attempt to compensate for the abrupt reduction in blood flow. The kidneys and brain are the organs with the most robust autoregulation [2, 3].

AP is regulated by several interrelated systems operating over the short and long term; specifically, baroreceptors at the level of the aortic arch and carotid sinus, and the renin-angiotensin-aldosterone system, which regulates blood volume. Baroreceptors in the carotid sinus and aortic arch transmit impulses to the autonomic nervous system with every change in blood pressure to maintain it within normal values, inducing arterial vasoconstriction or vasodilation. In fact, pressure-sensitive receptors are also located in the atria, ventricles, and pulmonary parenchyma, all contributing to this function [2, 3].

1.5 Mean Arterial Pressure (MAP)

MAP is used as a surrogate for organ perfusion pressure, although they are not the same. Central arterial pressure is not the same as organ perfusion pressure: the latter is the difference between inflow and outflow pressures. Inflow pressure may be lower than MAP, a condition that occurs when arterial resistance is high. The pressure in the hepatic artery is 20% lower than MAP because the hepatic vascular bed has high resistance. Blood flow in the coronary arteries occurs during diastole, while during systole, myocardial contraction interrupts circulation; therefore, coronary artery pressure is similar to diastolic pressure. Outflow pressure in the brain may be either intracranial pressure or the pressure in the venous circulation of the head, depending on which is higher. For the left ventricle, it will be either the diastolic pressure of the left ventricle itself or that in the right atrium, whichever is higher. In abdominal organs, it will be either intra-abdominal pressure or central venous pressure (CVP), depending on which is higher. For the kidneys, it will be intra-abdominal pressure, CVP, or intracapsular pressure, whichever is highest. All these forms of vis a tergo can vary under pathological conditions; defining a MAP threshold does not guarantee adequate perfusion pressure in different organs. In practice, MAP is a clinically available surrogate for perfusion pressure, but it must always be interpreted in light of organ-specific outflow pressure [2, 3, 11, 10]. In healthy individuals, cerebral blood flow is maintained constant for MAP values between 60 and 160 mmHg. Within 70–130 mmHg, renal blood flow is maximal; thus, glomerular filtration is optimal within this pressure range. Myocardial blood flow is autoregulated within certain limits of coronary perfusion pressure (CoPP), although myocardial perfusion is not maintained at a constant value; instead, it is adapted to the current myocardial O_2 demand. Although autoregulation of blood flow protects the brain, heart, and kidneys from hypoperfusion due to hypotension, AP is almost entirely responsible for the perfusion of other organs, particularly splanchnic organs such as the stomach, liver, and pancreas, which have a low capacity for autoregulation of blood flow [10]. In the presence of marked hypotension,

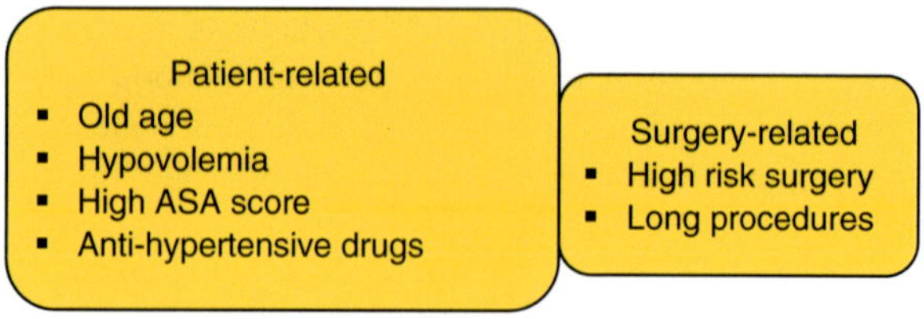

Fig. 1.3 Predictive factors for perioperative hypotension

local vasodilation can increase flow only if inflow pressure is adequate; if cardiac output is insufficient, this reflex will not meet the metabolic demands of the organs. Systemic hypotension is always a pathological event, as it results from the failure of regulatory systems to maintain adequate organ perfusion.

Blood pressure in healthy individuals varies significantly throughout the day, although it can be maintained within certain parameters. Patients undergoing surgery and the critically ill are more predisposed to experiencing marked hypotension (Fig. 1.3). Intraoperative hypotension in patients undergoing non-cardiac surgery under general anesthesia has been associated with a higher risk of postoperative mortality, myocardial injury after non-cardiac surgery (MINS), myocardial infarction, cardiogenic shock, acute kidney injury, delirium, and stroke [10].

Predictive factors for perioperative hypotension are related to the patient or the surgery, as shown in Fig. 1.3 [10, 12]. In elderly patients, a MAP <65 mmHg is strongly associated with postoperative death. Emergency procedures, high ASA scores, COPD, and general anesthesia further increase this risk. Admission to the PACU (post-anesthesia care unit), on the other hand, is a protective factor [12].

1.6 Hypotension and Perioperative Risk

The latest SIAARTI guidelines on perioperative hemodynamic management in patients undergoing non-cardiac surgery recommend the use of a risk stratification score/system, in particular the LEE index, developed to predict major adverse postoperative cardiovascular events, and the scoring system derived from the American College of Surgeons National Surgical Quality Improvement Program (ACS NSQIP) database, which, after entering the type of surgical procedure and 21 patient-related variables online, calculates the probability of mortality and morbidity. These scores can help us identify the most vulnerable patients and determine their perioperative management pathway [7].

In the perioperative period, it is recommended to continue therapy with betablockers and calcium channel blockers, while the use of ACE inhibitors and sartans (ACE-Is/ARBs) remains controversial. Their use may exacerbate intraoperative hypotension and prolong it throughout the perioperative period. There is no consensus among international guidelines on whether to continue or discontinue them. The European Society of Cardiology and the European Society of Anaesthesiology recommend discontinuing ACE-Is/ARBs 24 h before surgery if used for hypertension, and continuing them if prescribed for heart failure or left ventricular dysfunction.

Furthermore, if these latter patients are not taking ACE-Is/ARBs prior to surgery, the recommendations advise starting them 1 week before the surgical procedure. Intraoperative hypotension occurs in patients under both general and neuraxial anesthesia. The causes of perioperative hypotension are illustrated in Fig. 1.4 [10].

About one-third of perioperative hypotensive episodes occur in the period following induction of general anesthesia but before surgical incision and can be described as post-induction or pre-incision hypotension. While post-induction hypotension is caused exclusively by anesthesia management, hypotension occurring during surgery may be due to numerous factors related to both general anesthesia and the surgical procedure. Hypotension may, among other factors, be caused by vasodilation (anesthetic drugs, systemic inflammation), intravascular hypovolemia (bleeding), low cardiac output (bradycardia or low stroke volume), high intrathoracic pressure (mechanical ventilation), impairment of the sympathetic nervous system, or compromised baroreflex regulation [11].

The type of surgical procedure, together with various surgery-related events (e.g., changes in patient positioning, arterial clamping, bleeding), helps define the optimal blood pressure for an individual patient at a given time. For example, in patients undergoing surgery in the beach chair position, differences in hydrostatic pressure between the level of the heart and the level of the brain should be taken into account [2].

In patients with essential arterial hypertension, the reduction in organ blood flow occurs at higher MAP levels compared to healthy subjects, as the critical threshold for autoregulation is higher (Fig. 1.5). These patients may be more exposed to renal injury, stroke, and myocardial infarction, with a threshold value of MAP <65 mmHg. In these patients, postoperative mortality and the incidence of complications are higher for MAP values between 45 and 75 mmHg, even for shorter exposure times compared to patients without this condition [3, 5].

The INPRESS study, conducted in major surgery, is currently the only trial that has compared hemodynamic management of patients based on a generic intraoperative hypotension threshold value with hemodynamic management based on a patient-specific blood pressure threshold. In this multicenter study, patients in the standard treatment group received boluses of ephedrine for any SBP < 80 mmHg or less than 40% of the patient's resting SBP. Patients in the personalized treatment group received a continuous infusion of norepinephrine during surgery and for 4 h

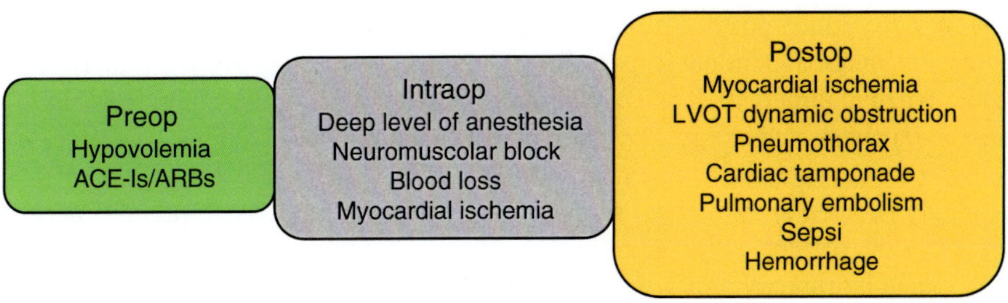

Fig. 1.4 The perioperative causes of hypotension

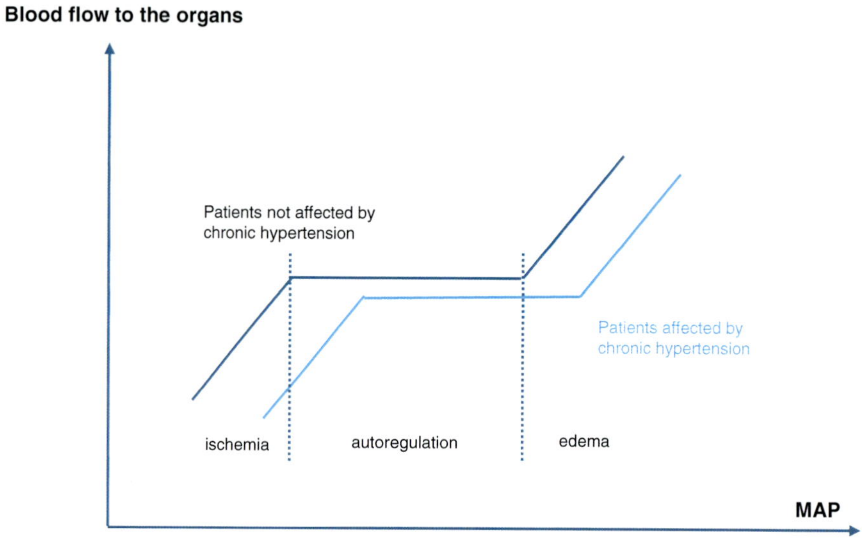

Fig. 1.5 Autoregulation of organ blood flow in normotensive and hypertensive patients

postoperatively, to maintain SBP within 10% of the baseline reference value. The use of personalized SBP values significantly reduced the risk of postoperative organ dysfunction. However, the INPRESS study has several limitations, including the use of two different drugs in the two study groups and the determination of baseline blood pressure values based on single, non-standardized measurements. A personalized blood pressure threshold could be key to a more appropriate approach for each individual patient undergoing surgery under general anesthesia. Blood pressure measured in the outpatient setting, rather than the day before surgery in the surgical ward or even before induction of anesthesia, appears to be a good method for defining the baseline blood pressure value. However, the timing, setting, and optimal technique for ambulatory blood pressure monitoring remain unclear [2, 4, 11].

1.7 Perioperative Optimization

The SIAARTI guidelines suggest adopting a GDT protocol for hemodynamic management to reduce postoperative mortality and morbidity in non-cardiac surgery, especially major abdominal surgery. The fundamental principle of GDT is to achieve hemodynamic targets such as DO_2, stroke volume/cardiac output, fluid responsiveness parameters, and oxygenation parameters, such as central venous oxygen saturation ($ScvO_2$), oxygen extraction ratio (O_2 ER), and lactate levels, which are typically pursued at the start of surgery and maintained in the postoperative period based on the patient's clinical condition. Measurement of central venous pressure (CVP) and pulmonary artery occlusion pressure (PAOP) (static parameters) is performed using a pulmonary artery catheter (PAC), which may expose patients to

Table 1.1 Limitations of dynamic variables

Clinical condition	Results
RR/RR < 3.6	*False negatives*
Arrhythmias	*False positives*
TV < 8 ml/kg IBW (ideal body weight)	*False negatives*
Abdominal hypertension	*False positives*
Open chest	*False negatives*
Spontaneous respiratory efforts	*False negatives and false positives*

complications related to placement and intravascular permanence. Moreover, CVP and PAOP accurately guide fluid therapy in only 50% of patients. Recent European guidelines on perioperative hemorrhage management clearly recommend avoiding the use of central venous pressure and pulmonary artery occlusion pressure as the sole variables to guide fluid therapy and preload optimization during severe hemorrhage, favoring dynamic assessment of fluid responsiveness (Table 1.1) and non-invasive measurement of cardiac output. However, dynamic variables have limitations that must be considered [7].

1.8 Blood Pressure Measurement

SIAARTI emphasizes the importance of avoiding hypotensive episodes with MAP <65 mmHg and using continuous (invasive and non-invasive) blood pressure monitoring; in particular, invasive blood pressure monitoring is recommended in high-risk patients to obtain oximetric and metabolic parameters [7]. The common approaches for measuring blood pressure are the intermittent non-invasive oscillometric method and continuous methods, both invasive intra-arterial and non-invasive using a finger cuff (volume clamp method). The intermittent oscillometric method is the most widely used but the least accurate and reliable: it performs measurements every 3–5 min; its performance depends on the selection of cuff size relative to limb circumference; at low pressures, its performance is poor. Continuous invasive blood pressure measurement via intra-arterial cannula remains the clinical gold standard. Complications after placement of radial, brachial, and femoral cannulas, such as ischemia, major bleeding, or infections, are rare. Radial artery pressure may overestimate central pressure due to pulse pressure amplification during wave propagation from the heart to the periphery, except in septic patients treated with vasopressors, liver transplant patients, and in cardiac surgery, where radial blood pressure measurement may be underestimated. The transducer must be zeroed and positioned at the level of the right atrium, the arterial waveform must be free of artifacts, and the dynamic response of the catheter/tubing/transducer must be adequate (damping). Blood pressure measurement via intravascular arterial catheter detects twice as many hypotensive episodes and triggers one third more vasopressor boluses compared to intermittent oscillometric measurements. The non-invasive finger cuff method, which uses the volume clamp technique—also known as vascular unloading technology—enables continuous monitoring without an intra-arterial catheter. These systems use finger cuffs equipped with an infrared photodiode and a light detector to estimate, via plethysmography, the blood volume in the digital arteries and its changes during the cardiac cycle. The system controls the finger cuff to maintain a constant blood volume in the digital arteries. The arterial flow curve is reconstructed from the cuff pressure required to maintain the blood volume in the digital arteries. A prerequisite is that blood flow in the fingers is pulsatile; therefore, this method cannot be used in cases of shock or with high doses of vasopressors. Studies comparing these techniques to the arterial catheter have yielded heterogeneous results, but in a pilot study, it proved superior to oscillometric measurement [2, 3].

1.9 Prevention of Hypotension

Anesthesia professionals regularly assess changes in blood pressure and attempt to predict when patients will become hypotensive. Intraoperative hypotension cannot be predicted based on patient characteristics or surgical procedure, which may be considered potential risk factors. Continuous arterial pressure monitoring can help us detect hypotensive episodes. Given the strong association between intraoperative hypotension and increased incidence of death, myocardial injury, and AKI, new scientific technologies have focused on enabling the anesthesiologist/intensivist to predict hypotensive episodes. A recent development is an artificial intelligence (AI) algorithm, developed through machine learning, that predicts an impending hypotensive episode from a complex analysis of the arterial waveform obtained via intra-arterial catheter or non-invasive monitoring. Machine learning involves the practical application of statistical techniques. Preventing hypotension, treating it, or both, is the application of this technology [2, 13]. Blood pressure management is guided by an index ranging from 0 to 100; a value equal to or greater than 85 alerts us 5–15 min before the hypotensive episode occurs. In addition, the system provides calculated secondary variables that allow us to assess preload (dynamic preload variables such as SVV and PPV), afterload (dynamic arterial elastance Ea_{dyn} given by the PPV/SVV ratio), and contractility (dP/dt_{max}), i.e., information necessary to determine the most appropriate treatment and to be integrated with other available clinical data [6, 8, 10, 14]. The algorithm was trained on arterial pressure waveforms from 1334 surgical or critically ill patients and externally validated in 204 surgical patients, demonstrating a sensitivity of 88% and a specificity of 87% in predicting hypotension 15 min before the event [2]. Naturally, the algorithm cannot predict hypotension resulting from clinical interventions, including hypotension caused by pressure on major vessels by surgeons or changes in patient positioning, such as reverse Trendelenburg [2]. The AI algorithm predicts an outcome based on statistical data from the literature, which is subject to considerable uncertainty, as evidenced by the numerous definitions of perioperative hypotension. At the same time, we know that low blood pressure values are associated with organ damage and death, so predicting and preventing a harmful event has potential in clinical practice. Further studies are needed to support such monitoring and its applicability in clinical practice, with a tangible improvement in patient prognosis [13].

1.10 Outcome

Roshanov et al. analyzed, in a retrospective study, the relationship between perioperative hypotension and perioperative cardiovascular events in patients with risk factors or a history of coronary artery disease undergoing major non-cardiac surgery. The study showed that hypotension was an independent risk factor for myocardial infarction or cardiovascular death, regardless of the presence or degree of coronary artery disease diagnosed by coronary CT [15]. Myocardial infarction and myocardial injury after non-cardiac surgery (MINS) appear to be due to a mismatch between oxygen supply and demand rather than plaque rupture as occurs preoperatively. Myocardial infarction is defined by elevated troponin levels and symptoms or signs of myocardial ischemia. MINS is defined by elevated troponin and includes both myocardial infarction and any other ischemic myocardial injury not meeting the definition of myocardial infarction. More than 90% of MINS and myocardial infarction cases occur within the first 2 postoperative days, and more than 90% are asymptomatic. Mortality among patients with elevated troponin without symptoms is almost as high as in symptomatic patients. In the absence of routine troponin screening, many cases of asymptomatic myocardial injury go undetected. A reasonable strategy would be to measure troponin preoperatively and for the first three postoperative days. From the VISION cohort study, postoperative hypotension is more strongly associated with myocardial infarction and/or death compared to intraoperative hypotension [14].

A retrospective study demonstrated an association between intraoperative hypotension, AKI, and postoperative myocardial injury. The risk of renal and myocardial injury was significantly increased with intraoperative MAP values below 55–60 mmHg. An intraoperative MAP <55 mmHg, even for a short duration (e.g., 1–5 min), was associated with AKI and myocardial injury, and the likelihood of these organ injuries increased with longer periods spent below this threshold [11]. Gregory et al. observed that a decrease in MAP <75 mmHg significantly increased the risk of requiring renal replacement therapy or dialysis, with a further increase in risk for every 5 mmHg decrease in MAP [1]. AKI is common after non-cardiac surgery, with stage II–III occurring in up to 1% of patients and up to 7.4% when including stage I. Exposure to a MAP <55 mmHg for less than 5 min is associated with an 18% increased risk of AKI. These studies confirm that both the degree and duration of hypotension are strongly associated with AKI [14]. The incidence of AKI after non-cardiac surgery, depending on the study, ranges from 2.9% to 57.4% based on the procedure. Approximately 0.3% of patients require postoperative dialysis. The etiology of AKI is multifactorial, but there is strong evidence that ischemia and hypoxia are the major factors. The kidney is at risk because the lower limit of autoregulation of renal blood flow is higher, similar to that of the brain. The perioperative MAP threshold value is still under discussion, but intervention to increase MAP is currently the best therapeutic approach to prevent or treat intraoperative hypotension [16].

Delirium is a common complication of cardiac surgery; in non-cardiac surgery, its incidence is about 10% and increases with age. The pathophysiology of delirium is multifactorial and likely includes inadequate cerebral perfusion. The threshold for cerebral autoregulation is unclear: it appears to be around 85 mmHg, but there is wide interindividual variability. Hypotension is associated with delirium and cognitive decline, but the data in the literature, especially for non-cardiac surgery, are inconsistent. Blood pressure fluctuations, rather than a relative or absolute blood pressure value, seem to be implicated in its onset. Perioperative hypotension, both intra- and postoperative, appears to increase the risk of delirium [14, 17]. The few studies in the literature have not shown a significant correlation between perioperative hypotension and the incidence of stroke, but the data remain inconsistent [17]. Gregory et al. reported a statistically significant correlation between hypotension and major adverse cardiac and cerebrovascular events, such as AMI or acute ischemic stroke (MACCE) [1].

1.11 Treatment of Hypotension

Based on the analysis of the literature, to prevent organ damage, it is important to anticipate hemodynamic changes through continuous monitoring of hemodynamic variables. Since perioperative hypotension has multiple causes, treatment should focus on the underlying causal mechanisms to the extent that they can be identified. This may include reducing the dose of vasodilatory anesthetics, treating vasodilation with vasopressors, increasing blood flow with inotropes, increasing heart rate with atropine, or treating intravascular hypovolemia with crystalloids, colloids, or blood products. At present, it remains unclear which vasopressors and types of fluids are most appropriate for perioperative hypotension [2].

Fluid administration should be guided by careful monitoring. Neither liberal nor restrictive fluid management has been shown to improve patient outcomes. Excessive fluid administration is associated with tissue edema, coagulation abnormalities, acidosis, and pulmonary edema. Excessive restriction, on the other hand, can lead to hypovolemia and hypoperfusion with oxygen debt (Fig. 1.6). SIAARTI recommendations suggest achieving a near-zero fluid balance in patients considered normovolemic at the start of surgery. A slightly positive fluid balance may be allowed in the first 24 h postoperatively to protect renal function [7].

Vasopressors are commonly used to treat hypotension during surgery. Phenylephrine is most commonly used in the United States, while norepinephrine is preferred in other countries. The former is a pure alpha-agonist, which increases blood pressure by raising vascular resistance, at the expense of a decrease in cardiac

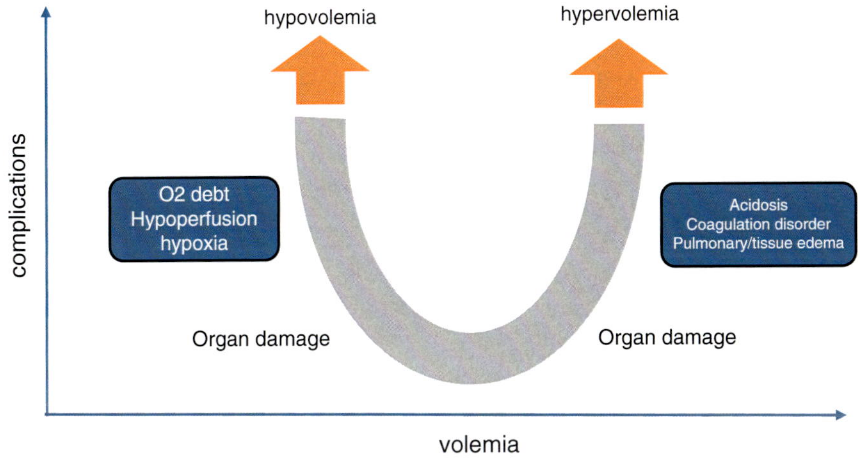

Fig. 1.6 Association between fluid therapy and postoperative complications

output. The latter is both a potent alpha-adrenergic agonist and a weak beta-adrenergic agonist, which should partially preserve cardiac output. Blood pressure is maintained by both agents, but phenylephrine reduces splanchnic blood flow and oxygen delivery (DO_2). Norepinephrine has not been shown to improve outcomes in surgical patients, despite the theoretical preservation of splanchnic circulation and DO_2 [14]. .Vasopressin is used as a second-line vasopressor in patients refractory to norepinephrine and to reduce the dosage of the latter, keeping it within a safe range. However, its efficacy and safety as a first-line agent are becoming increasingly evident, especially in vasoplegic syndrome after cardiac surgery and in septic shock. The use of vasopressin instead of norepinephrine in these cases appears to reduce the incidence of mortality or postoperative complications such as AKI [16]. The use of vasopressors and inotropes in the perioperative period to control blood pressure fluctuations, according to a recent review, seems to reduce postoperative complications and hospital length of stay in adults undergoing major abdominal surgery [17]. SIAARTI recommends the use of inotropic agents, vasoconstrictors, and vasodilators only when fluids alone are insufficient to optimize hemodynamics and increase $SV/CO/DO_2$ [7].

Inotropes are used to increase cardiac contractility and heart rate, thereby increasing cardiac output. They should be administered with awareness of potential adverse effects (increased myocardial O_2 consumption, arrhythmias, peripheral hypoperfusion, and, in the case of inodilators, vasodilation) and always guided by advanced hemodynamic monitoring. Adrenaline and dobutamine act as beta-adrenoceptor agonists. Other agents have a lusitropic effect, promoting ventricular relaxation during diastole. These are called inodilators; one example is levosimendan, which also has a vasodilatory effect [16].

1.12 Conclusions

Perioperative hypotension is associated with an increased risk of death, AKI, and myocardial injury. Following major surgical procedures, more than 30% of patients experience postoperative complications [7]. Perioperative hypotension is linked to longer hospital stays and higher healthcare costs [18]. There is no consensus in the scientific community on the definition of perioperative hypotension due to the heterogeneity of studies. A MAP threshold value below 65 mmHg, careful assessment of comorbidities that may modify this value, knowledge of patient- and surgery-related risk factors, and continuous blood pressure monitoring during the perioperative period may reduce the incidence of perioperative hypotension and the onset of postoperative complications that increase mortality. The use of advanced hemodynamic monitoring within GDT protocols in high-risk patients may improve outcomes.

For the treatment of hypotensive episodes, fluids, vasoconstrictors, and/or inotropes are available. Their use should be guided by careful analysis of hemodynamic variables, weighing the cost/benefit ratio. Predicting hypotensive episodes using artificial intelligence systems could improve perioperative hemodynamic management, but further studies are needed. Postoperative hypotension remains an underestimated problem due to inadequate monitoring in wards, but it also significantly affects mortality and postoperative complications [4, 14]. Randomized clinical trials are needed to confirm the data available in the literature.

References

1. Gregory A, Stapelfeldt WH, Khanna AK, Smischney NJ, Boero IJ, Chen Q, Stevens M, Shaw AD. Intraoperative hypotension is associated with adverse clinical outcomes after noncardiac surgery. Anesth Analg. 2021;132(6):1654–65. https://doi.org/10.1213/ANE.0000000000005250. PMID: 33177322; PMCID: PMC8115733.
2. Saugel B, Sessler DI. Perioperative blood pressure management. Anesthesiology. 2021;134(2):250–61. https://doi.org/10.1097/ALN.0000000000003610. PMID: 33206118.
3. Pinsky MR, Teboul JL, Vincent JL. Hemodynamic monitoring, Intensive Care Lessons. Antonio Delfino Editore; 2023.
4. Hoppe P, Kouz K, Saugel B. Perioperative hypotension: clinical impact, diagnosis, and therapeutic approaches. J Emerg Crit Care Med. 2019;4 https://doi.org/10.21037/jeccm.2019.10.12.
5. Wijnberge M, Schenk J, Bulle E, Vlaar AP, Maheshwari K, Hollmann MW, Binnekade JM, Geerts BF, Veelo DP. Association of intraoperative hypotension with postoperative morbidity and mortality: systematic review and meta-analysis. BJS Open. 2021;5(1):zraa018. https://doi.org/10.1093/bjsopen/zraa018. PMID: 33609377; PMCID: PMC7893468.
6. Vos JJ, Scheeren TWL. Intraoperative hypotension and its prediction. Indian J Anaesth. 2019;63(11):877–85. https://doi.org/10.4103/ija.IJA_624_19. Epub 2019 Nov 8. PMID: 31772395; PMCID: PMC6868662.
7. Italian Society of Anesthesia, Analgesia, Resuscitation and Intensive Care. Guidelines for perioperative hemodynamic management in adult patients undergoing non-cardiac surgery. SIAARTI; 2022. p. 1–42.

8. Szrama J, Gradys A, Bartkowiak T, Woźniak A, Kusza K, Molnar Z. Intraoperative hypotension prediction—a proactive perioperative hemodynamic management—a literature review. Medicina. 2023;59(3):491.
9. Wesselink EM, Kappen TH, Torn HM, Slooter AJC, van Klei WA. Intraoperative hypotension and the risk of postoperative adverse outcomes: a systematic review. Br J Anaesth. 2018;121(4):706–21. https://doi.org/10.1016/j.bja.2018.04.036. Epub 2018 Jun 20. PMID: 30236233.
10. Guarracino F, Bertini P. Perioperative hypotension: causes and remedies. J Anesth Analg Crit Care. 2022;17 https://doi.org/10.1186/s44158-022-00045-8.
11. Kouz K, Hoppe P, Briesenick L, Saugel B. Intraoperative hypotension: pathophysiology, clinical relevance, and therapeutic approaches. Indian J Anaesth. 2020;64(2):90–6. https://doi.org/10.4103/ija.IJA_939_19. Epub 2020 Feb 4. PMID: 32139925; PMCID: PMC7017666.
12. Zhao B, Chen X, Chen Q, Li G, Chen Z, Yang Z, Gu L, Xiao X, Wang Z, Ning J, Yi B, Lu K, Zhang H, Gu J. Intraoperative hypotension and related risk factors for postoperative mortality after noncardiac surgery in elderly patients: a retrospective analysis report. Clin Interv Aging. 2021;16:1757–67. https://doi.org/10.2147/CIA.S327311. PMID: 34621121; PMCID: PMC8491785.
13. Kappen T, Beattie WS. Perioperative hypotension 2021: a contrarian view. Br J Anaesth. 2021;127(2):167–70. https://doi.org/10.1016/j.bja.2021.03.015. Epub 2021 Apr 24. PMID: 33902915.
14. Daniel M, Sessler I. Perioperative hypotension. Anesthesia Patient Safety Foundation; 2021.
15. Roshanov PS, Sheth T, Duceppe E, Tandon V, Bessissow A, Chan MTV, Butler C, Chow BJW, Khan JS, Devereaux PJ. Relationship between perioperative hypotension and perioperative cardiovascular events in patients with coronary artery disease undergoing major noncardiac surgery. Anesthesiology. 2019;130(5):756–66. https://doi.org/10.1097/ALN.0000000000002654. PMID: 30870165.
16. Lankadeva YR, May CN, Bellomo R, Evans RG. Role of perioperative hypotension in postoperative acute kidney injury: a narrative review. Br J Anaesth. 2022;128(6):931–48. https://doi.org/10.1016/j.bja.2022.03.002. Epub 2022 Apr 22. PMID: 35465952.
17. Lizano-Díez I, Poteet S, Burniol-Garcia A, Cerezales M. The burden of perioperative hypertension/hypotension: a systematic review. PLoS One. 2022;17(2):e0263737. https://doi.org/10.1371/journal.pone.0263737. PMID: 35139104; PMCID: PMC8827488.
18. Stapelfeldt WH, Khanna AK, Shaw AD, Shenoy AV, Hwang S, Stevens M, Smischney NJ. Association of perioperative hypotension with subsequent greater healthcare resource utilization. J Clin Anesth. 2021;75:110516. https://doi.org/10.1016/j.jclinane.2021.110516. Epub 2021 Sep 15. PMID: 34536719.

Perioperative Hemodynamic Optimization

2

Sabino Scolletta

2.1 Introduction

Perioperative hemodynamic optimization is a strategy aimed at improving outcomes in patients undergoing surgical procedures, especially major surgeries, through the monitoring and active management of hemodynamic parameters. This approach focuses on maintaining adequate tissue perfusion and oxygenation, thereby preventing complications such as organ ischemia, infections, and multiple organ failure. The objectives of perioperative hemodynamic optimization, therefore, include stabilization of cardiac output and organ perfusion, as well as optimization of oxygen delivery. The key elements of perioperative hemodynamic optimization are the use of advanced hemodynamic monitoring, targeted fluid management, and the use of inotropic and vasopressor support. The various steps of perioperative hemodynamic optimization involve the preoperative phase, with correction of hypovolemia or pre-existing anemia; the intraoperative phase, with continuous hemodynamic monitoring to adjust volume status, cardiac output, and vascular tone for optimal circulatory conditions, using individualized protocols to avoid prolonged arterial hypotension; and finally, the postoperative phase, with continued monitoring in high-risk patients in step-down or intensive care and correction of any residual imbalances. The benefits of perioperative hemodynamic optimization include reduced postoperative complications, improved patient functional recovery, shorter hospital stays, and improved survival in high-risk patients.

S. Scolletta (✉)
Emergency-Urgency Department - Unit of Anesthesia and Intensive Care, Trauma and Organ Failure, Siena University Hospital – Santa Maria alle Scotte, Siena, Italy
e-mail: sabino.scolletta@unisi.it

D. Chiumello, A. De Gasperi (eds.), *Practical Trends in Anesthesia and Intensive Care 2026*, https://doi.org/10.1007/978-3-032-25721-5_2

2.2 Perioperative Hemodynamic Optimization

Scientific literature from the past 15 years has shown that overall perioperative mortality is approximately 4%, that high-risk surgical patients account for about 20% of the surgical population, but that this group contributes to the highest incidence of perioperative complications and mortality and to 80% of hospital costs [1].

Surgical intervention can induce a significant systemic inflammatory response that varies according to the patient's condition, the urgency of the surgical intervention, the type of procedure, and any potential volume of blood loss. Furthermore, perioperative physiological changes can lead to redistribution of body fluids, electrolyte imbalances, and significant metabolic alterations. Anesthetic procedures may cause arterial hypotension due to drug-induced peripheral vasodilation and reduced cardiac function, while the use of neuraxial anesthesia can result in vasodilation and, in more severe cases, persistent vasoplegia that is poorly responsive to treatment [2] (Fig. 2.1).

One of the most feared perioperative complications is low cardiac output syndrome, defined by the presence of a systolic blood pressure < 90 mmHg, a cardiac index <2.0 l/min/m^2, and signs and symptoms of tissue hypoperfusion due to reduced oxygen delivery to the tissues and an imbalance between oxygen delivery and consumption [3]. Moreover, the hemodynamic status of the surgical patient, especially those at high perioperative risk, can change rapidly; therefore, the use of perioperative hemodynamic monitoring can enable the anesthesiologist to estimate oxygen delivery and optimize it, implementing the best anesthetic management.

The assessment of tissue oxygen delivery is, in most cases, based on indirect and nonspecific signs, such as the occurrence of arterial hypotension, decreased urine output, the presence of cold and mottled skin, a positive capillary refill test, increased serum lactate levels, and, in the awake patient, changes in neurological status.

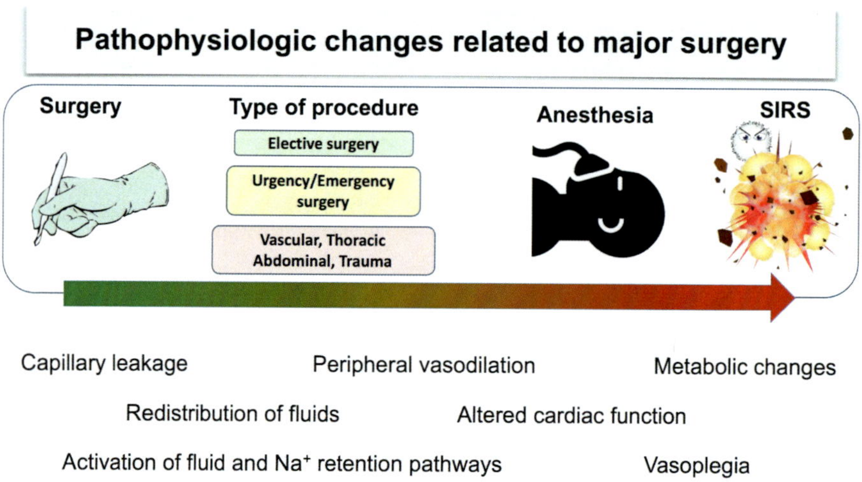

Fig. 2.1 Pathophysiologic changes related to major surgery

In high-risk surgical patients, "standard" vital signs, such as blood pressure and heart rate, which are routinely monitored in any type of surgical procedure using multiparametric systems, may not be sufficiently sensitive to guide the anesthesiologist toward a personalized pharmacological treatment, as these variables may remain stable even when intraoperative blood loss or fluid shifts result in a 30% reduction in circulating volume. Therefore, although these vital signs are essential, simple, and immediate for basic hemodynamic monitoring, their changes should primarily be interpreted as "alerts" for the anesthesiologist, who should then pay attention to other cardiovascular parameters and more advanced monitors, integrating the information obtained to estimate tissue oxygen delivery and consumption and to initiate appropriate treatment. This approach allows the clinician to optimize perioperative hemodynamics and ensure adequate organ perfusion for the patient [4].

Since oxygen delivery is determined by cardiac output and arterial oxygen content (the latter derived from arterial oxygen saturation and hemoglobin levels), it cannot be simply and indirectly estimated from blood pressure; rather, it requires not only the measurement of heart rate but also the calculation of stroke volume, which can only be obtained using more advanced hemodynamic monitoring systems.

The perioperative application of advanced hemodynamic monitoring techniques to guide the clinician toward optimal patient management defines the so-called "Hemodynamic Goal Directed Therapy (HGDT)," which, based on predefined hemodynamic targets, aims to optimize cardiovascular performance through the use of fluids, inotropes, and vasoactive agents. The ultimate goal is to ensure adequate tissue oxygenation and prevent low cardiac output syndrome. This anesthetic approach is a key element of many ERAS protocols [5].

2.3 How to Implement a Perioperative Hemodynamic Optimization Protocol

Over the years, the scientific literature has proposed various treatment protocols, some of which are quite simple, while others are rather complex and not reproducible or applicable in primary care centers or those with limited resources. Therefore, the aim is to simplify HGDT protocols to facilitate and expand their application in many centers. In this context, Saugel et al. proposed a simple and intuitive algorithm based on the application of the "5 Ts" [6].

2.4 A Practical Approach: The 5 Ts of Goal-Directed Therapy (Fig. 2.2)

2.4.1 The First T

The first T refers to the concept of *Target population*, that is, which type of patient should be considered for an HGDT protocol. Numerous studies have shown that

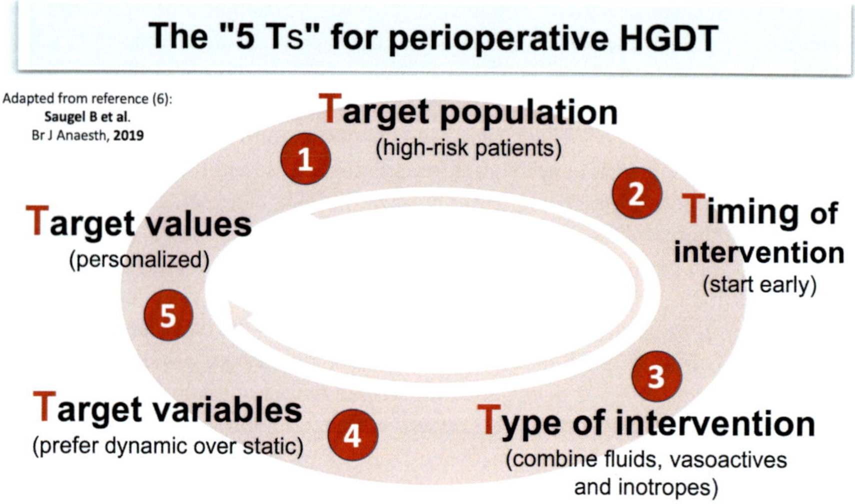

Fig. 2.2 The "5 Ts" for preoperative HGDT

Table 2.1 Patients and comorbidities associated with increased perioperative risk

Elderly patients
Diabetes
Malignancies
Chronic cardiovascular and renal diseases
Chronic obstructive pulmonary disease
Patients undergoing emergency surgery
Patients undergoing surgical procedures lasting more than 2 h with anticipated fluid and blood loss
Patients undergoing invasive surgery (gastrointestinal, orthopedic, neurosurgery, vascular, etc.)

appropriate anesthetic management can improve outcomes, provided that a given HGDT protocol is applied to patients or procedures at high surgical risk (e.g., elderly patients, individuals with systemic diseases and disabling comorbidities, emergency or urgent surgeries) (Table 2.1).

2.4.2 The Second T

The second T refers to the concept of *Timing of intervention*, that is, how promptly, at what moment and in what context of the perioperative course advanced hemodynamic monitoring should be used in high-risk patients. Hemodynamic monitoring can be useful in two key contexts. The first context, based on a "reactive" approach, occurs when a problem has already been identified (e.g., arterial hypotension); in this case, monitoring is applied after the problem arises to help us identify the underlying pathophysiological processes so that appropriate therapies can be selected. For example, a typical scenario is a patient in shock with arterial hypotension, for whom therapeutic options may include administration of fluids, vasopressors, or inotropic agents, depending on the hemodynamic assessment derived from the integration of multiple variables. In this case, advanced hemodynamic monitoring will help us understand the pathophysiological alterations and guide our treatment. However, as is easily understood, in this situation, we are "chasing" the hemodynamic problem that has already manifested, and then trying to correct it. The second context is more preventive, based on a "proactive" approach in which monitoring is applied early and allows for the detection of physiological changes in order to take preventive action, that is, before a significant problem occurs (e.g., by maintaining blood pressure and heart rate within a predetermined range). A typical example in this case is the perioperative patient, in whom monitoring can be used even before induction of anesthesia to detect early changes in volemic status and low oxygen delivery, allowing for timely corrective therapy [7]. Therefore, the application of advanced hemodynamic monitoring techniques in high-risk patients, for appropriate and early HGDT, should be implemented as soon as possible, even before surgery, and then continued throughout all perioperative phases.

2.4.3 The Third T

The third T refers to the concept of *type of therapeutic intervention*, that is, whether to optimize hemodynamic status with fluids, vasopressors, or inotropes.

It is well known that in cases of hemodynamic instability, the most common therapeutic intervention performed by anesthesiologists is the administration of fluids to optimize circulating volume and preload. However, about 20% of patients treated with fluid therapy may experience inappropriate volume overload. It is known that both hypovolemia and hypervolemia are associated with a proportional increase in postoperative complications, as represented by the characteristic "U shape curve" [8] (Fig. 2.3). The curve shows how the severity of hypovolemia or hypervolemia leads to progressive deterioration of organ function, which can result in multiorgan failure; in practice, tissue hypoperfusion due to low cardiac output (hypovolemia) or systemic microcirculatory dysregulation and generalized edema (hypervolemia) is responsible for reduced tissue oxygen delivery and consumption.

Perioperative fluid management aimed at hemodynamic optimization (HGD fluid management) is one of the cornerstones of ERAS protocols. With these protocols, in the preoperative phase, it is recommended to maintain a euvolemic state and good hydration, avoiding prolonged fasting and "mechanical" preparation of the gastrointestinal tract, while also correcting any anemia. The intraoperative phase involves individualized treatment, usually infusing 4–5 ml/kg/h of fluids to maintain euvolemia. Similarly, to the initial phase, the postoperative phase also aims to maintain a euvolemic state, so that at the end of surgery the three perioperative phases should result in a slightly positive and near-zero fluid balance for the patient [9] (Fig. 2.4). Therefore, before administering additional fluids to the patient, which

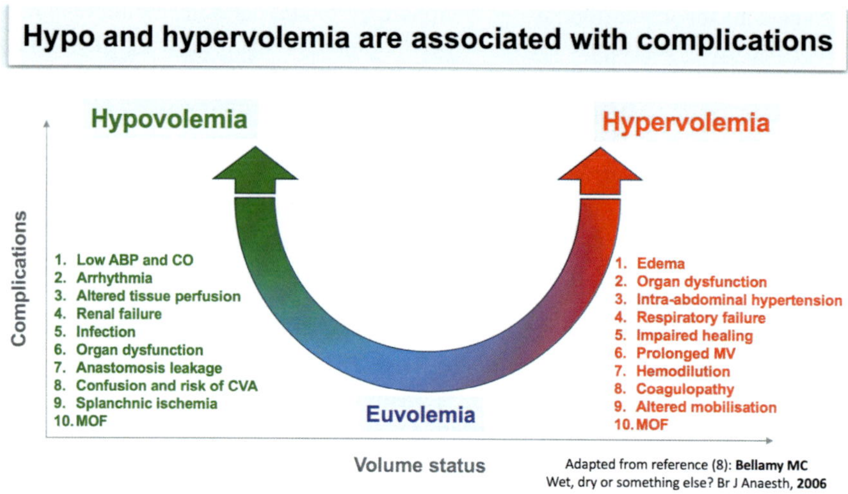

Fig. 2.3 Hypo and hypervolemia are associated with complications

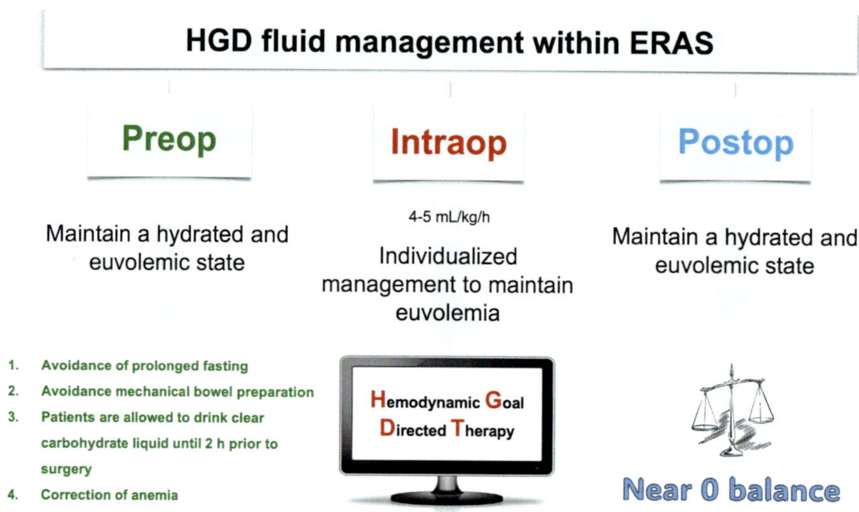

Fig. 2.4 HGD fluid management within ERAS

could result in a highly positive balance (hypervolemia), it is important to ensure that the hemodynamic problem encountered (e.g., arterial hypotension) can indeed be resolved by increasing volemia, venous return, preload, and thus cardiac output. Very often, the decision to administer perioperative fluids does not take into account some simple but fundamental rules. For example, applying the simple "TROL rule" allows the anesthesiologist to adopt a correct stepwise fluid management approach, as it considers the type of fluids to be administered (Type; e.g., crystalloids vs colloids), the rate of administration (Rate; e.g., 250 ml in 15 min), the objectives to be achieved (Objectives; e.g., increase in mean arterial pressure > 65 mmHg, reduction in heart rate < 90 bpm, increase in urine output >1 ml/kg/h, etc.), and finally the limits to be respected (Limits; e.g., not exceeding a certain individual volume load) [10]. The concept of "fluid salvage" (or fluid resuscitation) is different and should be applied in cases of severe hemodynamic instability due to shock, in which fluid management in subsequent steps includes optimization, stabilization, and de-escalation (or evacuation) (SODS and ROSE protocols) [11]. In these cases, the "fluid salvage/resuscitation" phase involves the administration of fluids over a few minutes and should be guided by monitoring dynamic variables of fluid responsiveness (see subsequent sections); conversely, the fluid optimization phase takes place over the following hours, still under dynamic monitoring guidance; stabilization and de-escalation (evacuation) occur over several days and should aim to achieve a neutral fluid balance by reducing fluid administration, potentially also through the use of diuretics.

2.4.4 When to Initiate Therapy with Vasoactive Drugs

Recommendations regarding the timing for starting continuous infusion of a vasoconstrictor suggest early initiation, generally when there is no response to volume expansion; in fact, it is preferable to start it concurrently with fluid therapy, before volume resuscitation is complete. Early use of vasopressors also reduces the amount of fluids administered, due to redistribution of blood from the "unstressed" to the "stressed" volume compartment. The most commonly used trigger for starting a vasopressor is the mean arterial pressure value, that is, when it falls below 65 mmHg despite optimized volume status. The vasopressor of choice remains norepinephrine, considered the first-line vasoactive amine for the treatment of arterial hypotension poorly responsive to fluid therapy, as it offers several advantages over other vasoconstrictors. Compared to adrenaline, norepinephrine does not act on β2-adrenergic receptors; therefore, it does not increase serum lactate levels, which can thus be used as markers of adequate or inadequate systemic tissue perfusion and to guide treatment toward hemodynamic optimization. Unlike dopamine and adrenaline, norepinephrine increases cardiac index without increasing heart rate, thus avoiding excessive myocardial oxygen consumption. In addition, it also acts on cardiac β1-adrenergic receptors and can therefore preserve and facilitate ventriculo-arterial coupling (V-A Coupling) [12]. Finally, by increasing systemic vascular resistance and arteriolar tone (afterload), norepinephrine reflexively increases cardiac inotropy (ANREP effect), which in turn improves blood pressure and organ perfusion [13]. The "threshold" dose of norepinephrine at which it is appropriate to add a second vasopressor is not clearly defined in the literature. However, it is reasonable to start a second vasopressor when the norepinephrine dose exceeds 0.25 mcg/kg/min. Adrenaline has been suggested as a second- or third-line vasopressor. However, with high-dose norepinephrine, α1 receptors may already be saturated and downregulated. For this reason, the use of adrenaline, which targets the same receptors as norepinephrine, may be of limited benefit. Conversely, in cases of arterial hypotension poorly responsive to norepinephrine, the next logical step in vasoconstrictor therapy would be the administration of vasopressin, which acts on different receptors (AVPR1a, AVPR1b, AVPR2). Other vasopressor agents, though less commonly used, may be added as third-line options in the absence of hemodynamic response to the second step, such as terlipressin, selepressin, angiotensin II, and methylene blue [14].

The dosage of vasoconstrictors should be reduced, and eventually discontinued, in the event of side effects (e.g., peripheral ischemia) and, above all, as soon as the hemodynamic status has stabilized, circulating volume and organ perfusion are adequate, and the patient's clinical condition has improved.

2.4.5 When to Initiate Therapy with Inotropic Agents

The use of inotropic agents should be considered only when low mean arterial pressure or decreased cardiac output is due to impaired myocardial contractile function; thus, reduced inotropy will result in tissue hypoperfusion. In practice, the optimal timing and decision to initiate inotropic therapy should be based on three questions: (a) assess whether it is truly necessary; (b) identify the most appropriate inotrope; (c) determine when it should be reduced and/or discontinued. The first question is answered by the presence of the following signs and symptoms: low systolic blood pressure (<90 mmHg), low cardiac index (<2.2 l/min/m^2), cold and mottled skin and periphery, oliguria (<30 ml/h or < 0.5 ml/kg/min), hyperlactatemia (>2 mmol/l), reduced venous oxygen saturation (<60%), and, in the awake patient, altered mental status (confusion, drowsiness). In addition, it is essential that intravascular volume has been thoroughly assessed and optimized beforehand, and that other treatable pathological conditions have been excluded (e.g., coronary artery disease, pulmonary embolism, arrhythmias, cardiac tamponade, valvular diseases). For the second question, it is crucial to evaluate several aspects, such as whether the patient is on chronic beta-blocker therapy, if left or right or biventricular heart failure is present, if the condition is acute or chronic ischemic heart disease, or if pulmonary arterial hypertension is present. Finally, the third question concerns the stabilization of the clinical picture and the improvement of symptoms, vital signs, biochemical markers of organ dysfunction, and the improvement of cardiac function as assessed by echocardiography.

The inotrope of choice remains dobutamine, considered the first-line amine for the treatment of low cardiac output due to reduced inotropy, while the use of dopamine is discouraged, mainly because of its arrhythmogenic potential. However, it should be remembered that among the side effects secondary to inotrope administration, there may be metabolic alterations (e.g., changes in blood glucose and insulin release), endocrine effects (e.g., dysregulation of prolactin and thyroid hormone production), and immunological effects (altered T cell function and levels of pro-inflammatory cytokines). Other inotropic drugs are used in specific cases, such as phosphodiesterase inhibitors (e.g., milrinone, enoximone) or calcium sensitizers (e.g., levosimendan) [15].

2.4.6 The Fourth T

The fourth T refers to the concept of *Target variables*, that is, the goal of achieving predefined (optimal) values for certain hemodynamic parameters that are associated with adequate organ perfusion. In this regard, mean arterial pressure (MAP) is certainly the most commonly measured hemodynamic variable, as restoring an adequate mean arterial pressure (>65 mmHg) ensures optimal tissue perfusion and, at the same time, maintains the autoregulation of blood flow to individual organs. It is well known that blood flow and perfusion pressure, which depend on MAP, are independent of each other when MAP exceeds 65 mmHg (mechanism of blood flow autoregulation). Conversely, when MAP falls below 60 mmHg, organ perfusion (blood flow) becomes "pressure-dependent" and is linearly correlated with MAP (loss of autoregulation), resulting in low oxygen delivery that worsens as arterial pressure decreases [16]. Recently, with the aim of preventing intraoperative arterial hypotension and tissue hypoperfusion, a straightforward hemodynamic variable has been introduced (hypotension prediction index, HPI) which, when correctly applied and interpreted, allows for the prediction, with a certain probability, that a given perioperative hemodynamic setting will soon lead to arterial hypotension (MAP <65 mmHg lasting at least 1 min). This alert enables the anesthesiologist to monitor the patient more closely, integrating various hemodynamic data and intervening proactively with appropriate therapeutic adjustments [17, 18].

Blood pressure measurement is straightforward, whereas the assessment of other target variables requires advanced monitoring systems (e.g., estimation of stroke volume and cardiac output, calculation of systemic vascular resistance, measurement of cardiac filling pressures and pulmonary arterial pressure, assessment of fluid responsiveness, etc.). Some advanced monitoring systems allow for the application of "hemodynamic goal-directed fluid therapy," based on the evaluation of dynamic indices of fluid responsiveness.

2.4.7 Estimation of Preload and Dynamic Indices of Fluid Responsiveness

It is common practice to estimate preload by measuring central venous pressure (CVP) using a central venous catheter (CVC). However, not all surgical patients have a CVC in place and, in various circumstances, CVP may not be useful due to numerous pathophysiological conditions that limit its applicability. For example, CVP values may over- or underestimate the patient's actual volume status when venous tone is altered by various factors, such as when venous vascular compliance is affected by specific conditions (cardiovascular diseases, medications), or in the presence of tricuspid valve disease (stenosis or insufficiency), cardiac rhythm disturbances, significant changes in intrathoracic pressure (e.g., excessive PEEP, pneumothorax), and in cases of right heart failure or cardiac tamponade. Despite these limitations, the use of CVP to guide resuscitation is straightforward and universally applicable, so it is wiser to consider these limitations rather than to disregard CVP values entirely, as they reflect the patient's cardiocirculatory status [19]. Similar considerations apply to monitoring pulmonary artery occlusion pressure (PAOP), which is even more invasive to measure, as it can only be obtained with a pulmonary artery catheter and inflation of its balloon.

Over the years, other hemodynamic variables have been proposed for estimating preload, such as measurement of ventricular end-diastolic volumes or areas (RVEDV or LVEDV, RVEDA or LVEDA), which obviously require echocardiographic expertise; or the estimation of intrathoracic blood volume (ITBV), global end-diastolic cardiac volume (GEDV), and extravascular lung water (EVLW), which can be obtained using more advanced monitoring techniques (transpulmonary thermodilution) [20]. It should be noted that PVC and PAOP pressures, being determined by end-diastolic volume, are naturally influenced by ventricular compliance and are therefore limited in their ability to reflect the actual volemic status. Furthermore, regarding GEDV and LVEDV volumes, since their relationship with stroke volume depends on ventricular contractility, they are poor predictors of fluid responsiveness in cases of impaired cardiac function; thus, they cannot be used as dynamic variables to assess response to a fluid bolus (fluid challenge). Therefore, rather than monitoring pressures and volumes, HGDT recommends evaluating the dynamic response of a patient to fluid administration, potentially predicting it using so-called dynamic indices of fluid responsiveness [21]. A parameter is considered a predictor of a positive response to a fluid challenge (recommended bolus of 3–5 ml/kg over 15–20 min) if there is a relationship between its baseline value and changes in stroke volume following volume expansion. In this context, a patient is defined as a "fluid responder" when their stroke volume increases by 10–15% after a fluid load, and such a response will prompt the anesthesiologist to administer additional fluids to optimize hemodynamic status and treat any hypotension or organ hypoperfusion. However, for the transition from volume expansion to resolution of hypoperfusion to occur, several conditions must be met, such as the absence of endothelial damage (capillary leak) and microcirculatory dysfunction [22]. Dynamic variables of fluid responsiveness can be obtained using monitoring techniques based on pulse contour analysis, or with ultrasonographic techniques (e.g., Doppler, M-mode echocardiography, etc.). The analysis of pulse wave variations in relation to respiratory cycles during spontaneous or mechanical ventilation forms the physiological basis of the so-called "heart-lung interaction." According to the Frank-Starling-Maestrini law, for every increase or decrease in volume (preload), within certain limits, the heart responds with a corresponding increase or decrease in stroke volume. During mechanical ventilation, as intrathoracic pressure becomes positive, the inspiratory phase will result in a reduction in venous return and preload, and consequently, stroke volume will also decrease. The opposite occurs during the expiratory phase. Therefore, oscillations in the pulse wave during mechanical ventilation can be used to estimate the degree of hypovolemia and the potential for a positive response to fluid loading. Dynamic variables derived from arterial waveform analysis include systolic pressure variation (SPV) and the percentage variation in pulse pressure (PPV). Additionally, pulse contour methods, by calculating stroke volume from the area under the arterial pressure curve, can also provide the percentage variation in stroke volume (SVV), which physiologically indicates the degree of influence (dynamic obstacle) that intrathoracic pressure exerts on venous return and preload. Generally, percentage variations in pulse pressure or stroke volume exceeding 13–15% indicate a potential hypovolemic state and the need for fluid administration to prevent arterial hypotension. Naturally, it is the clinician's responsibility to determine whether the patient truly requires fluids, as several patients with PPV or SVV values greater than 15% may not necessarily need volume treatment, since they may present with stable hemodynamics and adequate organ perfusion. Similarly, ultrasonographic techniques also allow for the assessment of certain dynamic variables of fluid responsiveness in relation to changes in venous return and preload during mechanical ventilation. These include Doppler-derived velocity variations estimated in the aorta (ΔVpeak, ΔVTIao), percentage variations in inferior vena cava distension (dIVC), or collapse of the superior vena cava (cSVC). Percentage variations in the systolic peaks of the plethysmographic waveform (SPVplet), measured with a simple pulse oximeter, can also indicate volume depletion and potential fluid responsiveness. This option is particularly useful in less complex surgical procedures for which continuous invasive monitoring with an intra-arterial catheter is not recommended [23, 24] (Table 2.2). Naturally, the application of dynamic indices of fluid responsiveness requires verification of certain conditions: adequate quality of the pulse waveform and acoustic window in the case of ultrasonographic techniques; a heart rate to respiratory rate ratio >3.6; absence of cardiac arrhythmias; ventilation with a tidal volume of at least 8 ml/kg; absence of intra-abdominal hypertension; closed chest; and absence of spontaneous breathing [25]. Therefore, these dynamic indices cannot be used in surgical patients undergoing abdominal hyperinflation, thoracic surgery, or procedures performed under sedation or in regional anesthesia, in patients presenting with bradycardia, and, finally, in those who cannot be ventilated with high volumes.

In the aforementioned cases, some authors suggest performing the passive leg raising (PLR) test, provided that this maneuver is feasible and not contraindicated in the surgical patient. PLR, conducted for a few minutes, improves venous return by recruiting blood from the lower limbs and, in fluid responders, will increase stroke volume [26]. Therefore, in the event of a positive response to PLR, the anesthesiologist can safely administer fluids to improve tissue perfusion.

Table 2.2 Dynamic variables of fluid responsiveness

SPV	Systolic pressure variation
PPV	Pulse pressure variation
SVV	Stroke volume variation
SPVplet	Systolic pressure variation by pulse oximetry
ΔVpeak	Variation in aortic flow peak velocity by Doppler
ΔVTIao	Variation in aortic velocity-time integral by Doppler
cSVC	Collapsibility of the superior vena cava
dIVC	Distensibility of the inferior vena cava

In theory, during surgery, fluid responsiveness tests could be automated on anesthesia machines and mechanical ventilators, allowing the anesthesiologist to regularly assess the patient's fluid responsiveness status at set intervals without any additional workload [27].

2.4.8 The Role of the Central Venous Catheter: Venous Saturation

For more complex surgical procedures, the anesthesiologist often needs to cannulate a central vessel using a central venous catheter (CVC). With this catheter, in addition to infusing fluids and administering drugs, it is possible to measure central venous pressure (CVP) and collect blood samples to assess central venous oxygen saturation ($ScvO_2$). $ScvO_2$ is an indicator of global tissue perfusion, as it reflects the overall oxygen extraction by all tissues. Although this information is more accurately obtained from mixed venous saturation in the pulmonary artery (SvO_2), $ScvO_2$ still represents its physiological significance and trend over time. Moreover, it does not require the insertion of a pulmonary artery catheter. Some hemodynamic techniques allow continuous measurement of $ScvO_2$ values using dedicated central venous catheters equipped with fiber optic sensors. International scientific societies, regardless of the patient's underlying condition, recommend maintaining an $ScvO_2$ of at least 65%, as this value indicates an oxygen extraction of less than 35% and, consequently, a normal relationship between oxygen delivery and consumption. For example, in some surgical procedures, significant blood loss may occur, leading to hypotension and reduced tissue oxygen delivery. In such cases, since tissue oxygen consumption must remain constant, cellular O_2 extraction will increase, resulting in a decrease in $ScvO_2$. Because $ScvO_2$ changes are quite rapid and occur within seconds, they can serve as an early alert for the anesthesiologist, indicating an alteration in the oxygen delivery/consumption relationship. The integrated assessment of other hemodynamic parameters will help to understand the ongoing pathophysiological changes and implement appropriate corrective therapies [28].

2.5 Which Hemodynamic Monitoring Techniques to Use

Effective perioperative hemodynamic monitoring should include, in addition to measurement of arterial and central venous pressure, estimation of stroke volume, cardiac output, dynamic variables of fluid responsiveness, oxygen delivery and extraction, and other cardiocirculatory variables, such as parameters that indirectly provide information on cardiac contractility and efficiency, vascular resistance, and volume overload [29].

Over the years, hemodynamic monitoring techniques have evolved, offering anesthesiologists increasingly less invasive systems that are easy to use and provide integrated, continuous information, often independently of operator intervention. Currently, advanced hemodynamic monitoring devices can be broadly classified according to the physiological method they use to estimate cardiocirculatory variables (algorithm) and their degree of invasiveness. Each device, depending on the specific algorithm applied, also provides specific and sometimes complex hemodynamic variables. However, the common feature of all hemodynamic monitoring techniques is the ability to estimate stroke volume and cardiac output, the latter being essential for calculating oxygen delivery [30].

Classic bolus thermodilution using a pulmonary artery catheter (PAC) is the technique that historically marked the beginning of advanced hemodynamic monitoring in anesthesia and intensive care; it remains the reference standard for clinical validation of other monitoring systems. It is based on the concept that the cooling/heating of blood (thermal variation) in the pulmonary artery, measured over time by a thermistor in the PAC, can represent the amount of blood ejected by the heart in 1 min, i.e., the cardiac output. However, factors such as lower surgical complexity and perioperative risk, the time and expertise required for PAC insertion, the sometimes non-intuitive interpretation of the parameters provided, and the potential complications associated with its invasiveness limit its use in non-cardiothoracic perioperative settings.

Transpulmonary thermodilution represents a less invasive method than the previous one, as it uses a central venous catheter instead of a PAC and, for detecting blood temperature changes, requires a dedicated arterial catheter to be inserted into a peripheral artery and equipped with a thermistor. This technique offers the advantage of being able to calculate certain special variables, such as GEDV, EVLW, and the cardiac function index (CFI). However, due to the same factors that limit the use of classical bolus thermodilution, this technique is also not recommended for less complex surgical procedures or for monitoring low-risk perioperative patients.

Pulse contour methods (PCM) derive hemodynamic data from the analysis of the pressure waveform via an arterial catheter and, therefore, provide continuous information; moreover, being less invasive, they are among the most widely used systems in the perioperative period, even in complex patients. Thanks to specific algorithms unique to each system, it is also possible to monitor certain hemodynamic variables related to vascular status (e.g., arterial elastance) and cardiovascular performance (cardiac function index, dP/dP, cardiac cycle efficiency, cardiac power output). As previously described, these systems are especially used to monitor dynamic variables of fluid responsiveness (PPV, SVV) and thus optimize perioperative volemic status. Some PCMs analyze the arterial signal in a completely non-invasive manner using small plethysmographic cuffs placed around the fingers. These can be used for hemodynamic monitoring in low-risk patients or those undergoing minor surgical procedures, for whom arterial cannulation is not required. However, several factors can reduce the accuracy and reliability of PCMs, such as suboptimal arterial signal quality due to vascular diseases (e.g., stenosis, atherosclerosis) or significant changes in arterial impedance (peripheral edema, vasoconstriction).

Ultrasound techniques use the Doppler effect to estimate cardiac output in the ascending aorta (transthoracic Doppler) or descending aorta (transesophageal Doppler). In addition, morphological changes in the Doppler signal provide more advanced hemodynamic information regarding arterial vascular status (afterload), cardiac function (contractility), and volemic status (preload). Thanks to their lower invasiveness (transesophageal) or complete non-invasiveness (transthoracic), Doppler methods can also be used in minor surgical procedures and in low-risk perioperative patients. However, their limitations should not be overlooked, some of which are related to operator dependency, the quality of the ultrasound signal, esophageal diseases, and discomfort (esophageal probe), which contraindicate their use in awake patients.

Bioreactance is a completely non-invasive hemodynamic technique that studies voltage changes over time of an electrical current; as this current passes through the thorax, it undergoes modifications related to systolic-diastolic variations in blood flow in the thoracic aorta. These variations indirectly reflect stroke volume and, therefore, cardiac output. Being completely non-invasive, bioreactance is widely used in less complex procedures and in the pre- and postoperative periods. However, its main limitation is its inapplicability in thoracic surgery.

From the brief description above of currently available hemodynamic monitoring techniques, it is clear that there is no ideal system for all situations, types of surgery, or patients, as each has its limitations. However, some of these systems offer the possibility of using platforms that can interface with other perioperative monitoring systems (e.g., depth of anesthesia) or can be extended according to a sort of "hemodynamic monitoring escalation," which becomes increasingly advanced and accurate in cases of surgical complexity and high perioperative risk (e.g., pulse contour method combined with transpulmonary thermodilution and central venous saturation) [7, 29, 30] (Table 2.3).

2.5.1 How to Choose the Hemodynamic Monitoring Technique in the Perioperative Period

The selection of a perioperative hemodynamic monitoring technique can be based on three fundamental elements: (a) the trade-off between accuracy and invasiveness; (b) the level of the hospital center; (c) perioperative risk and surgical complexity. In the first case, some less accurate techniques may be more useful for monitoring trends in variables rather than their absolute values (e.g., less invasive systems). The level of the hospital center will influence the choice of device based on clinicians' experience and budget availability. The third element, the most important, recommends the use of non-invasive techniques for low-risk patients/procedures (bioreactance, transthoracic Doppler, non-invasive PCM); suggests less invasive techniques for intermediate-complexity surgical procedures and patients at intermediate perioperative risk (esophageal Doppler, PCM combined with thermodilution, $ScvO_2$); and recommends more advanced technologies for major surgical procedures and patients at high perioperative risk (pulmonary artery catheter, SvO_2) (Fig. 2.5).

It should be emphasized that the choice of a specific monitor should also be based on the characteristics of the device itself, considering its accuracy and precision, response time (continuity of data provided, beat by beat), operator

Table 2.3 Main hemodynamic monitoring techniques

Method	Variables provided	Limitations
Bolus thermodilution	Cardiac output, pulmonary artery pressures, wedge pressure, central venous pressure, venous oxygen saturation	Invasive Not continuous
Transpulmonary thermodilution	Cardiac output, intracardiac total volume, extravascular lung water, cardiac function indices	Invasive Requires central venouos catheter
Pulse contour	Cardiac output, dynamic variables of fluid responsiveness, afterload, and conctractility indices	Requires an optimal arterial signal Reduced accuracy in the presence of vascular diseases or changes in arterial impedance
Doppler	Cardiac output, dynamic variables of fluid responsiveness, afterload and contractility indices	Operator dependent Requires an adequate ultrasound signal
Bioreactance	Cardiac output, dynamic variables of fluid responsiveness, afterload, and contractility indices	Not usable in thoracic surgery

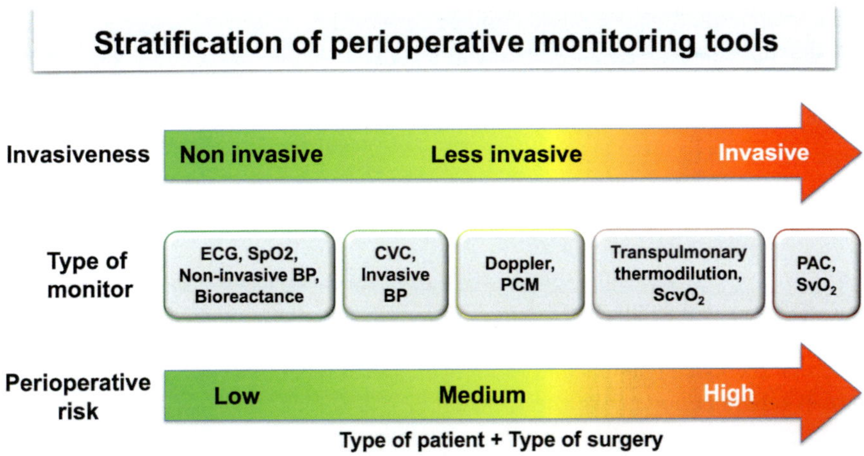

Fig. 2.5 Stratification of perioperative monitoring tools

independence and ease of use, costs, invasiveness and potential complications, the ability to provide more advanced information (afterload, preload, contractility), and the ability to deliver information useful for correctly applying a hemodynamic monitoring-guided treatment protocol (HGDT). The scientific literature reiterates the concept that it is not the monitor itself that improves patient outcomes but rather the perioperative management when it is appropriate and correctly tailored to the individual patient [7, 29, 30].

2.5.2 The Fifth T

The fifth and final T refers to the concept of *Target values*, that is, the goal of directing perioperative management to the individual patient, according to specific and personalized protocols that allow for the achievement of optimal hemodynamic variable values in each patient. In this regard, it is advisable for the anesthesiology team to establish perioperative decision-making algorithms based on the characteristics of their own center, the type of surgical pathway, and the patient population to be treated. An example might be as follows: after assessing mean arterial pressure, cardiac output, and dynamic indices of fluid responsiveness, in the case of suspected tissue hypoperfusion, one could intervene with a fluid bolus (fluid challenge) or with a PLR to determine if the patient is a fluid responder. Subsequently, if the response is positive, cardiac output should continue to be optimized with fluid therapy, whereas in the case of a negative response to the fluid challenge or PLR, it will be necessary to identify the hemodynamic problem and suspect possible vasoplegia and/or reduced contractility, initiating appropriate therapy with vasoconstrictors and/or inotropes. Therefore, a reasonable therapeutic sequence would be: fluids, vasoconstrictors, inotropes. It is important, therefore, to assess the individual response to each step of the decision-making algorithm rather than attempting to preemptively and necessarily bring hemodynamic variables that appear "abnormal" into a predetermined range. This proactive, yet reasoned and individualized approach prevents complications that may arise in certain patient groups, especially those with impaired cardiac function (e.g., fluid overload, pulmonary edema) [16].

2.6 Conclusions

Perioperative hemodynamic optimization is a fundamental intervention in anesthesia, especially in patients undergoing major surgery or at high risk of complications. A structured, reasoned, simple approach based on advanced monitoring and personalized protocols can significantly improve clinical outcomes, representing a standard of care in perioperative anesthesiology.

References

1. Fellahi JL, Futier E, Vaisse C, Collange O, Huet O, Loriau J, Gayat E, Tavernier B, Biais M, Asehnoune K, Cholley B, Longrois D. Perioperative hemodynamic optimization: from guidelines to implementation-an experts' opinion paper. Ann Intensive Care. 2021;11(1):58.
2. Desborough JP. The stress response to trauma and surgery. Br J Anaesth. 2000;85(1):109–17.
3. Vincent JL, De Backer D. Circulatory shock. N Engl J Med. 2013;369(18):1726–34.
4. Saugel B, Critchley LAH, Kaufmann T, Flick M, Kouz K, Vistisen ST, Scheeren TWL. Journal of Clinical Monitoring and Computing end of year summary 2019: hemodynamic monitoring and management. J Clin Monit Comput. 2020;34(2):207–19.

5. Dmytriiev D, Nazarchuk O, Melnychenko M, Levchenko B. Optimization of the target strategy of perioperative infusion therapy based on monitoring data of central hemodynamics in order to prevent complications. Front Med (Lausanne). 2022;9:935331.
6. Saugel B, Kouz K, Scheeren TWL. The '5 Ts' of perioperative goal-directed haemodynamic therapy. Br J Anaesth. 2019;123(2):103–7. https://doi.org/10.1016/j.bja.2019.04.048.
7. Vincent JL, Rhodes A, Perel A, Martin GS, Della Rocca G, Vallet B, Pinsky MR, Hofer CK, Teboul JL, de Boode WP, Scolletta S, Vieillard-Baron A, De Backer D, Walley KR, Maggiorini M, Singer M. Clinical review: update on hemodynamic monitoring–a consensus of 16. Crit Care. 2011;15(4):229.
8. Bellamy MC. Wet, dry or something else? Br J Anaesth. 2006;97(6):755–7.
9. French WB, Scott M. Fluid and hemodynamics. Anesthesiol Clin. 2022;40(1):59–71.
10. Vincent JL. Critical care medicine, vol. 2. Churcill Livingstone: Elsevier; 2009. p. 20–1.
11. Wiedermann CJ. Phases of fluid management and the roles of human albumin solution in perioperative and critically ill patients. Curr Med Res Opin. 2020;36(12):1961–73.
12. Levy B, Fritz C, Tahon E, Jacquot A, Auchet T, Kimmoun A. Vasoplegia treatments: the past, the present, and the future. Crit Care. 2018;22(1):52.
13. De Backer D, Pinsky M. Norepinephrine improves cardiac function during septic shock, but why? Br J Anaesth. 2018;120(3):421–4.
14. Russell JA. Vasopressor therapy in critically ill patients with shock. Intensive Care Med. 2019;45(11):1503–17.
15. Farmakis D, Agostoni P, Baholli L, Bautin A, Comin-Colet J, Crespo-Leiro MG, Fedele F, García-Pinilla JM, Giannakoulas G, Grigioni F, Gruchała M, Gustafsson F, Harjola VP, Hasin T, Herpain A, Iliodromitis EK, Karason K, Kivikko M, Liaudet L, Ljubas-Maček J, Marini M, Masip J, Mebazaa A, Nikolaou M, Ostadal P, Põder P, Pollesello P, Polyzogopoulou E, Pölzl G, Tschope C, Varpula M, von Lewinski D, Vrtovec B, Yilmaz MB, Zima E, Parissis J. A pragmatic approach to the use of inotropes for the management of acute and advanced heart failure: an expert panel consensus. Int J Cardiol. 2019;297:83–90.
16. Meng L, Yu W, Wang T, Zhang L, Heerdt PM, Gelb AW. Blood pressure targets in perioperative care. Hypertension. 2018;72(4):806–17.
17. Dong S, Wang Q, Wang S, Zhou C, Wang H. Hypotension prediction index for the prevention of hypotension during surgery and critical care: a narrative review. Comput Biol Med. 2024;170:107995.
18. Ackland GL, Abbott TEF. Hypotension as a marker or mediator of perioperative organ injury: a narrative review. Br J Anaesth. 2022;128(6):915–30.
19. De Backer D, Vincent JL. Should we measure the central venous pressure to guide fluid management? Ten answers to 10 questions. Crit Care. 2018;22(1):43.
20. Brienza N, Biancofiore G, Cavaliere F, Corcione A, De Gasperi A, De Rosa RC, Fumagalli R, Giglio MT, Locatelli A, Lorini FL, Romagnoli S, Scolletta S, Tritapepe L. Clinical guidelines for perioperative hemodynamic management of non cardiac surgical adult patients. Minerva Anestesiol. 2019;85(12):1315–33.
21. Heming N, Moine P, Coscas R, Annane D. Perioperative fluid management for major elective surgery. Br J Surg. 2020;107(2):e56–62.
22. Monnet X, Teboul JL. My patient has received fluid. How to assess its efficacy and side effects? Ann Intensive Care. 2018;8(1):54.
23. Monnet X, Shi R, Teboul JL. Prediction of fluid responsiveness. What's new? Ann Intensive Care. 2022;12(1):46.
24. Monnet X, Teboul JL. Assessment of fluid responsiveness: recent advances. Curr Opin Crit Care. 2018;24(3):190–5.
25. Michard F, Chemla D, Teboul JL. Applicability of pulse pressure variation: how many shades of grey? Crit Care. 2015;19(1):144.
26. Monnet X, Cipriani F, Camous L, Sentenac P, Dres M, Krastinova E, Anguel N, Richard C, Teboul JL. The passive leg raising test to guide fluid removal in critically ill patients. Ann Intensive Care. 2016;6(1):46.

27. Michard F, Biais M, Lobo SM, Futier E. Perioperative hemodynamic management 4.0. Best Pract Res Clin Anaesthesiol. 2019;33(2):247–55.
28. Marx G, Reinhart K. Venous oximetry. Curr Opin Crit Care. 2006;12(3):263–8.
29. Vincent JL, Pelosi P, Pearse R, Payen D, Perel A, Hoeft A, Romagnoli S, Ranieri VM, Ichai C, Forget P, Della Rocca G, Rhodes A. Perioperative cardiovascular monitoring of high-risk patients: a consensus of 12. Crit Care. 2015;19(1):224.
30. De Backer D, Hajjar L, Monnet X. Monitoring cardiac output. Intensive Care Med. 2024;50(11):1912–5.

Management of Direct Oral Anticoagulants (DOACs) in the Perioperative Period for Elective and Emergency Procedures: Discontinuation (If and When Necessary), Resumption, Reversal (If and When Necessary)—Update 2026

3

Andrea De Gasperi, Riccardo Giossi, Chiara Parati, Alessandro Squizzato, and Laura Petrò

3.1 Introduction

Direct oral anticoagulants (DOACs)—*dabigatran (D), rivaroxaban (R), apixaban (A), edoxaban (E)*—represent a major advance in oral anticoagulant therapy and are now largely replacing vitamin K antagonists (VKAs, warfarin, acenocoumarol) for both prophylaxis and antithrombotic treatment [1–6]. DOACs are also referred to as *non-vitamin K antagonist oral anticoagulants* (NOACs)), an acronym that will not be used in this article.

The main indications of DOACs include stroke prevention in patients with non-valvular atrial fibrillation (AF), and the treatment and prevention of deep venous

A. De Gasperi (✉)
Former Director AR2, Ospedale Niguarda Ca' Granda, Milano, Italy

R. Giossi
Clinical Chemistry Analysis Unit – Poison Control Center and Clinical Pharmacology Unit, ASST GOM Niguarda, Milan, Italy
e-mail: riccardo.giossi@ospedaleniguarda.it

C. Parati
Hospital Pharmacist – Pharmacy Unit – ASST GOM Niguarda, Milan, Italy
e-mail: chiara.parati@ospedaleniguarda.it

A. Squizzato
General Medicine Unit – Sant'Anna Hospital – Como – ASST Settelaghi, Como, Italy
e-mail: alessandro.squizzato@uninsubria.it

L. Petrò
Post-Transplant ICU, Ospedale Policlinico San Martino, Genoa, Italy

D. Chiumello, A. De Gasperi (eds.), *Practical Trends in Anesthesia and Intensive Care 2026*, https://doi.org/10.1007/978-3-032-25721-5_3

thrombosis (DVT) and pulmonary embolism (PE) [2, 4]. Recent data indicate that 1–2% of the general population is receiving long-term anticoagulant therapy. In the EU and USA, DOACs currently account for 68–79% of anticoagulant prescriptions [3]. Compared to VKAs, DOACs offer a more manageable, effective, and safer therapeutic option, owing to their more predictable pharmacodynamic (PD) and pharmacokinetic (PK) profiles, reduced need for laboratory monitoring, and a lower incidence of major bleeding events (2–3.6%). These characteristics substantially simplify both clinical and logistical management for physicians and patients [2, 4]. DOACs exert their anticoagulant effects by directly inhibiting specific factors in the coagulation phase of *hemostasis* ("cessation of bleeding"). Hemostasis is complex, tightly regulated, comprising four overlapping phases: vascular (vasoconstriction), platelet, coagulation, and fibrinolytic phases. Crosstalk among these components, together with the crucial role of the endothelium, maintains the complex balance between effective tissue repair (and thus "cessation of bleeding") and the restriction of clot formation to sites of vascular injury [7].

Antithrombotic therapy includes both antiplatelet agents (not discussed in this chapter) and anticoagulants. Anticoagulants can be classified according to their mechanism of action within the coagulation cascade:

- Unfractionated heparin (UF), low molecular weight heparins (LMWH), and fondaparinux, which exerts an indirect anticoagulant effect by binding to and activating antithrombin (AT).
- VKAs (warfarin and acenocoumarol), which inhibit hepatic synthesis of the vitamin K-dependent coagulation factors (II, VII, IX, and X) in their active form.
- DOACs [2, 4], which directly inhibit key coagulation enzymes, thrombin and factor Xa.

Among the four DOACs, dabiga*tr*an inhibits *tr*ombin (factor IIa), while rivaro*xa*ban, api*xa*ban, and edo*xa*ban inhibit *factor Xa*.

Due to their widespread use, emergency department (ED) physicians, anesthesiologists, and surgeons are increasingly required to manage DOAC therapy appropriately in both elective and urgent/emergency medical or surgical settings [8]. Approximately 20% of patients receiving DOACs will require surgery or invasive procedures during treatment, and 0.5–3.5% may experience intracranial hemorrhage (ICH) or major bleeding events [1–6]. In an *elective* surgical or interventional setting, DOAC management can be planned in a multidisciplinary setting, allowing for individualized risk assessment and optimized perioperative strategies. In contrast, *urgent or emergency* interventions or spontaneous hemorrhagic complications pose significant clinical challenges, particularly when dealing with the decision to reverse or not the anticoagulant [1–4, 8]. Up to 30% of patients on DOACs who present to the ED have no residual anticoagulant effect. Therefore, even in the presence of cerebral hemorrhage, drug reversal may not be required, as it could expose the patient to an increased risk of thromboembolic rebound [6]. Conversely, in patients with acute ischemic stroke who have taken a DOAC within the previous 48 h, the inability to reliably exclude residual anticoagulant activity using laboratory tests may lead to the inappropriate withholding of thrombolytic therapy in up to 28% of otherwise eligible cases [6, 9–11]. The key issues to be addressed, particularly in urgent and emergency settings, include (i) availability of methods to assess the presence or absence of DOAC-related anticoagulant activity; (ii) the safe management of patients undergoing elective procedures; (iii) the indication of DOAC reversal; and (iv) the optimal reverse strategies, including available agents and procedural approaches.

3.2 DOACs: Classification, Indications, and Contraindications

A recent review published in 2024 [12] proposed a "pragmatic" classification of DOACs based on safety and efficacy criteria derived from their approved or investigated indications across different clinical settings. According to this framework, DOACs were classified as:

(i) "*Preferred*" for the proposed indication
(ii) "*Under investigation*" when safety and efficacy have not yet been established for the indexed indication
(iii) "*Not to be used*"

3.2.1 Indications

The currently approved indications for the four DOACs include [1–4]:

- Prevention of stroke in patients with non-valvular atrial fibrillation (AF) (primary indication)
- Treatment and prevention of venous thromboembolism (VTE), including deep venous thrombosis (DVT) and pulmonary embolism (PE) (including the orthopedic surgery setting)
- Use in selected clinical scenarios, including:
  - Heparin-induced thrombocytopenia (HIT).
  - Patients with AF and concomitant coronary events and/or undergoing interventional procedures (e.g., coronary artery stenting), in whom a DOAC is combined with a single antiplatelet agent (usually Clopidogrel) after an initial 7–10 day course of dual antiplatelet therapy (DAPT). In these settings, the DOAC dosage should be adjusted according to the specific agent and indication (AF versus DVT), age (if >80 years), body weight (if <60 kg), renal function (estimated glomerular filtration rate, eGFR) <50 ml/min), and in presence of clinically relevant drug -drug interaction(s) (see below) [2].

3.2.2 Conditions in Which DOACs Are Still Under Investigation [1–4, 12]

The efficacy and safety of DOACs are still under investigation in several clinical conditions, including left ventricular thrombus, vascular catheter-associated DVT, splanchnic vein thrombosis, and cerebral venous thrombosis, and in patients with severe renal impairment, particularly those with eGFR <15 ml/min (for anti-Xa agents).

3.2.3 Conditions in Which DOACs Should Not Be Used [1–4, 12]

Several clinical conditions have been identified in which DOACs are (currently) considered less effective, less safe, or without clear clinical benefit compared with alternative antithrombotic strategies and therefore should not be used:

- Presence of mechanical heart valves.
- AF of rheumatic origin.
- Antiphospholipid antibody syndrome.
- Transcatheter aortic valve replacement (TAVR).
- Embolic stroke of undetermined origin, for which antiplatelet therapy is preferred.
- Advanced chronic kidney disease (stage IV, eGFR <30 mL/min), for which robust evidence supporting the efficacy and safety of A, R, and E remains limited; however, it should be noted that no formal contraindication is reported in the respective Summary of the product characteristics (SPCs).
- Severe hepatic insufficiency, particularly CHILD Class C patients (see below C*ontraindications*).

3.2.4 Contraindications

The following conditions are considered contraindications to DOAC therapy [12]:

- Moderate-to-severe hepatic impairment (CHILD Pugh class B and C): A is contraindicated in Child-Pugh C; R in Child-Pugh B and C; D in cases of significant enzyme elevation AST/ALT x 2 the upper limit of normal [5] (see below)
- Severe renal impairment (defined as eGFR <30 ml/min) for D
  - Regarding severe renal impairment, a recent patient-level meta-analysis (COMBINE-AF), which pooled data from completed randomized studies [13], demonstrated that in subjects with eGFR ≥25 ml/min, standard-dose DOACs were safer and more effective than warfarin.
- Pregnancy and breastfeeding due to placental transfer and excretion into breast milk, as well as the limited data available on the fetus and newborn

- Pregnancy: At present, the contraindication is primarily based on SPC recommendations and the limited clinical data available. In women receiving DOAC therapy who become pregnant, switching to heparin is mandatory. Warfarin is contraindicated during pregnancy, at least until week 12, due to the high risk of congenital malformations and warfarin embryopathy, intrauterine death, spontaneous abortion, and maternal and fetal hemorrhage [14]. Beyond the first trimester, the decision to resume warfarin or continue heparin should be guided by the patient's individual thromboembolic risk. Importantly, DOACs have not, to date, clear evidence of teratogenicity. The largest available study reported a rate of fetal abnormalities among live births exposed to DOACs during pregnancy (predominantly during the first trimester) of about 6.0%, with no consistent pattern identified and a spontaneous abortion rate comparable to the general population [15]. In a *worst-case scenario*, the proportion of major congenital defects was estimated at approximately 4.0%, while the overall incidence of DOAC embryotoxicity was around 2.0%. These findings are nonetheless considered reassuring and support the 2016 International Society of Thrombosis and Hemostasis (ISTH) recommendations, which do not regard inadvertent DOAC exposure during pregnancy as a medical reason for elective termination and switching to heparin [16]. Finally, isolated care reports describe the continuation of DOAC therapy throughout pregnancy in highly selected circumstances, such as the case of a woman with a history of HIT and antithrombin deficiency treated with A, resulting in a favorable maternal and neonatal outcome [17]. Nevertheless, any therapeutic decision involving anticoagulation during pregnancy should be undertaken within a multidisciplinary framework, ideally involving clinicians with specific expertise in this area or a perinatal toxicology/teratology information service (TIS) to ensure an individualized risk/benefit assessment.

3.3 DOACs: Pharmacokinetic and Pharmacodynamic Profiles (PK/PD)

An understanding of the PK/PD characteristics is essential for the appropriate perioperative management of DOACs and is therefore briefly reviewed here [2, 4, 18]. DOACs are administered orally at fixed doses and, unlike vitamin K antagonists (VKAs), do not require routine monitoring of coagulation times. In fact, INR values do not correlate with the degree of anticoagulation achieved with DOACs (see below) and are therefore unsuitable for clinical monitoring of their anticoagulant activity. DOACs are characterized by a relatively short half-life (8–14 h), a rapid onset of action (2–4 h), and peak activity occurring 2–3 h after administration. Renal excretion represents a major determinant of DOACs, although the extent varies substantially among different agents, ranging from 25% of A to 80% for D. Consequently, renal function plays a critical role in DOAC management, particularly in patients with chronic kidney disease (CKD) or acute renal impairment [2].

Among the PK variables of DOACs, the *elimination half-life,* $(t_{1/2})$h *plays* a pivotal role in determining the duration of effect and to guide the timing of drug discontinuation and resumption, particularly to avoid residual anticoagulant effect in case of invasive procedures. The four DOACs and their key pharmacokinetic characteristics are discussed below [2, 4, 5, 18, 19].

3.3.1 Apixaban (A)

A is a direct and reversible inhibitor of free and clot-bound *factor Xa*. A prolongs global coagulation times, including prothrombin time (PT)/international normalized ratio (INR) and activated partial thromboplastin time (aPTT), and indirectly inhibits thrombin-induced platelet aggregation [19]. A linear correlation exists over a wide dose range between anti-factor Xa activity and **A** plasma concentrations. From a kinetic perspective, absorption occurs in the small intestine, and food intake does not affect its bioavailability (close to 50%). Protein binding is high (>80%); volume of distribution (V_d) is small (21 liters), indicating predominant distribution within the extracellular fluid, with a limited impact on extremes of body weight on drug exposure. Peak plasma concentration is achieved 2.5–4 h after administration. Elimination occurs through both renal (approximately 25–30%) and hepatic pathways, with a plasma clearance of 3.3 L/h and a half-life ($t_{1/2}$ h) ranging from 9 to 11 h. Dose adjustment based on "standard" body weight is not required, although consideration may be required in case of severe obesity. Apixaban is not contraindicated in CHILD Pugh classes A and B patients but should be avoided in CHILD C patients. In patients with chronic renal failure (CRF), dose adjustment may be warranted, given the partial renal elimination (25–30%). In the UK and Europe, dose reduction is recommended for patients with AF and with a creatinine clearance of 15–29 mL/min or for those who meet at least two of the following three criteria: age ≥80 years, body weight ≤ 60 kg, or serum creatinine ≥133micromol/L. This dose reduction is not recommended for the treatment of VTE. Significant drug-drug interactions may occur with strong CYP3A4 and P-glycoprotein (P-gp) inducers or inhibitors (phenytoin, rifampicin, carbamazepine, and ketoconazole).

3.3.2 Edoxaban (E)

E is a selective and competitive inhibitor of *factor Xa*. It inhibits thrombin formation for up to 24 h following administration, resulting in prolongation of PT/INR and aPTT, and indirectly inhibits thrombin-induced platelet aggregation [19]. A linear relationship exists between plasma E levels and anti-factor Xa activity. E is absorbed in the small intestine, with a bioavailability of approximately 60%, and reaches peak plasma concentrations 1–2 h after administration, irrespective of food intake.

V_d is large (approximately 107 liters) and follows a two-compartment kinetic model. Protein binding is moderate (approximately 55%). Elimination occurs via both renal (approximately 50%) and non-renal routes, including biliary and hepatic excretion. Plasma clearance is 22 L/h and $t_{1/2}$ h ranges from 10 to 14 h. Dose reduction is required in patients with impaired renal function (eGFR 15–50 ml/min). Advanced age and body weight <60 kg may further reduce non-renal clearance. E undergoes metabolism through multiple hydrolytic pathways, conjugation, and oxidation. Co-administration with strong P-gp inhibitors (cyclosporine, dronedarone, erythromycin, and ketoconazole) requires dose reduction. No dose adjustment is required with CHILD class A and B liver disease patients, given the limited hepatic metabolism (10%). However, E has not been studied in CHILD class C patients. Notably, an eGFR >95 ml/min may be associated with increased renal clearance and a potential reduction in antithrombotic activity. This warning is included in the US SPC, but not in the EU or UK documents. PPIs (proton pump inhibitors) may slightly reduce drug exposure by lowering gastric pH.

3.3.3 Rivaroxaban (R)

R is a direct, specific, and competitive inhibitor of *factor Xa*. R inhibits thrombin formation for up to 24 h, allowing once-daily dosing. It prolongs PT/INR (with a linear correlation to plasma R concentration) and, to a lesser extent, aPTT, and indirectly inhibits thrombin-induced platelet aggregation [19]. Absorption occurs primarily in the stomach and is influenced by food intake, particularly at higher doses (15–20 mg). Bioavailability is high (80–100%), and peak concentrations (C_{max}) are reached 2–3 h after administration. Half-life ($t_{1/2}$ h) ranges from 9 to 11 h. Protein binding is high (95%), and V_d is moderate (approximately 55 L), with minimal impact of body weight on kinetics. *R* is eliminated through both renal and metabolic pathways, with approximately 33% excreted unchanged in urine and an additional 30% as metabolites. Hepatic metabolism via cytochrome P450 enzymes accounts for approximately 60% of total clearance, while fecal elimination contributes approximately 28%. Total clearance is about 10 L/h. In elderly subjects, increased drug exposure appears to be primarily related to age-associated declines in renal function rather than age itself. Strong CYP3A4 and P-gp inhibitors (azoles and protease inhibitors) may significantly increase R plasma concentrations, whereas inducers (Rifampicin, phenytoin, and carbamazepine) may reduce drug exposure up to a possible treatment failure. Given the role of hepatic clearance in R metabolism, the drug is indicated only in CHILD class A patients and is contraindicated in CHILD B and C class patients [4]. In patients with renal impairment, drug exposure and activity increase proportionally with declining renal function, concentration increases being reported in the range of 44–64%. Nonetheless, the significant contribution of non-renal clearance allows its use in selected patients with eGFR >15 ml/min.

3.3.4 Dabigatran (D)

D etexilate (a prodrug) is a direct competitive inhibitor of free and fibrin-bound thrombin. Its anticoagulant effect, achieved by blocking the conversion of fibrinogen to fibrin, is rapid and reversible. D prolongs PT/INR, aPTT, and ecarin clotting time (snake venom) and indirectly inhibits thrombin-induced platelet aggregation [19]. It is absorbed at the level of the stomach and small intestine; food does not affect its absorption. Peak plasma concentrations are reached 1.5 h after administration, with maximal anticoagulant activity approximately 2–3 h after administration, followed by a reduction of approximately 50% over the subsequent 12 h. Total clearance is high (70–140 liters/h), and $t_{1/2}$ h is approximately 12–14 h. Protein binding is low (35%), and V_d ranges from 60 to 70 L. The relatively large V_d may contribute to variable tissue distribution and, although not definitely established, may contribute to potential therapeutic failures in cases of obesity, particularly when treating DVT. Renal elimination accounts for approximately 80% of D clearance. Therefore, reduced renal clearance leads to a marked increase in drug exposure, ranging from 1.5 to 6 times, depending on the severity of renal failure. Metabolites are eliminated via the biliary route, and the 20% hepatic clearance warrants its cautious use in patients with moderate hepatic impairment, while it is contraindicated in CHILD class C patients (in the EU and UK) [4]. In the EU and UK, D is also contraindicated with eGFR <30 ml/min, and dose reduction is recommended if eGFR is between 30 and 50 ml/min. Age significantly influences plasma drug concentrations, and dose reduction is recommended in the EU and UK for elderly patients with AF. Concomitant use of P-gp inhibitors (ketoconazole, dronedarone, itraconazole, cyclosporine, and glecaprevir/pibrentasvir, and to a lesser extent verapamil) results in significant increases in drug exposure. Conversely, the use of P-gp inducers (rifampicin, carbamazepine, and phenytoin) has been associated with reduced D levels. PPIs (proton pump inhibitors) may slightly decrease drug exposure due to reduced gastric pH.

For readers interested in a more detailed discussion dealing with the interaction between hepatic function and DOACs' PK/PD profiles, the recent review by Douketis provides a comprehensive overview [4].

3.3.5 DOACs and Obesity

A brief note is warranted regarding the use of DOACs in obese patients, a still highly controversial area often debated in terms of contraindications or dose adjustment. A recent ISTH review reported that A and R demonstrated efficacy and safety profiles similar to warfarin in the treatment of DVT. On this basis, standard dosing for DVT may be considered even in individuals with BMI >40 and/or body weight >120 kg, supported by the evidence of comparable anti-Xa levels in both obese and normal BMI subjects [20].

For readers interested in a more comprehensive discussion on DOACs use in obesity (including controversies and available evidence), we suggest the recent in-depth review by Menichelli et al. [21]

3.3.6 Management of Drug-Drug Interactions (DDI) with DOACs

The management of drug-drug interactions (DDIs) involving DOACs represents a clinically relevant challenge. A comprehensive and detailed discussion is beyond the scope of this chapter; however, several key concepts should be addressed and applied on a case-by-case basis. Clinical decision-making should primarily rely on information provided in the SPCs of the interacting drugs, supplemented by guidelines, recommendations, available literature, and expert physician judgement/advice.

The main PK interaction pathways for DOACs involve CYP3A4 and the P-gp transporter. R and A undergo significant metabolization by CYP3A4, E is minimally metabolized by CYP3A4, and D is not metabolized via CYP-dependent pathways. Conversely, all four DOACs are substrates of P-gp, an efflux transporter that plays a major role in limiting intestinal absorption and promoting elimination of xenobiotics. Concomitant administration of CYP3A4 and P-gp inhibitors or inducers may result in clinically relevant increases or decreases in DOAC plasma concentrations. Therefore, R and A are particularly prone to interactions with moderate-strong inhibitors/inducers of both CYP3A4 and P-gp, whereas D and E are mainly affected by P-gp-mediated interactions.

The 2021 European Heart Rhythm Association (EHRA) guidelines provide a practical framework for the daily clinical assessment of relevant DDIs involving DOACs [22]. A color-coded table classifies potentially interacting drugs according to the specific DOAC involved

- *White*: no clinically relevant DDI expected
- *Yellow*: caution advice, particularly if two or more "yellow" drugs or bleeding risk factors are present (corresponding to mild-moderate inhibition of CYP3A4 and/or P-gp)
- *Orange*: dose reduction recommended for D and E according to SPC
- *Red*: contraindicated due to a marked increase in DOAC plasma concentrations (strong inhibition of CYP3A4 and/or P-gp)
- *Light blue*: caution advised, especially in cases of polypharmacy or when two or more light blue drugs are present due to reduced DOAC exposure (mild induction of CYP3A4 and/or P-gp)
- *Dark blue*: contraindicated due to reduction of DOAC plasma concentrations (moderate-to-strong induction of CYP3A4 and/or P-gp)

Based on combinations of interacting drugs and the extent and modifiability of bleeding risks, EHRA guidelines propose a management flowchart that includes possible dose adjustments. It should be emphasized that in the presence of red, orange, or multiple yellow factors, or when alternative DOACs or less interacting therapies are unavailable and bleeding risk is high, alternative strategies for stroke prevention should be considered. In experienced centers, strategies may include off-label dose reduction of DOACs (generally discouraged due to lack of RCT data) based on available PK information and/or measurements of DOACs plasma levels. In real-world clinical practice, patients are increasingly exposed to complex poly-pharmacy, including life-saving or non-modifiable therapies (e.g., oncological drugs, immunosuppressants, etc.). Should it be the case, rather than focusing on the effect of individual drugs, it may be more appropriate to assess the overall balance of inhibition and induction resulting from the combined pharmacological regimen. If and where available, repeated measurements of DOAC plasma concentrations, with timing and methods tailored to the PK/PD characteristics of the interacting agents, may further support clinical decision-making. For such a complex assessment, consultation with clinicians experienced in anticoagulation management and/or advice from a specialist in Clinical Pharmacology and Toxicology is strongly recommended.

3.4 DOACs: Mechanisms of Action and Interactions with the Coagulation Cascade [2–4]

Direct oral anticoagulants include the direct *thrombin* inhibitor (DTI, Dabiga*tr*an) and the direct *factor Xa* inhibitors (DXaIs) Api*xa*ban, Rivaro*xa*ban, Edo*xa*ban). These agents selectively block key procoagulant enzymes involved in fibrin clot generation. Each DOAC inhibits a single target enzyme, a feature reflected in the drug nomenclature, in which the inhibited factor is embedded in the drug name.

Thrombin—Thrombin (factor IIa) is the final effector enzyme of the coagulation cascade and is generated through the proteolytic cleavage of prothrombin by activated factor X (tenase). Thrombin plays a central role in hemostasis: it converts fibrinogen to fibrin, activates coagulation factors V, VIII, XI, and XIII, and promotes platelet activation through protease-activated receptors (PAR1 and PAR4) expressed on the platelet surface. In addition, thrombin interacts with endothelial cell receptors involved in natural anticoagulation pathways, including thrombomodulin, protein C, and protein S. Thrombin is biologically active both in the circulating phase and when bound to the clot. D, as a direct thrombin inhibitor, blocks the conversion of fibrinogen to fibrin in both free and clot-bound thrombin. In contrast, UF and LMWH inhibit thrombin indirectly, by potentiating AT activity (a natural anticoagulant and physiological inhibitor of the coagulation process) and are effective only against thrombin in the fluid phase [23].

Factor Xa: Factor Xa occupies a strategic position immediately upstream of thrombin in the coagulation cascade. It is generated through the proteolytic activation of Factor X by one of the two X-ase (tenase) complexes. Inhibition of Factor Xa effectively suppresses thrombin generation and amplification, a key aspect of the new *cell-based model* of hemostasis, which has replaced the intrinsic and extrinsic phases of the old model) [7]. Direct Factor Xa inhibitors (DXaIs, R, A, E) bind selectively and reversibly to the active site of Factor Xa, inhibiting the conversion of prothrombin to thrombin without the need for cofactors [24]. Similar to thrombin Factor Xa is active both in circulating clot-bound form, DXaIs being able to block both. In contrast, indirect Factor Xa inhibitors such as heparin and fondaparinux (a synthetic pentasaccharide) exert their effects through AT and inactivate Factor Xa only in the fluid phase.

Anticoagulation in Chronic Renal Failure (CRF) Patients

Given the relevance of renal dysfunction in anticoagulant management, a concise overview of recommended strategies for anticoagulation in patients with CRF is provided, tailored to different clinical settings [4]. Renal function should be estimated using the Cockcroft-Gault formula, preferably incorporating current body weight in accordance with methods used in DOAC registration trials [25].

- *Hospitalized* patients with CRF
  - UF or LMWH is generally used
- *Outpatients* with mild to moderate CRF (*eGFR ≥ 30 < 50 ml/min*)
  - Based on robust evidence, DOACs are considered valid alternatives to VKAs.
  - A 2019 meta-analysis cited by Douketis, including 34,000 patients (predominantly with AF), documented that compared to warfarin, DOACs were associated with a significant reduction in stroke risk, no increase in major bleeding (including intracranial bleeding), and a trend toward improved survival [4].
  - Dose adjustments may be required depending on the specific DOAC and patient characteristics ([2, 4)].
- *Outpatients* with severe CRF (eGFR <30 ml/min)
  - Despite emerging data suggesting acceptable efficacy and safety of certain DOACs, warfarin is generally preferred for long-term treatment.
  - A 2020 systematic review cited by Douketis et al. [4], including nine studies (two randomized trials) involving patients with severe CRF (including those on dialysis and indications such as AF or DVT, reported similar efficacy between DOACS. Notably, bleeding risk with A was comparable to that observed with warfarin.

3.5 DOACs: Effects on Coagulation Tests [1, 6, 9–11]

Despite the advantage of the predictable pharmacokinetics of DOACs, several clinical scenarios require assessment of their actual anticoagulant effect using laboratory testing. They include massive bleeding, intracranial hemorrhage, high-risk elective procedures, urgent/emergency interventions (including thrombolysis), complex comorbidities (renal failure, hepatic failure), suspected overdose, pathological overweight, or underweight. The "standard" screening coagulation tests (PT/INR, aPTT,

Thrombin Time (TT)) provide limited and often unreliable information regarding the anticoagulant activity of DOACs and lack specificity for the individual drugs. Interpretation of these tests requires precise knowledge of the drug assumed, the timing of the last dose, and the characteristics of the assay used [3]. Based on the available evidence, Tripodi et al. recommend [10] the following assays for a reliable measurement of DOAC plasma concentrations

- Dabigatran: dTT [diluted Thrombin Time] and ecarin-based assays [ECA]
- Rivaroxaban, Apixaban, Edoxaban: Anti-factor Xa activity

These assays can be calibrated using drug-specific standards, with results expressed in ng/ml [11]. Accurate interpretation depends on knowledge of the timing of the last drug administration. At present, no studies have conclusively defined therapeutic target plasma concentrations of DOACS, although median peak and trough levels are available, along with emerging correlations between plasma concentrations and thrombotic and bleeding events [11]. Tables 3.1 and 3.2 (adapted and modified from ([9–11]) summarize, respectively, the effects of DOACs on conventional (PT/aPTT) (Table 3.1) and on selected hemostatic tests (Table 3.2).

The diagnostic accuracy of coagulation assays may vary significantly in the presence of low plasma concentrations of DOACs. Moreover, the lack of availability of laboratory tests for DOACs on a 24/7 basis is still a critical issue not only in Spoke Hospitals but also in some Hub Centers. This limitation underscores the Società Italiana di Emostasi e Trombosi (SISET) recommendation to adequately expand/equip clinical laboratories with reliable assays for DOAC measurements, applicable in both elective and emergency settings [1, 10, 11].

International guidelines [25–28] indicate that *plasma drug concentrations >30 ng/ml* are associated with "clinically relevant" anticoagulant activity, whereas concentrations *<30 ng/ml* are generally considered safe to proceed with thrombolysis or surgical/interventional procedures, including neuraxial anesthesia [28]. These thresholds may also assist in scheduling elective procedures when PK criteria alone are insufficient or unreliable and in avoiding unnecessary or potentially harmful reversal strategies in cases of intracranial hemorrhage and/or other life-threatening bleeding.

Table 3.1 Effects of DOACS on conventional hemostatic tests (see text)

	Drug	Apixaban	Edoxaban	Rivaroxaban	Dabigatran
Test					
PT			⬆	⬆⬆	⬆
APTT					⬆⬆
DTT Diluted thrombin time		No activity	No activity	No activity	⬆⬆ ⬆⬆
Activity ANTI FXA		⬆⬆ ⬆	⬆⬆ ⬆	⬆⬆ ⬆	No activity

Modified from [9–11]

Table 3.2 Effects of DOACs on selected hemostatic parameters

Hemostatic parameters	Expected effect on activity or on coagulation factors in the presence of DOACS
Antithrombin (activity)	**Overestimation**
Protein C/protein S (activity)	**Underestimation**
Coagulation factors	**Underestimation**
Fibrinogen	**Underestimation**
Factor XIII	**Underestimation**

Modified from [9–11]

3.5.1 Measurement and Monitoring of the Anticoagulant Effect of DOACs

3.5.1.1 Anti-Xa Agents (R A E)

The anticoagulant effect of DXA can be reliably quantified using an anti-Xa (aXa) assay, specifically calibrated for the individual drug. When drug-specific calibration is available, an anticoagulant effect is generally considered undetectable at plasma concentrations <30 ng/mL. In settings where drug-specific calibrated aXa assays are not available, a chromogenic aXa test may be used as a surrogate. In this context, undetectable anticoagulant activity is usually defined as an aXa level <0.1 IU/mL. Close collaboration with the clinical laboratory is essential to determine the assays in use and to agree on locally validated cutoffs capable of reliably excluding clinically relevant anticoagulant activity.

3.5.1.2 Direct Thrombin Inhibitor (D)

The anticoagulant effect of Dabigatran can be assessed using the thrombin time (TT), a test extremely sensitive to the presence of the drug. However, due to this high sensitivity, even minimal D concentrations may result in a markedly prolonged TT, making it unsuitable for quantitative assessment of anticoagulant intensity. To overcome this limitation, diluted Thrombin Time (dTT) assays are preferred as they allow a more accurate estimation of D plasma levels. A D concentration <30 ng/mL is generally considered an appropriate cutoff level to exclude clinically relevant anticoagulant activity [1, 9–11, 28].

3.5.1.3 Pragmatic Cutoffs in Urgent and Semi-urgent Clinical Scenarios

In a recent review, Douketis et al. proposed a plasma DOAC concentration <50 ng/mL as a pragmatic threshold allowing urgent or semi-urgent procedures to be performed without the need for anticoagulant reversal. This recommendation is largely derived from the conclusions of the PAUSE study (see below) and reflects real-world perioperative decision-making [2]. However, in the same authoritative and updated review by Douketis et al. [2] (confirmed in 2025 UPTODATE recommendations) [4], it is emphasized that a DOAC dose has been assumed within the previous 48 h and laboratory testing is not available, anticoagulant reversal should be strongly recommended, as a high-risk situation [2–4]. Notably, the 2025 ASRA guidelines on DOACs and regional anesthesia recommend a more conservative value of 30 ng/mL when considering neuraxial or deep regional blocks, underscoring the need to tailor thresholds to the specific clinical context and to the bleeding risk [28].

3.5.2 Emergency Procedures (Surgical, Endoscopic, Radiological, etc.)

In urgent and emergency settings, it is imperative to determine whether clinically relevant anticoagulant activity of DOAC is present. As noted above, proposed—but not yet universally accepted clinical thresholds suggest that plasma concentrations <30 ng/mL or <50 ng/mL may be considered safe to proceed with invasive procedures. In selected urgent/emergency scenarios, such as observational studies of pharmacological thrombolysis for ischemic stroke, a higher cutoff value (<100 ng/mL) has also been used [5]. So far, no cutoff value derived from specific coagulation assays has been validated in RCTs and can therefore be considered "definitive." Moreover, urgent/emergency settings highlight the critical need for robust, reliable, and rapidly available tests, ideally including point-of-care (POC) methods able to identify DOAC plasma concentrations below critical relevant thresholds (<30 ng/mL or <50 ng/mL or even <100 ng/mL). Such testing would allow decision-making to be guided not only by pharmacokinetic considerations but also by objective laboratory data [4, 5, 28]. Currently, apart from the DOA SENSE DIPSTICK for urine, no reliable POC tests are commercially available. Consequently, recent proposed algorithms that partially incorporate laboratory testing are not (yet) fully applicable in routine clinical practice, despite their considerable conceptual interest [5]. Currently, only algorithm components based on blood levels above or below predefined thresholds (30 ng/mL, 50 ng/mL, 100 ng/mL) can realistically be used to guide treatment decision, including the need for anticoagulant reversal [5]. In this context, the availability of alternatives and more reliable POC solutions in the near future is eagerly awaited. Below are brief comments on the urinary dipstick (available and CE-marked) [5] and on viscoelastic tests (not yet commercially available) [29]. Given the risk false-positive/false-negative results with several coagulation assays used in clinical practice, reliance on validated and reliable tests is mandatory [5, 29]

1. *DOAC dipstick* (urine test—DOA SENSE, Heidelberg, Germany, CE marked, but not FDA approved)
   (a) This test detects traces of all DOACs (DRAE). When positive, sensitivity for plasma concentrations >30 ng/mL is reported to be between 95% and 100% for all DOACs.
   (b) Negative test can rule out plasma concentrations >14 ng/mL for RAE and >19 ng/mL for D. However, the method is not currently recommended for quantitative assessments of anticoagulant activity [5].

   (c) Specificity is relatively low in several studies, raising concerns regarding false-positive results [5].

2. *CLOT PRO* viscoelastic system (hemonetics)

   This viscoelastic platform uses dedicated reagents to assess DOAC activity [22]:

   (a) Ecarin-based assay (CLOTPRO—ECA) (ecarin is a snake venom) for D: the test shows a very high correlation with plasma D concentrations.
   (b) Russell's viper venom (RVV) (CLOTPRO - RVV) for Xa inhibitors.
   (c) The reported turnaround time is <10 min, although the system is not yet fully automated. CLOTPRO was studied between 2019 and 2021 and marketed in 2021; it was withdrawn from the market in 2024. It is expected (with high probability) to return to the market in 2026 [29].

3. Emerging role of dedicated viscoelastic tests (VETs)

   According to the most recent literature, there is a substantial interest in the use of VETs with *dedicated* cartridges (e.g., CLOT PRO and QUANTRA viscoelastic testing systems) to guide clinical management in both elective and urgent/emergency settings [29].
4. *Conventional VETs* (TEG6 HAEMONETICS and ROTEM SIGMA WERFEN) are not reliable for the clinical management of patients on DOACs, either in elective or emergency settings, and should not be used for this purpose [29].

3.6 Management of DOACs in Surgical Patients: Elective and Urgent/Emergency Settings

To address the management of DOACs in urgent/emergency conditions, the following key documents will be used: (i) the perioperative management guidelines proposed by Douketis et al. [2, 4] for elective surgical and interventional procedures; (ii) the 2024 ESAIC guidelines [8]; (iii) the 2021 ESC guidelines [22]; and (iv) the 2025 ASRA guidelines [21]. Recommendations regarding monitoring, strategies for planning interventional procedures, and the choice of reversal approaches (pharmacological or procedural) are summarized accordingly.

The need for invasive procedures—whether elective or urgent/emergent—or for the treatment of spontaneous bleeding in patients receiving DOACs increasingly places ED physicians, anesthesiologists, and surgeons at the forefront of managing these complex clinical scenarios. Among patients treated with DOACs: (i) the incidence of intracranial bleeding is low (0.3–0.5%); (ii) between 10% and 20% of patients treated with DOACs undergo surgical procedures or invasive interventions while treated; and (iii) indication for DOAC therapy is progressively expanding to include elderly patients, individuals with AF, and more and more frequently frail patients with multiple comorbidities [1, 2, 4, 8].

In the surgical patient, optimal management strategies must be clearly defined in the following clinical scenario.

- *Elective procedures*
  - (i) Whether or not perioperative interruption is necessary
  - (ii) Appropriate timing of drug discontinuation and resumption
- *Urgent/emergency procedures*
  - (i) Management of recent (<48 h) DOAC assumption
  - (ii) Indications for and safe implementation of DOAC reversal when required
- *Patient with spontaneous bleeding*
  - (i) Whether or not anticoagulation reversal is indicated
  - (ii) The choice and timing of reversal strategies as part of the emergency management

Therefore, the optimal perioperative and emergency management of patients receiving DOACs requires a thorough understanding of several key elements: (i) mechanisms of action and PK/PD properties of each agent; (ii) the availability and limitations of reliable drug-specific laboratory assays; (iii) the effect of DOACs on both "generic" and "specific" coagulation tests to avoid misinterpretation (see Tables 3.1 and 3.2); (iv) indications and contraindications for DOAC use; and (v) the availability, indications, contraindications, and clinical effects of reversal agents [1, 2, 4, 8].

3.6.1 DOACs in Patients Undergoing Elective Surgical Procedures (or Interventional Radiology, Endoscopy, or Other Procedures)

The clinical management of a patient receiving DOAC therapy who requires elective surgery or invasive procedures involves a careful decision on whether to temporarily interrupt or continue anticoagulation during the perioperative period. The aim is twofold: to minimize thrombotic risk, which may transiently increase when the drug is withheld, and to reduce the procedure-related bleeding, which depends on the intrinsic bleeding risk of the procedure. It should be recognized that periprocedural bleeding may require a prolonged interruption of anticoagulation, a longer suspension of anticoagulation, further increasing the thromboembolic risk. In patients treated with DOACs, PK/PD properties, in particular, the rapid onset of action, relatively short elimination half-life, and predictable clearance pathways allow for an easier periprocedural management compared with VKAs [2, 4, 18]. Specifically, DOAC therapy requires shorter interruption periods, faster postoperative resumption, obviating the need for *bridging* therapy with heparin in many cases. These considerations form the basis of management strategies primarily driven by PK/PD parameters—the so-called *pharmacokinetic strategy*. This approach, however, does not fully account for patient-specific factors and procedural issues.

3.6.1.1 Timing of DOAC Interruption Based on Procedural Bleeding Risk

For elective procedures, current recommendations suggest the following approach [1, 30].

Procedures with *low or moderate bleeding risk*

- DOAC therapy should be discontinued prior to the procedure for a period corresponding to two to three elimination half-lives.
- Anticoagulation may generally be resumed on the day following the procedure, provided adequate hemostasis has been achieved.

Procedures with *high bleeding risk*

- DOAC therapy should be discontinued for a period corresponding to approximately 4–5 elimination half-lives.
- Anticoagulation should be resumed no earlier than postoperative day (POD) 2 or 3, provided adequate hemostasis has been achieved, and always addressing patient-related issues.

3.6.1.2 A Patient- and Procedure-Tailored Approach

A more individualized and nuanced strategy has been proposed by Douketis [2, 4], integrating PK/PD issues with clinical and procedural variables. This approach emphasizes that decisions regarding the time of interruption, duration of suspension, and resumption of DOAC therapy should be based on the combined assessment of the following

- *Patient-related factors*
  - Presence of comorbidities and/or frailty able to influence drug clearance or bleeding risk
  - Conditions associated with altered PK/PD profiles (e.g., renal dysfunction)
  - Overall thromboembolic risk
- *Procedure-related bleeding risk* (see Table 3.3), which includes
  - Type of surgery/intervention
  - Nature of the procedure (elective vs urgent)
  - Classification of the bleeding risk as
    - *Minimal risk*
    - *Low risk*—bleeding within POD 2 between 0 and 2%
    - *High risk*—bleeding within POD 2 between 2 and 4%
  - *Notably, some classifications include "minimal risk" procedures within the "low-risk" category*
- *Severity and Clinical Relevance of Potential Bleeding*
  - *Major bleeding* is generally (though not universally) defined as (i) bleeding associated with a high risk of mortality; (ii) occurring at a critical anatomical

site (e.g., intracranial, pericardial, retroperitoneal, intramedullary, intraocular); (iii) requiring surgical/interventional treatment associated with a hemoglobin decrease $\geq$2 g/dL or requiring transfusion of $\geq$2 units of red blood cells.

This integrated framework allows for a more precise balance between bleeding and thrombotic risk and supports individualized perioperative decision-making in patients treated with DOACs.

3.6.1.3 Estimation of Thromboembolic Risk and Timing of DOAC Interruption

Assessment of thromboembolic risk represents a cornerstone of periprocedural management in patients receiving DOACs. Thromboembolic risk is multifactorial, being influenced by advanced age, presence of AF, mechanical heart valves, and history of arterial or venous thromboembolism, particularly DVT and PE. In this context, validated stratification tools, such as CHA_2 DS_2 VASc score for patients with AF and guideline-based indication for anticoagulant therapy in mechanical valve disease, venous thrombosis (VTE, venous thromboembolism), should systematically be applied. A general and widely accepted principle is that, whenever feasible, elective procedures should be postponed for three to 6 months following an acute thromboembolic event to minimize recurrence risk, highest during the first 4 weeks, substantially decreased after 3–4 months, and considered substantially low after 1 year.

Determining the Timing of DOAC Interruption The timing of DOACs discontinuation before a procedure should be defined through an integrated assessment based on PK/PD characteristics of each DOAC, renal and hepatic function, both of which can significantly impact drug clearance. Procedural bleeding risk, classified as minimal, low, and high (see Table 3.3).
For procedures associated with *minimal* bleeding risk (dental extractions, cataract surgery, skin biopsies), current recommendations generally advise *not to interrupt* DOAC therapy, provided local hemostatic measures are applied.

In parallel, thromboembolic risk should always be reassessed, with the aim of optimally scheduling the procedure when the risk is lowest, particularly if the thrombotic risk is high but transient. In selected high-risk scenarios, usually within 4 weeks of an acute venous thromboembolic event, temporary placement of a vena cava filter may be considered, although this strategy should be reserved for exceptional cases and carefully weighed against potential complications.

3.6.1.4 Pharmacokinetic Versus Laboratory-Based Strategies

While periprocedural management of DOACs has traditionally relied upon a "pharmacokinetic" -based strategy, several authors argue that this approach should be complemented by a "laboratory-based" strategy [1, 10, 11]. Such an approach could be particularly relevant in settings where reliance on PK criteria alone should be unsafe or insufficient, including, but not limited to, surgical intervention/invasive procedure with a high bleeding risk; adverse event (bleeding or thrombosis);

Table 3.3 Classification of surgical interventions/procedures according to the hemorrhagic risk

Lower risk procedures (infrequent bleeding/low clinical impact)
1. Dental and periodontal surgery, including implant placement
2. Cataract or glaucoma surgery
3. Endoscopy (without biopsy or resection)
4. Superficial surgery, skin biopsy, abscess incision, vaccination
5. Pacemaker or ICD implantation (except for complex procedures)
6. Electrophysiological study or catheter ablation (except for complex procedures)
7. Routine elective intervention on coronary/peripheral arteries (except complex procedures)
Low-risk procedures (infrequent bleeding and without serious clinical impact)
1. Complex dental procedures
2. Endoscopy with simple biopsy
3. Minor orthopedic surgery (foot, hand, arthroscopy)
High-risk procedures (frequent bleeding with significant clinical impact)
1. Neurosurgery
2. Cardiac surgery
3. Vascular surgery (aortic aneurysm repair, vascular bypass, including peripheral)
4. Thoracic surgery
5. Spinal or epidural anesthesia; diagnostic lumbar puncture
6. Complex interventional cardiology (e.g., lead extraction, epicardial ablation for VT, chronic total occlusion PCI, etc.)
7. Abdominal surgery
8. Liver biopsy
9. Major orthopedic surgery
10. Major urological surgery/biopsy /ESWL (extracorporeal shock wave lithotripsy)

decision-making in case of thrombolytic therapy in acute ischemic stroke; situations requiring urgent consideration of DOAC reversal. In these settings, measurement of plasma DOAC concentrations allows a more accurate assessment of residual anticoagulant activity, supporting personalized decisions (see Sect. 3.6). The availability of reliable, rapid, and ideally 24/7 plasma DOAC assays should be strongly advocated, providing clinicians with a powerful tool to optimize patient safety and improve periprocedural and emergency management. Such a combined pharmacokinetic and laboratory-based framework should represent the most rational and patient-centered approach to the perioperative management of DOAC therapy [1, 9–11].

3.6.2 Interruption of DOACs

Owing to their favorable PK/PD profiles, interruption of DOAC therapy generally requires only a short suspension period. B*ridging* with heparin is rarely indicated and avoided in a large part of the cases. Very selected exceptions may include an anticipated very slow recovery of gastrointestinal function (e.g., postoperative ileus) and inability to resume oral therapy. The most robust evidence supporting perioperative DOACs management (interruption/resumption) derives from the PAUSE study (Perioperative Anticoagulation Use for Surgery Evaluation), a large prospective cohort study that enrolled approximately 3000 patients receiving DOAC for AF who underwent elective surgery or invasive procedures [31, 32].. The study adopted a pragmatic, strictly pharmacokinetic-based strategy, with standardized DOAC interruption and resumption schedule, no coagulation testing, and no LMWH bridging. The clinical relevance and safety of this approach were demonstrated by (i) low rates of adverse outcomes (major bleeding <2%; ischemic stroke <0.5%); (ii) excellent protocol adherence (94%) to both preoperative interruption and postoperative resumption schedules; and (iii) high external validity and generalizability across different DOACs and procedural risk categories [32]. These results strongly support the rationale of a simplified standardized approach to DOAC interruption in elective surgery, particularly in low-risk conditions.

3.6.3 Management of DOACs in Elective Surgery/Procedures [2, 4] (According to Douketis et al. and Bleeding Risk as per Table 3.3) [2, 4, 22, 23]

1. Procedures with *minimal bleeding risk*

   DOAC therapy is not generally interrupted, with minor timing adjustments based on the schedule

   - DOACs administered twice daily
     - Omit the morning dose on the day of the procedure
     - Resume therapy with the evening dose
   - DOACs administered once daily
     - The DOAC is taken in the evening of the procedure
2. Procedures with *mild or moderate bleeding risk*
   - DOAC therapy should be temporarily suspended
     - *The day before* the procedure for *RAE*
     - *Two days before* the procedure for *D*
   - DOAC therapy is resumed
     - The day after the procedure, provided that adequate hemostasis has been achieved
3. Procedures with *high bleeding risk*
   - A longer interruption of DOAC therapy is required
     - *From day 2 before* the procedure for *RAE*
     - *From day 4 or 5* (depending on renal function) *before* the procedure for *D*
   - DOAC therapy is resumed 2–3 days after the procedure. However, in the presence of bleeding risk, the administration of DOACs is generally recommended on POD 3.

In cases of prolonged DOAC suspension (due either to postoperative ileus and/or to procedures precluding early gastrointestinal absorption and in patients with high thromboembolic risk, the use of prophylactic doses of LMWH (enoxaparin 40 mg once daily) may be considered as a temporary measure until oral anticoagulants can be reliably resumed. Interested readers are invited to access the original "visual" summary by Douketis et al. [2] of DOAC interruption and resumption strategies, stratified by procedural bleeding risk and renal function (for D).

Alongside the "*pharmacokinetic*" strategy, since as early as 2015, the need to use a "*laboratory-based*" strategy in specific, complex contexts/conditions has been increasingly recognized: this is well emphasized (and justified) by Squizzato et al. in the SISET 2022 document [1]. The need for two strategies—"*pharmacokinetic-based*" and "*laboratory-based*"—underscores how the PK criterion can be validated by the laboratory-based approach, which allows for "verification" of the appropriateness of the pragmatic pharmacological strategy. FCSA [1, 10] considers the measurement of plasma DOAC levels to be "*clinically necessary*" in patients:

- At "higher" risk of bleeding ("extremely high")
- Who, due to renal or hepatic function, age, body weight, or frailty, may be at high risk of elevated plasma DOAC levels
- At risk of severe bleeding complications

3.7 The Setting of Urgency/Emergency and the Issue of DOAC Reversal [8]

In the setting of surgical or interventional emergencies or in patients presenting with spontaneous bleeding while on DOAC therapy, several management strategies have been proposed over time. However, only recently has clinical practice been substantially modified by the availability of specific *direct* DOAC reversal agents, in addition to "*non-specific*" agents, such as prothrombin complex (PCC), activated prothrombin complex (aPCC), and recombinant activated Factor (rFVIIa). It is important to emphasize that no single optimal strategy exists, as emergency scenarios are heterogeneous and may require individualized decision-making. According to the 2024 ESAIC recommendations [8], several points should be highlighted:

(i) *Given the low to very low level of evidence available, most recommendations are weak.*
(ii) *Only a minority of recommendations are supported by high-quality evidence, underscoring the urgent need for future, well-designed prospective studies.*
(iii) *At the moment, no specific recommendations are available for special populations, such as pediatric patients or patients with traumatic brain injury.*

(iv) *The high to very high cost of direct reversal antagonists (particularly andexanet alfa) may (but should not!!) influence clinical decision-making. Therefore, it is mandatory to involve Hospital Administrations and Strategic/Health Management to ensure equitable access and to avoid restricting potentially life-saving therapies.*

When surgical or interventional procedures are to be performed on the same day of DOAC intake, reversal strategies may include the use of specific antagonists, non-specific procoagulant agents (largely off-label for this indication), or even dialysis techniques in case of D.

It should be emphasized that neuraxial techniques or deep peripheral blocks are absolutely contraindicated in patients on DOAC therapy presenting in emergency situations [28, 33]. The most recent ASRA 2025 guidelines explicitly contraindicate the use of reversal agents to perform neuraxial anesthesia or peripheral block *(grade IIC), recommending* general anesthesia when required [28].

3.7.1 Reversal of DOACs

The decision to reverse DOACs should be multidisciplinary and as prompt as possible (time sensitive) [2–8]. Both patient-related factors (age, comorbidities, renal function, and site and severity of bleeding) and procedural-related factors (urgency and bleeding risk of the intervention) must be carefully evaluated. A recent survey—conducted prior to the clinical availability of specific reversal agents—revealed several critical gaps in clinical practice: (i) only one third of hospitals had formal protocol for emergency DOAC reversal; (ii) fresh frozen plasma (FFP) was still administered in at least one third of case, despite the widespread dissemination of guidelines recommending restrictive indications for its use; (iii) in at least 60% of cases, a cardiologic and/or hematologic/coagulation consultation was obtained, and in roughly half of cases, a multidisciplinary consensus supported the use of PCC [34]. Indeed, multidisciplinary assessment involving surgeons, anesthesiologists, cardiologists, and hematologists serves a dual purpose: to consider whether the procedure can be postponed, even by 12–24 h; if the intervention is deemed non-deferrable, to guide the choice and timing of the most appropriate reversal strategy. As already emphasized, time since last DOAC intake and renal function are among the critical determinants of a residual anticoagulant effect, given the impact of PK/PD characteristics.

Specific reversal agents are currently available for DOAC—*idarucizumab* for D and *andexanet alpha* for anti-Xa agents, as well as *nonspecific agents with high hemostatic properties*, such as three- or preferably four-factor prothrombin complex concentrate [PCC], activated PCC [aPCC, FEIBA], recombinant activated factor VII [rFVIIa] [2–8].

3.7.2 Hemorrhagic Complications Associated with Anticoagulant Use

The most significant hemorrhagic complications with oral anticoagulants—both DOACs and VKAs—are intracranial hemorrhage (ICH) and gastrointestinal bleeding (GIB). As reported in the recent review by Pozzi et al. [3], *20%* of ICH cases are attributable to VKA therapy. In patients treated with DOACs, both morbidity and mortality are significantly lower compared to those treated with VKAs. Similar findings have been reported for GIB, with reduced transfusion requirements and fewer complications in DOAC-treated patients. Of particular interest in surgical patients—when balancing hemorrhagic and thrombotic risk is critical, -perioperative bleeding rate and transfusion requirements appear lower than in those receiving VKAs [3].

3.7.2.1 Guidelines and Future Perspectives

The discussion of DOAC reversal is based on the following key sources: ESC 2021 [22], ESAIC 2024 [8], ASRA 2025 [28]; and major contributions by Squizzato et al. [1], Tripodi et al. [9–11], Douketis et al. [2, 4], Pozzi et al. [3], Tran et al. [5], and Mbhor et al. [6] The clinical context includes patients requiring urgent or emergency surgery or interventional procedures—including central and deep peripheral nerve blocks—as well as those presenting to the emergency department with active bleeding while on DOAC therapy. Management considerations must address (i) the appropriate use of specific reversal agents (*idarucizumab, IDA, for D* and *andexanet alpha, Aα, for anti-Xa, RAE*) or available non-specific hemostatic agents and (ii) the clinical contexts in which their use is indicated or not (see Figure 9 page 1638 in ESC 2021) [22]. Although still debated, a promising near-future approach involves the integration of the pharmacokinetic-based strategies with an advanced "laboratory-based" assessment [1, 9–11], combining the quantitative plasma DOACs measurement with emerging VETs [29]. Such an integrated strategy could improve the process of decision-making regarding the antidotes us. This underlines the critical importance of reliable laboratory assays and validated POC tests, not only in *hub* centers but also in *spoke* hospitals, given the widespread use of DOACs in urgent clinical scenarios. The 2021 ESC strongly recommend the following [22]: "to develop a multidisciplinary hospital consultation strategy involving cardiologists, hemostasis experts, emergency physicians/intensive care specialists, anesthesiologists, and surgeons, with the involvement of the Laboratory and Medical Directorate and the preparation of a protocol that includes (i) availability for consultation 24/7; (ii) specific coagulation tests for DOACs available on an emergency basis; (iii) availability of direct or non-specific antagonists in easily accessible locations; (iii) instructions for their use."

This strategy should be widely disseminated, easily accessible (intranet site, emergency department, pocket guides, etc.), regularly reviewed, and, if necessary, subject to audit for complex cases. The interested readers are referred to the 2021 ESC guideline [22] operational protocol: to be underlined, that for D in case of a non-life-threatening scenario, and if IDA is not available, the use of dialysis techniques is to be considered.

3.7.3 Direct DOAC Antagonists [2, 4, 8]

3.7.3.1 Idarucizumab (IDA)

IDA is a humanized monoclonal antibody fragment directed against D with an affinity 350 times greater than that of thrombin. It produces immediate and sustained neutralization of D anticoagulant effects. Current recommendations are largely derived from the REVERSE-AD study, a prospective non-randomized trial, that formed the basis for EMA approval of IDA as a specific antidote for D in 2016 [8, 35, 36]. The study enrolled 503 patients: 301 with uncontrolled bleeding—predominantly gastrointestinal bleeding (GIB) and intracranial hemorrhage (ICH)—and 202 requiring urgent procedures. Laboratory assessment of anticoagulant reversal was performed in more than 90% of patients using diluted Thrombin Time (dTT), ecarin clotting time (ECT), both specific for D, as well as activated partial thromboplastin time (aPTT), non-specific but sensitive assay for D. Based on normalization of dTT and ECT, biochemical reversal was achieved in 100% of the cases. Clinical hemostasis within 24 h was achieved in 68% of patient cases, with a median time to hemostasis of 2.5 h. Thrombotic events occurred in 4.8% and 6.8% at 30 and 90 days, respectively, most within the first 5 days after administration, one-third occurring after resumption of anticoagulant therapy. Overall mortality ranged from 12.5% to 13.5%. Among the limitations of the REVERSE AD study ([8, 37, 38)] are (i) coagulation testing was performed (too) early after IDA administration (4 h), potentially overestimating sustained results; (ii) about 25% of the patients had measurable D plasma concentrations at 12–24 h after antidote administration. This phenomenon has been attributed to a "redistribution" of IDA from the extravascular to the intravascular space. In patients with renal impairment, instead, the prolonged D elimination could have resulted in incomplete antagonism following the standard dose (5 grams) of IDA, thus reflecting D pharmacokinetics rather than antidote failure [38].

3.7.3.2 Andexanet alfa (Aα)

A***α*** is a modified, recombinant, and catalytically inactive human FXa: this molecule reversibly binds RAE, thereby reducing their activity and restoring endogenous FXa availability. Administration consists of an initial intravenous slow bolus (15–30 min), followed by a continuous infusion for 2 h. The ANNEXA-4 study, a prospective single-cohort trial, evaluated Aα inpatients presenting with major acute bleeding within 18 h of intake of apixaban (54%), rivaroxaban (40%), or enoxaparin (6%), and with baseline anti-FXa activity ≥75 ng/mL [39, 40]. ICH accounted for 64% of patients and GIB for 26%. Treatment resulted in a 92% reduction in anti-FXa activity. Hemostatic efficacy at 12 h post-administration was rated "excellent" or "good" in 85% of patients with GIB and 80% of those with ICH. Thirty-day mortality was 14%. Thrombotic events occurred in 10% of patients, none of whom had resumed oral anticoagulant therapy at the time of the event. However, Aα also binds to tissue factor pathway inhibitor (TFPI), leading to increased thrombin generation, a mechanism that may at least in part explain the higher thromboembolic complications rate compared with other reversal strategies [34]. Consequently, dose selection should be individualized and discussed with a specialist, and based primarily on the timing of the last FXa inhibitor intake (< or >8 h) [22]. *Two dosing options are available: "Low dose"*—intravenous bolus of 400 mg (30 mg min^{-1}), followed by an infusion of 480 mg (4 mg min^{-1}). *"High dose"*—800 mg IV bolus, followed by 960 mg infusion (8 mg min^{-1}). Specialist consultation is mandatory when considering Aα for minor bleeding or for urgent high-risk surgery, as these scenarios have not yet been adequately studied. As with the REVERSE-AD study for IDA [35, 36], the ANNEXA-4 study for Aα [39, 40] was an uncontrolled and non-randomized study, with biomarker reduction and clinical hemostasis as co-primary endpoints. On this basis, EMA and FDA approved Aα for adult patients treated with A and R when reversal is required for *life-threatening* or uncontrolled/uncontrollable bleeding [8, 22]. The ESC 2021 guidelines emphasized that "*given the very similar mechanism of action of Aα on E (preliminary data from the ANNEXA-4 study, Benz* et al., *International Stroke Conference 2021), a similar reversal effect on E may be expected*" [22], even if the use of Aα for edoxaban remains *off-label* in several national guidelines, included NHS UK hospital guidelines [22].

For completeness, the randomized ANNEXA-I trial comparing *Andexanet with standard of care* (SOC) in ICH demonstrated superiority in limiting hematoma expansion [41]. Here again too, several caveats are to be raised: (i) 30-day neurological outcome were similar; (ii) the "hematoma expansion" as outcome was a surrogate; (iii) early trial termination may have overestimated benefit (thus not fully guaranteeing a true superiority); (iv) SOC was heterogeneous (at the discretion of the treating physician), and PCC dosing potentially suboptimal; and (v) inclusion criteria were modified after trial initiation, from "intracranial hemorrhage" to "intraparenchymal hemorrhage."

3.7.3.3 Hemostatic Interventions with Non-specific Agents (Prothrombin Complex Concentrate (PCC), Activated Prothrombin Complex Concentrate (aPCC, FEIBA), and rFVIIa)

Before the availability of specific DOAC antagonists, and still in selected circumstances, non-specific hemostatic agents—PCC, aPCC, and rFVIIa—have been used to manage severe bleeding associated with recent DOAC intake [8]. Although these agents do not directly inhibit DOACs, they may enhance the hemostatic capacity. SPCs of several DOACs mention PCC and aPCC as potential reversal strategies, leading some clinicians to consider their use as "in label" in clinical practice, despite PCC and aPCC products' label defining this indication as "*off label*."

PCCs are lyophilized human plasma-derived concentrates of vitamin K-dependent coagulation factors (FII, FVII, FIX, and FX); three-factor formulations lacking

FVII are also available. Dosing is standardized according to FIX content (approximately 500 IU per vial). Some preparations contain small amounts of protein C and protein S, AT, or heparin [12]. Even if off-label, PCC use in DOAC-associated bleeding is a well-established clinical practice [42–44].

aPCC (activated prothrombin complex) (*FEIBA, factor eight inhibitor bypass activity*) contains non-activated FII, FIX, and FX, and FVII, and small amounts of protein C and protein S. Originally developed for hemophilia patients with inhibitors, aPCC has been used off-label to manage perioperative bleeding in both hemophilic and non-hemophilic patients [45].

In the absence of specific antagonists—in particular for RAE when Aα is unavailable, PCC and aPCC may be considered as "non-specific" procoagulant therapies in cases of *life-threatening* bleeding, urgent surgery, or massive hemorrhage associated with DOACs (as well as in cases requiring rapid antagonization of VKAs) [42–46]. Their rationale differs by agent: (i) for RAE, increased levels of vitamin K-dependent factors and FX may partially overcome inhibition; and (ii) for D, increased prothrombin availability may enhance thrombin generation, even if IDA remains the actual standard of care.

PCC and aPCC remain clinically relevant, especially given the limited availability and high cost of Aα (to be noted, Aα has been approved in some Italian HUB hospitals for preoperative reversal in non-bleeding patients, even if still *off-label* at present). The use of PCC, aPCC, and rFVIIa is associated with a non-physiological and prolonged increase in thrombin generation, driven in part by the long half-life prothrombin (about 60 h). Consequently, the risk of thromboembolic complications represents the principal safety concern, particularly in surgical or trauma settings. Similarly, rFVIIa markedly enhances thrombin generation and FXa activity. In non-hemophilic patients, particularly with ICH, its use has been associated with an increased risk of arterial and venous thromboembolic events, limiting its use to highly selected rescue situations. The interested readers are invited to refer to the algorithm proposed by Douketis et al. [2], which includes both PK and laboratory parameters. To underline the use of a cutoff of plasma concentrations of ≤50 ng/mL to proceed to surgery without antagonization [2].

The conclusions of Douketis et al. [2]—together with the considerations proposed by the Italian authors [1, 3, 9–11]—should

- Serve as the foundation for a shared institutional-wide protocol, multidisciplinary in scope and widely implemented within the hospital
- Emphasize that

  1. In patients taking DOAC, who require *elective* surgical or non-surgical procedures, standardized management protocols can be safely applied without routine measurements of plasma DOAC level (pharmacokinetic strategy) and without heparin bridging, provided that renal function—particularly in patients treated with D is addressed.
  2. Specific clinical scenarios, patients' characteristics, or procedural context associated with *increased bleeding risk* justify, if not mandate, the measure-

ments of plasma DOAC levels in elective surgery, aiming at a reduction of perioperative risk. [1, 10, 11]

3. In patients requiring *urgent or emergency* procedures, the use of reversal agents may be appropriate when the last DOAC intake occurred within 48 h, and DOAC plasma concentrations are elevated (>30 ng/mL, or >50 ng/mL, this latter threshold, even if not yet universally accepted, has been proposed by Douketis et al.) [2] or when DOAC levels are not available.
4. There is a clear and currently unmet need to define widely accepted plasma concentration cutoff values, to be incorporated into institutional—and ideally regional—protocols. These thresholds should not be left to "individual" clinical discretion for both clinical robustness and obvious medico-legal reasons. These concepts are in line with ASRA 2025 guidelines [28] and with bleeding risk stratification proposed for endoscopic procedures (Endoscopy 2016) [47].

3.8 Pharmacological, Laboratory-Based, or Personalized Management?

To conclude the discussion on the clinical management of DOACs in urgent/emergency settings—while considering that similar principles may increasingly apply or become strongly recommended even in selected elective contexts—it is useful to revisit the role of "specific" coagulation testing including plasma DOAC levels and POC assays, such as urinary assays or (hopefully in the near future) dedicated viscoelastic methods (CLOTPRO and QUANTRA) [6, 28, 29] particularly in high-risk or complex scenarios. This topic remains debated, reflecting the coexistence of two strategies in the literature: a predominantly "pharmacokinetic-based" approach and a "laboratory-based" approach. While evidence-based recommendations provide an essential framework to manage DOAC-associated bleeding, real-word decision—making inevitably varies according to clinical scenarios and patient characteristics. In a patient on DOAC therapy presenting with a surgical emergency, there is no single optimal, universally effective, and risk-free management strategy. Patient comorbidities, frailty, and baseline thromboembolic risk are always to be addressed and integrated into decision-making. Hence, management requires a comprehensive clinical assessment, encompassing medical history, timing and modality of the last DOAC intake, site and severity of bleeding, and the anticipated thromboembolic risk following anticoagulant reversal. This represents a true individualized risk-benefit assessment for the reversal, whether reversal is achieved using specific or non-specific antagonists. Importantly, in urgent and emergency settings, the use of specific coagulation assays and plasma drug levels measurements—and in the near future, VETs and/or urinary tests should not be considered as an alternative to "pragmatic" decisions based on the PK/PD properties of DOACs, but rather as complementary [1, 3, 6, 9–11]. As emphasized by Mora [29], in line with the positions championed by Tripodi et al. [9–11], Squizzato et al. [1], and Pozzi et al. [3], specific coagulation assays expressed as plasma drug concentrations (and VETs when available) allow a rapid and comprehensive assessment of the coagulation phase. Their role is relevant not only in urgent/emergency scenarios but also in elective settings, where they become particularly valuable in moderate-to-high-risk conditions. Ideally, clinicians should "have access, as quickly as possible, to the most accurate available 'specific' monitoring method, including plasma assays, both in elective and emergency settings." [29] Conversely, it is increasingly evident that "conventional" (or "global") coagulation tests fail to provide useful and reliable information in patients treated with DOAC. Although tests of abnormality may sometimes suggest the presence of clinically relevant drug levels, such changes are inconsistent and insufficient for decision making [9–11]. Given the availability of plasma assays for DRAE— and, in part, of urinary detection tests—a major step forward would be the widest implementation of specific laboratory testing in both elective and emergency settings, both in hub and spoke hospitals. This approach consistent with the proposal by Mbhor et al. [6] would significantly enhance patient safety, quality, and appropriateness of care. Finally, according to Mora et al. [29], preliminary data suggest that the integration of VETs using DOAC-specific reagents may further improve clinical assessment. When combined with plasma drug level determination (e.g., anti-Xa for RAE), this strategy may represent the most advanced and potentially safest approach to individualized DOAC therapy.

3.9 Conclusions

In light of the clinical, technical, and organizational considerations discussed above, all hospital units involved in perioperative and emergency care should be fully aware of which assays are locally available to measure anticoagulant activity and the cutoff values used to define the absence of clinical anticoagulant effect—acknowledging that full standardization of these thresholds is pending but eagerly awaited. This requirement underscores the strategic relevance of a hospital- wide, shared, and continuously updated protocol. In this framework, Hospital Trusts, Administrative and Strategic Management, Medical Management, and Quality and Risk Management Offices must be actively involved in decision-making processes that carry relevant clinical implications. This is particularly relevant for the "comprehensive" management of DOAC-treated patients undergoing elective or emergency surgical or invasive procedures as well as for those presenting with spontaneous bleeding in urgent/emergency situations. Appropriate investments in resources able to influence outcomes in urgency/emergency scenarios—while simultaneously enabling meaningful qualitative and quantitative improvements in elective care—represent a substantial step forward in modern clinical medicine. Such investments align not only with patient safety priorities but also with principles of responsible and sustainable healthcare economics. As stated by Mora, "the integration of evidence-based recommendations into clinical workflows and the appropriate and widespread use of available resources can ultimately bridge the gap between guidelines and clinical care" (unpublished data, reported from *ESAIC Conference 2025, 27.5.25*).

In conclusion, targeted economic investment aimed at improving organizational readiness, diagnostic capabilities, and protocol implementation should be considered a true risk management strategy. If and when appropriately planned and implemented, such a strategy provides a substantial contribution to patient safety in modern perioperative and emergency medicine.

The interested readers are strongly encouraged to refer to

- Samama CM. How to manage safely direct oral anticoagulants in patients undergoing a neuraxial procedures? No definite answer yet! J Thromb Haemost. 2025;23:2112–2113.
- ASRA 2025 Evidence-based guidelines [28] for the detailed management of locoregional anesthesia (central and peripheral blocks) in patients under DOACs treatment.
- The PERIXa study by Lee et al. [49]
- The editorial written by Douketis and Spyropoulos in JAMA in 2025 [48] commenting on the PERIXa study.
- The ongoing PAUSE 2 study (ClinicalTrials.gov ID NCT06957366) [50].

References

1. Squizzato A, Poli D, Barcellona D, et al. Management of DOAC in patients undergoing planned surgery or invasive procedure: Italian Federation of Centers for the diagnosis of thrombotic disorders and the surveillance of the antithrombotic therapies (FCSA) position paper. Thromb Haemost. 2022;122:329–35.
2. Douketis JD, Spyropoulos AC. Perioperative management of patients taking direct oral anticoagulants. A review. JAMA. 2024;332:825-834.
3. Pozzi A, Lucà F, Gelsomino S, et al. Coagulation tests and reversal agents in patients treated with Oral anticoagulants: the challenging scenarios of life-threatening bleeding and unplanned invasive procedures. J Clin Med. 2024;13:2451.
4. Douketis JD, Lip GYH. Perioperative management of patients receiving anticoagulants. UPTODATE, 2025. Section Ed Leung LLK, Deputy Ed Tirnauer JS. Accessed Nov 2025.
5. Tran HS, Merriman E, Baker R, et al. 2025 Guidelines for direct oral anticoagulants: a practical guidance on the prescription, laboratory testing, and peri-operative and bleeding management. Intern Med J. 2025;55:1–10.
6. Mbroh J, Birschmann I, Ebner M, et al. Rapid assessment of direct oral anticoagulants in acute stroke—an educational systematic review. Eur Stroke J. 2025;10(1S):24–34.
7. Hoffman M, Monroe DM. A cell based model of Hemostasis. Thromb Haemost. 2001;85:958–65.
8. Grottke O, Afshari A, Ahmed A, et al. Clinical guideline on reversal of direct oral anticoagulants in patients with life threatening bleeding. Eur J Anaesthesiol. 2024;41:327–50.
9. Tripodi A. The laboratory and the direct oral anticoagulants. Blood. 2013;121:4031–5.
10. Tripodi A, Ageno W, Ciaccio M, et al. Position Paper on laboratory testing for patients on direct oral anticoagulants. A Consensus Document from the SISET, FCSA, SIBioC and SIPMeL. Blood Transfus. 2018;16:462–70.
11. Tripodi A, Marchetti M, Scalambrino E. Direct oral anticoagulant measurements: when is it necessary? Blood Transfus. 2024; https://doi.org/10.2450/BloodTransfus.942.
12. Bejjani A, Khairani CD, Assi A, et al. When direct oral anticoagulants should not be standard treatment. J Am Coll Cardiol. 2024;83:444–65.

13. Carnicelli A, Hong H, Giugliano R, et al. Individual Patient Data from the Pivotal Randomized Controlled Trials of Non-Vitamin K Antagonist Oral Anticoagulants in Patients with Atrial Fibrillation (COMBINE AF): Design and Rationale: From the COMBINE AF (A Collaboration between Multiple Institutions to Better Investigate Non-vitamin K Antagonist Oral Anticoagulant Use in Atrial Fibrillation) Investigators. Am Heart J. 2021;233:48–58.
14. Ferreira S, Costa R, Malveiro D, Vieira F, Tuna M. Warfarin embryopathy: Balancing maternal and fetal risks with anticoagulation therapy. Pediatr Neonatol. 2018;59(5):534–5. https://doi.org/10.1016/j.pedneo.2018.02.005. Epub 2018 Feb 8. PMID: 29501347.] [RCOG; Green-top Guideline No. 37a, April 2015. Reducing the risk of venous thromboembolism during pregnancy and the puerperium. https://www.rcog.org.uk/media/qejfhcaj/gtg-37a.pdf].
15. Beyer-Westendorf J, Tittl L, Bistervels I, Middeldorp S, Schaefer C, Paulus W, Thomas W, Kemkes-Matthes B, Marten S, Bornhauser M. Safety of direct oral anticoagulant exposure during pregnancy: a retrospective cohort study. Lancet Haematol. 2020;7(12):e884–91. https://doi.org/10.1016/S2352-3026(20)30327-6.
16. Cohen H, Arachchillage DR, Middeldorp S, Beyer-Westendorf J, Abdul-Kadir R. Management of direct oral anticoagulants in women of childbearing potential: guidance from the SSC of the ISTH. J Thromb Haemost. 2016;14:1673–6.
17. Komori M, Hayata E, Nakata M, Yuzawa H, Oji A, Morita M. Apixaban therapy in a pregnant woman with heparin-induced thrombocytopenia and venous thromboembolic events caused by congenital antithrombin deficiency: a case report. Case Rep Womens Health. 2020;27:e00200. https://doi.org/10.1016/j.crwh.2020.e00200. PMID: 32300539; PMCID: PMC7152699.
18. Hindley B, Lip GYH, McCloskey AP, Penson PE. Pharmacokinetics and pharmacodynamics of direct oral anticoagulants. Exp Op Drug Metab Toxicol. 2023;19:911–23.
19. Renda G, Bucciarelli V, Barbieri G, Lanuti P, Berteotti M, Malatesta G, Cesari F, Salvatore T, Giusti B, Gori AM, et al. Ex vivo antiplatelet effects of oral anticoagulants. J Cardiovasc Dev Dis. 2024;11(4):111.
20. Martin KA, Beyer-Westendorf J, Davidson BL, et al. Use of direct oral anticoagulants in patients with obesity for treatment and prevention of venous thromboembolism: updated communication from the ISTH SSC Subcommittee on Control of Anticoagulation. J Thromb Haemost. 2020;19:1874–82.
21. Menichelli D, Pannunzio A, Baldacci E, Cammisotto V, Castellani V, Mormile R, Palumbo IM, Chistolini A, Violi F, Harenberg J, Pastori D, Pignatelli P. Plasma concentrations of direct oral anticoagulants in patients with Nonvalvular atrial fibrillation and different degrees of obesity. Clin Pharmacokinet. 2025;64(3):453–62. https://doi.org/10.1007/s40262-025-01474-8. Epub 2025 Feb 12. PMID: 39937335; PMCID: PMC11954712.
22. Steffel J, Collins R, Antz M, Cornu P, Desteghe L, Haeusler KG, Oldgren J, Reinecke H, Roldan-Schilling V, Rowell N, Sinnaeve P, Vanassche T, Potpara T, Camm AJ, Heidbüchel H, External Reviewers. 2021 European Heart Rhythm Association Practical Guide on the Use of Non-Vitamin K Antagonist Oral Anticoagulants in Patients with Atrial Fibrillation. Europace. 2021;23(10):1612–76. https://doi.org/10.1093/europace/euab065. Erratum in: Europace. 2021;23(10):1676. 10.1093/europace/euab157. PMID: 33895845; PMCID: PMC11636576.
23. Di Nisio M, Middeldorp S, Buller HR. Direct thrombin inhibitors. N Engl J Med. 2005;353:1028.
24. Samama MM. The mechanism of action of rivaroxaban – an oral direct FXa inhibitor – compared to other anticoagulants. Thromb Haemost. 2011;127:497.
25. Ha JT, Neuen BL, Cheng LP, et al. Benefits and harms of oral anticoagulant use in chronic kidney disease: a systematic review and meta-analysis. Ann Inter Med. 2019;171:181.
26. Ahmed N, Audebert H, Turc G, et al. Consensus statements and recommendations from the ESO-Karolinska Stroke Update Conference, Stockholm 11–13 November 2018. Eur Stroke J. 2019;4:307–17.
27. Levy JH, Shaw JR, Castellucci LA, et al. Reversal of direct oral anticoagulants: guidance from the SSC of the ISTH. J Thromb Haemost. 2024;2024:0717. https://doi.org/10.1016/j.jtha.2024.07.00925.26.

28. Kopp SL, Vandermeulen E, McBane RD, et al. Regional anesthesia in patients receiving antithrombotic or thrombolytic therapy: American Society of Regional Anesthesia and Pain Medicine Evidence-Based Guidelines (fifth edition). Reg Anesth Pain Med. 2025:1–29. https://doi.org/10.1136/rapm-2024-105766.
29. Mora L, Poce-Pellicè L, Qiontana DM. Viscoelastic monitoring of direct oral anticoagulants (DOACs). Blood Transfus. 2025;23(1):59–63. https://doi.org/10.2450/BloodTransfus.867.
30. Spyropoulos AC, Brohi K, Caprini J, et al. SSC Subcommittee on Perioperative and Critical Care Thrombosis and Haemostasis of the International Society on Thrombosis and Haemostasis. Scientific and Standardization Committee Communication: guidance document on the periprocedural management of patients on chronic oral anticoagulant therapy: recommendations for standardized reporting of procedural/surgical bleeding risk and patient-specific thromboembolic risk. J Thromb Haemost. 2019;17(11):1966–72.
31. Douketis JD, Spyropoulos AC, Anderson JM, et al. The perioperative anticoagulant use for surgery evaluation (PAUSE) study for patients on a direct oral anticoagulant who need an elective surgery or procedure: design and rationale. Thromb Haemost. 2017;117:2415–24.
32. Douketis JD, Spyropoulos AC, Duncan J, et al. Perioperative management of patients with atrial fibrillation receiving a direct oral anticoagulant. JAMA Intern Med. 2019;179:1469–78.
33. Torrano V, Anastasi S, De Cassai A. Enhancing safety in regional anesthesia: guidelines from SIAARTI. J Anesth Analg Crit Care. 2025;5:26. https://doi.org/10.1186/s44158-025-00245-y.
34. Levy JH, Connors JM, Steiner, et al. Management of oral anticoagulants prior to emergency surgery or with major bleeding: a survey of perioperative practices in North America: communication from the Scientific and Standardization Committees on Perioperative and Critical Care Haemostasis and Thrombosis of the International Society on Thrombosis and Haemostasis. Res Pr Thromb Haemost. 2020;4:562–8.
35. Pollack C, Eikelboom J, Weitz J, et al. Initial results of the RE-VERSE AD trial: idarucizumab reverses the anticoagulant effects of dabigatran in patients in an emergency setting of major bleeding, urgent surgery or interventions. Emerg Med J. 2015;32(12):979–80.
36. Pollack CV, Reilly PA, vanRyn J, et al. Idarucizumab for dabigatran reversal – full cohort analysis. N Engl J Med. 2017;377(5):431–41.
37. Hegemann I, Ganter C, Widmer CC, et al. Ongoing redistribution of dabigatran necessitates repetitive application of idarucizumab. Br J Anaesth. 2018;121:505–8.
38. Simon A, Domanovits H, Ay C, et al. The recommended dose of idarucizumab may not always be sufficient for sustained reversal of dabigatran. J Thromb Haemost. 2017;15:1317–21.
39. Connolly SJ, Crowther M, Eikelboom JW, ANNEXA-4 Investigators, et al. Full study report of andexanet alfa for bleeding associated with factor Xa inhibitors. N Engl J Med. 2019;380:1326–35.
40. Carpenter E, Singh D, Dietrich E, et al. Andexanet alfa for reversal of factor Xa inhibitor-associated anticoagulation. Ther Adv Drug Saf. 2019;10:2042098619888133.
41. Connolly SJ, Sharma M, Cohen AT, Demchuk AM, Członkowska A, Lindgren AG, et al. Andexanet for Factor Xa Inhibitor–Associated Acute Intracerebral Hemorrhage. NEJM. 2024;390:1745–55.
42. Grottke O, Aisenberg J, Bernstein R, et al. Efficacy of prothrombin complex concentrates for the emergency reversal of dabigatran-induced anticoagulation. Crit Care. 2016;20:115.
43. Schulman S, Gross PL, Ritchie B, et al. Prothrombin complex concentrate for major bleeding on factor Xa inhibitors: a prospective cohort study. Thromb Haemost. 2018;118:842–51.
44. Grottke O, Schulman S. Four-factor prothrombin complex concentrate for the management of patients receiving direct oral activated factor X inhibitors. Anesthesiology. 2019;131:1153–65.
45. Bolliger D, Szlam F, Molinaro RJ, et al. Thrombin generation and fibrinolysis in antifactor IX treated blood and plasma spiked with factor VIII inhibitor bypassing activity or recombinant factor VIIa. Haemophilia. 2010;16:510–7.
46. Panos NG, Cook AM, John S, Neurocritical Care Society Pharmacy Study Group, et al. Factor Xa inhibitor-related intracranial hemorrhage: results from a multicenter, observational cohort receiving prothrombin complex concentrates. Circulation. 2020;141:1681–9.

47. Veitch AM, Vanbiervliet G, Gershlick AH, Boustiere C, Baglin TP, Smith LA, et al. Endoscopy in patients on antiplatelet or anticoagulant therapy, including direct oral anticoagulants: British Society of Gastroenterology (BSG) and European Society of Gastrointestinal Endoscopy (ESGE) guidelines. Endoscopy. 2016;48:1–18.
48. Spyropoulos AC, Douketis JD. Standardized management of direct oral anticoagulants for elective procedures. JAMA Netw Open. 2025;8:e2458739. https://doi.org/10.1001/jamanetworkopen.2024.58739.
49. Lee SR, Lee KY, Park JS, The PERIXa Investigators, et al. Perioperative factor Xa inhibitor discontinuation for patients undergoing procedures with minimal or low bleeding risk. JAMA Netw Open. 2024;8(2):e2458742.
50. Perioperative Anticoagulant Use for Surgery Evaluation -2 (PAUSE-2) Study Patients Receiving a Direct Oral Anticoagulant (DOACs—Dabigatran, Rivaroxaban, Apixaban or Edoxaban) and needing Elective High-Bleed-Risk Surgery or an Invasive Procedure (PAUSE 2 RCT) ClinicalTrials.gov ID NCT06957366.

Prediction of (Difficult) Airway Management: From Statistics to Clinical Practice and Artificial Intelligence

4

Daniele Salvatore Paternò, Luigi La Via, and Massimiliano Sorbello

The ability to foresee the future, the art of divination—from the Oracle of Delphi to tarot cards, from the prophecies of South American native peoples to those of the evangelists—has always represented a highly coveted utopia for humankind, yet it has continually inspired the search for the ability to interpret and intuit the value and meaning of premonitory signs.

While modern Medical Science is grounded in *Evidence-Based Medicine*, meta-analyses, and *systematic reviews* that seek to identify the scientific certainties necessary and preparatory for understanding and identifying criteria for anticipating events (whether errors, complications, or pathophysiological developments), it is clear that there are still areas in Medicine where *prediction* remains difficult and inextricably linked to a kind of divinatory art—the *clinical eye* described in classic medical and surgical semiotics texts.

The prediction of difficult airway management is probably among those clinical areas where science inevitably gives way to experience, to the ability to integrate information, and to sound judgment in order to prevent airway management incidents.

We will therefore analyze the evolution of the ability to predict difficult airway management through a purely mathematical-statistical approach, an *evidence-based*

D. S. Paternò
Department of Anesthesia and Intensive Care, Giovanni Paolo II Hospital, Ragusa, Italy

L. La Via
Department of General Surgery and Medical Surgical Specialties (CHIRMED), University of Catania, Catania, Italy
e-mail: luigi.lavia@unict.it

M. Sorbello (✉)
Department of Anesthesia and Intensive Care, Giovanni Paolo II Hospital, Ragusa, Italy

ARTID – University of Enna Kore, Enna, Italy
e-mail: massimiliano.sorbello@unikore.it

D. Chiumello, A. De Gasperi (eds.), *Practical Trends in Anesthesia and Intensive Care 2026*, https://doi.org/10.1007/978-3-032-25721-5_4

analysis of available data, interpretation of *auditing* and *incident reporting* data, without neglecting the possibilities offered by artificial intelligence and the interpretation of *big data*.

And, not least, the sound *art of medicine*.

4.1 The Dichotomy Between Predicted and Unpredicted Difficult Airways

The first Italian document analyzing the problem of difficult airway management, and the implications related to the ability to predict it and thus develop a consequent strategy, dates back to 1998 and was authored by Giulio Frova [1]. This document laid the foundation for what would later become, in 2005, the guidelines published by the Italian Society of Anesthesia Analgesia, Resuscitation and Intensive Care (SIAARTI), which still today serve as a scientific reference for the Italian anesthesiology community [2]. Both documents were based on a significant conceptual approach: the patient must be evaluated in advance, with analysis of medical history, anatomical, and clinical factors, and from this comprehensive assessment, a dichotomous outcome regarding the degree of difficulty should be determined. On one hand, there is unexpected difficulty (which becomes less likely the more careful, thorough, and multi-variable the analysis of predictive factors), and on the other, anticipated difficulty, which is further subdivided into "borderline" and "severe" difficulty, essentially based on the presence or absence of severe ventilation difficulty associated with anticipated severe intubation difficulty [2].

This approach, perhaps somewhat dogmatic, nonetheless represented a deliberate choice by a group of experts [3], partly aligned with the path chosen by the American Society of Anesthesiologists (ASA) in the guidelines published in 1993 [4], in 2003 [5], and, even more so, in 2022 [6].

Similarly, the guidelines promoted by the Indian Society of Anesthesiologists—All India Airway Management Association (AIDAA) [7] structured decision-making and planning based on the anticipation of difficulty, and even more distinctly, the Canadian guidelines, which traditionally were divided into two separate documents: one focused on the management of anticipated difficulty [8] and one on unanticipated difficulty [9].

In contrast, "traditionally," the British Difficult Airway Society, both in the 1998 and 2015 documents, referred exclusively to the management of unanticipated difficulty, almost taking for granted the anticipation of difficulty or, in any case, not emphasizing a preventive planning approach based on the assessment of difficult airway management.

This concept is also indirectly present in the recently published Awake Tracheal Intubation document [10], which, while detailing the approach to intubation with maintenance of spontaneous breathing, does not identify predictive criteria guiding this choice.

4.2 The Mathematical-Statistical Approach to Predicting Difficult Airway Management

Having clarified the importance of predicting difficult airway management, the next step is to understand which tools should be used to effectively achieve this goal.

In statistics, prediction follows mathematical rules, whose complexity increases as the goal is to minimize the proportion of unexpected events, which in statistical terms is expressed by positive and negative predictive value, and by the concepts of sensitivity and specificity.

Sensitivity and specificity are two criteria used to assess a test's ability to identify and distinguish, within a population sample, individuals who do and do not possess the characteristic of interest.

Sensitivity and specificity in the statistical sense differ from their clinical counterparts; to summarize the concept, the *sensitivity* of a statistical test answers the question, "How many of the subjects WITH difficult airway management who underwent the test were POSITIVE, that is, identified as having a difficult airway?" Conversely, again simplifying, the *specificity* in the statistical sense answers the question, "How many of the subjects WITHOUT difficult airway management who underwent the test were NEGATIVE, that is, identified as not having a difficult airway?" These questions were explored and analyzed by Yentis in a landmark editorial [11], aimed at determining whether the prediction of difficult airway management was truly useful or rather a *pointless ritual.* The author mathematically demonstrated that tests for predicting a difficult airway are unreliable, with sensitivity and specificity even lower than those of weather forecasts projected one week ahead (predictive power positive predictive value of about 19%); this is because, at first glance, the distribution of airway management difficulty does not follow a Gaussian distribution but rather results from the overlap of the "large" Gaussian of "easy" cases and the "small" Gaussian of "difficult" cases, with overlapping areas that explain why so many predicted difficulties turn out to be "false positives," and why some difficulties remain "unanticipated" despite testing.

This is a significant statistical truth, supported by a recent editorial [12], and it follows that as long as we apply predictive tests in a purely statistical sense, the results will not change, with a (fortunately small) proportion of difficulties escaping prediction, and a (larger) proportion of predicted difficulties that are not clinically confirmed.

Over time, various approaches have been attempted to improve sensitivity and specificity; one certainly successful strategy, as highlighted in the landmark work of Shiga [13] and in many subsequent analyses [14], is to combine tests: by increasing the number of predictive tests to which the patient is subjected, the predictive power regarding airway management difficulty improves. However, the intrinsic limitation of this approach is that it remains "quantitative" and not "qualitative," meaning it does not allow us to "weigh" one index against another in terms of severity, nor to analyze the (multiple) combinations of various anatomical parameter alterations used to predict difficulty.

The situation does not improve when using "scoring" tests, such as the well-known El-Ganzouri Risk Index [15]. This index, specifically, is effective in establishing quantitative cut-offs ("greater than or less than" indicating different management strategies), but provides little or no qualitative information. This is even more evident when simply analyzing one of the parameters, patient weight, which is not expressed in terms of body mass index, introducing a significant bias in the assessment (a weight of 110 kg is very different in an individual 180 cm tall compared to one 150 cm tall).

In light of these considerations, another aspect that gradually became apparent, also in view of adverse events, was the awareness that it was necessary to separate, in the assessment of difficulty and in the determinism of complications, the impact of a difficult laryngoscopy/intubation from that of difficult (mask/supraglottic) ventilation, since these involve different outcomes and required strategies.

The landmark study by the French group led by Langeron was the first to "quantify" the incidence of difficult mask ventilation, reporting a significant 5% [16], which was appropriately reduced to around 1% by the larger and methodologically more rigorous (with more precise definitions) studies by the groups of Kheterpal [17] and Norskov [18].

The recognized importance of this additional predictive need certainly complicated the task of "predictors," especially in light of the growing awareness of obstructive sleep apnea and its potential implications for difficult ventilation and laryngoscopy [19].

The subsequent response of the scientific community involved, on the one hand, the refinement of statistical methodologies, including the expansion of sample size, and on the other, the realization that it was necessary to somehow reduce the "weight" of the mathematical-statistical approach by moving toward a personalized approach.

4.3 Science and Art of Prediction

Analyses from the Danish Anesthesia Database [20], and data from the National Audit Project 4 (a large-scale, year-long audit conducted in England by the RCOA and AAGBI) [21] clearly indicate that there are still many incidents related to the fallibility of difficulty prediction, both directly and as a co-factor in the failure to plan an effective strategy.

The contribution of science to this situation can be identified in the two major meta-analyses/systematic reviews conducted independently by the groups of Detski [22] in America and Roth [23] in Europe. Both studies, independently, identified the *upper lip bite test* as the most sensitive and specific test for predicting laryngoscopic difficulty, thereby downplaying the significance—sometimes elevated to mythic status—of tests such as the Mallampati or thyromental distance.

Both studies, however, collect and analyze the results of other studies, which themselves were methodologically biased: six different definitions of difficult intubation, and the a priori exclusion of all "known" difficult patients, including those with an inter-incisor distance less than 2 cm, which, according to the studies by Detski and Roth, is not a predictive parameter for difficult laryngoscopy. This represents a scientific, but not clinical, reality—an outcome of excluding all patients with this characteristic and directing them to awake techniques.

Hence, the need for art.

This is what Heidegger and Pandit evoke in a famous editorial [24] that begins by paraphrasing Tolstoy's Anna Karenina. The difficult airway is multifactorial, multilayered, and arises from the infinite possible combinations of countless degrees of deviation from normality across multiple parameters. If every airway *is easy in the same way, every airway is difficult in its own way.*

This leads to a multiparametric analytical approach that must be individualized and contextualized for each patient, establishing a strategy not in pursuit of the perfect test, but built on the awareness of imperfection and favoring prudence over the precision of prognosis.

This important *paradigm shift* entails a reassessment in a new light, grounded in the understanding that no patient dies or suffers severe complications as a result of failed intubation, but rather from failed oxygenation [25].

This concept emerges even more forcefully when considering the fields of emergency and intensive care, where the INTUBE study [26] has revealed numbers and types of incidents that have long been underestimated and overlooked, and where making an accurate prediction of difficulty is even more challenging.

It has also highlighted the concept, new yet almost self-evident, of the *physiologically difficult airway*, in which the anatomical factor may be normal, or even if altered, becomes secondary to reduced apnea tolerance, hemodynamic instability, absence of reflexes, and the many issues of the critically ill patient [27].

Extending the challenge of predicting difficulty to the critically ill patient, it is therefore essential to consider these variables, in addition to the operator's experience: thus, the MACOCHA score was developed, introducing these variables into a scoring system for predicting difficulty [28] (Table 4.1).

Thus, an approach to predicting difficulty emerges that, from being purely anatomical, also becomes pathophysiological but still appears incomplete in light of a careful analysis of incident data.

The NAP4 [21], English medicolegal data [29], and the American Closed Claims Projects [30] all unanimously suggest that, in the genesis of incidents, the human

Table 4.1 MACOCHA score [28]

Category	Criterion (MACOCHA Acronym)	Points
Patient	**M**allampati (class III or IV)	5
	Obstructive sleep apnea (OSA)	2
	Cervical spine (reduced mobility)	1
	Opening of mouth (< 3 cm)	1
Pathology	**C**oma (reason for intubation)	1
	Hypoxia (severe hypoxemia <80%)	1
Operator	**A**nesthesiologist not experienced (non-anesthesiologist operator)	1

Total Score: From 0 (Easy intubation) to 12 (Very difficult intubation)

factor plays a predominant role. The absence of a strategy, of planning, of adequate communication, and cognitive biases—especially in emergencies—represent the common denominator of all documented incidents [31].

Just as the MACOCHA score introduces the role of the physician's experience in airway management, the experience of the team is also important (and a team of experts is not necessarily an expert team), as are planning and sharing the strategy, the available tools, and the ergonomics and logistics of the locations where airway management takes place.

The time is ripe to speak of *context-sensitive prediction of difficulty*.

4.4 The Modern Approach to Predicting Difficulty

At this point, it becomes clear that the concept of predicting a difficult airway is, in itself, outdated.

Instead, the focus should be on planning for all airways, not just the "difficult" ones, since even this approach introduces cognitive biases that lead to a dichotomous view of airway management as either easy or difficult.

Airway management difficulty exists on a *continuum* in which strategies and decisions must be tailored according to the ability to maintain patient oxygenation throughout the entire process leading to definitive airway acquisition [32].

This strategy should be developed taking into account the patient's medical history and anatomical conditions, underlying pathophysiological states, the region involved in any surgical procedure (surgical conflict), available resources, the expertise of the operator and team, the setting (including NORA, emergency department, out-of-hospital), and must include risk assessment and potential complications at extubation, also implying the definition of the post-procedural level of care (Table 4.2).

This approach, which could be defined as *context-sensitive*, becomes adaptable to all circumstances and various settings in which intervention is required, including patients with specific characteristics (pregnancy, trauma, endocrine surgery, airway surgery), and also provides a more definitive *perioperative* perspective, considering that airway management difficulties may arise at any point during the patient's care pathway.

The purpose of airway difficulty assessment should not be to place the patient at a specific and precise *moment* of risk, but rather to evaluate the constant availability of a *rescue* airway, a plan B to ensure oxygenation.

The question, therefore, shifts from "Will my patient be difficult to intubate?" to an awareness ("I need to define the strategy for managing this patient's airway") and to a new question: "Can I suppress the patient's spontaneous breathing?"

If the answer is yes, neuromuscular blockade becomes a consequential and unavoidable step in the strategy [33]. Conversely, if the only plan B is to maintain spontaneous breathing, the choice of device (laryngoscopy, videolaryngoscopy, flexible bronchoscope, tracheotomy/cricothyrotomy under local anesthesia, ECMO

Table 4.2 Multidimensional framework for context-sensitive airway assessment

Patient-related anatomical features	Patient-related physiological considerations	System and context factors
Mouth opening capacity (<3 cm interincisor gap)	Previous airway management difficulties	Clinical expertise of the airway manager
Mandibular protrusion capability, retrognathia	Baseline oxygen impairment, acute lung injury/ARDS	Institutional airway protocols, presence of airway leadership, standardized training programs
Oropharyngeal visualization (static and dynamic assessment), phonation-modified Mallampati classification, pathological lesions, cervicofacial scarring, absent dentition, dense facial hair, habitual snoring	Intrapulmonary shunting, circulatory shock states, myocardial dysfunction, reduced hemoglobin, systemic inflammatory response, elevated metabolic oxygen demands, late-term gestation	Clinical environment: operating theater, critical care unit, emergency department, remote anesthesia locations, monitored anesthesia care settings, prehospital environment
Anterior neck measurements (thyromental and sternomental distances)	Elevated body mass index	Point-of-care ultrasound capability and operator proficiency
Impalpable cricothyroid window	Sleep-disordered breathing (validated screening tools)	Rescue device accessibility
Cervical soft tissue dimensions, cervical spine range of motion	Deliberate preservation of neuromuscular function	Procedural skill competency
Post-surgical or post-radiation neck anatomy	Anticipated extubation-related risks	Interdisciplinary team capabilities

cannulation) becomes secondary to the priority of preserving the patient's spontaneous respiratory activity and airway muscle tone.

The "context-sensitive" approach thus allows for the identification of those "universal" parameters useful for assessing difficulty, both anatomically (upper lip bite test, Mallampati, interincisor distance, etc.) and physiologically (hemodynamic parameters, vascular volume status, P/F ratio, blood gases, etc.), which must then be interpreted in relation to the specific context.

A difficulty that is not critical in a healthy elective patient scheduled for a planned procedure may take on a completely different significance in a term pregnant woman requiring urgent cesarean section under general anesthesia. In this case, for the same anatomical difficulty, additional physiological challenges arise (increased oxygen consumption, tissue edema, higher Mallampati score), as well as contextual factors (time pressure of the emergency), and potentially issues related to devices and the team. Furthermore, a supraglottic device that may not be strictly necessary in the first scenario (the elective patient can be awakened after reversal and mask ventilation, with rescheduling using another technique) becomes essential in the term pregnant patient, being fundamental for possible rescue ventilation (second-generation supraglottic device) and for intubation with a flexible bronchoscope through the device [34].

Similarly, a roadside intervention for maxillofacial trauma may require that the context-sensitive assessment suggests cricothyrotomy under local anesthesia with spontaneous breathing as the first approach to airway control, if the risk of encountering a difficult airway is offset by the lack of valid rescue options [35].

Patients with obstructive sleep apnea must be evaluated both physiologically and anatomically, but the assessment must also consider the possibility of difficult extubation and, above all, the need to define an appropriate level of postoperative care, given the risk of airway-related complications occurring even some time after elective intubation/extubation [36].

Attention to extubation and anticipation of difficult extubation is automatic in all patients in whom a difficult airway was anticipated or encountered; however, it must always be considered, in a context-sensitive manner, that a patient with an easy airway may become a difficult extubation (and reintubation) case. This is commonly seen in head and neck surgery, supra-aortic vascular surgery, cervical spine stabilization, or in robotic surgery with steep and prolonged Trendelenburg position, and must be taken into account during perioperative airway management planning [37].

The NORA (Non-Operating Room Anesthesia) environment is an extremely important aspect in balancing the prediction of difficulty, planning of airway management (often underestimated), and the number of incidents (often underreported) [38]. The increasing number of procedures in NORA involves ever more complex patients undergoing procedures that require anesthetic assistance, sedation, and sometimes airway control, both electively and in emergencies. Anticipation and planning are perhaps even more important than in the operating room, precisely because the procedure takes place outside the anesthesiologist's natural environment. Knowing the available devices, using monitoring ($EtCO_2$, depth of anesthesia), and planning patient management are extremely important in this context, and follow the rules of context-sensitive prediction, as anatomical, physiological, logistical, device, and team-related difficulties are all involved (Figs. 4.1 and 4.2).

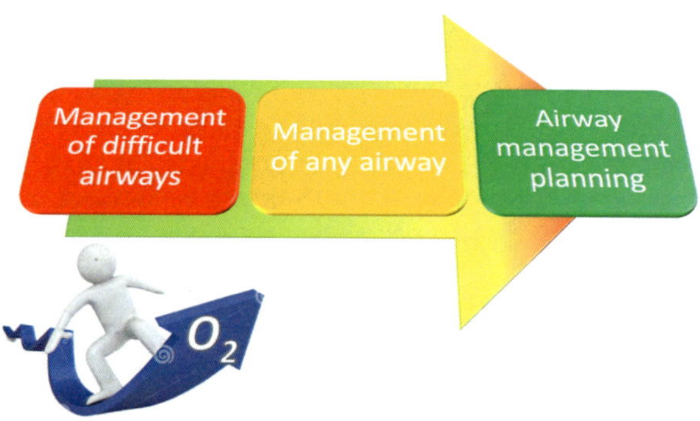

Fig. 4.1 From prediction of a difficult airway to airway planning

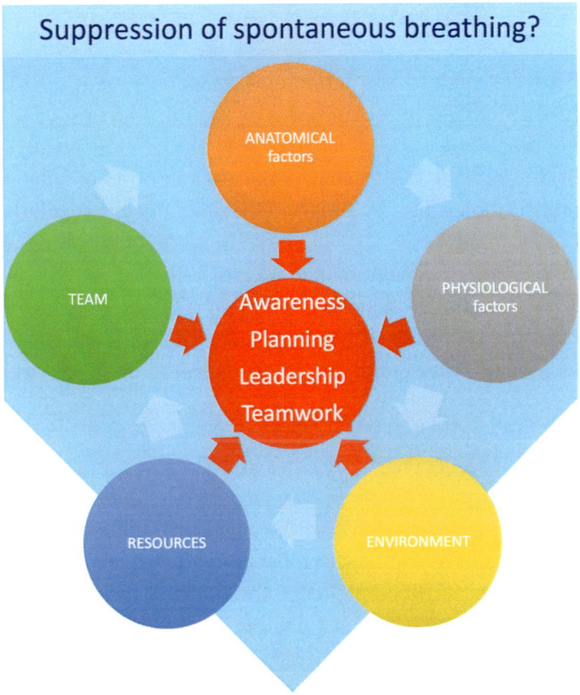

Fig. 4.2 The context-sensitive approach to airway management planning

Ultimately, airway planning must be

- Context-sensitive.
  - Anatomical, physiological, devices, setting, team.
- Anticipated.
  - A previously difficult airway can only become "more difficult."
  - A previously easy airway can become difficult.
- Multiparametric.
  - Upper lip bite test and all other anatomical predictors.
  - Physiological assessment.
  - Team briefing.
  - The greater the number of tests, the better the sensitivity and specificity.
- Multilevel.
  - All predictive parameters for ventilation/laryngoscopy/intubation/supraglottic ventilation/difficult cricothyrotomy.
  - All hemodynamic (oxiphoresis) and oxygenation parameters.
  - All context-specific parameters (obstetrics, trauma, emergency, ICU).

4.5 The Future and New Perspectives

The approach to predicting airway management difficulty has been fundamentally revolutionized in recent years by the introduction of videolaryngoscopes into clinical practice.

Introduced around the 2000s, after a period of slow and cautious adoption among anesthesiologists, videolaryngoscopes have, especially since the COVID-19 pandemic, become widely available in all hospitals and are now considered indispensable tools for airway management [39].

The recent systematic review by Hansel [40] has definitively established their efficacy and safety, from increasing first-pass success compared to the Macintosh, to reducing the incidence of desaturation and unrecognized accidental esophageal intubation.

Ultimately, they have changed the *pattern* of intubation difficulty [41].

Difficult laryngoscopy has now become much rarer, and many of the factors "classically" predictive of laryngoscopic difficulty have consequently become less relevant compared to direct laryngoscopy.

Conversely, we do not have evidence of specific predictive factors for videolaryngoscopic difficulty, except for reduced interincisor distance, logically, and new cut-offs for the values we were accustomed to measuring.

Several studies have highlighted that, specifically for videolaryngoscopes, experience with the device is certainly a predictor of success [42, 43], but clarifying studies are lacking, and above all, there is a lack of precise data regarding the *shift* in the site of difficulty observed with videolaryngoscopes, from laryngoscopy to tube passage into the trachea.

The use of these devices can also itself be a trigger for cognitive biases and decision-making errors, insofar as the awareness of a more effective tool may raise the threshold for caution and lower the perceived "weight" of prediction in particularly challenging but not predictably extremely difficult cases.

On the technological front, ultrasound is also gaining increasing popularity, along with greater availability and know-how among anesthesiologists.

Several studies have proposed its use as an instrumental adjunct in predicting laryngoscopic difficulty, but at present, the data are insufficient for a precise recommendation, also in light of the operator-dependent variability of the examination and the measurements obtained [44, 45]. The most reliable parameter, and the one that best correlates with laryngoscopic difficulty, appears to be the thickness of the pre-epiglottic space [46]; however, although already suggested in several guidelines, the use of ultrasound remains cautiously promising but not yet substantially validated [32].

Both virtual and "physical" endoscopy can be important tools for predicting difficulty, especially in certain specific surgical areas (head and neck and thoracic surgery), and are recommended by some guidelines [6], but their use does not constitute a universally adopted clinical routine [47].

New and interesting promises and perspectives arise from the growing development and exponential interest in artificial intelligence.

The ability to manage *big data* suggests that the analysis of large databases could improve the predictive power and cut-off values of traditional parameters and, quite possibly, help identify new ones.

Machine learning has been applied to the analysis of voice, facial morphology, vocal cord morphology, and the study of various anatomical interactions and morphological relationships. However, even in this case, the available results are still far from representing a validated technology and a reliable resource in airway management, although it cannot be excluded that this scenario may rapidly change, in line with the fast-paced evolution of technology and artificial intelligence algorithms [48–52].

4.6 Conclusions

The evolution of knowledge, incident analysis, technological advances, and the increasing complexity of patients requiring airway management have progressively and profoundly changed the approach to predicting airway management difficulties.

What was once a mere sequence of tests and measurements has shifted to an awareness of their poor specificity (thus preparing for a severe difficulty that may not actually exist) and sensitivity (failing to adequately prepare for an underestimated but actually difficult airway), even leading to the question of whether it is still "worthwhile" to perform these tests and the prediction of difficulty itself.

In light of the understanding that the prediction of difficulty, by its very nature an inherently fallible attempt, remains a fundamental step insofar as it prompts and leads to the development of a preprocedural strategy, efforts have been made to review its principles and cornerstones.

The prediction of a (solely) difficult airway becomes the planning of (every) airway; parameters evolve from being merely anatomical to also include physiological, structural, logistical, device-related, and team-related factors; planning and prediction become *context-sensitive* and as tailored as possible to the patient's specific anatomical and physiological characteristics and the team's resources.

The goal is no longer to preemptively identify and grade the difficult airway but to understand its specific implications, in order to answer the *simple* question of whether or not to suppress the patient's spontaneous breathing, keeping the primary objective (oxygenation) above the means or devices used to achieve it.

This remains valid and inseparable even in the modern approach with videolaryngoscopy, which has shifted the focus of difficulty from laryngoscopy to the passage through the vocal cords, but which, on the other hand, is an extremely versatile technique that is well suited to awake approaches, with maintenance of spontaneous breathing.

Finally, technological advances have provided the airway manager with versatile tools such as preprocedural endoscopy, whether virtual or physical, as well as techniques that are now ubiquitous, though still to be perfected and universally validated, such as airway ultrasonography.

The future will likely offer us access to the resources of artificial intelligence, big data analysis, and machine learning, which will probably enhance our predictive abilities and, at the same time, simplify their application, for example, through the analysis of voice or somatic features.

Until then, it will always be necessary to remember the Hippocratic *primum non nocere* and the old adage that *prevention is better than cure,* where our best preventive medicine is always to ensure patient oxygenation.

References

1. Frova G. Difficult intubation and the problem of airway control in adults [The difficult intubation and the problem of monitoring the adult airway. Italian Society of Anesthesia, RESUSCITATION, and Intensive Therapy (SIAARTI)]. Minerva Anestesiol. 1998;64(9):361–71.
2. Petrini F, Accorsi A, Adrario E, Agrò F, Amicucci G, Antonelli M, et al. SIAARTI study group "difficult airways"; IRC and SARNePI; task force. Recommendations for airway control and difficult airway management. Minerva Anestesiol. 2005;71(11):617–57.
3. Frova G, Sorbello M. Algorithms for difficult airway management: a review. Minerva Anestesiol. 2009;75(4):201–9.
4. Practice guidelines for management of the difficult airway. A report by the American Society of Anesthesiologists Task Force on Management of the Difficult Airway. Anesthesiology. 1993;78(3):597–602.
5. American Society of Anesthesiologists Task Force on Management of the Difficult Airway. Practice guidelines for management of the difficult airway: an updated report by the American Society of Anesthesiologists Task Force on Management of the Difficult Airway. Anesthesiology. 2003;98(5):1269–77. https://doi.org/10.1097/00000542-200305000-00032.
6. Apfelbaum JL, Hagberg CA, Connis RT, Abdelmalak BB, Agarkar M, Dutton RP, et al. 2022 American Society of Anesthesiologists Practice Guidelines for Management of the Difficult Airway. Anesthesiology. 2022;136(1):31–81. https://doi.org/10.1097/ALN.0000000000004002.
7. Myatra SN, Shah A, Kundra P, Patwa A, Ramkumar V, Divatia JV, et al. All India Difficult Airway Association 2016 guidelines for the management of unanticipated difficult tracheal intubation in adults. Indian J Anaesth. 2016;60(12):885–98. https://doi.org/10.4103/0019-5049.195481.
8. Law JA, Duggan LV, Asselin M, Baker P, Crosby E, Downey A, et al. Canadian Airway Focus Group. Canadian Airway Focus Group updated consensus-based recommendations for management of the difficult airway: part 2. Planning and implementing safe management of the patient with an anticipated difficult airway. Can J Anaesth. 2021;68(9):1405–36. https://doi.org/10.1007/s12630-021-02008-z.
9. Law JA, Duggan LV, Asselin M, Baker P, Crosby E, Downey A, et al. Canadian Airway Focus Group. Canadian Airway Focus Group updated consensus-based recommendations for management of the difficult airway: part 1. Difficult airway management encountered in an unconscious patient. Can J Anaesth. 2021;68(9):1373–404. https://doi.org/10.1007/s12630-021-02007-0.
10. Ahmad I, El-Boghdadly K, Bhagrath R, Hodzovic I, McNarry AF, Mir F, O'Sullivan EP, Patel A, Stacey M, Vaughan D. Difficult airway society guidelines for awake tracheal intubation (ATI) in adults. Anaesthesia. 2020;75(4):509–28. https://doi.org/10.1111/anae.14904.
11. Yentis SM. Predicting difficult intubation—worthwhile exercise or pointless ritual? Anaesthesia. 2002;57(2):105–9. https://doi.org/10.1046/j.0003-2409.2001.02515.x.

12. Heidegger T, Pandit JJ. Difficult airway management: from the power of prediction to the art of management. Anesth Analg. 2025;140(2):290–4. https://doi.org/10.1213/ANE.0000000000007202.
13. Shiga T, Wajima Z, Inoue T, Sakamoto A. Predicting difficult intubation in apparently normal patients: a meta-analysis of bedside screening test performance. Anesthesiology. 2005;103(2):429–37. https://doi.org/10.1097/00000542-200508000-00027.
14. Vannucci A, Cavallone LF. Bedside predictors of difficult intubation: a systematic review. Minerva Anestesiol. 2016 Jan;82(1):69–83.
15. el-Ganzouri AR, McCarthy RJ, Tuman KJ, Tanck EN, Ivankovich AD. Preoperative airway assessment: predictive value of a multivariate risk index. Anesth Analg. 1996;82(6):1197–204. https://doi.org/10.1097/00000539-199606000-00017.
16. Langeron O, Masso E, Huraux C, Guggiari M, Bianchi A, Coriat P, Riou B. Prediction of difficult mask ventilation. Anesthesiology. 2000;92(5):1229–36. https://doi.org/10.1097/00000542-200005000-00009.
17. Kheterpal S, Han R, Tremper KK, Shanks A, Tait AR, O'Reilly M, Ludwig TA. Incidence and predictors of difficult and impossible mask ventilation. Anesthesiology. 2006;105(5):885–91. https://doi.org/10.1097/00000542-200611000-00007.
18. Lundstrøm LH, Rosenstock CV, Wetterslev J, Nørskov AK. The DIFFMASK score for predicting difficult facemask ventilation: a cohort study of 46,804 patients. Anaesthesia. 2019;74(10):1267–76. https://doi.org/10.1111/anae.14701.
19. Corso RM, Sorbello M, Buccioli M, Carretta E, Nanni O, Piraccini E, Merli G, Petrini F, Guarino A, Frova G. Survey of knowledge and attitudes about obstructive sleep Apnoea among Italian Anaesthetists. Turk J Anaesthesiol Reanim. 2017;45(3):146–52. https://doi.org/10.5152/TJAR.2017.51423.
20. Nørskov AK. Preoperative airway assessment – experience gained from a multicentre cluster randomised trial and the Danish Anaesthesia Database. Dan Med J. 2016;63(5):B5241.
21. Cook TM, Woodall N, Frerk C, Fourth National Audit Project. Major complications of airway management in the UK: results of the Fourth National Audit Project of the Royal College of Anaesthetists and the Difficult Airway Society. Part 1: anaesthesia. Br J Anaesth. 2011;106(5):617–31. https://doi.org/10.1093/bja/aer058.
22. Detsky ME, Jivraj N, Adhikari NK, Friedrich JO, Pinto R, Simel DL, Wijeysundera DN, Scales DC. Will this patient be difficult to intubate?: the rational clinical examination systematic review. JAMA. 2019;321(5):493–503. https://doi.org/10.1001/jama.2018.21413.
23. Roth D, Pace NL, Lee A, Hovhannisyan K, Warenits AM, Arrich J, Herkner H. Airway physical examination tests for detection of difficult airway management in apparently normal adult patients. Cochrane Database Syst Rev. 2018;5(5):CD008874. https://doi.org/10.1002/14651858.CD008874.pub2.
24. Pandit JJ, Heidegger T. Putting the 'point' back into the ritual: a binary approach to difficult airway prediction. Anaesthesia. 2017;72(3):283–8. https://doi.org/10.1111/anae.13720.
25. Sorbello M, Afshari A, De Hert S. Device or target? A paradigm shift in airway management: implications for guidelines, clinical practice and teaching. Eur J Anaesthesiol. 2018;35(11):811–4. https://doi.org/10.1097/EJA.0000000000000893.
26. Russotto V, Myatra SN, Laffey JG, Tassistro E, Antolini L, Bauer P, et al.; INTUBE Study Investigators. Intubation practices and adverse Peri-intubation events in critically ill patients from 29 countries. JAMA. 2021;325(12):1164–72. https://doi.org/10.1001/jama.2021.1727.
27. Karamchandani K, Nasa P, Jarzebowski M, Brewster DJ, De Jong A, Bauer PR, et al. Society of Critical Care Anesthesiologists (SOCCA) Physiologically Difficult Airway Task Force. Tracheal intubation in critically ill adults with a physiologically difficult airway. An international Delphi study. Intensive Care Med. 2024;50(10):1563–79. https://doi.org/10.1007/s00134-024-07578-2.

28. De Jong A, Molinari N, Terzi N, Mongardon N, Arnal JM, Guitton C, et al. AzuRéa Network for the Frida-Réa Study Group. Early identification of patients at risk for difficult intubation in the intensive care unit: development and validation of the MACOCHA score in a multicenter cohort study. Am J Respir Crit Care Med. 2013;187(8):832–9. https://doi.org/10.1164/rccm.201210-1851OC.
29. Oglesby FC, Ray AG, Shurlock T, Mitra T, Cook TM. Litigation related to anaesthesia: analysis of claims against the NHS in England 2008-2018 and comparison against previous claim patterns. Anaesthesia. 2022;77(5):527–37. https://doi.org/10.1111/anae.15685.
30. Joffe AM, Aziz MF, Posner KL, Duggan LV, Mincer SL, Domino KB. Management of Difficult Tracheal Intubation: a closed claims analysis. Anesthesiology. 2019;131(4):818–29. https://doi.org/10.1097/ALN.0000000000002815.
31. Stiegler MP, Tung A. Cognitive processes in anesthesiology decision making. Anesthesiology. 2014;120(1):204–17. https://doi.org/10.1097/ALN.0000000000000073.
32. Lamperti M, Romero CS, Guarracino F, Cammarota G, Vetrugno L, Tufegdzic B, et al. Preoperative assessment of adults undergoing elective noncardiac surgery: updated guidelines from the European Society of Anaesthesiology and Intensive Care. Eur J Anaesthesiol. 2025;42(1):1–35. https://doi.org/10.1097/EJA.0000000000002069.
33. Fuchs-Buder T, Romero CS, Lewald H, Lamperti M, Afshari A, Hristovska AM, et al. Peri-operative management of neuromuscular blockade: a guideline from the European Society of Anaesthesiology and Intensive Care. Eur J Anaesthesiol. 2023;40(2):82–94. https://doi.org/10.1097/EJA.0000000000001769.
34. Mushambi MC, Athanassoglou V, Kinsella SM. Anticipated difficult airway during obstetric general anaesthesia: narrative literature review and management recommendations. Anaesthesia. 2020;75(7):945–61. https://doi.org/10.1111/anae.15007.
35. Rudolph SS, Root CW, Tvede MF, Fedog T, Wenger P, Gellerfors M, Apel J, Ünlü L. Confined space airway management: a narrative review. Scand J Trauma Resusc Emerg Med. 2025;33(1):79. https://doi.org/10.1186/s13049-025-01357-8.
36. Petrini F, Di Giacinto I, Cataldo R, Esposito C, Pavoni V, Donato P, et al. Obesity Task Force for the SIAARTI Airway Management Study Group. Perioperative and periprocedural airway management and respiratory safety for the obese patient: 2016 SIAARTI Consensus. Minerva Anestesiol. 2016;82(12):1314–35.
37. Sorbello M, Frova G. When the end is really the end? The extubation in the difficult airway patient. Minerva Anestesiol. 2013;79(2):194–9.
38. Bhavani SS, Abdelmalak B. Nonoperating room anesthesia: anesthesia in the gastrointestinal suite. Anesthesiol Clin. 2019;37(2):301–16. https://doi.org/10.1016/j.anclin.2019.01.010.
39. Saracoglu A, Saracoglu K, Sorbello M, Çakmak G, Greif R. The influence of the COVID-19 pandemic on videolaryngoscopy: a cross-sectional before-and-after survey. Anaesthesiol intensive Ther. 2023;55(2):93–102. https://doi.org/10.5114/ait.2023.129278.
40. Hansel J, Rogers AM, Lewis SR, Cook TM, Smith AF. Videolaryngoscopy versus direct laryngoscopy for adults undergoing tracheal intubation: a Cochrane systematic review and meta-analysis update. Br J Anaesth. 2022;129(4):612–23. https://doi.org/10.1016/j.bja.2022.05.027.
41. Lundstrøm LH, Nørskov AK, Kjeldgaard LD, Wetterslev J, Rosenstock CV. Implementation of video laryngoscopes and the development in airway management strategy and prevalence of difficult tracheal intubation: A national cohort study. Acta Anaesthesiol Scand. 2023;67(2):159–68. https://doi.org/10.1111/aas.14165.
42. Aziz MF, Bayman EO, Van Tienderen MM, Todd MM; StAGE Investigator Group; Brambrink AM. Predictors of difficult videolaryngoscopy with GlideScope® or C-MAC® with D-blade: secondary analysis from a large comparative videolaryngoscopy trial. Br J Anaesth. 2016;117(1):118–23. https://doi.org/10.1093/bja/aew128.
43. Amalric M, Larcher R, Brunot V, Garnier F, De Jong A, Moulaire Rigollet V, Corne P, Klouche K, Jung B. Impact of Videolaryngoscopy Expertise on First-Attempt Intubation Success in Critically Ill Patients. Crit Care Med. 2020;48(10):e889–e896. https://doi.org/10.1097/CCM.0000000000004497.

44. Carsetti A, Sorbello M, Adrario E, Donati A, Falcetta S. Airway Ultrasound as Predictor of Difficult Direct Laryngoscopy: A Systematic Review and Meta-analysis. Anesth Analg. 2022;134(4):740–50. https://doi.org/10.1213/ANE.0000000000005839.
45. Lazar AE, Gherghinescu MC. Airway Ultrasound for Anesthesia and in Intensive Care Patients-A Narrative Review of the Literature. J Clin Med. 2022;11(21):6327. https://doi.org/10.3390/jcm11216327.
46. Falcetta S, Sorbello M. Bats, Dracula and Batman: the sixth sense in airway management. Minerva Anestesiol. 2021;87(4):387–90. https://doi.org/10.23736/S0375-9393.21.15577-4.
47. Marchis IF, Negrut MF, Blebea CM, Crihan M, Alexa AL, Breazu CM. Trends in Preoperative Airway Assessment. Diagnostics (Basel). 2024;14(6):610. https://doi.org/10.3390/diagnostics14060610.
48. La Via L, Maniaci A, Gage D, Cuttone G, Misseri G, Lentini M, Paternò DS, Pappalardo F, SORBELLO M. Exploring the potential of artificial intelligence in airway management, Trends Anaesth Crit Care. 2024;59. https://doi.org/10.1016/j.tacc.2024.101512.
49. Zhang X, Xiong Z, Zhou Y, Zeng X. Artificial intelligence in imaging for obstructive sleep apnea: A comprehensive review. Sleep Med. 2025;137:108662. https://doi.org/10.1016/j.sleep.2025.108662.
50. Demir Senoglu G, Kara Timucin E, Kırısoglu S. Evaluation of anthropometric and ultrasonographic measurements with different machine learning methods in predicting difficult intubation: a prospective observational study. BMC Anesthesiol. 2025;25(1):496. https://doi.org/10.1186/s12871-025-03370-x.
51. Lonsdale H, Gray GM, Ahumada LM, Matava CT. Machine Vision and Image Analysis in Anesthesia: Narrative Review and Future Prospects. Anesth Analg. 2023;137(4):830–40. https://doi.org/10.1213/ANE.000000000000667.
52. Matava C, Pankiv E, Ahumada L, Weingarten B, Simpao A. Artificial intelligence, machine learning and the pediatric airway. Paediatr Anaesth. 2020;30(3):264–68. https://doi.org/10.1111/pan.13792.

Anesthesia for Cesarean Section

5

Gaetano Draisci and Stefano Catarci

5.1 Introduction

Anesthetic management of cesarean section is particularly important to reduce maternal and neonatal mortality and comorbidity, due to the unique characteristics and physiological changes of the obstetric population compared to the general population.

A multidisciplinary approach and clear communication with the mother are fundamental to ensure a safe and satisfactory childbirth experience. Continuous education and training are essential for anesthesiologists to provide high-quality care and contribute to the well-being of both mother and newborn.

5.2 Preoperative Assessment

The American Society of Anesthesiologists (ASA) guidelines for obstetric anesthesia recommend that pregnant women scheduled for cesarean section undergo a specific medical history and physical examination by an anesthesiologist [1].

The medical history should include a review of past medical history, obstetric history, current medical therapy, assessment of allergies, and a specific history of any issues during previous anesthetics; a physical examination must also be performed. Evaluation of the cardiovascular and respiratory systems, airway, and spine (for neuraxial anesthesia) is an integral part of the physical examination. For patients undergoing elective cesarean section, appropriate preoperative laboratory testing is

G. Draisci · S. Catarci (✉)
Department of Emergency, Anesthesiology and Intensive Care Sciences, Fondazione Policlinico Universitario A. Gemelli IRCCS, Rome, Italy
e-mail: gaetano.draisci@policlinicogemelli.it; stefano.catarci@policlinicogemelli.it

D. Chiumello, A. De Gasperi (eds.), *Practical Trends in Anesthesia and Intensive Care 2026*, https://doi.org/10.1007/978-3-032-25721-5_5

required, with particular attention to complete blood count, coagulation profile, serum electrolytes and metabolites, and electrocardiogram.

Additional preoperative laboratory tests should be individualized based on the patient's clinical situation and local institutional protocols. Pregnant women generally undergo blood group and antibody screening as part of routine prenatal care; it is advisable to repeat blood group and antibody screening prior to surgery in patients at high risk of intra- and postoperative hemorrhage.

5.3 Preparation for Cesarean Section

Preparation for anesthesia includes placement of one or more intravenous cannulas, administration of prophylaxis against aspiration of gastric contents, and standard monitoring as recommended by the American Society of Anesthesiologists (ASA).

Term pregnant women are at increased risk of aspiration of gastric contents due to delayed gastric emptying and incompetence of the lower esophageal sphincter. It should be noted that guidelines for preoperative fasting and aspiration prophylaxis are based more on expert consensus than on robust scientific evidence, as there are no randomized trials demonstrating that pharmacological interventions improve maternal outcomes.

- For elective cesarean section, it is advisable to observe 4 h of fasting for clear liquids and 8 h for solids.
- Clinical practice varies regarding the administration of pharmacological agents prior to scheduled and emergency cesarean section. American Society of Anesthesiologists (ASA) guidelines [1] state that timely administration of non-particulate antacids, H_2 receptor antagonists, and/or metoclopramide should be considered prior to surgical procedures in pregnant patients [2]. Similarly, the American Society of Anesthesiologists' guidelines for preoperative fasting recommend considering proton pump inhibitors in pregnant patients undergoing surgery.

Options for pharmacological prophylaxis include non-particulate antacids (e.g., sodium citrate-citric acid 30 ml orally), proton pump inhibitors (e.g., pantoprazole 40 mg intravenously), H_2 receptor antagonists (e.g., famotidine 20 mg intravenously), and prokinetic agents (e.g., metoclopramide 10 mg intravenously over one to 2 min). Metoclopramide has a dual action, promoting gastric emptying as a prokinetic and increasing lower esophageal sphincter tone, which can be particularly useful in term pregnant women who often exhibit lower esophageal sphincter dysfunction due to hormonal and anatomical factors.

Oral sodium citrate-citric acid solution increases gastric pH for approximately 1 h after administration, while the other prophylactic drugs have an onset of about 30–40 min.

It is important to note that a combination of antacid drugs may be more effective than single agents: in a meta-analysis of 22 randomized studies on pharmacological prophylaxis of gastric content aspiration in women undergoing general anesthesia for cesarean section, combined administration of antacids with H_2 antagonists was more effective in reducing gastric acidity than antacids alone and more effective than placebo [3].

- About antibiotic prophylaxis.
- Unlike other surgical procedures, sedatives are generally not administered as premedication before cesarean section, as these drugs cross the placental barrier and may affect the newborn at birth and cause some degree of maternal amnesia regarding the birth event. Reassurance and verbal support from the anesthesiologist often provide sufficient anxiolysis for most patients. However, in particularly anxious patients, premedication can be safely administered to facilitate neuraxial block placement or to help the patient tolerate the surgical procedure while conscious and under neuraxial anesthesia. In a randomized study, administration of midazolam (0.02 mg/kg IV) plus fentanyl (0.1 mcg/kg IV) before spinal anesthesia for cesarean section resulted in Apgar scores, neonatal pulse oximetry, and neurobehavioral scores not significantly different from placebo. Furthermore, no difference was reported in the mother's ability to recall the moment of delivery [4, 5].

5.4 Multiparametric Monitoring

Standard monitoring as defined by the American Society of Anesthesiologists includes pulse rate, noninvasive blood pressure measurement, electrocardiography, oxygen saturation monitoring by pulse oximetry, and temperature monitoring when significant changes in body temperature are anticipated. If sedatives are administered, end-tidal carbon dioxide ($EtCO_2$) should also be monitored.

Fetal heart rate should preferably be documented before and after the administration of neuraxial anesthesia. If possible, laboring patients who have been monitored in the labor room should continue to undergo cardiotocographic monitoring after transfer to the operating room when the procedure is significantly delayed (e.g., while establishing an epidural block with a catheter already in place for labor analgesia) or when clinically indicated.

5.5 Choice of Anesthetic Technique

Anesthesia options for cesarean section include neuraxial block (i.e., spinal anesthesia, epidural anesthesia, and combined spinal-epidural anesthesia) and general anesthesia.

The choice of anesthetic technique should be based on the urgency of the surgical procedure, maternal and fetal clinical status, the presence of maternal comorbidities, and whether an epidural catheter has previously been placed for labor analgesia.

The preferred technique for most patients undergoing cesarean section is neuraxial block rather than general anesthesia.

In fact, neuraxial block is currently the most widely used technique in over 95% of cesarean sections in the United States [6].

The advantages of regional anesthesia over general anesthesia include:

- Reduced risk of airway management: airway management is by definition more challenging in term pregnant women, who should be considered as "full stomach" patients (delayed gastric emptying) and who have an increased risk of difficult intubation (1:390) and "can't oxygenate, can't intubate" scenarios compared to the general population.
- Reduced use of systemic drugs before delivery and decreased transfer of drugs to the fetus.
- Use of neuraxial opioids for postoperative analgesia, ensuring better autonomic stability and minimizing the need for systemic opioids (opioid sparing effect).
- Optimization of maternal experience and the birth event. In the literature, general anesthesia for cesarean section is associated with an increased risk of awareness (1:670 compared to 1:18,000 in other surgical procedures under general anesthesia); moreover, neuraxial anesthesia may be associated with a reduced risk of severe postpartum depression. In a retrospective study of a database of over 400,000 cesarean sections, the use of general anesthesia was associated with an increased risk of postpartum depression requiring hospitalization, suicidal ideation, and self-inflicted injury [7]. It should be noted, however, that since the clinical circumstances requiring general anesthesia may be a confounding factor (for example, emergency or urgent situations), further studies are needed to accurately define this association.

Regarding the choice of anesthetic technique, it is appropriate to refer to the classification of the degree of urgency of cesarean section according to Lucas [8].

This system divides cesarean sections into categories according to their urgency. The aim of this classification is to provide a clear and systematic approach for the obstetric-anesthesia team, facilitating clinical decision-making and improving communication among healthcare team members.

Category I—Emergency cesarean section: by definition, there is an immediate threat to the life of the mother or fetus. Delivery must occur as quickly as possible.

Category II—Urgent cesarean section: there is maternal compromise or fetal distress (without immediate threat to the life of the mother or fetus).

Category III—Urgent cesarean section: delivery is required, but there is no maternal or fetal compromise.

Category IV—Elective cesarean section: this type of cesarean is scheduled in advance and may be performed for known clinical conditions or pre-existing maternal conditions.

In light of the above, neuraxial anesthesia should be considered an appropriate option even for urgent cesarean sections (types 2 and 3), particularly for patients at higher risk associated with general anesthesia (for example, anticipated difficult airway management on physical examination, recent oral intake of solids or liquids).

General anesthesia should be considered a reserved option for emergency cesarean sections (type 1). However, some experts note that a single-attempt spinal anesthesia performed by an experienced provider does not require significantly more time than induction of general anesthesia. The obstetrician and anesthesiologist should collaborate to determine the degree of urgency, so that the anesthesiologist can select the safest anesthetic technique for the patient.

Mortality directly related to anesthesia during cesarean section is currently very rare. According to data from the Pregnancy Mortality Surveillance System, mortality related to general anesthesia has decreased over the years, while mortality associated with regional anesthesia increased from 1979 to 2002 [9].

Scientific evidence on the neonatal effects of anesthetic technique (regional versus general) for cesarean section is not conclusive. Apgar scores and umbilical blood pH may be influenced by variables unrelated to the choice of anesthesia, including the indication for cesarean section itself (e.g., fetal distress), vasopressors administered during anesthesia (e.g., phenylephrine versus ephedrine), surgical technical issues, and other variables. A meta-analysis of 22 randomized studies including 1,800 patients undergoing cesarean section found no difference in umbilical artery or vein pH during elective cesarean section in patients receiving neuraxial or general anesthesia. In particular, mean Apgar scores at 1 min were higher with epidural block, but there was no difference in 5 min Apgar scores between general anesthesia and any type of neuraxial anesthesia [10].

In any case, neonatal exposure to anesthetic drugs (propofol, opioids, halogenated agents) during induction and maintenance of general anesthesia may potentially cause depression in the early neonatal period and the neonatal team should be informed of all drugs administered to the mother during induction of general anesthesia and prior to delivery.

5.6 Neuraxial Anesthesia

Options for neuraxial anesthesia include spinal anesthesia, epidural anesthesia, and combined spinal-epidural anesthesia.

To perform a cesarean section using a neuraxial technique, it is necessary to achieve sensory block from the sacral dermatomes up to thoracic level T4.

5.7 Spinal Anesthesia

Spinal anesthesia is the most commonly used neuraxial block technique for cesarean section. Spinal anesthesia is usually performed more rapidly than epidural anesthesia and provides a rapid onset of dense, bilateral, and reliable anesthesia using a very low dose of local anesthetic, with minimal risk of maternal toxicity or fetal drug transfer. The duration of anesthesia is limited after a single spinal injection, with no possibility to extend the anesthetic block if needed.

It is performed at the L3–L4 intervertebral level or, less frequently, at L2–L3 or L4–L5, using small-caliber atraumatic needles (25 gauge, 27 gauge), with a technique based on anatomical landmarks or ultrasound guidance.

Continuous spinal anesthesia may be performed to allow slow titration of spinal anesthesia in parturients with certain comorbidities (e.g., significant cardiac disease) or in patients in whom epidural catheter placement may be difficult or ineffective due to anatomical reasons (e.g., patients with extensive spinal surgery). Continuous spinal anesthesia is also a reasonable option after inadvertent dural puncture during an attempt at epidural catheter placement. All members of the nursing, obstetric, and anesthesia teams must be informed of the presence of the catheter in the intrathecal space, and the catheter must be appropriately labeled. On the other hand, it should be considered that in obstetric patients, the risk of post-dural puncture headache is high when using large-bore continuous spinal catheters, which limits the routine use of continuous spinal anesthesia.

For spinal anesthesia for cesarean section, a combination of local anesthetic and opioid administered into the subarachnoid space is commonly used.

Bupivacaine is the most commonly used local anesthetic for spinal anesthesia, due to its adequate duration of action for most cesarean sections, low incidence of transient radicular irritation, low cost, and wide availability. Other options include ropivacaine, levobupivacaine, and chloroprocaine.

Bupivacaine (hyperbaric 0.5%–0.75%–1%) is typically used at a dose of 8–12 mg and combined with an opioid (e.g., fentanyl, sufentanil, or morphine). The onset time of bupivacaine is 5–8 min. The effective dose for 95% of patients (ED95) of intrathecal hyperbaric bupivacaine for spinal anesthesia in cesarean section is 11.2 mg.

Obesity does not appear to affect the ED95 of hyperbaric bupivacaine. However, the ED95 of bupivacaine in extremely obese parturients (i.e., with a body mass index [BMI] greater than 50 kg/m ^{2}) has not been well defined [11–15].

Hyperbaric bupivacaine is preferred for its rapid onset and the ability to modify the spinal level by changing the position of the operating table. Within 1.5 h, the mid-thoracic sensory level will have regressed, although the total duration of action extends beyond 2.5 h.

Ropivacaine is available in an isobaric formulation. Therefore, if a hyperbaric solution is desired, dextrose (from 5% to 8.25%) must be added. Ropivacaine is approximately 40% less potent than bupivacaine. The duration of surgical anesthesia is shorter compared to bupivacaine. The dosing range for ropivacaine is 15–20 mg. In a comparative dose study, the ED50 (effective dose for 50% of patients) and ED90 of intrathecal ropivacaine in non-twin pregnant patients were 11.2 mg (95% CI 10.2–12.0) and 15.7 mg (95% CI 14.4–18.3), respectively. Regarding duration of action at equivalent doses, ropivacaine provides a sensory block similar to bupivacaine and may result in faster recovery of motor block [16–19].

Lidocaine (60–100 mg) is rarely used for spinal anesthesia due to the relatively high risk of transient neurologic symptoms in the non-obstetric population. For this reason, intrathecal lidocaine is usually avoided for anesthesia in cesarean section [20, 21].

Opioids may be added as adjuvants to the local anesthetic in spinal anesthesia to improve both intraoperative and postoperative analgesia. The addition of a lipophilic opioid is particularly useful to reduce discomfort from visceral manipulation (e.g., uterine manipulation). A meta-analysis including over 800 patients undergoing spinal anesthesia for cesarean section with and without various intrathecal opioids found that the need to supplement intraoperative analgesia with other drugs decreased from 24% to 4% with the addition of intrathecal opioid to the local anesthetic [22].

Liposoluble opioids such as fentanyl (10–15 mcg) and sufentanil (2.5–5 mcg) are commonly added to enhance intraoperative analgesia.

Liposoluble opioids provide minimal postoperative analgesia due to their short duration of action and, within clinical dosages, are not associated with delayed respiratory depression Pruritus is a common dose-related side effect of intrathecal fentanyl and sufentanil [23].

A 2020 meta-analysis of 14 randomized studies (700 patients) on the effects of adding fentanyl to bupivacaine for spinal anesthesia concluded that intrathecal fentanyl (10–15 mcg) reduces the need for supplemental intraoperative analgesia (4.5% vs. 29.6%, RR 0.18, 95% CI 0.11–0.27) and the incidence of intraoperative and postoperative nausea and vomiting [24]. The incidence of pruritus increased sixfold with the addition of fentanyl. Similar results were observed when fentanyl was added to a combination of bupivacaine and morphine. The optimal dose of intrathecal fentanyl cannot be determined, although doses between 10 and 12.5 mcg reduced the need for intraoperative analgesia and resulted in low rates of intraoperative nausea, vomiting, and pruritus.

Hydrophilic opioids (e.g., intrathecal morphine 75–100 mcg) are used as adjuvants primarily to provide postoperative analgesia as part of a multimodal opioid-sparing postoperative analgesic regimen.

The authors do not recommend the use of other intrathecal adjuvants (epinephrine, clonidine, neostigmine) due to the potential for increased maternal side effects.

5.8 Epidural Anesthesia

Epidural anesthesia is a continuous catheter-based technique that allows titration of the block and extension of duration with incremental dosing. Ongoing epidural analgesia during labor can be converted to epidural anesthesia if necessary, and is the preferred technique when a functioning epidural catheter is already in place (effective analgesia). Epidural anesthesia tends to be less dense than spinal anesthesia and has a slower onset.

It is performed at the L3–L4 intervertebral level or, less frequently, at L2–L3 or L4–L5, using an 18-gauge or 16-gauge Tuohy needle, with either the loss-of-resistance to saline or air technique. The saline technique is associated with a lower incidence of dural puncture.

Epidural anesthesia can be performed with ultrasound guidance in patients in whom the technique may be challenging (e.g., obesity, spinal abnormalities such as rotoscoliosis, lumbar spondylolisthesis, etc.).

Commonly used epidural local anesthetics include lidocaine, ropivacaine, and bupivacaine.

A mixture of 2% lidocaine 15–25 ml with epinephrine 1:200,000 and sodium bicarbonate 1–2 mEq results in a more rapid onset of sensory block and a lower risk of anesthesia failure compared to the local anesthetic alone. The addition of epinephrine allows detection of inadvertent intravascular catheter placement, while sodium bicarbonate increases the onset speed of the anesthetic mixture. Before any administration through the epidural catheter, aspiration should be performed to check catheter function and exclude intrathecal or intravascular migration. If possible, repeated boluses of the anesthetic mixture should be administered and the sensory level assessed, rather than administering the entire mixture rapidly.

The authors recommend the use of a mixture of 2% lidocaine with epinephrine (1:200,000 dilution) and 1–2 mEq sodium bicarbonate. Fifteen to twenty-five milliliters of 2% lidocaine with epinephrine (1:200,000) and bicarbonate are injected in 5 ml aliquots after a test dose of 3–5 ml. Onset of anesthesia generally occurs within 5–10 min.

Alkalinization of epidural lidocaine with epinephrine in patients with an epidural catheter in situ during labor reduced the time from epidural bolus to achievement of T4 sensory block from 9.7 to 5.2 min [25].

In a meta-analysis of 24 randomized studies evaluating the onset speed of various local anesthetics administered epidurally for cesarean section, the fastest onset of anesthetic block was achieved with 2% bicarbonate-buffered lidocaine [26]. The order of onset speed, from fastest to slowest, was 2% bicarbonate-buffered lidocaine >2% lidocaine >0.75% ropivacaine >0.5% bupivacaine. None of the study mixtures contained epinephrine or opioids.

Bupivacaine is not routinely used for anesthesia epidural in cesarean section due to the risk of cardiovascular complications following intravascular injection and its slow onset. The onset of the block occurs in approximately 20 min, and the duration of action (regression of two dermatomes) ranges from 120 to 240 min [27].

Epidural ropivacaine is approximately 40% less potent than bupivacaine, with a similar onset and a slightly shorter duration of action. Therefore, higher doses of ropivacaine may be required to achieve equivalent anesthesia compared to bupivacaine. Ropivacaine may have a greater safety margin than bupivacaine. However, animal and human studies comparing the cardiotoxicity of the two drugs have reported conflicting results: some have shown cardiac conduction abnormalities at lower doses of bupivacaine compared to ropivacaine, while others have found no difference between the two local anesthetics [28–32].

Opioids can be administered epidurally to increase the speed of onset of local anesthetics, improve the quality of anesthesia, and provide postoperative analgesia. Lipophilic opioids (fentanyl or sufentanil) are mainly used for intraoperative analgesia and are generally administered at the start of epidural anesthesia (before surgical incision). Hydrophilic opioids (i.e., morphine and hydromorphone) are used for postoperative analgesia and are generally administered after fetal extraction. Commonly administered opioid doses in the epidural space are fentanyl 25 mcg and sufentanil 10 mcg. Preservative-free morphine 2–3 mg may be administered as a single dose for postoperative analgesia after fetal extraction. The usual epidural dose ranges from 2 to 3 mg, providing adequate postoperative analgesia for 18–24 h as part of a multimodal pain management regimen [33–37].

5.9 Combined Spinal-Epidural Anesthesia

Combined spinal-epidural anesthesia offers the advantages of spinal anesthesia (rapid onset) and, in addition, the possibility to extend and prolong the anesthetic block via the epidural catheter. It can be used in patients in whom it is beneficial to minimize the hemodynamic impact of neuraxial block caused by vasoplegia (such as patients with heart disease).

The drugs used for combined spinal-epidural anesthesia are the same as those used for spinal and epidural anesthesia.

There are several options for performing the combined technique: needle-through-needle technique, with a Whitacre needle (usually 27 gauge) inside a Tuohy needle (18 gauge), or at different levels.

Similarly, a full dose of intrathecal drug can be administered, followed by epidural administration only if necessary, or a partial intrathecal dose with epidural administration (sequential technique).

In the first case (full intrathecal drug dose), the same initial doses and combinations of spinal drugs as in single-shot spinal anesthesia are administered. The first epidural drug dose is then given when the sensory level drops below T4. At that point, after negative aspiration from the catheter for blood and cerebrospinal fluid, a test dose of 3 ml of 2% lidocaine with epinephrine 1:200,000 is administered. In this context, this bolus serves as a test dose for intravascular injection (i.e., tachycardia would occur with intravascular injection of epinephrine). Since the patient already has a spinal block with motor block, the bolus is not a test for intrathecal injection. Therefore, it is always good practice to fractionate the local anesthetic dose (i.e., administer 3–5 ml at a time).

The test dose often restores a surgical level of anesthesia above T4. Subsequently, the sensory level should be checked every 20 min and fractionated doses of 2% lidocaine with epinephrine (3–5 ml) administered, according to the level of the block.

In the sequential technique, a lower amount of intrathecal local anesthetic is administered (e.g., 5–7 mg of bupivacaine), followed by subsequent epidural injections (e.g., 3–5 ml of 2% lidocaine with epinephrine), titrated to achieve an adequate sensory block up to T4.

Sequential techniques result in less hemodynamic impact with fewer hypotensive events and may provide greater safety regarding correct epidural catheter placement [38–40].

5.10 Ultrasound-Assisted Neuraxial Blocks

The incidence of difficult neuraxial blocks in obstetrics is estimated to be about 4%.

In general, the success of these techniques depends on the ability to locate the epidural or intrathecal space. Traditionally, neuraxial blocks are performed using anatomical landmarks, which are often difficult to locate or palpate in patients with obesity, back edema, underlying spinal deformity, or those who have undergone spinal surgery. It should be noted, however, that even in patients without these issues, a given intervertebral space is accurately identified in only 30% of cases, and anesthesiologists very often mistakenly identify a higher space than intended. This error is amplified by obesity and by attempts to locate an intervertebral space at higher spinal levels. Therefore, Tuffier's line, a widely used surface anatomical landmark, is not a reliable reference point.

The use of ultrasound reduces the number of attempts, is associated with a lower incidence of failed anesthesia, and increases patient satisfaction.

In obese pregnant patients, the use of ultrasound increases the number of successful first-attempt neuraxial blocks performed by experienced anesthesiologists and decreases the time required to perform the block [41].

Figure 5.1 shows parasagittal and transverse ultrasound scans in a pregnant patient undergoing ultrasound-assisted spinal anesthesia. In particular, the transverse scan allows visualization of the distance from the posterior complex to the skin.

5.11 High Neuraxial Block

High neuraxial block is reported to occur in 1/4336 anesthetics [40]. Assessment of handgrip strength is a quick way to determine whether the block involves the cervical nerve roots. If the patient is unable to maintain adequate oxygenation, rapid sequence induction with orotracheal intubation should be evaluated.

5.12 General Anesthesia

General anesthesia may be indicated for cesarean section in the following cases:

- Emergency cesarean section (category 1 urgency according to the Lucas classification), with insufficient time to perform a neuraxial block or to achieve a surgical level of anesthesia via an already placed epidural catheter.
- Maternal refusal or inability to cooperate with neuraxial anesthesia.
- Inadequate sensory level of the anesthetic block or failed neuraxial anesthesia.
- Severe maternal aortic stenosis or maternal hemodynamic instability.
- Relative or absolute contraindications to neuraxial block (e.g., coagulopathy, severe hypovolemia, infection at the epidural or spinal catheter insertion site, increased intracranial pressure).

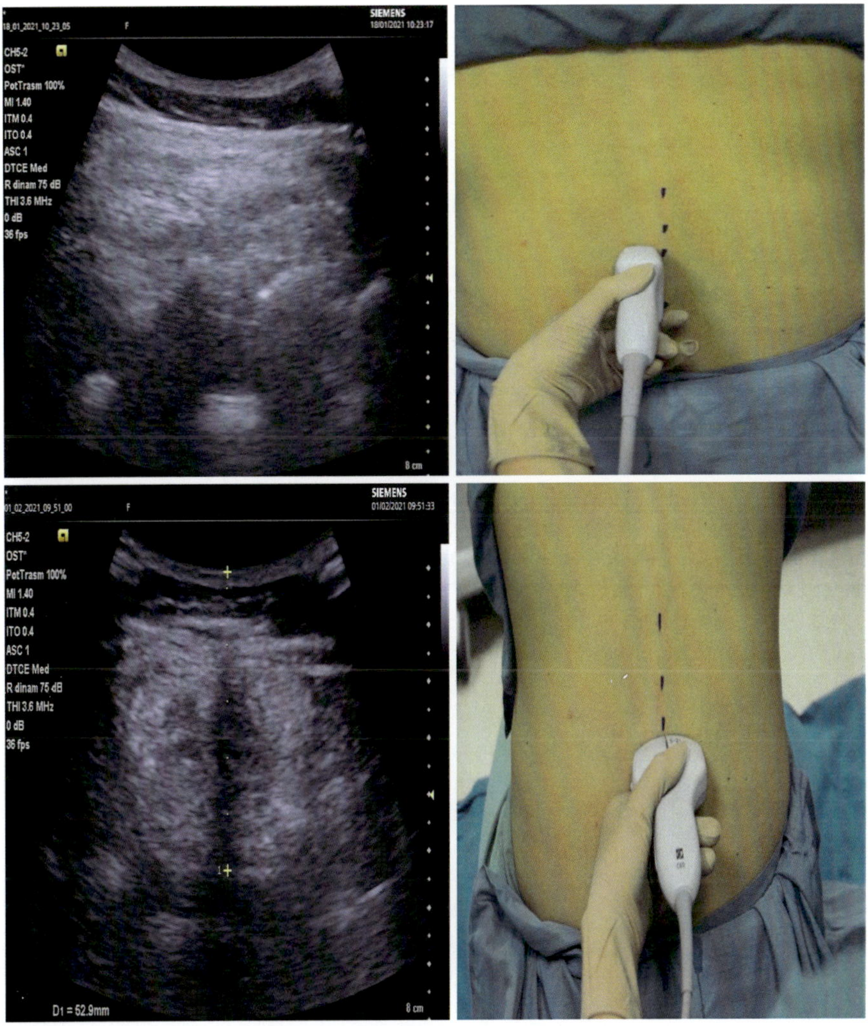

Fig. 5.1 Parasagittal and transverse ultrasound scans of the lumbar spine

Pregnant women undergoing general anesthesia are at higher risk of airway management difficulties and awareness compared to non-pregnant patients undergoing other types of surgery. The incidence of awareness during general anesthesia for obstetric patients can be as high as 1:212, compared to 1:19,600 for other types of surgery [41–45].

The incidence of airway management difficulties necessitates appropriate local institutional protocols for obstetric patients. The difficult airway management flowchart for pregnant women from the Obstetric Anaesthetists' Association is particularly useful [45].

Before general anesthesia, the pregnant patient is positioned on the operating table with a right lateral wedge (or left tilt) to shift the uterus to the left and avoid aortocaval compression, with the head and neck optimally positioned for intubation (sniffing position).

The patient's abdomen is generally prepared and disinfected before induction of anesthesia to minimize the time between induction and delivery and to reduce fetal exposure to anesthetics. The obstetrician performs the surgical incision only after the anesthesiologist has secured the airway with tracheal intubation.

Rapid sequence induction and intubation is the standard induction technique for cesarean section.

Preferred induction agents are propofol (2–2.5 mg/kg intravenously) or etomidate (0.3–0.5 mg/kg intravenously), although ketamine may be used in hemodynamically unstable or hypovolemic patients. All intravenous induction agents are lipophilic and therefore cross the placenta to reach the fetus. Neuromuscular blocking agents do not cross the placenta and are thus not associated with neonatal weakness.

Because pregnant patients generally do not receive pharmacological premedication and have a larger volume of distribution, full induction doses should be administered for general anesthesia.

For most patients, we avoid intravenous opioid administration until after fetal delivery, except in preeclamptic or cardiac patients. In a meta-analysis of 17 randomized, placebo-controlled trials on the use of alfentanil, remifentanil, or fentanyl during induction of anesthesia for cesarean section, no significant differences were found in Apgar scores at one or 5 min after administration of alfentanil or remifentanil [44]. In patients with preeclampsia, opioids and other medications are administered during induction to prevent hypertension during laryngoscopy and intubation, such as remifentanil.

A neuromuscular blocking agent such as succinylcholine (0.8–1 mg/kg) has historically been used during induction as part of the rapid sequence induction protocol.

Alternatively, rocuronium bromide can be used at maximal doses (1.2 mg/kg).

After induction and intubation, high-dose volatile anesthetics (e.g., sevoflurane, desflurane) may be administered with high oxygen flows to rapidly achieve an adequate end-tidal anesthetic concentration (1 MAC) and minimize the risk of intraoperative awareness.

It should be noted, however, that volatile anesthetics produce dose-dependent uterine relaxation [45], which can theoretically cause uterine atony and hemorrhage. After delivery, once fetal drug transfer is no longer possible, midazolam (1–2 mg) and an intravenous opioid (e.g., fentanyl or sufentanil) may be administered; 50% N_2O can be added to allow a reduction in the volatile anesthetic dose to 0.5–0.75 MAC or to replace the volatile agent with a propofol infusion.

Ventilation should be controlled or assisted to achieve an end-tidal CO_2 of approximately 30 mmHg, which should correspond to a normal partial pressure of carbon dioxide ($PaCO_2$) of 30–32 mmHg at term pregnancy.

5.13 Intraoperative Management

Immediately after performing the neuraxial block or before induction of general anesthesia, patients should be positioned with left tilt or right lateral wedge (left uterine displacement) to minimize the risk of aortocaval compression.

Traditionally, 15 degrees of left uterine displacement has been recommended for all pregnant patients with a visibly gravid uterus or more than 20 weeks' gestation. Two studies have examined the cardiovascular effects of a 15-degree tilt in patients undergoing spinal anesthesia [46]. Although these studies did not demonstrate a difference in fetal pH at birth, significant fluid and vasopressor administration was used in both studies to correct maternal hypotension, which may have influenced the results.

In one study, 100 healthy term parturients with singleton pregnancies were randomly assigned to either a 15-degree left lateral tilt or supine positioning after spinal anesthesia. Maternal blood pressure was maintained with simultaneous intravenous fluid co-loading and a phenylephrine infusion targeted to maintain baseline systolic blood pressure. No difference was found in neonatal acid–base status between groups. Systolic blood pressure and cardiac output were significantly lower in the supine group, despite increased phenylephrine administration [47].

In another study, noninvasive cardiac output monitoring was used during spinal anesthesia for cesarean delivery in 80 healthy parturients who were randomly assigned to either the supine position or a 15-degree left lateral tilt [48]. No differences were found between groups in systolic blood pressure, mean arterial pressure, cardiac index, nausea and vomiting, or neonatal Apgar scores.

Another study compared MRI images of inferior vena cava volume during 15 and 30 degrees of right and left lateral tilt in pregnant women between 31 and 39 weeks of gestation. Inferior vena cava compression was reduced with a 30-degree left lateral tilt, but not with a 15-degree left lateral tilt or with 15 or 30 degrees of right lateral tilt [49].

MRI assessment of aortic and vena cava volumes in pregnant and nonpregnant women demonstrated that the volume of the vena cava, but not the aorta, is influenced by the patient's position; specifically, a left lateral tilt of at least 30 degrees is required to improve the volume of the vena cava [50].

Most healthy parturients do not require supplemental oxygen during or after neuraxial anesthesia.

Nausea commonly occurs after neuraxial anesthesia. Prophylaxis for intraoperative and postoperative nausea and vomiting can be administered, particularly 4 mg intravenous ondansetron after delivery for the prevention of postoperative nausea and vomiting; other options described in the literature include metoclopramide to facilitate gastric emptying and dexamethasone (4–8 mg intravenously).

There are several possible causes of nausea and vomiting during cesarean section, including the following:

- Hypotension is the most common cause of nausea and usually resolves with restoration of baseline mean arterial pressure using vasopressors (e.g., phenylephrine or ephedrine).
- Visceral manipulation (e.g., exteriorization or reinsertion of the uterus) can cause nausea despite adequate neuraxial anesthesia.
- Uterotonic drugs, especially if administered rapidly, can cause nausea.

5.14 Treatment of Hypotension

Neuraxial block causes sympathetic blockade and vasodilation, which can result in hypotension that should be treated with vasopressors.

The goal should be to maintain mean arterial pressure within 10–20% of baseline values. To this end, vasopressor boluses can be administered to patients whose mean arterial pressure falls below 20% of baseline and to those who become symptomatic with nausea or vomiting.

A meta-analysis of 109 randomized studies on various strategies to prevent arterial hypotension during cesarean section found that vasopressors are more effective than fluid loading, leg compression, or other types of drugs [51]. One measure that can be used to temporarily increase venous return during vasopressor administration is the Trendelenburg position while the patient is supine, with leftward uterine displacement.

Phenylephrine, a direct alpha-adrenergic agonist, and ephedrine, an indirect alpha- and beta-adrenergic agonist, are both effective in treating hypotension resulting from spinal anesthesia in pregnant women.

Commonly used vasopressor doses for the treatment of hypotension include phenylephrine 50–100 mcg intravenous bolus or 25–100 mcg/min by intravenous infusion and ephedrine 5–10 mg intravenous bolus or 1–5 mg/min by intravenous infusion.

Phenylephrine is associated with a lower incidence of intraoperative nausea and vomiting and a lower incidence of fetal acidosis (umbilical artery pH), whereas ephedrine may be associated with an increased risk of fetal acidosis [52–55].

It has been suggested that the relative fetal acidosis occurs because ephedrine crosses the placenta, increasing the fetal metabolic rate. However, it should be noted that phenylephrine can cause reflex maternal bradycardia.

In cases of fetal compromise, it is unclear which vasopressor is preferable; a retrospective review of patients with preeclampsia undergoing cesarean section found no differences in umbilical artery pH between those who received ephedrine and those who received phenylephrine to treat spinal hypotension [56]. In another study in which preeclamptic patients were randomly assigned to prophylactic infusion of phenylephrine or ephedrine during spinal anesthesia, no difference in umbilical artery pH was found between the groups [57].

In a 2014 systematic review, prophylactic infusion of phenylephrine (with fluid loading) in parturients undergoing spinal anesthesia reduced the incidence of hypotension by about 60% before and after delivery (RR = 0.36) and decreased the incidence of nausea and vomiting (RR = 0.39) compared to no prophylaxis or ephedrine infusion [58]. No differences were found in other maternal or fetal endpoints or outcomes. The available studies for analysis were limited and included variable dosing regimens.

Several studies suggest that norepinephrine may be as effective as phenylephrine and may cause less maternal bradycardia [49–61]. Existing studies have used different dosing and administration protocols. A 2019 meta-analysis of three studies (294 patients) comparing norepinephrine with phenylephrine for the prevention of hypotension after spinal anesthesia for cesarean section found similar rates of hypotension and Apgar scores between groups, and a lower incidence of bradycardia with norepinephrine [56].

In another study, involving 82 parturients randomly assigned to receive prophylaxis for spinal-induced hypotension with a fixed dose of norepinephrine 4 mcg/min or phenylephrine 50 mcg/minute, the incidence of bradycardia was lower (4.8% versus 31.7%), and fetal pH was slightly higher in the norepinephrine group (7.35 [95% CI 7.33–7.37] versus 7.34 [95% CI 7.26–7.36]) [62]. Apgar scores, incidence of hypotension, and use of rescue vasopressors were similar.

5.15 Intraoperative Fluid Management: Crystalloids and Colloids

Regarding fluid management, a rapid intravenous bolus of crystalloids is usually administered at the time of spinal anesthesia induction (co-load), together with vasopressors as needed or prophylactically. Typically, during neuraxial block placement, a bolus of 500–1000 ml of crystalloids can be given intravenously.

Crystalloid solutions are more commonly used than colloid solutions during cesarean section.

To prevent fetal hypoglycemia, glucose-containing solutions should be avoided.

As in other surgical settings, it is important to maintain normothermia to reduce complications associated with hypothermia (coagulopathy, cardiovascular and metabolic risks, infectious complications). Providers should aim to maintain normothermia in both mother and newborn by keeping the ambient temperature at 22–23 °C and, if necessary, using warmed fluids [63–68].

5.16 Administration of Uterotonics

Uterine contraction is the main mechanism for reducing uterine bleeding after delivery. The uterus is massaged and oxytocin is administered as the first-line uterotonic agent.

Protocols for oxytocin infusion vary by center but should include the administration of small, slow intravenous bolus doses (i.e., <5 units IV) or controlled infusion.

Rapid administration of oxytocin can cause hypotension, nausea and vomiting, chest pain with electrocardiogram changes, and even acute cardiovascular events

[69–72]. The incidence of side effects is directly related to the rate of administration.

Therefore, the minimum effective dose of oxytocin should be used.

The optimal dose and route of administration (i.e., bolus or infusion) of oxytocin during cesarean section are not clear. In a prospective, double-blind study, 60 patients were randomly assigned to receive either bolus doses of oxytocin, 3 units over 15 s IV, or oxytocin infusion during elective cesarean section under spinal anesthesia. Uterine tone was assessed by the obstetrician at 3 min intervals, with additional oxytocin boluses given as needed. Patients in the bolus group required less oxytocin to achieve adequate uterine tone compared to those in the infusion group (mean 4 versus 8.4 IU), although there were no differences in systolic or diastolic blood pressure, heart rate, side effects, or total blood loss between the two groups [72].

If a bolus injection is given after cesarean section, some studies suggest that adding an oxytocin infusion reduces delayed blood loss and the need for blood transfusion and/or additional uterotonic agents compared to bolus injection alone [73, 74].

Women who receive oxytocin during labor may develop desensitization and require higher doses of oxytocin to achieve a uterotonic effect. In one study, the bolus dose of oxytocin required to achieve adequate uterine tone in 90% of patients (ED90) who had received 10 h of oxytocin during labor was 2.99 (95% CI 2.32–3.67) units, compared to an ED90 of 0.35 (95% CI 0.18–0.52) units in patients undergoing elective cesarean section [75, 76].

Similarly, the ED90 for oxytocin infusion is about 15 units/hour for elective cesarean sections but may increase to 44 units/h in patients who were previously in labor with oxytocin augmentation [77, 78].

Patients at high risk of hemorrhage may benefit from prolonged postpartum infusions to reduce the risk of delayed hemorrhage.

Other uterotonic agents that may be used include carbetocin 100 mcg over 1 min and, as second-line agents, sulprostone 0.5 mg in 250 ml saline over 15 min or rectal prostaglandins.

5.17 Postoperative Analgesia

Multimodal postoperative analgesia should be used to promote rapid recovery and minimize the need for opioids in the postoperative period. The pain management strategy after cesarean section should consist of neuraxial opioids and non-opioid analgesics opioids scheduled at fixed intervals (paracetamol and nonsteroidal anti-inflammatory drugs), reserving systemic opioids for breakthrough pain. Enhanced recovery protocols, similar to those used in other types of surgery, have been developed. The ERAC (enhanced recovery after cesarean) protocol consists of multidisciplinary best practices and includes recommendations covering the entire perioperative period (pre-, intra-, and postpartum) [79–82].

Abdominal wall blocks, although less effective than intrathecal morphine, should be considered in patients undergoing general anesthesia; various wall block

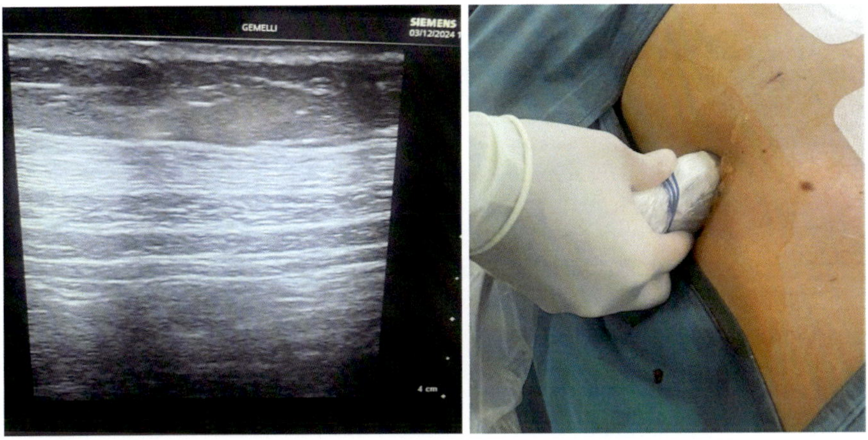

Fig. 5.2 Ultrasound-guided TAP block at the end of cesarean section

techniques are described in the literature: transversus abdominis plane (TAP) block, ilioinguinal and iliohypogastric nerve block, quadratus lumborum block (QLB2 block), erector spinae plane (ESP) block, and wound infiltration [83–85]. Figure. 5.2 shows an example of an ultrasound-guided TAP block at the end of a cesarean section.

5.18 Conclusions

- Women undergoing cesarean section should receive a targeted medical history and physical examination by an anesthesiologist.
- For patients undergoing cesarean section, pharmacological prophylaxis for aspiration of gastric contents should be considered. Options include sodium citrate-citric acid, 30 mL orally immediately before anesthesia, an H_2 receptor antagonist (e.g., famotidine 20 mg IV) or a proton pump inhibitor (e.g., pantoprazole 40 mg IV) administered 40–60 min before induction, and metoclopramide 10 mg IV given at least 30 min before induction.
- The choice of anesthetic technique should be based on maternal and fetal status, comorbidities, expected duration of the procedure, and the presence or absence of an epidural catheter in situ. If a functioning epidural catheter is present, it can be used to convert analgesia to anesthesia. For most patients, neuraxial anesthesia is the technique of choice for cesarean section rather than general anesthesia.
- For spinal anesthesia, the drugs administered include a local anesthetic (e.g., hyperbaric bupivacaine 8–12 mg), a lipophilic opioid (e.g., sufentanil 5 mcg) to enhance intraoperative anesthesia, and/or a hydrophilic opioid (e.g., preservative-free morphine 75–150 mcg) for postoperative analgesia.
- For epidural anesthesia, the epidural solution generally includes a local anesthetic (e.g., 2% lidocaine with epinephrine 1:200,000 and sodium bicarbonate),

a lipophilic opioid (e.g., sufentanil 10 mcg) to enhance intraoperative anesthesia, and a hydrophilic opioid (e.g., preservative-free morphine 2–3 mg) for postoperative analgesia.

- For general anesthesia, rapid sequence induction and intubation should be performed. After induction, a high concentration of volatile anesthetic (e.g., sevoflurane or desflurane) is administered to rapidly achieve 1 MAC of end-tidal anesthetic and minimize the risk of awareness.
- After performing the neuraxial block or before induction of general anesthesia, significant uterine displacement should be achieved with a right lateral wedge or left tilt to avoid aortocaval compression.
- After performing the anesthetic block, administration of phenylephrine, ephedrine, or norepinephrine should be considered to prevent and treat neuraxial block-induced hypotension, aiming to maintain maternal mean arterial pressure within 20% of baseline.

References

1. Practice Guidelines for Obstetric Anesthesia: an updated report by the American Society of Anesthesiologists Task Force on Obstetric Anesthesia and the Society for Obstetric Anesthesia and Perinatology. Anesthesiology. 2016;124:270.
2. Practice guidelines for preoperative fasting and the use of pharmacologic agents to reduce the risk of pulmonary aspiration: application to healthy patients undergoing elective procedures: an updated report by the American Society of Anesthesiologists Task Force on Preoperative Fasting and the use of pharmacologic agents to reduce the risk of pulmonary aspiration. Anesthesiology. 2017;126:376.
3. Paranjothy S, Griffiths JD, Broughton HK, et al. Interventions at caesarean section for reducing the risk of aspiration pneumonitis. Cochrane Database Syst Rev. 2010;2010:CD004943.
4. Frölich MA, Burchfield DJ, Euliano TY, Caton D. A single dose of fentanyl and midazolam prior to cesarean section have no adverse neonatal effects. Can J Anaesth. 2006;53:79.
5. Manouchehrian N, Bakhshaei MH. Nitrous oxide effect on relieving anxiety and pain in parturients under spinal anesthesia for caesarean section. Anesth Pain Med. 2014;4:e16662.
6. Bucklin BA, Hawkins JL, Anderson JR, Ullrich FA. Obstetric anesthesia workforce survey: twenty-year update. Anesthesiology. 2005;103:645.
7. Guglielminotti J, Li G. Exposure to general anesthesia for cesarean delivery and odds of severe postpartum depression requiring hospitalization. Anesth Analg. 2020;131:1421.
8. Lucas N, Nel MR, Robinson PN. The anaesthetic classification of caesarean sections. Anaesthesia. 1996;51(8):791–2. https://doi.org/10.1111/j.1365-2044.1996.tb07900.x. PMID: 8795329
9. Hawkins JL, Chang J, Palmer SK, et al. Anesthesia-related maternal mortality in the United States: 1979-2002. Obstet Gynecol. 2011;117:69.
10. Afolabi BB, Lesi FE. Regional versus general anaesthesia for caesarean section. Cochrane Database Syst Rev. 2012;10:CD004350.
11. Ginosar Y, Mirikatani E, Drover DR, et al. ED50 and ED95 of intrathecal hyperbaric bupivacaine coadministered with opioids for cesarean delivery. Anesthesiology. 2004;100:676.
12. Carvalho B, Collins J, Drover DR, et al. ED(50) and ED(95) of intrathecal bupivacaine in morbidly obese patients undergoing cesarean delivery. Anesthesiology. 2011;114:529.
13. Lee Y, Balki M, Parkes R, Carvalho JC. Dose requirement of intrathecal bupivacaine for cesarean delivery is similar in obese and normal weight women. Rev Bras Anestesiol. 2009;59:674.

14. Heng Sia AT, Tan KH, Sng BL, et al. Hyperbaric versus plain bupivacaine for spinal anesthesia for cesarean delivery. Anesth Analg. 2015;120:132.
15. Sng BL, Han NLR, Leong WL, et al. Hyperbaric vs. isobaric bupivacaine for spinal anaesthesia for elective caesarean section: a Cochrane systematic review. Anaesthesia. 2018;73:499.
16. McDonald SB, Liu SS, Kopacz DJ, Stephenson CA. Hyperbaric spinal ropivacaine: a comparison to bupivacaine in volunteers. Anesthesiology. 1999;90:971.
17. Gautier P, De Kock M, Huberty L, et al. Comparison of the effects of intrathecal ropivacaine, levobupivacaine, and bupivacaine for caesarean section. Br J Anaesth. 2003;91:684.
18. Mei Z, Ngan Kee WD, Sheng ZM, et al. Comparative dose-response study of hyperbaric ropivacaine for spinal anesthesia for cesarean delivery in singleton versus twin pregnancies. J Clin Anesth. 2020;67:110068.
19. Malhotra R, Johnstone C, Halpern S, et al. Duration of motor block with intrathecal ropivacaine versus bupivacaine for caesarean section: a meta-analysis. Int J Obstet Anesth. 2016;27:16.
20. Philip J, Sharma SK, Gottumukkala VN, et al. Transient neurologic symptoms after spinal anesthesia with lidocaine in obstetric patients. Anesth Analg. 2001;92:405.
21. Aouad MT, Siddik SS, Jalbout MI, Baraka AS. Does pregnancy protect against intrathecal lidocaine-induced transient neurologic symptoms? Anesth Analg. 2001;92:401.
22. Dahl JB, Jeppesen IS, Jørgensen H, et al. Intraoperative and postoperative analgesic efficacy and adverse effects of intrathecal opioids in patients undergoing cesarean section with spinal anesthesia: a qualitative and quantitative systematic review of randomized controlled trials. Anesthesiology. 1999;91:1919.
23. Belzarena SD. Clinical effects of intrathecally administered fentanyl in patients undergoing cesarean section. Anesth Analg. 1992;74:653.
24. Uppal V, Retter S, Casey M, et al. Efficacy of intrathecal fentanyl for cesarean delivery: a systematic review and meta-analysis of randomized controlled trials with trial sequential analysis. Anesth Analg. 2020;130:111.
25. Lam DT, Ngan Kee WD, Khaw KS. Extension of epidural blockade in labour for emergency caesarean section using 2% lidocaine with epinephrine and fentanyl, with or without alkalinisation. Anaesthesia. 2001;56:790.
26. Reschke MM, Monks DT, Varaday SS, et al. Choice of local anaesthetic for epidural caesarean section: a Bayesian network meta-analysis. Anaesthesia. 2020;75:674.
27. Hillyard SG, Bate TE, Corcoran TB, et al. Extending epidural analgesia for emergency caesarean section: a meta-analysis. Br J Anaesth. 2011;107:668.
28. Lefrant JY, de La Coussaye JE, Ripart J, et al. The comparative electrophysiologic and hemodynamic effects of a large dose of ropivacaine and bupivacaine in anesthetized and ventilated piglets. Anesth Analg. 2001;93:1598.
29. Schwoerer AP, Scheel H, Friederich P. A comparative analysis of bupivacaine and ropivacaine effects on human cardiac SCN5A channels. Anesth Analg. 2015;120:1226.
30. Ngan Kee WD, Ng FF, Khaw KS, et al. Determination and comparison of graded dose-response curves for epidural bupivacaine and ropivacaine for analgesia in laboring nulliparous women. Anesthesiology. 2010;113:445.
31. Santos AC, DeArmas PI. Systemic toxicity of levobupivacaine, bupivacaine, and ropivacaine during continuous intravenous infusion to nonpregnant and pregnant ewes. Anesthesiology. 2001;95:1256.
32. Dony P, Dewinde V, Vanderick B, et al. The comparative toxicity of ropivacaine and bupivacaine at equipotent doses in rats. Anesth Analg. 2000;91:1489.
33. Hong JY, Jee YS, Jeong HJ, et al. Effects of epidural fentanyl on speed and quality of block for emergency cesarean section in extending continuous epidural labor analgesia using ropivacaine and fentanyl. J Korean Med Sci. 2010;25:287.
34. Cherng CH, Wong CS, Ho ST. Epidural fentanyl speeds the onset of sensory block during epidural lidocaine anesthesia. Reg Anesth Pain Med. 2001;26:523.
35. Singh SI, Rehou S, Marmai KL, Jones PM. The efficacy of 2 doses of epidural morphine for postcesarean delivery analgesia: a randomized noninferiority trial. Anesth Analg. 2013;117:677.

36. Vora KS, Shah VR, Patel B, et al. Postoperative analgesia with epidural opioids after cesarean section: comparison of sufentanil, morphine and sufentanil-morphine combination. J Anaesthesiol Clin Pharmacol. 2012;28:491.
37. Marroquin B, Feng C, Balofsky A, et al. Neuraxial opioids for post-cesarean delivery analgesia: can hydromorphone replace morphine? A retrospective study. Int J Obstet Anesth. 2017;30:16.
38. Thorén T, Holmström B, Rawal N, et al. Sequential combined spinal epidural block versus spinal block for cesarean section: effects on maternal hypotension and neurobehavioral function of the newborn. Anesth Analg. 1994;78:1087.
39. Fan SZ, Susetio L, Wang YP, et al. Low dose of intrathecal hyperbaric bupivacaine combined with epidural lidocaine for cesarean section—a balance block technique. Anesth Analg. 1994;78:474.
40. Choi DH, Ahn HJ, Kim JA. Combined low-dose spinal-epidural anesthesia versus single-shot spinal anesthesia for elective cesarean delivery. Int J Obstet Anesth. 2006;15:13.
41. Van de Putte P, Vernieuwe L, Bouchez S. Point-of-care ultrasound in pregnancy: gastric, airway, neuraxial, cardiorespiratory. Curr Opin Anaesthesiol. 2020 Jun;33(3):277–83.
42. D'Angelo R, Smiley RM, Riley ET, Segal S. Serious complications related to obstetric anesthesia: the serious complication repository project of the Society for Obstetric Anesthesia and Perinatology. Anesthesiology. 2014;120:1505.
43. Pandit JJ, Andrade J, Bogod DG, et al. 5th National Audit Project (NAP5) on accidental awareness during general anaesthesia: summary of main findings and risk factors. Br J Anaesth. 2014;113:549.
44. Odor PM, Bampoe S, Lucas DN, et al. Incidence of accidental awareness during general anaesthesia in obstetrics: a multicentre, prospective cohort study. Anaesthesia. 2021;76:759.
45. Mushambi MC, Kinsella SM, Popat M, Swales H, Ramaswamy KK, Winton AL, Quinn AC, Obstetric Anaesthetists' Association; Difficult Airway Society. Obstetric Anaesthetists' Association and Difficult Airway Society guidelines for the management of difficult and failed tracheal intubation in obstetrics. Anaesthesia. 2015;70(11):1286–306.
46. Cluver C, Novikova N, Hofmeyr GJ, Hall DR. Maternal position during cesarean section for preventing maternal and neonatal complications. Cochrane Database Syst Rev. 2013;2013:CD007623.
47. Lee AJ, Landau R, Mattingly JL, et al. Left lateral table tilt for elective cesarean delivery under spinal anesthesia has no effect on neonatal acid-base status: a randomized controlled trial. Anesthesiology. 2017;127:241.
48. Tsai SE, Yeh PH, Hsu PK, et al. Continuous hemodynamic effects of left tilting and supine positions during cesarean section under spinal anesthesia with a noninvasive cardiac output monitoring system. Eur J Anaesthesiol. 2019;36:72.
49. Fujita N, Higuchi H, Sakuma S, et al. Effect of right-lateral versus left-lateral tilt position on compression of the inferior vena cava in pregnant women determined by magnetic resonance imaging. Anesth Analg. 2019;128:1217.
50. Higuchi H, Takagi S, Zhang K, et al. Effect of lateral tilt angle on the volume of the abdominal aorta and inferior vena cava in pregnant and nonpregnant women determined by magnetic resonance imaging. Anesthesiology. 2015;122:286.
51. Fitzgerald JP, Fedoruk KA, Jadin SM, et al. Prevention of hypotension after spinal anesthesia for cesarean section: a systematic review and network meta-analysis of randomized controlled trials. Anaesthesia. 2020;75:109.
52. Ngan Kee WD, Khaw KS, Ng FF, Lee BB. Prophylactic phenylephrine infusion for preventing hypotension during spinal anesthesia for cesarean delivery. Anesth Analg. 2004;98:815.
53. Allen TK, George RB, White WD, et al. A double-blind, placebo-controlled trial of four fixed rate infusion regimens of phenylephrine for hemodynamic support during spinal anesthesia for cesarean delivery. Anesth Analg. 2010;111:1221.
54. Siddik-Sayyid SM, Taha SK, Kanazi GE, Aouad MT. A randomized controlled trial of variable rate phenylephrine infusion with rescue phenylephrine boluses versus rescue boluses alone on physician interventions during spinal anesthesia for elective cesarean delivery. Anesth Analg. 2014;118:611.

55. George RB, McKeen DM, Dominguez JE, et al. A randomized trial of phenylephrine infusion versus bolus dosing for nausea and vomiting during cesarean delivery in obese women. Can J Anaesth. 2018;65:254.
56. Xu S, Shen X, Liu S, et al. Efficacy and safety of norepinephrine versus phenylephrine for the management of maternal hypotension during cesarean delivery with spinal anesthesia: a systematic review and meta-analysis. Medicine (Baltimore). 2019;98:e14331.
57. Higgins N, Fitzgerald PC, van Dyk D, et al. The effect of prophylactic phenylephrine and ephedrine infusions on umbilical artery blood pH in women with preeclampsia undergoing cesarean delivery with spinal anesthesia: a randomized, double-blind trial. Anesth Analg. 2018;126:1999.
58. Ituk US, Cooter M, Habib AS. Retrospective comparison of ephedrine and phenylephrine for the treatment of spinal anesthesia induced hypotension in preeclamptic patients. Curr Med Res Opin. 2016;32:1083.
59. Wei C, Qian J, Zhang Y, et al. Norepinephrine for the prevention of spinal-induced hypotension during cesarean delivery under combined spinal-epidural anesthesia: randomized, double-blind, dose-finding study. Eur J Anaesthesiol. 2020;37:309.
60. Heesen M, Hilber N, Rijs K, et al. A systematic review of phenylephrine vs. norepinephrine for the management of hypotension associated with neuraxial anesthesia in women undergoing cesarean section. Anaesthesia. 2020;75:800.
61. Ngan Kee WD, Lee SWY, Ng FF, Khaw KS. Prophylactic norepinephrine infusion for preventing hypotension during spinal anesthesia for cesarean delivery. Anesth Analg. 2018;126:1989.
62. Theodoraki K, Hadzilia S, Valsamidis D, Stamatakis E. Prevention of hypotension during elective cesarean section with a fixed-rate norepinephrine infusion versus a fixed-rate phenylephrine infusion. A double-blinded randomized controlled trial. Int J Surg. 2020;84:41–9.
63. Loubert C. Fluid and vasopressor management for cesarean delivery under spinal anesthesia: continuing professional development. Can J Anaesth. 2012;59:604.
64. McDonald S, Fernando R, Ashpole K, Columb M. Maternal cardiac output changes after crystalloid or colloid coload following spinal anesthesia for elective cesarean delivery: a randomized controlled trial. Anesth Analg. 2011;113:803.
65. Tawfik MM, Tarbay AI, Elaidy AM, et al. Combined colloid preload and crystalloid coload versus crystalloid coload during spinal anesthesia for cesarean delivery: a randomized controlled trial. Anesth Analg. 2019;128:304.
66. Chooi C, Cox JJ, Lumb RS, et al. Techniques for preventing hypotension during spinal anesthesia for cesarean section. Cochrane Database Syst Rev. 2020;7:CD002251.
67. Park SK, Park DN, Kim YW, et al. Colloid coload versus crystalloid coload to prevent maternal hypotension in women receiving prophylactic phenylephrine infusion during cesarean delivery: a randomized controlled trial. Int J Obstet Anesth. 2022;49:103246.
68. Grylack LJ, Chu SS, Scanlon JW. Use of intravenous fluids before cesarean section: effects on perinatal glucose, insulin, and sodium homeostasis. Obstet Gynecol. 1984;63:654.
69. Jonsson M, Hanson U, Lidell C, Nordén-Lindeberg S. ST depression at cesarean section and the relation to oxytocin dose. A randomized controlled trial. BJOG. 2010;117:76.
70. May A. The confidential enquiries into maternal deaths 1997-1999: what can we learn? Int J Obstet Anesth. 2002;11:153.
71. Langesaeter E, Rosseland LA, Stubhaug A. Hemodynamic effects of repeated doses of oxytocin during cesarean delivery in healthy parturients. Br J Anaesth. 2009;103:260.
72. Kovacheva VP, Soens MA, Tsen LC. A randomized, double-blinded trial of a "rule of threes" algorithm versus continuous infusion of oxytocin during elective cesarean delivery. Anesthesiology. 2015;123:92.
73. Güngördük K, Asicioglu O, Celikkol O, et al. Use of additional oxytocin to reduce blood loss at elective cesarean section: a randomized controlled trial. Aust N Z J Obstet Gynaecol. 2010;50:36.
74. Sheehan SR, Montgomery AA, Carey M, et al. Oxytocin bolus versus oxytocin bolus and infusion for control of blood loss at elective cesarean section: double blind, placebo controlled, randomised trial. BMJ. 2011;343:d4661.

75. Balki M, Ronayne M, Davies S, et al. Minimum oxytocin dose requirement after cesarean delivery for labor arrest. Obstet Gynecol. 2006;107:45.
76. Carvalho JC, Balki M, Kingdom J, Windrim R. Oxytocin requirements at elective cesarean delivery: a dose-finding study. Obstet Gynecol. 2004;104:1005.
77. George RB, McKeen D, Chaplin AC, McLeod L. Up-down determination of the ED(90) of oxytocin infusions for the prevention of postpartum uterine atony in parturients undergoing cesarean delivery. Can J Anaesth. 2010;57:578.
78. Lavoie A, McCarthy RJ, Wong CA. The ED90 of prophylactic oxytocin infusion after delivery of the placenta during cesarean delivery in laboring compared with nonlaboring women: an up-down sequential allocation dose-response study. Anesth Analg. 2015;121:159.
79. Wilson RD, Caughey AB, Wood SL, et al. Guidelines for antenatal and preoperative care in cesarean delivery: enhanced recovery after surgery society recommendations (part 1). Am J Obstet Gynecol. 2018;219:523.e1.
80. Caughey AB, Wood SL, Macones GA, et al. Guidelines for intraoperative care in cesarean delivery: enhanced recovery after surgery society recommendations (part 2). Am J Obstet Gynecol. 2018;219:533.
81. Sultan P, Sharawi N, Blake L, Carvalho B. Enhanced recovery after cesarean delivery versus standard care studies: a systematic review of interventions and outcomes. Int J Obstet Anesth. 2020;43:72.
82. Bollag L, Lim G, Sultan P, et al. Society for Obstetric Anesthesia and Perinatology: consensus statement and recommendations for enhanced recovery after cesarean. Anesth Analg. 2021;132:1362.
83. Patel SD, Sharawi N, Sultan P. Local anesthetic techniques for post-cesarean delivery analgesia. Int J Obstet Anesth. 2019 Nov;40:62–77.
84. Ryu C, Choi GJ, Jung YH, Baek CW, Cho CK, Kang H. Postoperative analgesic effectiveness of peripheral nerve blocks in cesarean delivery: a systematic review and network Meta-analysis. J Pers Med. 2022;12(4):634.
85. Wang P, Chen X, Chang Y, Wang Y, Cui H. Analgesic efficacy of ultrasound-guided transversus abdominis plane block after cesarean delivery: a systematic review and meta-analysis. J Obstet Gynaecol Res. 2021 Sep;47(9):2954–68.

6 Perioperative Management of Patients Undergoing Oncologic Pulmonary Resection Surgery

Federico Piccioni and Fabio Piccirillo

6.1 Introduction

Thoracic anesthesia for oncologic resection surgery can be considered a subspecialty due to the numerous specific features that characterize every phase of the patient's perioperative course. The thoracic anesthesiologist must possess the skills to guide appropriate preoperative risk assessment and stratification, develop specific technical approaches, and have the pathophysiological knowledge required to manage surgery that significantly impacts both the respiratory and hemodynamic systems. Over the past 20 years, several aspects of anesthetic management in thoracic surgery have been revised, and clinicians must now be familiar with these updates to minimize the risk of perioperative complications [1]. This text summarizes the most important aspects of managing this patient population, referencing the 2018 guidelines of the Enhanced Recovery After Surgery (ERAS) Society and the 2019 Italian Consensus on perioperative management of patients undergoing thoracic resection surgery (PACTS), developed by a multidisciplinary group of experts from the Italian Society of Anesthesia, Analgesia, Resuscitation and Intensive Care (SIAARTI), the Italian Society of Thoracic Surgery (SICT), the Italian Society of Thoracic Endoscopy (SIET), the Italian Society of Surgery (SIC), the Italian Society of Pulmonology (SIP), and the Italian Association of Hospital Pulmonologists (AIPO) [2–4].

F. Piccioni (✉) · F. Piccirillo
Anesthesia and Perioperative Medicine Unit, IRCCS Humanitas Research Hospital, Rozzano, Italy
e-mail: federico.piccioni@humanitas.it; fabio.piccirillo@humanitas.it

D. Chiumello, A. De Gasperi (eds.), *Practical Trends in Anesthesia and Intensive Care 2026*, https://doi.org/10.1007/978-3-032-25721-5_6

6.2 Preoperative Assessment

Preoperative evaluation of patients undergoing oncologic thoracic surgery is essential to estimate perioperative risk and optimize anesthetic management. These patients often present with comorbidities such as pulmonary diseases (chronic bronchitis and emphysema), cardiovascular diseases, or reduced functional reserve due to previous oncologic treatments (such as chemotherapy or radiotherapy). In addition to a thorough medical history, careful cardiovascular and respiratory assessment is crucial and should be tailored to the planned procedure.

6.2.1 Cardiovascular Assessment

Cardiological evaluation can be considered the first step in risk stratification, as the cardiovascular system is always subject to a certain degree of impact depending on the extent of planned parenchymal resection. The pulmonary circulation and right heart constitute a low-pressure system that, in the perioperative phase, must always counteract a level of pulmonary hypertension proportional to the extent of the resection performed. According to the 2022 guidelines of the European Society of Cardiology (ESC), thoracic surgery procedures are considered to carry an intermediate or high risk of postoperative cardiovascular complications [5]. Ideally, patients should be referred for specialist cardiology evaluation in the presence of cardiovascular risk factors. In this regard, the use of a risk assessment tool such as the Revised Cardiac Risk Index (RCRI) is recommended to identify patients at higher risk of cardiovascular complications and those who would benefit from preoperative cardiology evaluation [6]. A specific version of the RCRI has been developed for thoracic surgery, in which major resective procedures are given greater weight (ThRCRI) [7]. Several large observational studies have confirmed the validity of this tool, showing an association between a score greater than two and an increased incidence of postoperative complications. Specific cardiological assessments should therefore be performed according to ESC guidelines, regardless of whether the patient is undergoing thoracic surgery. It is important, when indicated, to use instrumental tests such as echocardiography and, if necessary, second-level investigations in cases of high risk for cardiovascular complications. It should be noted that several guidelines recommend perioperative monitoring of cardiac biomarkers based on preoperative risk assessment [5, 8, 9]. Measurement of high-sensitivity troponins (hs-cTnT and hs-cTnI) and B-type natriuretic peptide (BNP) can be valuable tools for individualized risk stratification and for early detection of myocardial injury after surgery. The 2025 ESAIC Updated guidelines suggest using natriuretic peptides as biological markers in high-risk patients (RCRI >2) undergoing high-risk surgery [8].

In addition to cardiovascular risk factors, it is important to assess the patient's functional capacity, which is also useful for evaluating cardiorespiratory reserve. A rough estimate of metabolic equivalents (METs) based on general information about daily activities is often imprecise. In this context, the use of a tool such as the

Duke Activity Status Index (DASI) questionnaire, which through 12 questions allows a more accurate estimation of METs, has proven useful [10]. In the authors' experience, the DASI score correlates with the number of steps taken by the patient during the day as measured by a wearable wrist device and, even more importantly, with the results obtained from the 6-min walking test (6MWT) [11].

6.2.2 Pulmonary Function Assessment

Adequate assessment of pulmonary function is essential in a context where surgery will have a negative impact on the patient's respiratory function. Through global spirometry and measurement of the alveolar-capillary diffusion capacity for carbon monoxide (DLCO), it is possible to evaluate respiratory function from both a mechanical and parenchymal perspective. The measurements obtained for forced vital capacity (FVC), forced expiratory volume in 1 s (FEV1), and DLCO can be compared with the predicted values for age and anthropometric parameters, and their variation after bronchodilator administration can be calculated. Most importantly, these measurements serve as the starting point for estimating postoperative residual function by calculating predicted postoperative values ($ppoFEV_1$ and ppoDLCO), based on the number of pulmonary segments expected to be resected. Predicted postoperative $ppoFEV_1$ and ppoDLCO values greater than 60% are considered permissive for the proposed surgery [3]. Values between 40% and 60% require further functional assessment using low-complexity tests such as the six minute walking test (6MWT) or the Stair Climb Test (SCT) [3, 12]. Insufficient results on these tests or $ppoFEV_1$ and ppoDLCO values below 40% require cardiopulmonary exercise testing (CPET) [3]. Several algorithms have been proposed in the literature for standardized assessment following this pathway [13–15], and as an example, Fig. 6.1 shows the algorithm developed and adopted at the authors' center.

CPET provides numerous parameters useful for evaluating exercise tolerance from both a cardiac and pulmonary perspective [3, 13–15]. The most widely considered parameter for assessing a patient's suitability for thoracic surgery is the peak oxygen consumption achieved (VO_2 Max), which decreases with age but is normally above 20 ml/kg/min even in untrained individuals. To better understand the value of VO_2 Max, it is useful to consider its relationship with METs. Each MET corresponds to an oxygen consumption of 3.5 ml/kg/min; therefore, when referring to a value of four METs as the minimum threshold for assessing a patient's functional reserve, this corresponds to a VO_2 Max of approximately 14 ml/kg/min. From this perspective, patients with a VO_2 Max of at least 15 ml/kg/min are considered operable. A value between 10 and 15 ml/kg/min should be considered as an increased risk of postoperative complications is assessed together with spirometric data, comorbidities, age, and any degree of patient frailty. A VO_2 Max value below 10 ml/kg/min should be considered prohibitive for surgery and should prompt consideration of alternative treatment strategies, such as reducing the extent of pulmonary resection or referring the patient for local disease control (e.g., radiotherapy, percutaneous ablation with radiofrequency or microwaves), with or without systemic

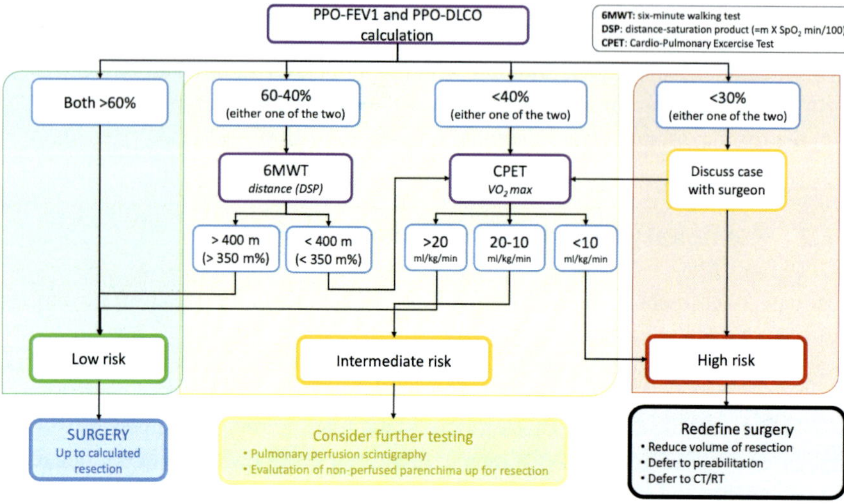

Fig. 6.1 Algorithm for the assessment of respiratory function tests in patients scheduled for thoracic surgery

therapy. Another very useful parameter from CPET is the slope of the relationship between ventilatory volume and carbon dioxide production (VE/VCO_2 slope) [16]. This index estimates respiratory efficiency, that is, the adequacy of ventilation in response to increasing CO_2 production during exertion. Normal values for the VE/VCO_2 slope range from 20 to 30 but increase in cases of ventilation-perfusion mismatch, pulmonary hypertension, and heart failure. VE/VCO_2 slope values above 34 are associated with a worse prognosis, regardless of whether VO_2 Max is less than or greater than 15 ml/kg/min, and in both patients with and without chronic obstructive pulmonary disease. An interesting algorithm has thus been proposed for risk stratification that specifically considers the VE/VCO_2 slope in patients with a VO_2 Max between 10 and 20 ml/kg/min [17].

6.2.3 Risk Assessment Scores

The main guidelines for preoperative assessment of patients undergoing non-cardiac surgery recommend the use of scoring systems that allow for better and more objective stratification of the risk of postoperative complications [8, 9]. Several such tools have been proposed in thoracic surgery. The Thoracoscore, developed and validated in France in 2007, is based on nine variables, including age, sex, ASA class, type of surgical procedure, degree of dyspnea, and performance status, and estimates the risk of in-hospital mortality [18]. In 2017, Brunelli, analyzing data from over 45,000 patients from the European Society of Thoracic Surgeons (ESTS) database, developed the Eurolung 1 and 2 scores, which are useful for assessing the risk of in-hospital cardiopulmonary complications and 30-day postoperative mortality [19].

Another score proposed for this surgical context is the CARDOT score (COPD, ASA PS, Right-side operation, Duration of surgery, Oxygen saturation, Thoracotomy), which, based on six variables, estimates the risk of respiratory complications with good discriminatory power [20]. From this perspective, the widely used ARISCAT (Assess Respiratory risk in Surgical Patients in Catalonia) score, mainly employed in the assessment of patients undergoing abdominal surgery, can also be helpful in stratifying the risk of postoperative pulmonary complications [21]. Unfortunately, every risk score has its limitations and, according to the results of a 2023 retrospective observational study from the United States based on a cohort of 2104 patients, none of the scoring systems demonstrated adequate discriminatory power to predict PPCs among patients undergoing pulmonary resection [22]. The authors therefore concluded that it is necessary to develop an alternative risk score to better predict patients at risk of PPC after thoracic surgery. For this reason as well, functional assessment should be integrated with an evaluation of the patient's degree of frailty, using tools such as the Clinical Frailty Scale (CFS), the Tilburg Frailty Indicator (TFI), and the modified Frailty Index (mFI). The prevalence of frailty in thoracic surgery is reported in the literature to be around 12–15%, depending on the populations considered and the assessment tools used (most commonly the mFI) [23–26]. This evaluation is important in the overall assessment of the patient because frailty and the presence of geriatric syndromes increase the risk of postoperative complications and mortality.

Prehabilitation in thoracic surgery is an approach aimed at optimizing the patient's physical, nutritional, and psychological condition prior to surgery, in order to improve postoperative outcomes [4]. It can be particularly useful in patients with chronic obstructive pulmonary disease or reduced functional reserve. Multimodal prehabilitation, which includes smoking cessation, respiratory rehabilitation, nutritional optimization, and physical exercise, is more effective than unimodal prehabilitation and, to be effective, should begin at least 3 weeks before surgery.

6.3 Intraoperative Anesthetic Management

6.3.1 Airway Management

Airway management is unique in thoracic surgery due to the need to use devices that allow for exclusion of the ventilation of the lung on the side of surgery. The double-lumen tube is the first-choice device for this purpose because, by enabling lung separation, it provides optimal control of ventilation and allows for effective suctioning of secretions or blood from both lungs [3, 27]. If lung separation is not the primary objective, a single-lumen tube combined with a bronchial blocker can be used. This device, equipped with an inflatable cuff at its distal end, allows for isolation of the downstream portion of the lung [3]. This combination is recommended for patients with difficult airways.

The use of videolaryngoscopy for tracheal intubation with a double-lumen tube improves glottic visualization and first-attempt success rates, reducing both the difficulty and time required for placement [28, 29]. Videolaryngoscopy can be employed in cases of unexpected difficult intubation.

The use of a flexible bronchoscope is recommended to verify the position of the lung separation or isolation device. Flexible bronchoscopy should always be available, and the thoracic anesthesiologist must possess adequate bronchoscopy skills to manage these devices.

6.3.2 Maintenance of Anesthesia

Maintenance of anesthesia in thoracic surgery is a topic of great interest among clinicians, who are divided between proponents of balanced anesthesia with halogenated agents and those favoring total intravenous anesthesia (TIVA). In the past, several studies have investigated the potential inhibitory effect of halogenated agents on the mechanism of hypoxic pulmonary vasoconstriction [30]. This effect has been demonstrated for halothane and isoflurane at doses higher than those used in clinical practice [30, 31]. For sevoflurane, the most commonly used halogenated agent today, such an inhibitory effect has not been demonstrated. On the contrary, interesting data suggest that it may exert a protective function on the endothelial glycocalyx at the capillary level, with potential benefits in reducing the risk of postoperative pulmonary complications [32]. A drawback of using halogenated agents in thoracic anesthesia is the increased risk of occupational exposure, especially in cases of complex airway device management or air leaks from anatomical structures during surgery. From this perspective, TIVA offers greater safety, including in terms of environmental sustainability, as suggested by the European Society of Anaesthesiology and Intensive Care (ESAIC) [33]. Furthermore, recent data suggest that propofol may have an immunomodulatory effect, potentially reducing the risk of cancer recurrence after surgery, although the magnitude of this effect is difficult to estimate [33]. Table 6.1 summarizes the comparison between halogenated anesthesia and TIVA in thoracic surgery.

The ERAS guidelines also recommend a multimodal approach to promote rapid postoperative recovery by reducing the use of opioids and long-acting drugs [2]. In this context, protocols have been proposed to reduce or eliminate the use of these drugs starting from the intraoperative phase. It is therefore possible to implement multimodal anesthesia protocols that are *opioid-sparing* or *opioid-free*, based on the use of adjuvant drugs as reported in several recent studies [34–38]. These protocols rely on loco-regional techniques and the administration of ketamine, dexmedetomidine, magnesium sulfate, intravenous lidocaine, and anti-inflammatory agents. A 2022 meta-analysis based on six studies reported several outcomes in favor of the *opioid-free* strategy, such as reduced opioid consumption, better pain control in the first 48 h after surgery, fewer postoperative complications, and earlier hospital discharge [39]. These results are certainly of great interest but require confirmation in adequately designed multicenter randomized trials.

Table 6.1 Comparison between anesthesia with halogenated agents or TIVA with respect to various aspects in thoracic surgery

	Halogenated agents	Total intravenous anesthesia
Effect on hypoxic pulmonary vasoconstriction	Possible inhibition, documented for halothane and isoflurane at high doses	No known effect
Effect on endothelial glycocalyx	Sevoflurane may have a protective effect	No known effect
Immunomodulatory effects	No known effect	Propofol may reduce the risk of tumor recurrence
Induction and emergence times	Typically faster	May require more careful management of emergence times
Indications for cases of complex ventilation	Risk of leakage in cases of double-lumen tube or bronchial blocker ventilation	Safer in these cases
Safety for healthcare personnel	Risk of exposure to inhaled agents, especially in the event of air leaks	Safer in these cases
Environmental impact	Halogenated agents are considered atmospheric pollutants	More environmentally friendly
Cost and availability	Generally less expensive in small doses	May be more expensive, but sustainable in the long term

6.3.3 One-Lung Ventilation

The main distinctive feature of thoracic anesthesia is one-lung ventilation (OLV), which, by collapsing the lung to be operated on, is essential to facilitate the surgical procedure, whether performed via thoracotomy, video-assisted, or robotic approaches. Hypoxemia during OLV is caused by an increase in the venous shunt fraction of the non-ventilated lung and by areas with a low ventilation-perfusion (V/Q) ratio [30, 40]. Therefore, during OLV, while the collapsed lung inevitably creates a shunt, the ventilated lung may also contribute to venous admixture through shunt and low V/Q areas. This occurs mainly in the presence of atelectatic regions of the lung caused by hypoventilation and the lateral decubitus position, due to the weight of the mediastinum, diaphragmatic compression by abdominal organs, and reduced compliance of the chest wall. The ventilation strategy should therefore ideally minimize perfusion of the collapsed lung and areas of low V/Q in the ventilated lung. In the past, the main objectives of OLV were to prevent atelectasis to counteract hypoxemia and to ensure carbon dioxide elimination. This was achieved by maintaining the minute ventilation during OLV equal to that used in two-lung ventilation, with a tidal volume of 8–10 mL/kg, which carried the risk of alveolar overdistension. In this context, the addition of positive end-expiratory pressure (PEEP) was approached cautiously, both because it could potentially increase the shunt fraction in the ventilated lung and due to its possible hemodynamic impact, with decreased venous return and cardiac output. The main intervention to counteract hypoxemia was therefore the use of a high fraction of inspired oxygen, which, however, becomes less effective as the level of venous shunt exceeds 30% and is also harmful at the endothelial level due to oxidative effects. Since the late 1990s, the importance of a lung-protective ventilation approach has gradually emerged, both in the management of critically ill patients and in those undergoing surgery. In thoracic anesthesia, numerous studies first demonstrated the relationship between high tidal volume ventilation and acute respiratory distress syndrome (ARDS), and then showed how OLV, based on tidal volumes of 5–6 mL/kg of ideal body weight, can be optimized to reduce hypoxemia and the risk of lung injury through the use of alveolar recruitment maneuvers and personalized PEEP titration [40]. Alveolar recruitment maneuvers are useful for aerating atelectatic areas and improve lung compliance and arterial oxygenation. The application of appropriate PEEP levels helps maintain ventilation above the closing capacity, thus keeping the recruited areas ventilated and reducing atelectrauma, that is, the injury associated with the cyclic opening and closing of alveoli. The search for the optimal PEEP value can be performed, after an alveolar recruitment maneuver, using the decremental test. This maneuver involves gradually increasing PEEP during the recruitment maneuver up to a value usually of 15 cmH_2O, which is then gradually reduced while observing at which value the lowest driving pressure is achieved; this represents the distending pressure calculated as the difference between plateau pressure and PEEP. While the application of these principles for better physiological management of OLV is now well established, it remains unclear which regimen may be most effective in minimizing the risk of postoperative pulmonary complications (PPC), including ARDS. Recent studies have not clarified whether, compared to tidal volumes of 5–6 mL/kg during OLV, PPCs can be reduced by combining recruitment maneuvers with even lower tidal volumes (4 mL/kg) or by titrating ventilation to maintain a driving pressure below the safety threshold identified in critically ill patients, namely 15 cmH_2O [41, 42]. This is partly due to the multifactorial etiology of PPCs (Fig. 6.2), which includes, in addition to the ventilation mode, intrinsic patient factors (age, preoperative inflammatory status, neoadjuvant chemotherapy, smoking, chronic obstructive pulmonary disease, cardiac conditions), as well as other anesthetic (fluid management) and surgical aspects (extent of parenchymal resection, complexity and duration of the procedure).

The above highlights the need for careful monitoring of respiratory parameters during OLV, namely airway pressures, ventilation flows, and exhaled carbon dioxide. Observing the curves related to these parameters is useful for the rapid identification of displacement of the device used for OLV, for detecting air leaks from anatomical structures undergoing surgery, and for optimizing ventilation and avoiding harmful ventilation modes. From this perspective, there has been debate over which mode of mechanical ventilation may be more advantageous during OLV. Volume-controlled ventilation (VCV) and pressure-controlled ventilation (PCV) regimens have been compared in several studies without demonstrating the superiority of one mode over the other. A meta-analysis of six studies reported

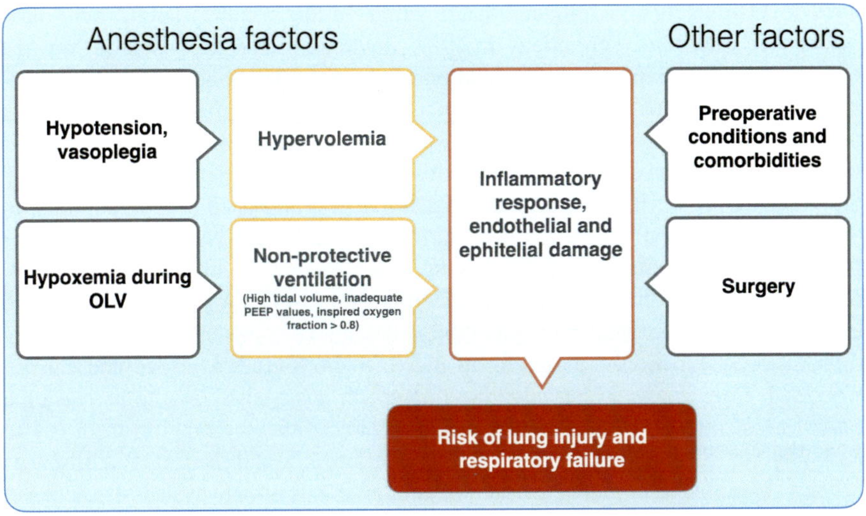

Fig. 6.2 Etiology of lung injury during one-lung ventilation (OLV). Potentially harmful anesthetic factors include hypervolemia, which is promoted by indiscriminate fluid administration to counteract hemodynamic alterations, and non-protective one-lung ventilation to address hypoxemia. There are also factors that are less modifiable, such as patient characteristics and comorbidities, as well as surgical aspects like the extent of parenchymal resection, complexity, and duration of the procedure. All these factors contribute to lung injury

better oxygenation and lower peak airway pressures with PCV [43]. No differences were observed in compliance, plateau, and mean airway pressure, $PaCO_2$, tidal volume, heart rate, and blood pressure, nor in postoperative complications. VCV is the most commonly used mode and allows delivery of a set tidal volume and, by establishing an adequate end-inspiratory pause, easy monitoring of driving pressure. The main disadvantage of this mode lies in the anesthesia machine's limited ability to compensate for air leaks. PCV allows better compensation for air leaks and enables adjustment of ventilation parameters to avoid increases in driving pressure. The limitation of this mode is the potential for hypoventilation in the event of increased airway resistance due to surgical manipulation or the presence of secretions or blood. More advanced modes, such as those based on PCV with guaranteed tidal volume, are now available in the most modern anesthesia machines. In a small randomized study in 2020 involving 16 patients, PCV with guaranteed volume, compared to VCV, reduced airway pressure in patients undergoing thoracotomy and decreased the release of plasma neutrophil elastase [44].

6.3.4 Fluid Therapy and Hemodynamic Management

Hemodynamic management is of utmost importance during thoracic surgery because the effects of anesthesia, hypoxic pulmonary vasoconstriction, the lateral decubitus position, surgical manipulation of the mediastinum, and great vessels all have direct impacts on cardiovascular function. In this context, careful fluid management is particularly important. In 1984, Zeldin, an American surgeon, was the first to analyze in a small study the relationship between the volume of fluids administered and pulmonary edema after pneumonectomy, concluding, among other things, that: "...the most important thing we can do to recognize the problem [hypervolemia] is to observe how our anesthesiologists load the patient with fluids" [45]. Subsequently, Marc Licker documented that a liberal approach to fluid administration, both intraoperatively and postoperatively, increases the risk of complications [46, 47]. From a pathophysiological perspective, accurate fluid management helps to protect the pulmonary circulation, which is characterized by low resistance and low pressure and is particularly vulnerable—especially in patients with pre-existing right heart dysfunction—to significant increases in volume overload and cardiac workload. Conversely, a restrictive fluid approach has been shown to increase the risk of renal injury, with an incidence after thoracic surgery ranging from 6% to 33% [48–50]. Several authors, the ERAS guidelines [2], and the PACTS consensus [4] now recommend targeting euvolemia, though this is not always easy to achieve. The use of goal-directed hemodynamic protocols, which have been shown to reduce complications and mortality in high-risk patients undergoing major surgery, is challenging to implement in thoracic anesthesia. These protocols partly base their decisions on dynamic indices such as pulse pressure variation (PPV) and stroke volume variation (SVV), which allow assessment of a patient's responsiveness to volume loading in terms of increased cardiac output. Unfortunately, these parameters are not reliable in the context of OLV during open-chest surgery, as they are based on the effects of mechanical ventilation on hemodynamics under conditions of a closed chest and two-lung ventilation with a tidal volume of 8 ml/kg [51]. Some recent studies have proposed using, for this purpose, the hemodynamic effects on stroke volume and dynamic indices of alveolar recruitment maneuvers [52], changes in PEEP values from 0 to 10 cmH_2O, [53] and changes in tidal volume from 5 to 8 ml/kg [54] with promising results, though further validation studies are needed.

Cardiac output monitoring, now easily performed in the operating room using systems based on arterial pressure waveform analysis, is useful in helping the anesthesiologist maintain cardiac output within the normal range, especially in high-risk patients. This is also essential for optimal management of OLV: extreme values of cardiac output negatively affect arterial oxygenation. Low cardiac output increases systemic oxygen extraction, resulting in reduced venous oxygenation and making adequate pulmonary re-oxygenation difficult. Excessively high cardiac output, on the other hand, may increase the venous shunt fraction and thus the proportion of blood flow that does not participate in alveolar gas exchange, resulting in hypoxemia [30].

Transesophageal echocardiography (TEE) is now increasingly used outside the traditional setting of cardiac surgery. The use of TEE in thoracic surgery is limited to specific patients and/or high-risk procedures such as lung transplantation or complex mediastinal surgery. As in other perioperative settings, TEE can therefore be a valuable tool for assessing ventricular function and cardiac filling volume, providing real-time information on cardiac performance and response to fluids or vasoactive drugs. TEE can also be helpful in clarifying the causes of acute hemodynamic instability of unknown origin or in managing patients with severe heart disease or major valvular defects.

6.3.5 Intraoperative Monitoring and Invasive Devices

Monitoring of patients undergoing thoracic surgery is essential to maintain homeostasis and ensure patient safety. Mechanical ventilation and hemodynamic monitoring have already been discussed in previous sections. Along with electrocardiographic monitoring, noninvasive blood pressure, and peripheral oxygen saturation, temperature and neuromuscular function monitoring should be considered standard. Maintenance of normothermia is recommended by SIAARTI and the PACTS consensus in all patients undergoing procedures lasting more than 30 min, with the goal of maintaining a core temperature of at least 36 °C [4, 55]. Maintaining normothermia is often a critical aspect in thoracic surgery because the lateral position and the related supports make it more difficult to optimally position active warming systems such as forced-air blankets or mattresses. In this regard, it is always useful to also employ fluid warming systems, although these are not very effective unless high-flow infusions are required. Neuromuscular monitoring is also recommended by SIAARTI Good Clinical Practice and ESAIC guidelines [56, 57]. This monitoring allows for the optimization of muscle relaxant administration to ensure paralysis of the diaphragm, which, due to its greater resistance to these drugs, can significantly interfere with surgical activity and contribute to ventilation difficulties. Ensuring complete recovery from neuromuscular blockade at the end of the procedure is the most important aspect of this type of monitoring. Patients undergoing thoracic surgery are at risk of PPC, for which residual postoperative paralysis (PORC) is a known risk factor. Neuromuscular monitoring, therefore, ensures complete recovery from residual blockade at the end of the procedure and, if necessary, allows for accurate titration of the reversal agent used. It should be emphasized that, when using rocuronium, sugammadex provides a faster recovery even in this context, and according to ESAIC and ASA guidelines, neostigmine administration should be reserved for superficial levels of residual blockade (train-of-four ratio >0.2) [57, 58]. A recent randomized study confirmed that, as in other surgical settings, in thoracic surgery as well, reversal of residual neuromuscular blockade is faster with sugammadex for both deep and superficial blockade [59].

The use of depth of anesthesia monitoring through electroencephalogram processing has not been specifically investigated in the context of thoracic anesthesia. The PACTS consensus suggests its use to improve anesthesia monitoring, enable individualized titration of anesthetics, and thus promote faster recovery at the end of surgery, although available studies have reached inconsistent conclusions regarding its impact on postoperative delirium and cognitive dysfunction [4]. The use of nociception monitoring systems in thoracic anesthesia is anecdotal, but these systems could have important implications in a surgical context where loco-regional techniques are widely used and, from an ERAS perspective aimed at reducing opioid administration to promote postoperative recovery, could allow for a more objective assessment of the anesthetic plan and precise titration of analgesic drugs [60].

Regarding the use of urinary catheters and nasogastric tubes, reference should be made to ERAS guidelines, which recommend minimizing their use and, if used, promoting early removal (typically on the first postoperative day for the former and at the end of surgery for the latter) [2, 4]. This strategy aims to reduce patient discomfort and promote mobilization and the spontaneous resumption of physiological functions.

6.3.6 Pain Management and Loco-regional Techniques

Effective postoperative pain control in thoracic surgery is crucial to promote patient recovery, facilitate respiratory rehabilitation, and reduce the risk of postoperative complications. Pain management is based on various strategies that combine loco-regional techniques and multimodal analgesic protocols. Loco-regional techniques are recommended both for their proven efficacy in improving postoperative pain control and for reducing the need for opioids, thereby promoting faster postoperative recovery [2, 4]. In a multimodal context, it is also important to ensure the administration of drugs with systemic analgesic effects such as steroids, nonsteroidal anti-inflammatory drugs, and paracetamol [4]. The use of these drugs should begin intraoperatively and continue after surgery, with a transition from intravenous to oral administration as soon as possible (typically from the first postoperative day).

Among loco-regional techniques, epidural analgesia, long considered the gold standard for pain control after thoracic surgery, is now generally reserved for procedures performed via thoracotomy [4]. Drugs are administered through a catheter placed in the thoracic epidural space (T5-T6 and T6-T7 levels), providing excellent analgesia with minimal impact on respiratory function. The role of this technique has been strongly questioned by a meta-analysis published in 2016 [61]. The study indicated that thoracic paravertebral block (TPVB) is a non-inferior alternative to epidural analgesia, but in the absence of strong evidence due to significant heterogeneity among the studies considered and a modest total number of patients. In the meantime, no randomized studies have been conducted to clarify which of the two techniques is superior in the context of open surgery, but in the authors' opinion, epidural analgesia is more effective, although more difficult to manage postoperatively, mainly due to the higher risk of hypotension and side effects, as suggested by a more recent meta-analysis [62]. Thoracic paravertebral block has become widely used because it is considered simpler and safer than epidural analgesia. It can be performed using a single-shot technique, with or without subsequent continuous infusion of local anesthetic via catheter. This block represents the most effective alternative to epidural analgesia, and the ultrasound-guided technique is now the most widely adopted approach, as it offers greater safety by allowing verification of correct access to the paravertebral space. More recently, other fascial plane blocks such as the erector spinae plane block (ESPB) and the serratus anterior plane block (SAPB) have become widely used in clinical practice due to their ease of execution and low risk of complications. These types of blocks, along with intercostal nerve blocks and surgical wound infiltration, are mainly employed for pain management following procedures performed with minimally invasive techniques, both video- and robot-assisted. Several studies have been published in recent years comparing these techniques, often with conflicting results. Some meta-analyses have attempted to synthesize the available literature. Balzani et al. confirmed that the use of locoregional techniques reduces morphine consumption, with moderate evidence for TPVB and ESPB and low evidence for SAPB and intercostal block [63]. Two studies have demonstrated the superiority of TPVB over other techniques [64, 65]. Another meta-analysis, however, suggested that ESPB may be the most effective and safest method for relieving pain after thoracic surgery, reducing both hospital length of stay and the incidence of postoperative complications [66]. The difficulty in determining which type of locoregional technique may be superior in this context is related to multiple factors, including differences in the execution of the technique itself (level and number of injections, single injection vs. catheter placement for continuous infusion, choice of drugs, analgesic protocol, surgical technique). It is therefore important for centers to adopt standardized protocols tailored to the specific clinical context, but there is also a clear need for well-designed multicenter studies to help define the best strategies in terms of both efficacy and safety, as well as their potential impact on major outcomes. Fig. 6.3 presents a possible algorithm that reflects current literature findings combined with the authors' experience.

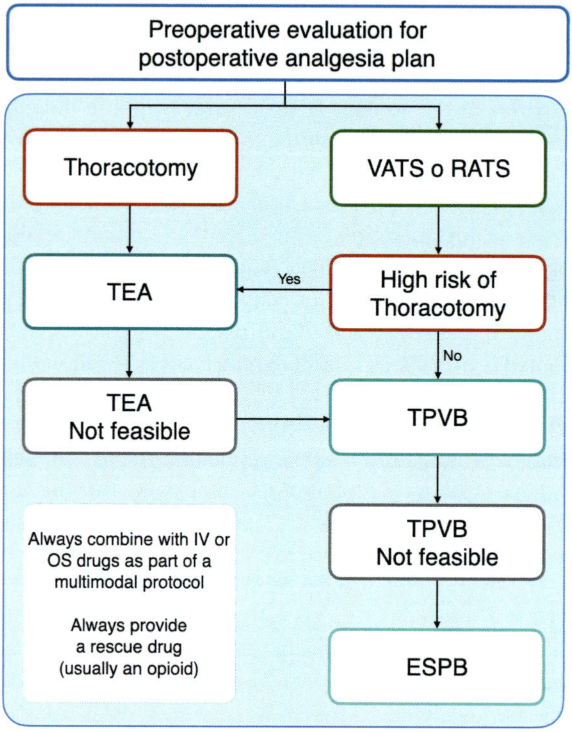

Fig. 6.3 Algorithm for selecting the loco-regional technique to be used in thoracic anesthesia. After preoperative assessment of the patient and the planned surgical procedure, thoracic epidural analgesia (TEA) and thoracic paravertebral block (TPVB) are considered first-line options for thoracotomy and minimally invasive approaches (video-assisted—VATS or robotic—RATS), respectively. If TEA cannot be used (or the technique fails), TPVB is chosen. The erector spinae plane block (ESPB) is an additional option when TPVB cannot be performed. Loco-regional techniques should always be part of a systemic multimodal approach, and it is mandatory to always provide a rescue medication to be used if the planned therapy is inadequate. The algorithm does not include less effective techniques such as the serratus anterior plane block (SAPB) and intercostal nerve block (ICNB), which may still be used if TEA, TPVB, and ESPB are not feasible

6.4 Postoperative Management

The postoperative phase following thoracic surgery should focus on optimal pain control and early patient mobilization to ensure a rapid return to autonomy and full recovery. Postoperative analgesia should be based on modern multimodal principles, leveraging the benefits of regional techniques combined with other analgesic drugs. Early mobilization from bed, physiotherapy programs, and the resumption of normal physiological functions should be primary objectives, achievable not only through adequate pain control but also by prompt removal of the nasogastric tube, urinary catheter, and chest drain [4]. The latter is a crucial element in the postoperative course of patients undergoing lung resection, with a significant impact on recovery and hospital length of stay. Although drainage is often indispensable, it can cause pain, limit pulmonary function, and reduce mobility, regardless of the surgical technique used. A meta-analysis of nine studies involving 918 patients who underwent lung resection via VATS found that about 50% of patients did not have a chest drain placed [67]. In these patients, postoperative pain scores and hospital length of stay were significantly lower compared to patients with chest drainage, with no differences in 30-day morbidity or re-intervention rates between the two groups. These results suggest that omitting chest drainage is a safe and feasible practice in selected patients; however, in current practice, chest drainage is commonly used, although there is now a tendency to use a single tube and digital drainage systems, which allow for better management and more rapid removal [4].

Postoperative pulmonary complications occur in 15–40% of patients undergoing major thoracic surgery and are associated with prolonged hospital stays and unfavorable long-term outcomes [13, 68, 69]. Although VATS procedures are associated with a lower incidence of postoperative pulmonary complications compared to thoracotomy, such complications remain a significant cause of short-term morbidity and mortality [68]. In many centers, especially those with low surgical volumes. Many preoperative factors influence the likelihood of postoperative intensive care admission in patients undergoing lung resection. These include open thoracotomy versus VATS, more extensive resections, and impaired preoperative pulmonary function or the presence of pulmonary comorbidities such as chronic obstructive pulmonary disease (COPD) [70–74]. However, there is evidence that routine admission of patients undergoing thoracic surgery to intensive care does not reduce mortality rates and may result in inappropriate admissions, higher healthcare costs, delayed mobilization, and an increased risk of nosocomial infections [13, 75].

To date, no studies have compared outcomes in patients undergoing thoracic surgery admitted to intensive care units, high-dependency units, or surgical wards, nor are there available data to identify which patients may benefit from postoperative intensive care admission or to determine the appropriate level of care required for each case. Identification of high-risk patients and management of their postoperative course should therefore be planned by considering patient characteristics as well as the resources available in each center. The ERS/ESTS task force recommendations suggest that patients undergoing lung resection should be managed in dedicated thoracic surgery units or in wards with respiratory expertise, where available [13]. Admission to intensive care should be reserved for patients requiring organ support.

Although noninvasive ventilation (NIV) has the potential to improve lung function, reduce muscle workload, postoperative hypoxemia, and atelectasis, randomized controlled trials have not shown consistent evidence that the use of NIV or continuous positive airway pressure (CPAP) in addition to standard medical therapy provides significant benefits. In a 2019 Cochrane review of eight clinical trials involving a total of 486 patients undergoing thoracic surgery, no significant differences were found between patients receiving NIV and control groups in terms of pulmonary complications, intubation rates, mortality, length of stay in intensive care, or overall hospital stay [76]. Therefore, it now appears more appropriate to use this type of support for the treatment of postoperative respiratory failure. An emerging alternative to NIV and CPAP for respiratory support in high-risk patients is high-flow nasal cannula (HFNC) oxygen therapy, which delivers high inspiratory flows, up to 60 L/min, capable of meeting the patient's oxygen demands. HFNC therapy offers several advantages, including the application of a moderate level of CPAP with a positive effect on oxygenation, a moderate contribution to carbon dioxide clearance, and proper airway humidification. In addition, it significantly reduces respiratory effort, improving tolerance and overall management of therapy. A post hoc analysis of a randomized trial in obese patients undergoing major thoracic surgery compared the efficacy of HFNC with NIV. The results showed that HFNC is not inferior to NIV in terms of treatment failure rates, intensive care mortality, or length of stay in intensive care or hospital [77]. HFNC therapy is also associated with a lower incidence of skin lesions compared to NIV. A 2024 meta-analysis based on the results of five studies suggests that the preventive use of HFNC instead of conventional oxygen therapy in patients extubated after lung resection surgery may significantly improve the oxygenation index within the first 12 h after extubation, but does not appear to have a significant impact on the incidence of postoperative hypoxemia, reintubation rates, escalation of respiratory support, postoperative PaCO2 differences, or length of hospital and intensive care stay.

6.5 Conclusions

Anesthesia for thoracic surgery requires a multidisciplinary approach from risk assessment to perioperative and postoperative management. The choice of anesthesia, technique for lung separation/isolation, monitoring of airway pressures, vital signs, hemodynamics, neuromuscular blockade, and anesthetic depth are fundamental to ensuring optimal outcomes. In the postoperative period, multimodal analgesia, including regional techniques, is essential for effective pain control. Decisions regarding postoperative intensive care, management of chest drainage, and personalized interventions complete the care pathway. Ongoing research continually updates clinical practice, drawing attention to details once overlooked that are now central to modern anesthesia.

References

1. Licker M, Triponez F, Diaper J, Ellenberger C, Tschopp JM, Bridevaux PO. Impact of thoracic anesthesia and analgesia on perioperative outcome. Anesthesiol Clin. 2010;29:691–703.
2. Batchelor TJP, Rasburn NJ, Abdelnour-Berchtold E, Brunelli A, Cerfolio RJ, et al. Guidelines for enhanced recovery after lung surgery: recommendations of the Enhanced Recovery After Surgery (ERAS) Society and the European Society of Thoracic Surgeons (ESTS). Eur J Cardiothorac Surg. 2019;55:91–115.

3. Piccioni F, Droghetti A, Bertani A, Coccia C, Corcione A, Corsico AG, et al. Recommendations from the Italian intersociety consensus on Perioperative Anesthesia Care in Thoracic surgery (PACTS) part 1: preadmission and preoperative care. Perioper Med (Lond). 2020;9:37.
4. Piccioni F, Droghetti A, Bertani A, Coccia C, Corcione A, Corsico AG, et al. Recommendations from the Italian intersociety consensus on Perioperative Anesthesia Care in Thoracic surgery (PACTS) part 2: intraoperative and postoperative care. Perioper Med (Lond). 2020;9:31.
5. European Society of Cardiology (ESC). Guidelines on cardiovascular assessment and management of patients undergoing non-cardiac surgery. Eur Heart J. 2022;43:2805–925.
6. Lee TH, Marcantonio ER, Mangione CM, Thomas EJ, Polanczyk CA, Cook EF, et al. Derivation and prospective validation of a simple index for predicting cardiac risk in major noncardiac surgery. Circulation. 1999;100:1043–9.
7. Brunelli A, Rocco G. The Thoracic Revised Cardiac Risk Index (ThRCRI) for perioperative risk stratification in thoracic surgery. J Thorac Cardiovasc Surg. 2010;140:1134–40.
8. Lamperti M, Romero C, Guarracino F, Cammarota G, Vetrugno L, Boris T, et al. Preoperative assessment of adults undergoing elective noncardiac surgery: updated guidelines from the European Society of Anaesthesiology and Intensive Care. Eur J Anaesthesiol. 2025;42:1–35.
9. Thompson A, Fleischmann KE, Smilowitz NR, de Las FL, Mukherjee D, Aggarwal NR, et al. 2024 AHA/ACC/ACS/ASNC/HRS/SCA/SCCT/SCMR/SVM guideline for perioperative cardiovascular management for noncardiac surgery: a report of the American College of Cardiology/American Heart Association Joint Committee on Clinical Practice Guidelines. Circulation. 2024;150:e351–442.
10. Hlatky MA, Boineau RE, Higginbotham MB, Lee KL, Mark DB, Califf RM, et al. A brief self-administered questionnaire to determine functional capacity (the Duke Activity Status Index). Am J Cardiol. 1989;64:651–4.
11. Greco M, Angelucci A, Avidano G, Marelli G, Canali S, Aceto R, et al. Wearable health technology for preoperative risk assessment in elderly patients: the WELCOME Study. Diagnostics. 2023;13:630.
12. Brunelli A, Refai M, Xiumé F, Salati M, Marasco R, Sciarra V, et al. Carbon monoxide lung diffusion capacity improves risk stratification in candidates for lung resection. Ann Thorac Surg. 2007;83:77–84.
13. Brunelli A, Charloux A, Bolliger CT, Rocco G, Sculier JP, Varela G, et al. European Respiratory Society and European Society of Thoracic Surgeons joint task force on fitness for radical therapy. ERS/ESTS clinical guidelines on fitness for radical therapy in lung cancer patients (surgery and chemo-radiotherapy). Eur Respir J. 2009;34:17–41.
14. Licker M, Triponez F, Diaper J, Karenovics W, Bridevaux PO. Preoperative evaluation of lung cancer patients. Curr Anesthesiol Rep. 2014;4:124–34.
15. Della Rocca G, Vetrugno L, Coccia C, Pierconti F, Badagliacca R, Vizza CD, et al. Preoperative evaluation of patients undergoing lung resection surgery: defining the role of the anesthesiologist on a multidisciplinary team. J Cardiothorac Vasc Anesth. 2016;30:530–8.
16. Rushwan A, Stefanou D, Tariq J, Drosos P, Chaudhuri N, Milton R, et al. Increased minute ventilation-to-carbon dioxide slope during cardiopulmonary exercise test is associated with poor postoperative outcome following lung cancer resection. Eur J Cardiothorac Surg. 2024;65(3):ezad337.
17. Salati M, Brunelli A. Risk stratification in lung surgery. Curr Surg Rep. 2016;4:37.
18. Falcoz PE, Conti M, Brouchet L, Chocron S, Puyraveau M, Mercier M, et al. The thoracic surgery scoring system (Thoracoscore): risk model for in-hospital death in 15,183 patients requiring thoracic surgery. J Thorac Cardiovasc Surg. 2007;133:325–32.
19. Brunelli A, Salati M, Rocco G, Varela G, Van Raemdonck D, Decaluwe H, et al. European risk models for morbidity (EuroLung1) and mortality (EuroLung2) to predict outcome following anatomic lung resections: an analysis from the European Society of Thoracic Surgeons database. Eur J Cardiothorac Surg. 2017;51:490–7.
20. Pipanmekaporn T, Bunchungmongkol N, Punjasawadwong Y, Lapisatepun W, Tantraworasin A, Saokaew S. A risk score for predicting respiratory complications after thoracic surgery. Asian Cardiovasc Thorac Ann. 2019;27:278–87.

21. Kaybal O, İncekara F, Alagöz A. The effectiveness of ARISCAT Risk Index, other scoring systems, and parameters in predicting pulmonary complications after thoracic surgery. Medicine (Baltimore). 2022;101:e29723.
22. Zorrilla-Vaca A, Grant MC, Rehman M, Sarin P, Mendez-Pino L, Urman RD, Varelmann D. Performance comparison of pulmonary risk scoring systems in lung resection. J Cardiothorac Vasc Anesth. 2023;37:1734–43.
23. Beckert AK, Huisingh-Scheetz M, Thompson K, Celauro AD, Williams J, Pachwicewicz P, et al. Screening for frailty in thoracic surgical patients. Ann Thorac Surg. 2017;103:956–61.
24. Sayan M, Artiran B, Ozturk F, Fattahov M, Akarsu I, Aslan MT, et al. The prognostic significance of modified frailty index-5 in patients undergoing pneumonectomy for lung cancer. Interdiscip Cardiovasc Thorac Surg. 2024;39:ivae179.
25. Lee ACH, Madariaga MLL, Lee SM, Ferguson MK. The risk analysis index is an independent predictor of outcomes after lung cancer resection. PLoS One. 2024;19:e0303281.
26. Wada H, Suzuki H, Sakairi Y, Tanaka K, Sata Y, Toyoda T, et al. Can modified frailty index predict postoperative complication after lung cancer surgery? Gen Thorac Cardiovasc Surg. 2024;72:176–82.
27. Langiano N, Fiorelli S, Deana C, et al. Airway management in anesthesia for thoracic surgery: a "real life" observational study. J Thorac Dis. 2019;11:3257–69.
28. Liu TT, Li L, Wan L, et al. Videolaryngoscopy vs. Macintosh laryngoscopy for double-lumen tube intubation in thoracic surgery: a systematic review and meta-analysis. Anaesthesia. 2018;73:997–1007.
29. Kim YS, Song J, Lim BG, et al. Different classes of videoscopes and direct laryngoscopes for double-lumen tube intubation in thoracic surgery: a systematic review and network meta-analysis. PLoS One. 2020;15(8):e0238060.
30. Lumb AB, Slinger P. Hypoxic pulmonary vasoconstriction physiology and anesthetic implications. Anesthesiology. 2015;122:932–46.
31. Jenkins SA, Bennett JR. Pulmonary vasoconstriction and volatile anesthetics: mechanisms and clinical implications. Anesth Analg. 2020;131:846–57.
32. Cho YH, Lee H, Song H. Protective effects of sevoflurane on the endothelial glycocalyx during thoracic surgery. J Cardiothor Vasc Anesth. 2019;33:931–9.
33. Buhre W, De Robertis E, Gonzalez-Pizarro P. The Glasgow declaration on sustainability in anaesthesiology and intensive care. Eur J Anaesthesiol. 2023;40:461–4.
34. Bello M, Oger S, Bedon-Carte S, Vielstadte C, Leo F, Zaouter C, Ouattara A. Effect of opioid-free anaesthesia on postoperative epidural ropivacaine requirement after thoracic surgery: a retrospective unmatched case-control study. Anaesth Crit Care Pain Med. 2019;38:499–505.
35. Devine G, Cheng M, Martinez G, Patvardhan C, Aresu G, Peryt A, et al. Opioid-free anesthesia for lung cancer resection: a case-control study. J Cardiothorac Vasc Anesth. 2020;34:3036–40.
36. Larue A, Jacquet-Lagrèze M, Ruste M, Tronc F, Fellahi JL. Opioid-free anaesthesia for video-assisted thoracoscopic surgery: a retrospective cohort study with propensity score analysis. Anaesth Crit Care Pain Med. 2022;41:101089.
37. Wang X-r, Jia X-y, Jiang Y-y, Li Z-p, Zhou Q-h. Opioid-free anesthesia for postoperative recovery after video-assisted thoracic surgery: a prospective, randomized controlled trial. Front Surg. 2023;9:1035972.
38. Mena GE, Zorrilla-Vaca A, Vaporciyan A, Mehran R, Lasala JD, Williams W, et al. Intraoperative dexmedetomidine and ketamine infusions in an enhanced recovery after thoracic surgery program: a propensity score matched analysis. J Cardiothorac Vasc Anesth. 2022;36:1064–72.
39. D'Amico F, Barucco G, Licheri M, Valsecchi G, Zaraca L, Mucchetti M, et al. Opioid free anesthesia in thoracic surgery: a systematic review and meta analysis. J Clin Med. 2022;11:6955.
40. Bernasconi F, Piccioni F. One-lung ventilation for thoracic surgery: current perspectives. Tumori. 2017;103:495–503.
41. Piccioni F, Langiano N, Bignami E, Guarnieri M, Proto P, D'Andrea R, et al. One-lung ventilation and postoperative pulmonary complications after major lung resection surgery. A multicenter randomized controlled trial. J Cardiothorac Vasc Anesth. 2023;37:2561–71.

42. Park M, Yoon S, Nam JS, Ahn HJ, Kim H, Kim HJ, et al. Driving pressure-guided ventilation and postoperative pulmonary complications in thoracic surgery: a multicentre randomised clinical trial. Br J Anaesth. 2023;130:e106–18.
43. Kim KN, Kim DW, Jeong MA, Sin YH, Lee SK. Comparison of pressure-controlled ventilation with volume-controlled ventilation during one-lung ventilation: a systematic review and Meta-analysis. BMC Anesthesiol. 2016;16:72.
44. Yao W, Yang M, Cheng Q, Shan S, Yang B, Han Q, et al. Effect of pressure-controlled ventilation-volume guaranteed on one-lung ventilation in elderly patients undergoing thoracotomy. Med Sci Monit. 2020;26:e921417.
45. Zeldin RA, Normandin D, Landtwing D, Peters RM. Postpneumonectomy pulmonary edema. J Thorac Cardiovasc Surg. 1984;87:359–65.
46. Licker M, de Perrot M, Spiliopoulos A, Robert J, Diaper J, Chevalley C, et al. Risk factors for acute lung injury after thoracic surgery for lung cancer. Anesth Analg. 2003;97:1558–65.
47. Licker M, Fauconnet P, Villiger Y, Tschopp JM. Acute lung injury and outcomes after thoracic surgery. Curr Opin Anaesthesiol. 2009;22:61–7.
48. Licker M, Cartier V, Robert J, Diaper J, Villiger Y, Tschopp JM, et al. Risk factors of acute kidney injury according to RIFLE criteria after lung cancer surgery. Ann Thorac Surg. 2011;91:844–50.
49. Ishikawa S, Griesdale DE, Lohser J. Acute kidney injury after lung resection surgery: incidence and perioperative risk factors. Anesth Analg. 2012;114:1256–62.
50. Yu Y, Xu S, Yan B, Tang X, Zhang H, Pan C, et al. Incidence and associations of acute kidney injury after general thoracic surgery: a system review and meta-analysis. J Clin Med. 2022;12:37.
51. Piccioni F, Bernasconi F, Tramontano GTA, Langer M. A systematic review of pulse pressure variation and stroke volume variation to predict fluid responsiveness during cardiac and thoracic surgery. J Clin Monit Comput. 2017;31:677–84.
52. Kimura A, Suehiro K, Juri T, Fujimoto Y, Yoshida H, Tanaka K, et al. Hemodynamic changes via the lung recruitment maneuver can predict fluid responsiveness in stroke volume and arterial pressure during one-lung ventilation. Anesth Analg. 2021;133:44–52.
53. Jun IJ, Chung MH, Kim JE, Lee HS, Son JM, Choi EM. The influence of Positive End-Expiratory Pressure (PEEP) in predicting fluid responsiveness in patients undergoing one-lung ventilation. Int J Med Sci. 2021;18:2589–98.
54. Zhang Y, Ding Y, Zhang J, Huang T, Gao J. Tidal volume challenge-induced hemodynamic changes can predict fluid responsiveness during one-lung ventilation: an observational study. Front Med (Lausanne). 2023;10:1169912.
55. SIAARTI Good Clinical Practice – Perioperative Normothermia. 2017. https://www.siaarti.it/media_center/file/c9e9e92f-3cbc-43e3-8738-995e269623cc.
56. SIAARTI Good Clinical Practice – Muscle Relaxation, Neuromuscular Monitoring and Reversal. 2018. https://www.siaarti.it/media_center/file/da366d6b-1198-4915-b497-5c4380ad9652.
57. Fuchs-Buder T, Romero CS, Lewald H, Lamperti M, Afshari A, Hristovska AM, et al. Perioperative management of neuromuscular blockade: a guideline from the European Society of Anaesthesiology and Intensive Care. Eur J Anaesthesiol. 2023;40:82–94.
58. Thilen SR, Weigel WA, Todd MM, Dutton RP, Lien CA, Grant SA, et al. 2023 American Society of Anesthesiologists practice guidelines for monitoring and antagonism of neuromuscular blockade: a report by the American Society of Anesthesiologists Task Force on Neuromuscular Blockade. Anesthesiology. 2023;138:13–41.
59. Piccioni F, Rosboch GL, Coccia C, Donati I, Proto P, Ceraolo E, et al. Decurarization After Thoracic Anesthesia using sugammadex compared to neostigmine (DATA trial): a multicenter randomized double-blinded controlled trial. J Anesth Analg Crit Care. 2024;4:9.
60. Sadowska D, Bialka S, Palaczynski P, Czyzewski D, Smereka J, Szelka-Urbanczyk A, et al. Opioid-free anaesthesia effectiveness in thoracic surgery—objective measurement with a skin conductance algesimeter: a randomized controlled trial. Int J Environ Res Public Health. 2022;19:14358.

61. Yeung JH, Gates S, Naidu BV, Wilson MJ, Gao SF. Paravertebral block versus thoracic epidural for patients undergoing thoracotomy. Cochrane Database Syst Rev. 2016;2:CD009121.
62. Xu M, Hu J, Yan J, Yan H, Zhang C. Paravertebral block versus thoracic epidural analgesia for postthoracotomy pain relief: a meta-analysis of randomized trials. Thorac Cardiovasc Surg. 2022;70:413–21.
63. Balzani E, Rosboch GL, Ceraolo E, Lyberis P, Filippini C, Piccioni F, et al. The effect of peripheral regional analgesia in thoracic surgery: a systematic review and a meta-analysis of randomized-controlled trials. Tumori. 2023;109:6–18.
64. Sandeep B, Huang X, Li Y, Xiong D, Zhu B, Xiao Z. A comparison of regional anesthesia techniques in patients undergoing video-assisted thoracic surgery: a network meta-analysis. Int J Surg. 2022;105:106840.
65. Pang J, You J, Chen Y, Song C. Comparison of erector spinae plane block with paravertebral block for thoracoscopic surgery: a meta-analysis of randomized controlled trials. J Cardiothorac Surg. 2023;18:300.
66. Li J, Sun Q, Zong L, Li D, Jin X, Zhang L. Relative efficacy and safety of several regional analgesic techniques following thoracic surgery: a network meta-analysis of randomized controlled trials. Int J Surg. 2023;109:2404–13.
67. Li P, Shen C, Wu Y, Lai Y, Zhou K, Che G. It is safe and feasible to omit the chest tube postoperatively for selected patients receiving thoracoscopic pulmonary resection: a meta-analysis. J Thorac Dis. 2018;10:2712–21.
68. Agostini PJ, Lugg ST, Adams K, Smith T, Kalkat MS, Rajesh PB, et al. Risk factors and short-term outcomes of postoperative pulmonary complications after VATS lobectomy. J Cardiothorac Surg. 2018;13:28.
69. Gómez-Hernández MT, Forcada C, Gómez F, Iscan M, Fuentes MG, Rivas CE, et al. Early outcomes of robotic versus video-thoracoscopic anatomical segmentectomy: a propensity score-matched real-world study. Eur J Cardiothorac Surg. 2024;66:ezae389.
70. Dulu A, Pastores SM, Park B, Riedel E, Rusch V, Halpern NA. Prevalence and mortality of acute lung injury and ARDS after lung resection. Chest. 2006;130:73–8.
71. Brunelli A, Ferguson MK, Rocco G, Pieretti P, Vigneswaran WT, Morgan-Hughes NJ, et al. A scoring system predicting the risk for intensive care unit admission for complications after major lung resection: a multicenter analysis. Ann Thorac Surg. 2008;86:213–8.
72. Cywinski JB, Xu M, Sessler DI, Mason D, Koch CG. Predictors of prolonged postoperative endotracheal intubation in patients undergoing thoracotomy for lung resection. J Cardiothorac Vasc Anesth. 2009;23:766–9.
73. McCall PJ, Macfie A, Kinsella J, Shelley BG. Critical care after lung resection: CALoR 1, a single-centre pilot study. Anaesthesia. 2015;70:1382–9.
74. Pinheiro L, Santoro IL, Perfeito JA, Izbicki M, Ramos RP, Faresin SM. Preoperative predictive factors for intensive care unit admission after pulmonary resection. J Bras Pneumol. 2015;41:31–8.
75. Brunelli A, Pieretti P, Al Refai M, Lacava N, Xiume' F, Boaron M, et al. Elective intensive care after lung resection: a multicentric propensity-matched comparison of outcome. Interact Cardiovasc Thorac Surg. 2005;4:609–13.
76. Torres MF, Porfírio GJ, Carvalho AP, Riera R. Non-invasive positive pressure ventilation for prevention of complications after pulmonary resection in lung cancer patients. Cochrane Database Syst Rev. 2019;3:CD010355.
77. Stéphan F, Bérard L, Rézaiguia-Delclaux S, Amaru P, BiPOP Study Group. High-flow nasal cannula therapy versus intermittent noninvasive ventilation in obese subjects after cardiothoracic surgery. Respir Care. 2017;62:1193–202.

Management of Allergies in Surgical Patients

7

Davide Chiumello, Tommaso Pozzi, and Arianna Ciabattoni

7.1 Introduction

The perioperative period encompasses the phases immediately before, during, and shortly after a surgical procedure performed under local or general anesthesia. During this time, exposure to various substances, both pharmacological and non-pharmacological, within a limited timeframe can trigger adverse reactions, including hypersensitivity reactions of immunological origin, which must be distinguished from reactions secondary to direct histamine release.

Since the most dangerous manifestation of a hypersensitivity reaction is anaphylaxis, physicians must be prepared to diagnose and manage the potentially life-threatening cardiopulmonary dysfunction that may occur. However, diagnosis in the perioperative setting is often challenging, as patients are under the effects of general or regional anesthesia and may have other causes of hypotension. Furthermore, due to its low incidence, anaphylaxis is an unexpected event, which may delay identification and treatment, resulting in increased mortality.

D. Chiumello (✉)
Department of Anesthesia and Intensive Care, ASST Santi Paolo e Carlo, San Paolo University Hospital, Milan, Italy

Department of Health Sciences, University of Milan, Milan, Italy

Coordinated Research Center on Respiratory Failure, University of Milan, Milan, Italy
e-mail: davide.chiumello@unimi.it

T. Pozzi · A. Ciabattoni
Department of Anesthesia and Intensive Care, ASST Santi Paolo e Carlo, San Paolo University Hospital, Milan, Italy
e-mail: tommaso.pozzi@asst-santipaolocarlo.it; arianna.ciabattoni@asst-santipaolocarlo.it

D. Chiumello, A. De Gasperi (eds.), *Practical Trends in Anesthesia and Intensive Care 2026*, https://doi.org/10.1007/978-3-032-25721-5_7

The management of such reactions is therefore extremely complex and should involve collaboration between anesthesiologists, who are responsible for acute management, and allergists, who are involved in diagnosis and confirmation of the causative agent.

7.2 Incidence

According to the NAP 6 report, in the United Kingdom over 1 year (November 2015–November 2016), among 3,126,067 anesthetic procedures, the incidence of perioperative anaphylaxis was approximately 1:11,752 anesthetics, likely underestimated as some cases were excluded due to missing data.

Since the incidence of perioperative anaphylaxis may vary depending on the population's environmental exposure to triggers, it is possible that the incidence is increasing as a result of growing sensitization to antibiotics, to the extent that antibiotics have surpassed neuromuscular blocking agents as the most frequent triggers [1].

The incidence of latex-induced anaphylaxis is steadily decreasing, likely due to the effectiveness of primary prevention measures and reduced exposure in various aspects of daily life.

The incidence of anaphylaxis due to dyes and chlorhexidine is currently increasing, while anaphylactic reactions to colloids have remained relatively stable (around 4%) [2].

Allergic reactions to local anesthetics, despite their frequent use, remain quite rare, accounting for less than 1% of possible adverse reactions [3].

7.3 Pathophysiology

Hypersensitivity is a pathological response to antigenic stimuli, with symptoms developing after a second exposure following a sensitization period during which an immunological response is generated.

Hypersensitivity reactions are mediated by two mechanisms:

1. Immunological mechanisms

Four categories are recognized based on the pathogenic mechanism:

Type I Reaction: Anaphylactic or Immediate This accounts for 60% of all allergic reactions.

It is characterized by a biphasic onset.

Initially, there is a sensitization phase with activation of TH2 lymphocytes and B lymphocytes, and production of specific IgE antibodies. The constant region of these antibodies binds to high-affinity receptors on the cell membranes of mast cells and basophils. Upon subsequent exposure to the sensitizing agent, which binds the variable regions of the specific IgE, mediators such as histamine and chemotactic factors are released. Neutrophils and eosinophils, proteolytic enzymes, leading to the development of the immediate reaction. In some cases, the hypersensitivity reaction occurs after the first exposure, as a consequence of cross-reactivity with other substances to which the patient is already sensitized.

A delayed phase follows, peaking 6–12 h after the immediate response, characterized by the presence and activation of neutrophils, eosinophils, and macrophages, resulting in destruction of the surrounding tissue.

In drug reactions, this phase plays a minor role.

Degranulation of mast cells and basophils in the skin leads to vasodilation and thus rash with pruritus; in the airways, vasodilation and increased vascular permeability result in edema and bronchoconstriction, causing shortness of breath and air trapping. Anaphylaxis occurs when the effects of the allergic reaction are evident in two different organ systems, most commonly associated with hypotension [4].

In rare circumstances, immunological reactions are not IgE-mediated.

Type II Reaction: Antibody Mediated A delayed reaction characterized by cytotoxic effects mediated by IgG. This type of pathological response involves the development of a new antigenic compound. Small, low-molecular-weight peptides (haptens) bind to the surface of cells, leading to the formation of autoantibodies against host cell components, with subsequent destruction of the antigen by neutrophils and macrophages through opsonization. In addition, the constant regions of these immunoglobulins can activate the complement pathway, a non-antigen-specific immune response, resulting in the formation of membrane pores and subsequent cell lysis [4].

The drugs most commonly causing type II reactions are beta-lactams, sulfonamides, isoniazid, and antiepileptics. The predominant manifestations are cutaneous (e.g., drug-induced pemphigus, thrombocytopenic purpura) and hemolytic anemia.

Type III Reaction: Immune Complex Mediated Reactions characterized by localized or systemic accumulation of immune complexes (antigen-IgG) and activation of the complement system.

Immune complexes trigger cellular damage through the same mechanism as type II hypersensitivity reactions, in addition to platelet activation, promoting thrombus formation [4]. These complexes tend to accumulate in postcapillary venules and therefore involve organs with rich vascularization (kidneys, skin, joints, and lungs), triggering drug-induced vasculitis and serum sickness. Symptoms may be limited to the skin (e.g., palpable purpura) or related to end-organ damage such as pulmonary hemorrhage or glomerulonephritis.

Type IV Reaction: Cell Mediated T lymphocytes (CD4+/CD8+) are inappropriately activated following the formation of new antigenic components via the previously described hapten model, resulting in necrosis of antigen-presenting cells. Histological evaluation reveals a marked lymphocytic infiltrate. The reaction has a delayed onset. Clinical manifestations are observed 24–72 h after initial exposure to the antigen.

The most common manifestations are contact dermatitis and toxic epidermal necrolysis [5].

2. Non-immunological mechanisms

Non-immunological reactions are caused by direct stimulation of mast cells and basophils, resulting in degranulation [6], and therefore do not require prior exposure [7]. These reactions are generally milder than those mediated by the immune system [8].

7.4 Clinical Presentation

Anaphylaxis is a rapidly developing, potentially life-threatening systemic hypersensitivity reaction. In most cases, it is IgE-mediated, but IgG-mediated immunological reactions or those involving immune complexes can also cause anaphylaxis.

Perioperative anaphylaxis has clinical features similar to anaphylaxis from other causes but also possesses distinctive features [1, 9, 10]:

- Early identification and management due to the presence of personnel specialized in resuscitation.
- The patient is often unconscious and therefore unable to report prodromal symptoms.
- The patient is covered by the surgical drapes.
- The majority of triggers are administered intravenously, thus having the potential for severe and rapid reactions.
- Many drugs are administered almost simultaneously.
- Many clinical manifestations may be nonspecific and resemble symptoms of other problems that can occur during anesthesia [11]; for example, anaphylactic reactions cause alterations in vascular permeability with extravasation of intravascular volume into the interstitial space, resulting in hypotension, but most anesthetic agents used for induction also cause cardiovascular changes such as hypotension up to hemodynamic instability in hypovolemic patients, due to direct and indirect effects on the heart, vascular system, and adrenergic responses.

Hence, the importance of performing a differential diagnosis (Table 7.1).

For the diagnosis of anaphylaxis, physicians rely on the appearance of specific signs and symptoms (Table 7.2) following exposure to an antigen within a time frame compatible with the route of exposure.

The clinical features of severe anaphylaxis are very similar regardless of whether the reaction is allergic or non-allergic.

Table 7.1 Differential diagnosis

Other causes of hypotension/vasoplegia
Arrhytmias
Cardiac tamponade
Cardiogenic shock
Hemorrhage
Overdose of vasoactive drugs
Partial sympathectomy from spinal/epidural anesthesia
Pulmonary embolus
Sepsis
Vasovagal reaction
Venous air embolism
Other causes of respiratory or airway symptoms
Acute bronchospasm / asthmatic reaction
Air embolism
Aspiration
Endotracheal tube malposition
Post extubation stridor
Pulmonary edema
Tension pneumothorax
Transfusion-related acute lung injury (TRALI)

Table 7.2 Signs and symptoms of perioperative anaphylaxis

System	Symptoms	Signs
Cardiovascular	Diaphoresis Dizziness Palpitations	Cardiac arrest Hypotension or cardiovascular collapse Decrease in $EtCO_2$ Tachycardia/bradycardia Dysrhythmias
Respiratory	Acute hoarseness Chest discomfort Short of breath Wheezing	Acute respiratory failure Bronchospasm/increased inspiratory pressures during ventilation Decreased pulmonary compliance Laryngeal edema Stridor
Mucosa/skin	Burning Itching Tingling	Flushing Diffuse erythema Cutaneous/mucosal edema Urticaria
Neurologic	Malaise Sense of impending doom	Confusion Loss of consciousness
Gastrointestinal	Nausea Abdominal cramps	Vomiting Diarrhea

7.4.1 Cardiovascular Signs

- Severe hypotension (46% of cases): initiate cardiopulmonary resuscitation with chest compressions if blood pressure <50 mmHg. More common in men than in women, possibly related to the presence of coronary artery disease (24% vs 8.4%), use of beta-blockers (27% vs 11%), and ACE inhibitors (21.2% vs 15.2%).
- Tachycardia (9.8% of cases): may rapidly progress to severe arrhythmias and cardiovascular collapse if not treated immediately.
- Bradycardia (3% of cases): may be an early sign of anaphylaxis, often mistaken for a non-allergic effect of anesthesia, especially in patients on beta-blocker therapy.
- Acute cardiopulmonary dysfunction with desaturation and hemodynamic instability, with varying degrees of hypotension up to cardiac arrest in intubated and unconscious patients. A decrease in $EtCO_2$ indicates reduced cardiac output as well as decreased tissue perfusion and correlates well with the severity of the reaction.
- Of all cardiac arrests, the majority (34) were PEA, and all were fatal, followed by (4) pulseless VF/VT and (2) asystole. Only six patients developed an arrhythmia prior to cardiac arrest, specifically four with bradycardia and two with VT. No cases of AF or supraventricular tachycardia.
- Kounis syndrome: a rare manifestation, consisting of acute coronary events associated with an immediate hypersensitivity reaction, such as that caused by the release of mediators from cardiac mast cells [12, 13].

7.4.2 Respiratory Signs

These are less frequent, observed in only about half of patients, particularly those with asthma [13].

In 1.5% of cases, there is isolated respiratory involvement [1].

- Bronchospasm or decreased oxygen saturation [14]: bronchospasm is the most common presentation in obese individuals and asthmatic patients, more frequent in women because more women have asthma (25% vs 16%).
- Laryngeal edema: only one patient required front-of-neck access for management [1].

7.4.3 Cutaneous Signs

- Rash, urticaria, and angioedema: observed in 66–70% of IgE-mediated reactions and > 90% of non-IgE-mediated reactions [15]. Rash is rarely a presenting feature.
- Cutaneous manifestations such as rash may be entirely absent, especially in severe hypersensitivity reactions, due to compromised skin perfusion, and may only appear secondarily after restoration of systemic perfusion.

Mild cutaneous manifestations may resolve spontaneously and thus go unnoticed, especially as the patient is covered by surgical drapes, which may result in re-exposure leading to a more severe and potentially life-threatening reaction [16].

7.4.4 Other Signs

- Rare but include coagulation abnormalities [17], pulmonary edema, and rhabdomyolysis. These are generally associated with prolonged anaphylactic shock, pre-existing cardiac disease, or the use of beta-blockers or ACE inhibitors.

Several classification systems have been proposed to assess the severity of reactions occurring during anesthesia (Table 7.3).

The factors influencing the severity of anaphylaxis are [18, 19]:

- Advanced age.
- Comorbidities: cardiac and respiratory diseases.
- Systemic mastocytosis or elevated baseline tryptase levels [20].
- Ongoing therapies: drugs that alter the response to amines: beta-blockers, ACE inhibitors, angiotensin II receptor antagonists, MAO inhibitors, tricyclic antidepressants, serotonin reuptake inhibitors.
- Route of administration: reactions are more rapid and severe with intravenous administration.
- Initial presentation: reactions with vascular collapse or cardiorespiratory arrest.
- Speed of clinical course: rapid reactions are associated with greater severity and mortality.
- Delay in administration of adrenaline: delay worsens outcomes in severe cases [21, 22].

The onset of the reaction may be:

<5 min: immediate onset: 66% of cases, mainly IgE-mediated reactions
<10 min: 83% of cases
<15 min: 88% of cases
<30 min: 95% of cases [1]

Table 7.3 Severity grading of anaphylactic reactions according to the modified Ring and Messmer scale

Grade of severity	Clinical signs
Grade I	Mucocutaneous signs: generalized erythema ± urticaria ± angioedema
Grade II	Not life-threatening signs: mucocutaneous signs ± hypotension ± tachycardia ± cough ± dyspnea ± digestive signs
Grade III	Life-threatening signs: cardiovascular collapse ± tachycardia or bradycardia, ± arrhytmias ± bronchospasm ± digestive signs
Grade IV	Cardiac or respiratory arrest

Distribution and timing of events:
58% of anaphylactic events occur in the operating room.

- 3% before induction
- 81% immediately after induction, mainly due to antibiotics, neuromuscular blockers, and hypnotic agents
- 13% during surgery
- 3% after surgery [1]

7.5 Management of Perioperative Allergic Reactions

The anesthesiologist plays a key role in both the prevention and treatment of hypersensitivity reactions.

7.5.1 Preventive Measures

These are based on identifying patients at risk.

A thorough medical history is essential. Investigate:

- A history of allergies or perioperative allergic reactions, all existing medical conditions, and current therapies.
- Risk factors: female sex, advanced age, multiple surgical procedures, history of asthma or atopy, frequent short-term use of antibiotics.

7.5.2 Step-by-Step Treatment

1. Recognition of the allergic reaction. Interpret the patient's signs and determine whether they are indicative of anaphylaxis, and if possible, hypothesize the likely trigger.
2. Removal of the causative agent.
3. Immediate treatment of the reaction.

First-line treatment:

Adrenaline. The drug of choice for the treatment of anaphylaxis. In severe reactions, delayed administration is associated with a worse prognosis. Adjust the dosage according to clinical severity.

Mild and slow-progressing forms:

- Intramuscular or subcutaneous route 0.3–0.5 mg, repeatable every 5–10 min.
- Aerosol route 1–4 mg if laryngeal stridor and/or bronchospasm.

Severe forms with marked laryngospasm or anaphylactic shock:

- Intravenous route 0.01 mg/kg (1:10,000 solution): If there is no response, administer 0.1–0.2 mg/kg intravenously over 3 min to avoid cardiac arrhythmias.
- Intravenous bolus 1 mg if cardiac arrest.

In patients taking beta-blockers or with heart disease, other vasoactive agents may be administered (norepinephrine, ephedrine, phenylephrine, and dopamine) [23]. Glucagon is used as a rescue treatment in patients on beta-blockers who may not respond to adrenaline [19, 24]. Methylene blue, useful for its ability to interfere with nitric oxide action at the level of vascular smooth muscle, should be administered in combination with adrenaline [25–27].

- Oxygen therapy after ensuring airway patency.

  Administer 100% oxygen and maintain SpO2 above 92%.

- Fluid infusion. In cases of severe hypotension, proceed with fluid infusion (preferably.

  Ringer's lactate). Start with 1–2 L of solution, repeat if necessary (Fig. 7.1).
  Second-line treatment:

- Antihistamines and corticosteroids.

  Used to prevent late symptoms and in grade I reactions [27, 28].
  They should not replace first-line drugs in severe anaphylactic reactions.

- Salbutamol if bronchospasm or lack of response to adrenaline.
- Atropine in cases of severe bradycardia refractory to adrenaline and/or fluid therapy, and in patients on beta-blockers as they may develop cardiac arrest in the early stages of anaphylaxis.

7.5.3 Post-treatment Actions

- Measurement of serum tryptase [29]. Determination of histamine and methylhistamine in urine is not routinely recommended due to measurement difficulties and low sensitivity [30, 31].
- Continuation with the surgical procedure.

The decision to proceed with surgery after an anaphylactic reaction is individualized and depends on the severity of the reaction, cardiorespiratory stability, and the urgency of the surgical procedure.

Grade 1–2 reactions: it may be possible to proceed with surgery.

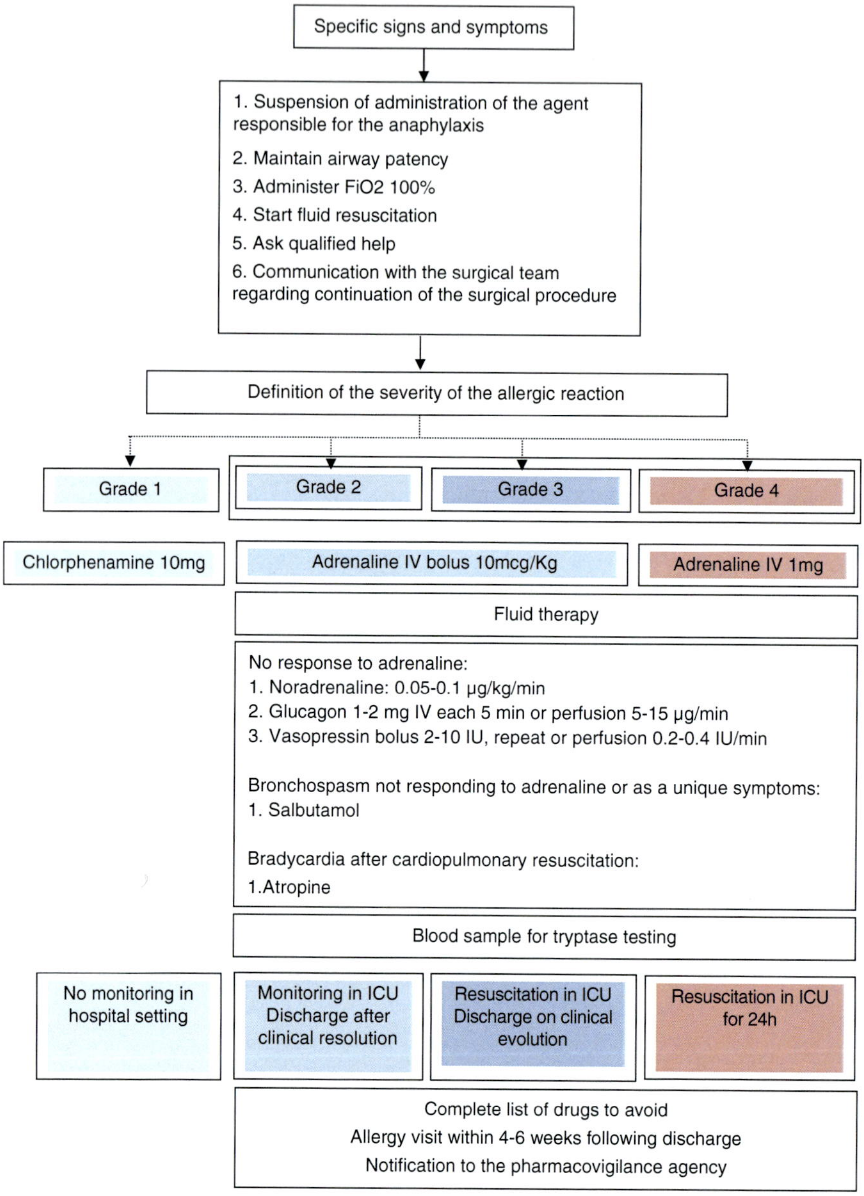

Fig. 7.1 Flowchart of allergic reaction management

Grade 3–4 reactions: decision based on stability and urgency.

If the patient is stabilized after the reaction, it may be beneficial to proceed with the surgical procedure in order to avoid a subsequent anesthesia. No differences have been reported between cases in which surgery was performed and those in which it was postponed [35].

Discharge

Grade 1–2 reactions: discharge upon resolution of symptoms.

Grade 3–4 reactions: observation for at least 24 h, in a ward or preferably in intensive care.

Before discharge, provide the patient with a clinical report containing all relevant information regarding the reaction: severity, treatment administered, possible causative agent, and refer the patient for an allergy evaluation. The anesthesiologist should contact the allergist to ensure all correct information regarding the event is provided.

To standardize the diagnosis and management of anaphylactic reactions, it is advisable to have a ready-to-use flow chart in all anesthesia departments [32–34] containing the following information:

- Algorithm for the treatment of anaphylaxis with drug dosages and routes of administration.
- Instructions for obtaining biological samples (type of tube and reference laboratory).
- A standardized data collection form to be sent to the allergy department [33].

7.6 Diagnostic Tests

Patients at risk of perioperative hypersensitivity, or those with an unclear or poorly defined history of allergic reaction, should be referred for an allergy evaluation to identify potential risk agents or causative agents.

Investigative tests are selected depending on whether the reaction is IgE-mediated or non-IgE-mediated.

- In vitro tests are performed during the acute phase of the reaction or hours after the reaction has been controlled.

The most obvious benefit of in vitro tests is that they can be performed without putting the patient at risk.

Serum Tryptase Measurement is recommended by guidelines, with high sensitivity. Peak occurs 1–2 h after the onset of the allergic reaction and levels remain elevated for several hours [35, 36], making it possible to collect samples once the patient is stabilized. Compare with subsequent baseline values. Elevated baseline tryptase levels correlate with more severe anaphylactic reactions [37].

Specific IgE Levels increase in the first weeks/months after the allergic reaction and subsequently decline over time [38], so they are not useful as a screening tool for the risk of allergic reaction [39]. Optimal timing is 1–2 months after the reaction.

A negative result may occur if the sample is collected too early at the time of the reaction or years after the allergic reaction without further exposure [38].

A negative specific IgE result can never be used to rule out an allergy [38, 40].

The determination of allergen-specific IgE levels is useful when interpreted in combination with skin test results [41].

Quantification tests for specific IgE are available in clinical practice for a limited number of drugs and substances used in the perioperative setting [39, 42].

With a few exceptions, for most drugs, the sensitivity and specificity are relatively low [43].

Basophil Activation Test (BAT) This test can be used with any substance that can be put into solution. It is a functional test that mimics in vitro the contact between allergens and basophil granulocytes, leading to their activation and subsequent expression of markers (CD63 and CD203c) on the cell membrane, which can be detected and quantified by flow cytometry.

CD63 is a marker of degranulation, and CD203c is a marker of cellular activation.

Specificity >90% and relatively high sensitivity (50–90%) when performed in specialized centers [44].

- In vivo tests

Performed after the reaction has resolved.

- Skin tests

First-line tests recommended for perioperative allergies. They should be performed 4–6 weeks after the onset of the allergic reaction to avoid false negatives due to cutaneous anergy following massive mast cell degranulation.

If the kinetics of the reaction, drugs, and agents administered are known - > skin tests are mandatory for all agents used, plus latex and chlorhexidine [45].

If information about the episode is unclear - > the agents to be tested depend on the type of surgery, anesthesia, and the severity of the reaction.

For each drug used in the perioperative period, the optimal concentrations to be used have been determined in order to avoid false positives (positivity due to high concentration or nonspecific histamine-releasing action on cutaneous mast cells) and false negatives (concentrations that are too low) [46].

- Skin prick test (SPT)

Useful for identifying IgE-mediated hypersensitivity.

Place a drop of antigen extract on the skin, followed by scarification with a lancet. Use the diluent alone as a negative control and histamine as a positive control.

Antihistamines and corticosteroids should be temporarily discontinued before performing the test to ensure accurate results.

The test is considered positive when the wheal formed in response to the allergen has a mean diameter >3 mm and is surrounded by erythema, and when the negative control is indeed negative [47, 48].

This test is easy to perform but has low sensitivity; therefore, if the result is negative or equivocal but clinical suspicion of allergy remains high, it should be followed by an intradermal test.

- Intradermal test (IDT)

Injection of a small amount of allergen under the skin, followed by measurement of the mean diameter of the wheal after 15–20 min or 24–72 h in the case of delayed hypersensitivity reactions. If the wheal increases by >3 mm compared to the baseline diameter of the initial wheal obtained with the prick test, the test is considered positive.

Higher sensitivity than the prick test but with a greater risk of IgE-mediated anaphylaxis and a higher risk of both false positives (most often attributable to drugs that cause skin irritation) and false negatives (if the test concentration is too low), thus affecting the specificity and sensitivity of the test [47, 48].

- Provocation Tests

Gold standard for the diagnosis of drug hypersensitivity reactions.

Administration of incremental doses of the drug of interest at regular intervals until a reaction occurs or the therapeutic dose is reached. The aim is to reproduce hypersensitivity symptoms in a controlled environment, under close supervision by trained personnel.

Indications:

- Ambiguous clinical history of previous reaction
- Unclear or unavailable allergy test results
- Exclusion of cross-reactivity between structurally homologous compounds
- Identification of safe alternatives to the implicated agents

Contraindications:

- Elderly patients
- Presence of comorbidities (heart failure, liver failure, renal failure, immunodeficiencies, malignancies)
- Pregnancy
- Uncontrolled asthma
- Ongoing acute infection
- Severe hypersensitivity to the drug (e.g., toxic epidermal necrolysis, Stevens-Johnson syndrome, systemic vasculitis)
- Circumstances that could prevent adequate management of the induced reaction

In the context of perioperative allergies, this test is generally not performed due to:

1. Inability to reach the full dose with all perioperative drugs, such as neuromuscular blockers, anesthetic agents, and opioids, due to their pharmacological effects and adverse events.
2. Lack of standardized provocation tests for substances such as latex and chlorhexidine.
3. Sensitivity and specificity are not 100%, so a negative test cannot always exclude an allergy.
4. Resource-intensive procedure, as the test involves many drugs and substances.
5. High-risk procedure that may cause anaphylaxis, thus requiring backup from the emergency team.

In the perioperative setting, it is not possible to identify the culprit drug simply based on the timing of administration and symptom onset, as many drugs are administered within a very short time frame.

Proposed diagnostic criteria for anaphylaxis:

1. Allergic Anaphylaxis:
   - Onset: within 60 min.
   - Tryptase: evidence of mast cell release.
   - Specific IgE: positive skin or serum tests.
   - Criteria for diagnostic certainty:
     • High certainty: four positive criteria.
     • Intermediate certainty: three positive criteria.

   Positivity for specific IgE is essential in both certainty categories.
2. Non-Allergic Anaphylaxis:
   - Onset: within 60 min.
   - Tryptase: evidence of mast cell activation.
   - Specific IgE: negative skin or serum tests.
   - Criteria for diagnostic certainty:
     • High certainty: four positive criteria.
     • Intermediate certainty: three positive criteria.

Following completion of the diagnostic workup, a medical report should be produced, including:

- Risk factors identified from the clinical history.
- Drugs tested and the results of the allergy tests performed.
- Any hypersensitivity reactions: unexpected reactions, signs and symptoms of the resulting reaction, severity, drugs administered, and the time required for symptom resolution.
- Recommendations for future patient management.
- Previously, uninvestigated hypersensitivity events during the perioperative period are a risk factor for the development of future potentially life-threatening allergic reactions [49].

7.7 Causative Agents

The prevalence of allergic reactions caused by different agents varies between countries due to differences in clinical practice. For example, in reports from the United States, antibiotics are the most frequent cause of perioperative anaphylaxis, a situation similar to the United Kingdom, whereas in European reports, neuromuscular blocking agents are most frequently implicated.

7.7.1 Antibiotics

They are the leading cause of perioperative hypersensitivity reactions. For most surgical procedures, antibiotic prophylaxis is required and is administered before, sometimes during, or after anesthesia. When administered after, hypotension resulting from anaphylaxis is exacerbated by general or neuraxial anesthesia.

Administration before induction of anesthesia is associated with several potential benefits:

- Less severe physiological imbalance caused by anaphylaxis
- Easier identification of the cause of anaphylaxis since few drugs have been administered
- Earlier identification and treatment

The antibiotics most frequently involved are those containing the beta-lactam ring.

Given the similar molecular structure between penicillins and cephalosporins, it is recommended to avoid cephalosporins in the presence of penicillin allergy; however, it has been suggested that the potential for cross-reactivity among penicillins is related to similarities in the R1 side chains rather than the beta-lactam ring itself.

If a patient has a history of hypersensitivity reaction to penicillins, the best choice is to select an alternative antibiotic with a different molecular structure [1, 41].

7.7.2 Neuromuscular Blocking Agents and Reversal Agents

Neuromuscular blocking agents are the first or second leading cause of anaphylaxis in many countries.

In France, they are responsible for about 60% of IgE-mediated perioperative anaphylaxis.

NAP 6 reports neuromuscular blocking agents as the allergic trigger in 64 cases (25%), including 32% of cases resulting in cardiac arrest or death.

The overall incidence of neuromuscular blocker-induced anaphylaxis was 5.3/100,000 exposures.

The highest incidence was seen with succinylcholine: 11.1/100,000.

95% of reactions occur within 5 min.

The suspected culprit is the tertiary or quaternary ammonium group, which is therefore associated with a high probability of cross-reactivity.

The risk of allergic reaction is highest with rocuronium (42% of cases), atracurium (35% of cases), succinylcholine (22% of cases), and lowest with cisatracurium.

Regarding reversal agents, Sugammadex has been shown to cause anaphylaxis in 1:64,000 exposures [1].

7.7.3 Chlorhexidine

An antiseptic agent is used for skin preparation at the surgical site. In NAP 6, 18 cases of anaphylaxis induced by chlorhexidine, accounting for 9% of anaphylaxis cases. The incidence of anaphylaxis is 0.78 per 100,000 exposures.

These reactions are also frequent in Belgium, Australia, and Denmark, while they remain rare in France, likely due to the predominant use of povidone-iodine in operating rooms.

Patients may become sensitized through the use of antiseptic mouthwashes, topical solutions, or previous use of antiseptics.

Cutaneous reactions to chlorhexidine are slower and milder compared to those caused by other agents.

7.7.4 Patent Blue

Dyes, mainly used by surgeons during surgical procedures (e.g., sentinel lymph node mapping), are the third most common cause of perioperative anaphylaxis in France. In the latest report, patent blue was responsible for 5.4% of all perioperative anaphylactic reactions [50, 51]. In the United Kingdom, 9 cases (3.4%) of anaphylaxis were induced by patent blue.

Incidence: 14.6 per 100,000 administrations.

Reactions often occur during or at the end of the procedure, depending on the route of administration.

Onset is slower than with other triggering agents, mostly occurring more than 15 min to over 60 min after administration.

Hypotension is the most common clinical manifestation, in some cases with systolic blood pressure dropping below 50 mmHg.

7.7.5 Latex

Allergic reactions to latex were much more frequent in the 1990s, when the HIV epidemic led to the widespread and continuous use of latex gloves. Due to high demand, these gloves were often made from lower-quality latex with higher protein content, resulting in increased sensitization among patients and healthcare staff.

The implementation of primary and secondary prevention measures, as well as the use of powder-free and higher-quality latex gloves, has led to a significant reduction in perioperative hypersensitivity reactions in recent years.

In sensitized patients, however, latex remains a serious concern.

In the operating room, systemic reactions to latex can result from exposure to latex proteins through various routes:

- Skin contact with anesthesia ventilation masks, tourniquets, ECG electrodes, adhesive tapes, elastic bandages, catheters, and ostomy bags.
- Contact with the mucous membranes of the mouth, vagina, urethra, or rectum.
- Contact with the peritoneum.
- Inhalational exposure via anesthesia equipment.

Prevention is key to the successful management of these patients.

For elective procedures, there is time to investigate this allergy in advance through:

- Targeted medical history. High-risk patients include those with multiple allergies, atopy, occupational exposure, those requiring intermittent catheterization, or those undergoing multiple procedures (e.g., reconstructive urologic surgery or repeated esophageal dilations for strictures). Information on reactions to bananas, avocados, kiwis, and other fruits, such as pineapple, is also important due to possible cross-reactivity.
- Allergy testing.

The skin prick test is performed with a standardized latex extract. It is the test of choice due to its high sensitivity (93%) and specificity (100%). If the test cannot be performed or is negative despite a high clinical suspicion, the allergy can be investigated by measuring specific IgE levels.

If both tests are negative but suspicion remains high, a provocation test may be performed.

Once high-risk patients are identified, particularly those with a history of grade 3 or 4 anaphylactic reactions, they should follow a latex-safe protocol:

- Schedule elective procedures preferably on Monday mornings or at least 6 h after the last procedure to allow for adequate air exchange and thorough cleaning of surfaces (e.g., first case of the operating session).
- Alert the intensive care unit and ensure the availability of a latex-safe bed.
- Inform all staff involved in the procedure about latex-safe protocols.
- Place signs at the entrance to the operating suite and within the clean pathway indicating "latex-safe protocol in effect"; post a sign at the entrance to the operating room indicating "latex-allergic patient".
- Only essential personnel should enter the operating room, and they should preferably remain inside until the end of the procedure to avoid inadvertent contamination.

- All staff must use latex-free surgical gloves (nitrile, neoprene).
- All personnel must use only certified latex-free devices, equipment, and supplies.
- Remove from the operating room any materials and equipment not required for the procedure;
- Cover non-replaceable and/or non-removable latex components (cables, mattresses, wheels) with plastic or aluminum food wrap, or with cotton or non-woven fabric drapes.
- In the absence of contraindications, use the operating room thus prepared also as the preparation and recovery area.

In the case of emergency procedures and known latex allergy, if the hospital facility is not equipped as required and the patient can be transferred, arrangements should be made to transport the patient to a better-equipped facility. If the patient cannot be transferred, procedures for managing this type of patient must be applied, and latex-free materials and instruments from the dedicated cart must be used.

In the case of emergency procedures and previously unknown latex allergy, in the event of an allergic reaction, initiate emergency treatment and use latex-free materials and instruments from dedicated carts, which must be available in every hospital facility [52].

7.8 Conclusions

Perioperative anaphylaxis is a rare complication of anesthesia but can be associated with significant morbidity and mortality. Immediate recognition of the reaction and early administration of adrenaline and fluid resuscitation are the cornerstones of management. Blood sampling for tryptase can help support the diagnosis of mast cell activation. It is advisable to perform allergy testing after the reaction to identify the causative agent and provide guidance for future anesthetics.

References

1. Harper NJN, Cook TM, Garcez T, et al. Anaesthesia, surgery, and life-threatening allergic reactions: epidemiology and clinical features of perioperative anaphylaxis in the 6th National Audit Project (NAP6). Br J Anaesth. 2018;121(1):159–71.
2. Harboe T, Guttormsen AB, Irgens A, et al. Anaphylaxis during anesthesia in Norway: a 6-year single-center follow-up study. Anesthesiology. 2005;102:897–903.
3. McClimon B, Rank M, Li J. The predictive value of skin testing in the diagnosis of local anesthetic allergy. Allergy Asthma Proc. 2011;32:95–8.
4. Kishiyama JL. Clinical immunology. In: LaDou J, Harrison RJ, editors. Current diagnosis & treatment: occupational & environmental medicine. 5th ed. New York: McGraw-Hill Education; 2014.
5. Heelan K, Sibbald C, Shear NH. Cutaneous reactions to drugs. In: Kang S, Amagai M, Bruckner AL, et al., editors. Fitzpatrick's dermatology. 9th ed. New York: McGraw-Hill Education; 2019.

6. Doenicke AW, Czeslick E, Moss J, Hoernecke R. Onset time. Endotracheal intubating conditions, and plasma histamine after Cisatracurium and Vecuronium administration. Anesth Analg. 1998;87:434–8.
7. Mertes PM, Alla F, Trechot P, Auroy Y, Jougla E. Anaphylaxis during anesthesia in France: an 8-year national survey. J Allergy Clin Immunol. 2011;128:366–73.
8. Mertes PM, Laxenaire M-C, Alla F, Peranesthesiques GdaEdRA. Anaphylactic and anaphylactoid reactions occurring during anesthesia in France in 1999–2000. Anesthesiology. 2003;99:536–45.
9. Mertes PM. Anaphylactic reactions during anaesthesia—let us treat the problem rather than debating its existence. Acta Anaesthesiol Scand. 2005;49:431–3.
10. Khan D, Solensky R. Drug allergy. J Allergy Clin Immunol. 2010;125:S126–37.
11. Ewan PW, Dugu EP, Mirakian R, Dixon TA, Harper JN, Nasser SM. BSACI guidelines for the investigation of suspected anaphylaxis during general anaesthesia. Clin Exp Allergy. 2010;40:15–31.
12. Franco Hernandez JA, Garcia Hernandez A, Lahoz Rodriguez D. Kounis syndrome secondary to an allergic reaction to metamizole. Rev Esp Anestesiol Reanim. 2012;59:217–9.
13. Michavila Gomez AV, Belver Gonzalez MT, Alvarez NC, Drug allergy Work Group of the Spanish Society of Paediatric Allergy I, et al. Perioperative anaphylactic reactions: Review and procedure protocol in paediatrics. Allergol Immunopathol (Madr). 2015;43:203–14.
14. Fisher MM, Ramakrishnan N, Doig G, Rose M, Baldo B. The investigation of bronchospasm during induction of anaesthesia. Acta Anaesthesiol Scand. 2009;53:1006–11.
15. Mertes PM, Laxenaire M-C. Allergy and anaphylaxis in anaesthesia. Minerva Anestesiol. 2004;70:285–91.
16. Malinovsky J-M, Decagny S, Wessel F, et al. Systematic follow-up increases the incidence of anaphylaxis during adverse reactions in anesthetized patients. Acta Anaesthesiol Scand. 2008;52:175–81.
17. De Souza RL, Short T, Warman GR, Maclennan N, Young Y. Anaphylaxis with associated fibrinolysis, reversed with tranexamic acid and demonstrated by thrombelastography. Anaesth Intensive Care. 2004;32:580–7.
18. Mertes PM, Malinovsky JM, Jouffroy L, et al. Reducing the risk of anaphylaxis during anesthesia: 2011 updated guidelines for clinical practice. J Investig Allergol Clin Immunol. 2011;21:442–53.
19. Dewachter P, Mouton-Faivre C, Emala CW. Anaphylaxis and anesthesia: controversies and new insights. Anesthesiology. 2009;111:1141–50.
20. Mirone C, Preziosi D, Mascheri A, et al. Identification of risk factors for severe hypersensitivity reactions in general anesthesia. Clin Mol Allergy. 2015;13:11.
21. Garvey LH, Belhage B, Krigaard M, et al. Treatment with epinephrine (adrenaline) in suspected anaphylaxis during anesthesia in Denmark. Anesthesiology. 2011;115:111–6.
22. Escolano F, Valero A, Huguet J, et al. Prospective epidemiologic study of perioperative anaphylactoid reactions occurring in Catalonia (1996-7). Rev Esp Anestesiol Reanim. 2002;49:286–93.
23. Kemp AM, Kemp SF. Pharmacotherapy in refractory anaphylaxis: when intramuscular epinephrine fails. Curr Opin Allergy Clin Immunol. 2014;14:371–8.
24. Campbell RL, Li JT, Nicklas RA, Sadosty AT, Members of the Joint Task Force. Practice Parameter Workgroup. Emergency department diagnosis and treatment of anaphylaxis: a practice parameter. Ann Allergy Asthma Immunol. 2014;113:599–608.
25. Lo JC, Darracq MA, Clark RF. A review of methylene blue treatment for cardiovascular collapse. J Emerg Med. 2014;46:670–9.
26. Zheng F, Barthel G, Collange O, et al. Methylene blue and epinephrine: a synergistic association for the treatment of anaphylactic shock. Crit Care Med. 2013;41:195–204.
27. Sheikh A, Ten Broek V, Brown SG, et al. H1-antihistamines for the treatment of anaphylaxis: Cochrane systematic review. Allergy. 2007;62:830–7.

28. Choo KJL, Simons FER, Sheikh A. Glucocorticoids for the treatment of anaphylaxis. Cochrane systematic review. Allergy. 2010;65:1205–11.
29. Berroa F, Lafuente A, Javaloyes G, et al. The usefulness of different plasma histamine and tryptase cut-off points in the diagnosis of peri-anaesthetic hypersensitivity reactions. Clin Exp Allergy. 2014;44:270–7.
30. Soar J, Pumphrey R, Cant A, Working Group of the Resuscitation C, et al. Emergency treatment of anaphylactic reactions—guidelines for healthcare providers. Resuscitation. 2008;77:157–69.
31. Sadleir PHM, Clarke RC, Bozic B, et al. Consequences of proceeding with surgery after resuscitation from intra-operative anaphylaxis. Anaesthesia. 2018;73:32–9.
32. Whitaker DK, Bratteb G, Smith AF, et al. The Helsinki declaration on patient safety in Anaesthesiology: putting words into practice. Best Pract Res Clin Anaesthesiol. 2011;25:277–90.
33. Schwartz LB. Diagnostic value of tryptase in anaphylaxis and mastocytosis. Immunol Allergy Clin N Am. 2006;26:451–63.
34. Harper NJ, Dixon T, Dugue P, et al. Suspected anaphylactic reactions associated with anaesthesia. Anaesthesia. 2009;64:199–211.
35. Krishna MT, York M, Chin T, et al. Multi-centre retrospective analysis of anaphylaxis during general anaesthesia in the United Kingdom: aetiology and diagnostic performance of acute serum tryptase. Clin Exp Immunol. 2014;178:399e404.
36. Kroigaard M, Garvey LH, Gillberg L, et al. Scandinavian Clinical Practice Guidelines on the diagnosis, management and follow-up of anaphylaxis during anaesthesia. Acta Anaesthesiol Scand. 2007;51:655e70.
37. Mirone C, Preziosi D, Mascheri A, et al. Identification of risk factors for severe hypersensitivity reactions during general anesthesia. Clin Mol Allergy. 2015;13:11.
38. Opstrup MS, Poulsen LK, Malling HJ, et al. Dynamics of plasma levels of specific IgE in chlorhexidine-allergic patients with and without accidental re-exposure. Clin Exp Allergy. 2016;46:1090e8.
39. Caffarelli C, Stringari G, Miraglia M, et al. Prevention of allergic reactions in anesthetized patients. Int J Immunopathol Pharmacol. 2011;24:S91–9.
40. Hjortlund J, Mortz CG, Stage TB, et al. Positive serum specific IgE has a short half-life in patients with penicillin allergy and its disappearance does not always indicate tolerance. Clin Transl Allergy. 2014;4:34.
41. Laguna JJ, Archilla J, Dona I, et al. Practical guidelines for perioperative hypersensitivity reactions. J Investig Allergol Clin Immunol. 2018;28:216e32.
42. World Allergy Organization. Drug allergies. Available at: https://www.worldallergy.org/education-and-programs/education/allergic-disease-resource-center/professionals/drug-allergies. Accessed 8 June 2020.
43. Anderson J, Rose M, Green S, et al. The utility of specific IgE testing to chlorhexidine in the investigation of perioperative adverse reactions. Ann Allergy Asthma Immunol. 2015;114:425–426.e1.
44. Ebo DG, Faber M, Elst J, et al. In vitro diagnosis of immediate drug hypersensitivity during anesthesia: a review of the literature. J Allergy Clin Immunol Pract. 2018;6:1176e84.
45. Caimmi S, Caimmi D, Cardinale F, et al. Perioperative allergy: uncommon agents. Int J Immunopathol Pharmacol. 2011;24:S61–8.
46. Bernardini R, Cardinale F, Franceschini F, et al. Perioperative allergies. Bologna: Ed Editeam; 2009. p. 89–94.
47. Kranke B, Aberer W. Skin testing for IgE-mediated drug allergy. Immunol Allergy Clin. 2009;29:503e16. https://doi.org/10.1016/j.iac.2009.04.003.
48. Brockow K, Romano A, Blanca M, et al. General considerations for skin test procedures in the diagnosis of drug hypersensitivity. Allergy Eur J Allergy Clin Immunol. 2002;57:45–51.
49. Dewachter P, Mouton-Faivre C, Castells MC, et al. Anesthesia in patients with multiple drug allergies: are all allergies the same? Curr Opin Anaesthesiol. 2011;24(3):320e5.

50. Tacquard C, Collange O, Gomis P, et al. Anaesthetic hypersensitivity reactions in France between 2011 and 2012: the 10th GERAP epidemiologic survey. Acta Anaesthesiol Scand. 2017;61:290–9.
51. Mertes PM, Malinovsky JM, Mouton-Faivre C, et al. Anaphylaxis to dyes during the perioperative period: reports of 14 clinical cases. J Allergy Clin Immunol. 2008;122:348–52.
52. Guidelines of the Lombardy Region for the prevention of latex allergic reactions in patients and healthcare workers.

8 New ESAIC Guidelines on Neuromuscular Blockade

Edoardo De Robertis, Rachele Simonte, and Enrico Bertoli

8.1 Introduction

Curare originated as a hunting poison in the heart of the Amazon rainforest. In 1577, Diego de Ortegón observed, in the upper Rio Napo region of the Amazon basin, blowguns and arrows coated with herbs that "once in the blood, kill rapidly," but it was not until 1596, with Lawrence Keymis leading an expedition in Guyana, that the term ourari (or k-urary, "where it comes, one dies") was first recorded.

In 1608, the Franciscan Fray Pedro de Aguado reported "small scratches without remedy, because the poison carried in the blood reaches the heart within twenty-four hours, causing tremors and loss of reason, to the point of uttering atrocious and desperate phrases."

In 1850, Pelouze and Bernard demonstrated that curare, the poison used by some South American indigenous tribes, abolished the effect of nerve stimulation on muscle without affecting the excitability of either the nerve or the muscle. It was initially believed that curare and nicotine acted directly on the muscles, rather than on the nerve endings, until it was shown that stimulation of the vagus nerve produced a substance, later identified as acetylcholine (ACh), the neurotransmitter at the neuromuscular junction of voluntary muscle.

In 1942, in Montreal, H.R. Griffith and E. Johnson used a preparation based on d-tubocurarine during anesthesia, in combination with tracheal intubation and mechanical ventilation, which was already being used successfully by the end of World War II. However, the practice of curarization was not immediately well

E. De Robertis (✉) · R. Simonte · E. Bertoli
Section of Anesthesia, Intensive Care, Critical Care and Pain Management, Department of Medicine and Surgery, University of Perugia, Perugia, Italy
e-mail: edoardo.derobertis@unipg.it; rachele.simonte@unipg.it; enrico.bertoli@studenti.unipg.it

D. Chiumello, A. De Gasperi (eds.), *Practical Trends in Anesthesia and Intensive Care 2026*, https://doi.org/10.1007/978-3-032-25721-5_8

received: the president of the French Society of Anesthesiology condemned it as a sacrilegious act, stating that "God gave man breath, and only God has the right to take it away."

In 1961, Dam and Goldman [1] highlighted that the most frequent cause of postoperative respiratory problems was the *use and misuse* of neuromuscular blocking agents. In 1979, the acronym PORC, *postoperative residual curarization,* was coined, and in the following years, increasing evidence suggested that residual neuromuscular blockade was among the risk factors for the development of pulmonary complications, with a direct impact on patient outcomes [2].

In 2019, after 40 years, Naveen [3] reported that 20.5% of patients still experienced postoperative residual neuromuscular blockade, which tripled the likelihood of admission to intensive care. Moreover, in a survey of 1629 anesthesiologists in 80 countries, only 57% of responses regarding neuromuscular blockade were correct.

Also in 2019, the results of the POPULAR study [4], commissioned by the then European Society of Anaesthesiology, were of great interest. The study concluded that the use of neuromuscular blocking agents was associated with an increase in postoperative complications and that the use of reversal agents did not reduce this risk. In reality, the study reveals a sobering snapshot of how neuromuscular blocking agents were being used, which deserves closer examination. The study was conducted in 221 hospitals across 28 European countries, including 17,150 patients who had received neuromuscular blocking agents. As many as 10,282 patients (59.9%) did not undergo neuromuscular block monitoring, and 8355 (47.8%) did not receive a reversal agent. Extubation was performed based on clinical criteria in 68.7% of cases, and only 16.5% were extubated with a TOFR$\geq$0.9.

Unfortunately, this is a rather disheartening picture, despite irrefutable evidence of the importance of monitoring and the need for careful and proper management of neuromuscular blockade.

Residual neuromuscular blockade (rNMB) remains today one of the major postoperative complications encountered, despite advances in neuromuscular monitoring techniques and the types and dosages of reversal agents for neuromuscular blockers. Even now, routine use of neuromuscular monitoring is limited and inadequate, resulting in an unacceptable risk of residual neuromuscular blockade and potentially life-threatening complications. As highlighted in the POPULAR study, neuromuscular monitoring is often unavailable, and peripheral nerve stimulation is used in less than 50% of cases in patients receiving neuromuscular blockade.

A large number of practitioners continue to rely on clinical assessments, but the truth is that there are no clinical tests that can reliably predict either the achievement of an adequate level of neuromuscular blockade, adequate recovery from blockade, or, even less so, are sufficiently sensitive to detect residual neuromuscular blockade.

In conclusion, the archaic practice known as "guided by experience" should have no place in modern anesthesiology or intensive care practice.

8.2 ESAIC Guidelines

In light of this complex yet scientifically clear situation, the European Society of Anaesthesiology and Intensive Care (ESAIC) sought to review the latest evidence in the literature and publish guidelines on the management of perioperative neuromuscular blockade [5], in order to provide recommendations for good clinical practice and improve the overall management of patients receiving neuromuscular blocking agents.

Specifically, the recently published European guidelines address eight different areas of practice in adult surgical patients, including both routine and rapid sequence induction and intubation scenarios, examining the depth of blockade according to surgical requirements and the use of specific reversal agents in particular clinical situations.

The ESAIC guidelines were developed by 14 experts from 9 different countries and follow the publication of other national society guidelines. The ESAIC guidelines addressed three main clinical questions:

1. Is the use of muscle relaxants necessary to facilitate intubation in adult patients?
2. Does the intensity of neuromuscular blockade influence outcomes in abdominal surgery?
3. What are the strategies for the diagnosis and treatment of residual neuromuscular paralysis?

Following a rigorous and well-defined ESAIC methodology, a thorough review of the literature was conducted, which, through various steps, led to the analysis and review of 88 scientific studies and the following main recommendations:

1. Intubation conditions are poor in 27% of non-relaxed patients compared to 3% of patients who received neuromuscular blocking agents.
2. Routine use of deep blockade is not necessary; a personalized approach is preferable.
3. The use of sugammadex is effective in reversing deep, moderate, or superficial blockade.
4. Sugammadex is preferable to neostigmine for deep, moderate, and superficial neuromuscular blockade induced by rocuronium.
5. Neostigmine may be used as an alternative to sugammadex for minimal neuromuscular blockade (TOF ratio from 0.4 to less than 0.9) induced by rocuronium.
6. Consider neostigmine for blockades deeper than minimal, based on clinical judgment but within the context of quantitative monitoring, with the clear understanding that deep blockades require more time to achieve a TOF ratio greater than or equal to 0.9.
7. It is impossible to accurately predict the depth of neuromuscular blockade using clinical tests or qualitative assessment.

8. Objective confirmation of a TOF of 0.9 or higher, obtained using quantitative methods, is essential before tracheal extubation.
9. Use ulnar nerve stimulation and quantitative neuromuscular monitoring with thumb monitoring.

In particular, the guidelines emphasize that there is compelling evidence that residual paralysis and pulmonary complications associated with neuromuscular blockade are less frequent after pharmacological reversal with sugammadex compared to neostigmine. Furthermore, the use of quantitative neuromuscular blockade monitoring is the main prerequisite for any appropriate perioperative management strategy of neuromuscular blockade.

The need for quantitative monitoring is not new and has been discussed extensively over the years. Most calls for its adoption have largely been ignored, and the actual number of anesthesiologists routinely using quantitative monitoring remains inadequate, resulting in unacceptably high rates of postoperative residual neuromuscular blockade (RNMB). The ESAIC guidelines on neuromuscular blockade management are the first to incorporate an explicit implementation strategy and to propose practical tools for its application.

By combining principles of quality and evidence-based medicine, good clinical practices can be implemented in daily care. However, to truly achieve this goal and put it into practice, all members of the anesthesia team must be actively involved, and their behavior must be guided by fundamental safety principles. Within a given department, it is essential that the guidelines are disseminated among anesthesiologists to help improve their theoretical and practical knowledge of neuromuscular monitoring and the appropriate use of drugs. ESAIC is committed to supporting the development of educational tools dedicated to the practical dissemination of knowledge, but beyond knowledge dissemination, it will be necessary to analyze barriers to guideline implementation related to the attitudes and beliefs of anesthesiologists. Clearly, the new ESAIC guidelines provide clinicians with an additional tool for the proper management of neuromuscular blockade, suggesting clear behavioral strategies and indicating their respective levels of evidence.

Finally, one last point deserves consideration. Simultaneously with the ESAIC guidelines, the American Society of Anesthesiologists (ASA) also published guidelines on neuromuscular blockade [6].

The two guidelines, developed completely independently but following the same rigorous methodological approach, present entirely overlapping recommendations. The task forces established by ASA and ESAIC chose recognized and transparent approaches, as well as a reproducible methodology to develop their respective recommendations. Neither task force was aware of the other's existence. Both acted independently (also due to the COVID-19 pandemic). Nevertheless, the published guidelines are in fact almost identical, further strengthening both the methodologies applied and the set of recommendations developed [7].

The ESAIC guidelines have some limitations, the main ones being:

- Pediatric patients are also at risk of RNMB, but the current guidelines do not address the pediatric population.
- The guidelines focus on perioperative management of neuromuscular blockade and do not consider NMB in the ICU.
- Monitoring sites other than the ulnar nerve/adductor pollicis muscle are not examined.
- Studies on how to manage emergency reintubation immediately after sugammadex reversal are lacking.
- Further studies are needed to better understand the clinical situations in which deep NMB may be beneficial.

In order to further explore the topics analyzed in the ESAIC guidelines, the following pages will focus on the following points:

- Reversing neuromuscular blockade with the aim of reducing residual neuromuscular blockade (TOFr <0.9) and related complications.
- Guiding clinicians toward appropriate monitoring.
- Using the most suitable reversal agent, also based on the depth of neuromuscular blockade.
- Recommendations for the implementation of QUANTITATIVE monitoring.

Topics related to the appropriate use of neuromuscular blocking agents in the management of difficult airways and issues concerning intraoperative NMB management aimed at optimizing intubation and surgical management will not be addressed.

8.3 Neuromuscular Blocking Agents and Antagonists

Neuromuscular blocking agents are drugs that interfere with the function of the motor endplate by acting on the cholinergic receptor nicotinic. The introduction of muscle relaxants into clinical practice marked a milestone in the history of anesthesia, improving intraoperative surgical conditions and facilitating the procedure of orotracheal intubation.

All drugs that block neuromuscular transmission are structurally similar to acetylcholine (ACh) and are mono- or bis-quaternary amines with low lipid solubility. This, combined with high ionization, results in an inability to cross membranes and a limited volume of distribution. These drugs are highly polar, and the ED95 expresses, in mg/kg, the effective dose required to achieve a 95% blockade of receptors, specific for each drug. Duration of action and receptor competition follow the law of mass action; onset time is calculated from drug administration to the point of maximum effect, while duration is measured from administration to recovery of

25% up to 100% of receptor function. Monitoring neuromuscular function, therefore, allows for appropriate dosing and titration of this class of drugs.

Neuromuscular blocking agents are divided into depolarizing agonists and non-depolarizing antagonists.

Among the depolarizing agents, succinylcholine is notable for its short duration of action, due to rapid hydrolysis—less than 10 minutes—by plasma and hepatic pseudocholinesterases. It acts at the nicotinic receptor site with an effect similar to ACh, mimicking its actions such as depolarization and generalized contraction of multiple muscle motor units (phase I block). Indeed, paralysis is preceded by transient fasciculations, which cause the release of serum K+. Repeated doses of succinylcholine may lead to receptor desensitization due to ineffective ACh action at the receptor, resulting in failure of repolarization (phase II block).

Non-depolarizing muscle relaxants act on the nicotinic receptor by competing with ACh. At high doses, they can penetrate the ion channel of the receptor and block prejunctional Na + channels, causing an even more intense blockade. They are antagonists of the nicotinic receptor and prevent the endogenous neurotransmitter from binding to the receptor.

Larger muscles such as the diaphragm are more resistant to blockade and recover more rapidly; this is not the case for the muscles involved in swallowing, which explains why clinical monitoring of neuromuscular recovery can be misleading, giving a false impression of restored respiratory capacity when the patient may not have fully regained control of the upper airway.

There are two families within this class of curare derivatives. The steroidal agents, such as Pancuronium, Vecuronium, Rocuronium, and Pipecuronium, are metabolized hepatically and renally. Atracurium, Cisatracurium, and Mivacurium are benzylisoquinolinium agents, metabolized in plasma via the Hoffmann elimination, a non-enzymatic pathway dependent on blood pH and physiological temperature.

These molecules differ in their pharmacokinetics and can be antagonized by acetylcholinesterase inhibitors.

Anticholinesterases Acetylcholinesterase is the target of these drugs, which, through hydrolysis, break the covalent acetyl-enzyme bond, increasing endogenous ACh concentration. Neostigmine, Edrophonium, and Pyridostigmine differ only in their pharmacokinetic properties, and their clinical parasympathomimetic effects are due to increased nicotinic neurotransmitter levels. As a result, bradycardia, vasodilation, hypotension, bronchoconstriction, increased gastric motility, and increased gastric and salivary secretions may occur. All these effects are counteracted by atropine, an agonist of the cholinergic receptor. Reversal of the block is achieved with a mixture of neostigmine (0.04/0.07 mg/kg IV) and atropine (0.3/0.6 mg/kg).

Sugammadex This is a gamma-cyclodextrin composed of eight oligosaccharide molecules forming a cyclic structure with a hydrophilic exterior and a hydrophobic central cavity. The diameter of the cavity adapts to the size of the molecule to be encapsulated, while the depth determines the binding strength. The structure is suitable for accommodating large molecules such as aminosteroidal muscle relaxants (Rocuronium, Vecuronium), whose quaternary ammonium groups stabilize the binding. The stable curare-sugammadex complex reduces the free concentration of curare in the central compartment, creating a concentration gradient that allows the release of nicotinic receptors at the postsynaptic level. The speed of this process depends on the timing of administration, drug kinetics, and concentration.

Just as it is important to ensure adequate anesthesia, it is also essential to verify that the clinical effects of muscle relaxants have worn off upon patient awakening, to avoid residual paralysis, which can cause postoperative pulmonary comorbidities. Therefore, reversal of neuromuscular block—whether with neostigmine, sugammadex, or spontaneous resolution—must be appropriately monitored.

8.4 Neuromuscular Monitoring

In the safety recommendations for the operating room issued by the Ministry of Labor, Health, and Social Policies in October 2009, section 4.5: "preventing anesthesia-related harm by ensuring vital functions," it is clearly stated that "neuromuscular transmission monitoring must always be available."

Neuromuscular monitoring is based on the use of a acceleromyograph that measures, using a piezoelectric transducer, the acceleration of isotonic muscle contraction. The depth of the block is primarily assessed by measuring the contraction of the adductor pollicis muscle elicited by stimulating the ulnar nerve (other monitoring sites include the posterior tibial or facial nerve).

The stimulus used to evoke contraction usually has a rectangular waveform with a duration of 0.2 milliseconds. In clinical practice, two main stimulation modalities are employed:

1. Single-twitch: supramaximal electrical stimulus at 0.1–1 Hz, useful for assessing the exact onset time of a neuromuscular block (onset time), when the muscle response to single-twitch is below 20%.
2. TOF (train-of-four) stimulation: delivery of 4 supramaximal stimuli every 0.5 seconds at a frequency of 2 Hz. In the presence of a non-depolarizing block, a sequential reduction in twitch amplitude is observed. The TOF ratio is the ratio between the fourth and the first contraction. The TOF ratio is useful intraoperatively and provides information on the need for additional drug dosing, when to administer the antagonist, and when to extubate the patient, considering the neuromuscular block resolved when the TOF ratio is >0.9.
3. Tetanic stimulation: used in conjunction with TOF when an adequate depth of neuromuscular block has been achieved and the TOF response is abolished. Tetanic stimulation at 50 Hz for 5 seconds induces acetylcholine release and sustained contraction during the stimulus, known as post-tetanic facilitation. A post-tetanic count (PTC) is obtained by applying, 3 seconds after the tetanus, a 1 Hz

stimulation every 15 seconds and counting the responses. The PTC is useful for determining the onset of neuromuscular block recovery and distinguishing between deep and moderate block.

Over the course of the history of neuromuscular block management, monitoring of peripheral nerve stimulation has been refined, with the introduction in 1970 of the TOF concept [8] (TOF 2 Hz, duration 2″).

In the study published by Viby-Mogensen [9], the concept of residual neuromuscular block is defined as a TOFr <0.7, as it was observed that a TOFr of approximately 0.7 corresponded to vital capacity and inspiratory capacity similar to physiological values.

With further research, the lower limit of the TOFr was raised to 0.9. This finding has been supported by several authors who demonstrated that a TOFr <0.9 may be associated with the appearance of symptoms such as:

- Weakness.
- Impaired hypoxic ventilatory response.
- Upper airway obstruction.
- Increased risk of aspiration.
- Prolonged stay in the PACU.

There is broad consensus that recovery from neuromuscular block occurs at a TOFr > = 0.9; such monitoring is performed on the adductor pollicis muscle after ulnar nerve stimulation.

The electrodes used should not have a diameter greater than 7–11 mm and should be positioned at a distance of 2.5–4 cm from each other.

This is because the use of inappropriate electrodes and/or incorrect positioning may result in inadequate nerve stimulation and compromise monitoring, with consequences for the assessment of neuromuscular block recovery.

Since the study by Viby-Mogensen, published in 1979 [9], and in subsequent studies, it has been shown that residual neuromuscular block at the end of the surgical procedure and/or in the PACU is common following the use of non-depolarizing neuromuscular blockers, with an incidence of 64% [10, 11].

But what are the factors contributing to this high incidence?

I. Variability in the action of neuromuscular blocking agents (there is no specific time that can guarantee adequate spontaneous recovery from the block [12, 13]).
II. Use of clinical assessments of neuromuscular block (head lift, inspiratory strength and pattern, tongue protrusion, tidal volume, handgrip strength).
III. Widespread use of peripheral nerve stimulation to assess the block, with the erroneous belief that four equal twitches or a sustained tetanic response indicate complete recovery.
IV. Proper use of neuromuscular blocker antagonists, which depends on accurate monitoring of block depth.

It should be noted that the "fixed dose and blind"; however, while the use of Sugammadex has drastically reduced the incidence of residual blockade, the problem persists with Neostigmine.

When discussing neuromuscular blockade monitoring, we can distinguish between different types of monitoring, although, as previously stated, some types of monitoring cannot provide a true indication of residual NMB [pulmonary complications (respiratory failure, hypoxia, pulmonary edema, atelectasis, bronchospasm, aspiration pneumonia) and/or other adverse events]:

- Clinical assessment (head lift, tongue protrusion, tidal volume, inspiratory strength, handgrip strength, etc.)
- QUALITATIVE assessment (peripheral nerve stimulation).
- QUANTITATIVE monitoring (TOFr).

It can be stated that QUANTITATIVE monitoring results in a lower incidence of residual neuromuscular blockade compared to qualitative or clinical assessment. This difference is significant and substantial.

8.5 Recommendations

1. *When QUANTITATIVE monitoring is used, it is strongly recommended to achieve a TOFr > = 0.9 before extubation.*

By analyzing residual NMB, the following incidences can be defined:

Outcome	Incidence of residual NMB
Sugammadex	
Confirmed TOFr	0.5%
TOFr not confirmed	2.2%
Qualitative assessment	13.8%
Clinical assessment	8.9%
Neostigmine	
Confirmed TOFr	5.3%
TOFr not confirmed	44.9%
Qualitative assessment	6.5%
Clinical assessment	24.9%

2. *What are the common issues encountered during monitoring?*

One of the issues that may arise with the acceleromyograph (specifically developed for routine quantitative neuromuscular monitoring because it is easy to use and provides reliable results) is the calibration of the TOFr baseline, which often exceeds a value of 1.0.

Therefore, it is clear that, in the context of NMB assessment, baseline calibration is of fundamental importance, in addition to the correct use and placement of electrodes.

3. *What factors influence QUANTITATIVE monitoring?*

So far, we have confirmed that with a TOFr > = 0.9, the the risk of residual NMB is minimal, but there are several factors that influence its measurement, one of which is the choice of the muscle being stimulated.

Specifically, when stimulating the adductor pollicis muscle, the time required to achieve a TOFr > = 0.9 is longer compared to:

- Corrugator supercilii muscle (facial nerve).
- Orbicularis oculi muscle (facial nerve).
- Flexor hallucis brevis muscle (posterior tibial nerve).

4. *Sugammadex or Neostigmine?*

The premise regarding the reversal of neuromuscular blocking agents is that, in this context, with the introduction of Sugammadex (a gamma-cyclodextrin derivative that inactivates rocuronium by encapsulating free molecules and forming a stable complex), the incidence of residual NMB and the recovery time from NMB, compared to the administration of Neostigmine, have been clearly reduced. The analysis to be performed in this context concerns the efficacy and safety of non-depolarizing NMB antagonists in order to achieve recovery from blockade.

Patients who received a neuromuscular blocking agent (especially rocuronium) and were reversed with Sugammadex experience a faster recovery (complete/moderate/shallow/minimal) and a lower risk of residual NMB compared to those reversed with Neostigmine.

For this reason, the use of Sugammadex is recommended over Neostigmine for deep or moderate NMB, while Neostigmine remains a reasonable alternative for minimal NMB (TOFr from 0.4 up to less than 0.9).

Some studies have reported an incidence of anaphylaxis of 1.6/10,000 in patients who received Sugammadex [14–16]. In one of these, a case of hypersensitivity was reported after administration of Sugammadex at 8.4 mg/kg, with symptoms including paresthesia of the hand and face, moderately blurred vision, dysgeusia, nausea, tachycardia, and epigastric pain.

No significant differences in bradycardia, tachycardia, or arrhythmias have been observed between sugammadex and neostigmine.

Similarly, no substantial differences in pulmonary complications have been reported, except for one study [17], which described a case of re-intubation after administration of N.

Regarding PONV, the incidence is lower with Sugammadex.

5. *What is the appropriate dosage for sugammadex?*
   - 2 mg/kg for a TOF of 2 up to a TOFr <0.9
   - 4 mg/kg for a PTC of 1 up to TOF 1
   - 16 mg/kg for immediate reversal of a single dose of rocuronium 1.2 mg/kg

   Overdose:

- 32 mg/kg (2× the maximum therapeutic dose).
- There have been case reports of administration of 40 mg/kg.

  Adverse events related to overdose:

- Dysgeusia 66.7%.
- Nausea 16.7%.
- Fatigue 16.7%.
- Laryngopharyngeal pain 16.7%.
- Headache 16.7%.
- Postural vertigo 8.3%.
- Abdominal pain 8.3%.
- Urinary urgency 8.3%.

6. *"Fixed Dose and Blind" Approach*

An important issue encountered during the reversal phase of neuromuscular blockade is the frequent use of the "fixed dose and blind" approach (Neostigmine 5 mg or Sugammadex 200 mg without first accurately assessing the depth of the block), which, however, does not imply full recovery.

The dosage of Neostigmine is 30 mcg/kg for minimal NMB, with maximal effect occurring in approximately <10 min. When Neostigmine has reached its peak but the TOFr<0.9, we have three options:

1. Allow continued spontaneous recovery.
2. Administer Sugammadex at the appropriate dose.
3. If a low initial dose of Neostigmine was given, an additional dose may be administered (up to a maximum of 50 mcg/kg; higher doses have not shown any additional effect).

7. *How to choose the reversal agent.*

   Several factors must be considered when selecting a reversal agent:

1. The type of NMB used.
2. Depth of the block.
3. Efficacy of the reversal agent on the NMB.

4. Side effects of the reversal agent.
5. Time required to achieve complete reversal.

Analyzing the depth of NMB and the choice of reversal agent, we see that the dose of Neostigmine that should be used for minimal NMB should not exceed 40 mcg/kg. When the TOFr exceeds 0.6–1.5, the appropriate dose is 30 mcg/kg.

A higher dose of Neostigmine (>30 mcg/kg) may result in the paradoxical effect of weakness after spontaneous recovery and TOFr> = 0.9. This can be avoided if quantitative monitoring is used [15].

When quantitative monitoring is not available and greater certainty is desired during extubation, a 10-minute interval should be observed after Neostigmine administration, whereas with monitoring, extubation can proceed when TOFr> = 0.9.

8. *How to reverse a benzylisoquinolinium NMB?*

To avoid residual NMB after administration of drugs such as atracurium or cisatracurium when using qualitative monitoring, the following is recommended:

1. Use Neostigmine at minimal NMB depth (Sugammadex has no effect).
2. In the absence of quantitative monitoring (which should be avoided), wait 10 minutes after reversal before proceeding with extubation.
3. If qualitative monitoring is used, extubation can proceed when a TOFr> = 0.9 is confirmed.

9. *How to monitor a succinylcholine-induced NMB?*

The only way to monitor NMB induced by succinylcholine (whether with normal or abnormal pseudocholinesterase function) is by measuring the single twitch height and using the percentage of that single twitch to assess the return of strength. When the regression of the block does not fall within the normal range, this may indicate abnormal pseudocholinesterase activity.

NM monitoring is recommended for extubation when there are clinical signs of delayed recovery from succinylcholine-induced NMB.

8.6 Conclusions

In summary, the benefits of complete recovery include greater patient satisfaction, shorter PACU stays, fewer pulmonary complications, and reduced mortality.

For safe and high-quality practice, the available evidence is unequivocal in supporting the need for quantitative NMB monitoring and the correct use of the drugs at our disposal.

Scientific societies provide clinicians with the tools to improve daily clinical practice. Is this enough? Certainly not. Guidelines must be implemented, and to achieve this, educational efforts are needed at all levels to ensure widespread adoption of the best clinical practices recommended. It is important to use every means to promote its understanding and acceptance, and consequently its dissemination and implementation in all anesthesia departments. The role of scientific societies is fundamental; in addition to providing scientific tools based on EBM, they must also help eliminate all barriers that may prevent clinicians from having the necessary resources to apply the recommendations in the best possible way.

References

1. Dam WH, Guldmann N. Inadequate postanesthetic ventilation. Curare, anesthetic, narcotic, diffusion hypoxia. Anesthesiology. 1961;22:699–707.
2. Fuchs-Buder T. Residual neuromuscular blockade and postoperative pulmonary outcome: the missing piece of the puzzle. Eur J Anaesthesiol. 2014;31:401–3.
3. Naveen N. Of confidence and consequence: outcomes and knowledge of postoperative residual neuromuscular blockade. Anesth Analg. 2019;28(6):1055.
4. Kirmeier E, Eriksson LI, Lewald H, Fagerlund MJ, Hoeft A, Hollmann M, Meistelman C, Hunter JM, Ulm K, Blobner M; POPULAR Contributors. Post-anaesthesia pulmonary complications after use of muscle relaxants (POPULAR): a multicentre, prospective observational study. Lancet Respir Med. 2019;7:129–40.
5. Fuchs-Buder T, Romero CS, Lewald H, Lamperti M, Afshari A, Hristovska AM, Schmartz D, Hinkelbein J, Longrois D, Popp M, de Boer HD, Sorbello M, Jankovic R, Kranke P. Perioperative management of neuromuscular blockade: a guideline from the European Society of Anaesthesiology and Intensive Care. Eur J Anaesthesiol. 2023;40(2):82–94.
6. Thilen SR, Weigel WA, Todd MM, Dutton RP, Lien CA, Grant SA, Szokol JW, Eriksson JL, Yaster M, Grant MD, Agarkar M, Marbella AM, Blanck JF, Domino KB. 2023 American Society of Anesthesiologists practice guidelines for monitoring and antagonism of neuromuscular blockade: a report by the American Society of Anesthesiologists task force on neuromuscular blockade. Anesthesiology. 2023;138:13–41.
7. Fuchs-Buder T, De Robertis E, Thilen SR, Champeau MW. Joint letter to the editor from the American Society of Anesthesiologists and the European Society of Anaesthesiology and Intensive Care on Management of Neuromuscular Blockade. Anesthesiology. 2023;139(3):366–7.
8. Ali HH, Utting JE, Gray C. Stimulus frequency in the detection of neuromuscular block in humans. Br J Anaesth. 1970;42:967–78.
9. Viby-Mogensen J, Jørgensen BC, Ording H. Residual curarization in the recovery room. Anesthesiology. 1979;50:539–41.
10. Fortier LP, McKeen D, Turner K, de Médicis E, Warriner B, Jones PM, Chaput A, Pouliot JF, Galarneau A. The RECITE Study: a Canadian prospective, multicenter study of the incidence and severity of residual neuromuscular blockade. Anesth Analg. 2015;121:366–72.
11. Saager L, Maiese EM, Bash LD, Meyer TA, Minkowitz H, Groudine S, Philip BK, Tanaka P, Gan TJ, RodriguezBlanco Y, Soto R, Heisel O. Incidence, risk factors, and consequences of residual neuromuscular block in the United States: the prospective, observational, multicenter RECITE-US study. J Clin Anesth. 2019;55:33–41.
12. Caldwell JE. Reversal of residual neuromuscular block with neostigmine at one to four hours after a single intubating dose of vecuronium. Anesth Analg. 1995;80:1168–74.
13. Debaene B, Plaud B, Dilly MP, Donati F. Residual paralysis in the PACU after a single intubating dose of nondepolarizing muscle relaxant with an intermediate duration of action. Anesthesiology. 2003;98:1042–8.

14. Horrow JC, Li W, Blobner M, Lombard J, Speek M, DeAngelis M, Herring WJ. Actual versus ideal body weight dosing of sugammadex in morbidly obese patients offers faster reversal of rocuronium- or vecuronium-induced deep or moderate neuromuscular block: a randomized clinical trial. BMC Anesthesiol. 2021;21:62.
15. Burbridge MA. Incidence of anaphylaxis to sugammadex in a single-center cohort of 19,821 patients. Anesth Analg. 2021;132:93–7.
16. Miyazaki Y, Sunaga H, Kida K, Hobo S, Inoue N, Muto M, Uezono S. Incidence of anaphylaxis associated with sugammadex. Anesth Analg. 2018;126:1505–8.
17. Lee TY, Jeong SY, Jeong JH, Kim JH, Choi SR. Comparison of postoperative pulmonary complications between sugammadex and neostigmine in lung cancer patients undergoing video-assisted thoracoscopic lobectomy: a prospective double-blinded randomized trial. Anesth Pain Med (Seoul). 2021;16:60–7.

Anesthetic Management of Pregnant Women with Neuromuscular Disorders

9

Fabrizio Racca, Elena Conti, and Giulia Racca

9.1 Introduction

Advances in the management of neuromuscular disorders (NMDs) have improved both the survival rate and the quality of life of patients affected by these conditions [1–3]. As a consequence, a gradual increase in the prevalence of pregnancies among women with NMDs has been observed [4]. NMDs vary in their risk of developing respiratory complications [3]. A significant subgroup of women with NMDs is at high risk of developing pulmonary complications (PCs) during pregnancy and labor [4–8]. Respiratory muscle weakness leading to alveolar hypoventilation and ineffective cough is the main cause of PCs in pregnant women with NMDs [4–8]. During pregnancy, the growing fetus reduces diaphragmatic excursion and increases the load on the respiratory muscles, raising the risk of alveolar hypoventilation, ineffective cough, and PCs, particularly in the third trimester of pregnancy and at the time of delivery [4, 9–11]. Additionally, the need of cesarean section constitutes another risk factor for PCs, often required by abdominal and trunk muscle weakness, which is common among women with NMDs [12]. Consequently, pregnancy in patients with NMD is associated with a significant risk of morbidity [8, 13].

F. Racca · E. Conti (✉) · G. Racca
Division of Anesthesia and Critical Care Medicine, Azienda Ospedaliera Ordine Mauriziano, Turin, Italy
e-mail: fracca@mauriziano.it; econti@mauriziano.it

D. Chiumello, A. De Gasperi (eds.), *Practical Trends in Anesthesia and Intensive Care 2026*, https://doi.org/10.1007/978-3-032-25721-5_9

Identifying women at risk of respiratory complications and implementing noninvasive ventilation (NIV) combined with mechanical insufflation–exsufflation (MI-E) during the peripartum period can allow the safe completion of pregnancy, even in NMD patients with severe respiratory impairment [14, 15]. The combined use of noninvasive ventilation (NIV) and MI-E during the peripartum period can effectively prevent and treat alveolar hypoventilation and airway secretion retention in patients with NMDs, thereby reducing the risk of PCs, prolonged tracheal intubation, and tracheostomy [13, 16–19].

This chapter aims to provide a practical approach to the anesthetic and respiratory management of the neuromuscular patients during childbirth. In particular, it will examine the respiratory pathophysiology of pregnancy, respiratory complications, delivery strategies, and the appropriate anesthetic and respiratory protocols for managing pregnant patients affected by NMDs.

9.2 Respiratory Complications of Neuromuscular Disorders

NMDs represent a heterogeneous group of disorders characterized by alterations affecting one component of the motor unit—namely, the motor neuron, the peripheral nerve, the neuromuscular junction, or the skeletal muscle. These conditions may be either acquired or inherited, and they are characterized by variability in age at symptom onset and clinical presentation. They also differ significantly in terms of clinical progression and prognosis. A unifying feature of all NMDs is the presence of impaired striated skeletal muscle function.

NMDs are classified according to the component of the motor unit affected, distinguishing four main categories: (i) motor neuron diseases, (ii) neuropathies, (iii) neuromuscular junction disorders, and (iv) myopathies. The classification of the main NMDs is provided in Table 9.1.

Respiratory muscle weakness—defined as the inability of these muscles at rest to generate normal pressure and flow during inspiration and expiration—is a common feature in many patients with NMDs and represents the pathophysiological basis for the development of PCs [20]. Depending on the specific disorder, patients with NMDs may exhibit varying degrees and combinations of inspiratory, expiratory, and/or bulbar muscle weakness [3].

The risk of respiratory impairment varies among different NMDs. Some neuromuscular diseases may be associated with severe respiratory dysfunction, while others may show only mild alterations in respiratory function or none at all [21–24] (Table 9.2).

Inspiratory muscle weakness compromises the pump function of the respiratory system, reduces the strength of the expiratory muscles, impairs the effectiveness of cough in clearing bronchial secretions, and decreases the tone of bulbar muscles, which may compromise upper-airway patency during sleep and/or

Table 9.1 Neuromuscular disorders

Motoneuron diseases	Amiotrofic Amyotrophic lateral sclerosis Spinal muscular atrophy (type 1, type 2, type 3, type 4) Bulbospinal muscular atrophy Poliomyelitis, post-polio syndrome
Peripheral neuropathies	Guillain-Barré syndrome Charcot-Marie-Tooth disease Chronic Inflammatory Demyelinating Polyneuropathy
Disorders of neuromuscular junction	Myasthenia Gravis Congenital myasthenic syndromes Lambert-Eaton syndrome
Myopathies	*Progressive muscular dystrophies* Dystrophinopathies (Duchenne muscular dystrophy, Becker muscular dystrophy) Myotonic dystrophy (type 1, type 2) Limb-girdle muscular dystrophy Facioscapulohumeral muscular dystrophy Oculopharyngeal muscular dystrophy *Congenital muscular dystrophies* Ullrich congenital muscular dystrophy Emery-Dreifuss congenital muscular dystrophy Merosin-deficient congenital muscular dystrophy *Congenital myopathies* Centronuclear myopathy Nemaline myopathy Myofibrillar myopathy *Metabolic myopathies* Glycogen storage myopathies Mitochondrial encephalomyopathies *Inflammatory myopathies* Polymyositis Dermatomyositis

swallowing [3]. These alterations can lead to the following pulmonary complications: (i) hypercapnia due to alveolar hypoventilation, initially nocturnal and later diurnal, resulting from diaphragm and/or intercostal muscle weakness (pump failure); (ii) hypoxemia caused by the formation of bronchial plugs with or without macro-atelectasis secondary to retention of bronchial secretions due to impaired cough; (iii) nocturnal apneas leading to hypoxemia during sleep; and (iv) aspiration of saliva and food leading to aspiration pneumonia due to bulbar muscle weakness [21, 22]. The key components leading to respiratory failure in NMDs are shown in Fig. 9.1.

Table 9.3 illustrates the varying incidence of swallowing impairment across different NMDs [25, 26]. The association of cough impairment together with dysphagia increases the risk of choking, aspiration pneumonia, and the development of pulmonary fibrosis [25, 27–29]. The presence of severe scoliosis—occurring mainly

Table 9.2 Respiratory complications in neuromuscular disorders

Rate of occurrence of respiratory complications	Diseases
Unavoidable	Amyotrophic lateral sclerosis Spinal muscular atrophy type 1 Duchenne muscular dystrophy Some limb-girdle muscular dystrophies (e.g., sarcoglycanopathies) Some myofibrillar myopathies
Frequent	Spinal muscular atrophy type 2 Guillain–Barré syndrome Myasthenia gravis Myotonic dystrophy type 1 Some limb-girdle muscular dystrophies (e.g., calpainopathy) Some congenital muscular dystrophies (e.g., Ullrich congenital muscular dystrophy) Some congenital myopathies (e.g., centronuclear, nemaline, myofibrillary myopathy) Congenital myasthenic syndromes Glycogen storage myopathies (e.g., late-onset Pompe disease) Mitochondrial encephalomyopathies
Occasional	Spinal muscular atrophy type 3 Facioscapulohumeral muscular dystrophy Becker muscular dystrophy Some congenital myopathies Some mitochondrial diseases Inflammatory myopathies
Rare	Charcot–Marie–Tooth disease Chronic inflammatory demyelinating polyneuropathy Oculopharyngeal muscular dystrophy

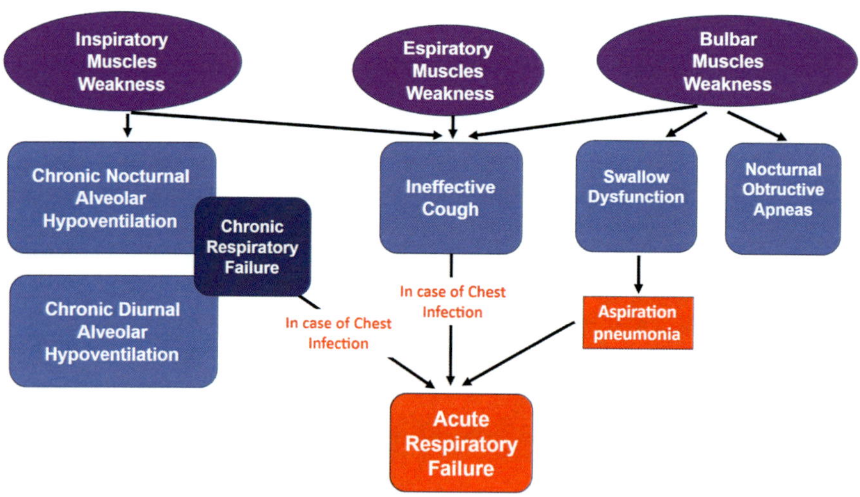

Fig. 9.1 Physiopathology of chronic and acute respiratory failure in neuromuscular disorders

Table 9.3 Swallowing difficulties in neuromuscular disorders

Rate of occurrence of swallowing difficulties	Diseases
Always present	Spinal muscular atrophy type 1 Duchenne muscular dystrophy (in the late stages of the disease)
Very frequent	Spinal muscular atrophy type 2 Amyotrophic lateral sclerosis Myotonic dystrophy type 1
Frequent	Mitochondrial encephalomyopathies In some type of glycogen storage myopathies (infantile-onset Pompe disease) In some subtypes of CMD, in some subtypes of congenital myopathies
Occasional	Spinal muscular atrophy type 3 Charcot-Marie-Tooth disease Becker muscular dystrophy Limb girdle muscular dystrophy Facioscapulohumeral muscular dystrophy

in patients with NMDs who lose independent ambulation before adulthood—further increases the risk of PCs [3, 30–32].

Therefore, NMDs may lead to the development of chronic hypercapnic respiratory failure and cough impairment, with or without dysphagia, which can become further complicated by episodes of acute respiratory failure (ARF) [3, 33]. Infections of the upper and lower airways, such as influenza-like illnesses and pneumonias, account for more than 90% of hospitalizations for ARF in patients with NMDs [34]. When cough impairment is present, airway infections promote the formation of endobronchial mucus plugs, which in turn cause hypoxemia due to altered ventilation–perfusion matching. Moreover, the accumulation of airway secretions and the consequent increase in respiratory workload—together with significant inspiratory muscle weakness—can induce marked changes in the breathing pattern, triggering rapid and shallow respiration, alveolar hypoventilation, and the onset or worsening of hypercapnia, resulting in the typical picture of acute hypoxemic–hypercapnic respiratory failure [3, 22, 33, 35]. In the presence of pneumonia, the possibility of aspiration pneumonia must always be considered [3, 21, 22]. If no evidence of upper or lower airway infection is found, other noninfectious causes that may lead to ARF in patients with NMDs should be considered. These include atelectasis, pneumothorax, depression of respiratory drive due to medications (such as benzodiazepine or opioid overdose, or residual effects of systemic anesthetics or neuromuscular blockers after general anesthesia), fat embolism in the setting of lower-limb fractures, or acute gastric or colonic distension causing diaphragmatic elevation [3, 21, 22]. Finally, in the case of a myopathy, left-sided heart failure—related to a hypokinetic cardiomyopathy or to a cardiac rhythm or conduction disorder—should also be considered among the possible triggers of ARF [36].

9.3 Respiratory Management of Patients with Neuromuscular Disorders

The use of NIV, combined with manual or mechanical cough-assist techniques, corrects alveolar hypoventilation and bronchial secretion retention, thereby reducing the rates of hospital admissions, tracheal intubations, and tracheostomies for ARF [3, 22, 37–40].

When positive-pressure mechanical ventilation is indicated for chronic hypercapnic respiratory failure, NIV is considered the first-line option [41]. NIV is preferred over invasive mechanical ventilation (IV) via tracheostomy because tracheostomy may impair phonation and is associated with greater morbidity [42]. In addition, compared with IV, NIV has the advantage of being used "on demand," resulting in less discomfort and a lower impact on social life. Therefore, tracheostomy is indicated only in the presence of one of the following criteria [3]: (i) severe bulbar disfunction; (ii) failure to wean from mechanical ventilation when intubation is necessary for an acute event; (iii) intolerance or failure of NIV in the management of chronic respiratory failure; and (iv) failure to manage bronchial secretions with MI-E. It is still a matter of debate whether the inability to tolerate more than 30 min off NIV represents an additional indication for tracheostomy.

In cases of ineffective cough, the use of cough-assist techniques is indicated, either manual (air-stacking techniques and expiratory assist maneuvers) or mechanical (mechanical insufflation–exsufflation).

Manual cough-assist techniques increase the amount of inspired air prior to cough initiation and/or assist the expiratory phase of the cough, both of which enhance the expiratory flow generated during coughing. The physiological mechanism of cough is characterized by an initial phase of deep inspiration. If the patient is unable to generate an adequate deep breath, this can be compensated by using an Ambu bag or a mechanical ventilator in volume-controlled mode to deliver a series of two or more consecutive inspiratory breaths—with no expirations in between—followed by a single cough effort (intrathoracic air-stacking techniques) [43]. A third inspiratory-assist technique is the glossopharyngeal breath, which enables the patient to autonomously generate small consecutive boluses of air—without the use of any device—by employing the glossopharyngeal muscles, resulting in a significant increase in intrathoracic air volume. The second phase of the cough is characterized by the contraction of the abdominal and intercostal expiratory muscles, preceded and followed, respectively, by the closure and opening of the glottis. Manual cough-assist involves compression of the abdomen and/or the chest by the caregiver [43]. This compression is applied when the patient contracts the abdominal muscles and the glottis opens.

The MI-E is an electromedical device (Fig. 9.2) [44] that provides cough assistance during both the inspiratory and expiratory phases. It delivers a series of positive pressure (+30–40) each followed by negative pressure (−30 to −40 cmH_2O). Together, they generate a pressure gradient between the mouth and the main bronchi of 60–80 cmH_2O, producing an expiratory flow similar to that generated by effective cough. This flow exceeds 270 ml/min and allows bronchial and tracheal

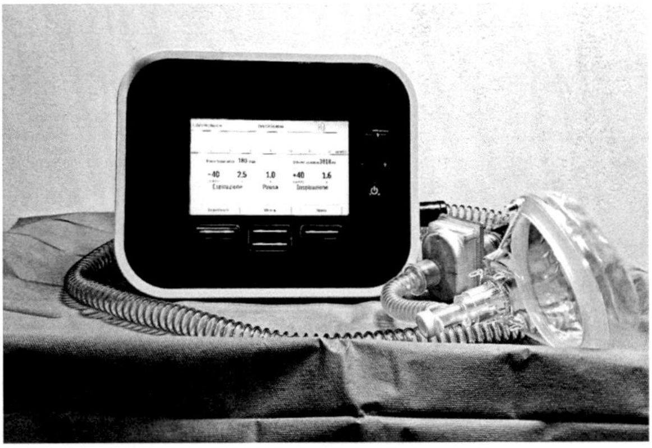

Fig. 9.2 Mechanical insufflation-exsufflation device. It allows for noninvasive airway clearance. This device removes secretions by applying a positive pressure to airway (insufflation), then rapidly shifting to negative pressure (exsufflation). The rapid shift in pressure produces a high expiratory flow of 360–660 L/min simulating a natural cough

secretions to reach the pharynx. MI-E device is usually well tolerated and can be administered either through an oro-nasal mask or through an endotracheal tube [3, 45].

Home use of MI-E and NIV, combined with pulse oximetry to monitor treatment effectiveness, is recommended in case of acute respiratory episodes as part of a home-management protocol of respiratory exacerbations. This approach showed a significant reduction of hospitalizations, respiratory complications, and mortality rates in patients with NMDs [35, 38].

Identifying individuals at high risk of developing respiratory complications—who may require the implementation of respiratory support (NIV and/or MI-E)—is essential to prevent severe respiratory events [38, 43, 46, 47]. Early recognition of at-risk patients, before any complications arise, is crucial. The easiest and most useful parameter to monitor both inspiratory and expiratory respiratory muscle strength is the forced vital capacity (FVC). Patients with an FVC below 50% of the predicted value are at risk of alveolar hypoventilation and ineffective cough. These patients, together with their caregivers, should be trained in the home-management protocol for respiratory exacerbations [40, 48].

In addition, when FVC is below 50% of the predicted value, additional instrumental assessments (overnight respiratory studies) and laboratory tests should be performed to determine the optimal time to initiate nocturnal NIV and cough assistance. Daytime hypercapnia is diagnosed via arterial or capillary blood gas analysis. Since nocturnal desaturations can result from either nocturnal hypercapnia or OSA, overnight pulse oximetry serves as a first-line screening tool for sleep-disordered breathing in patients with NMDs. Second-level sleep studies, such as polysomnography and transcutaneous CO_2 monitoring, are then used to diagnose OSA and nocturnal hypercapnia, respectively [3, 49]. Starting nocturnal NIV is indicated in the presence of symptoms of nocturnal hypoventilation or when daytime or nighttime

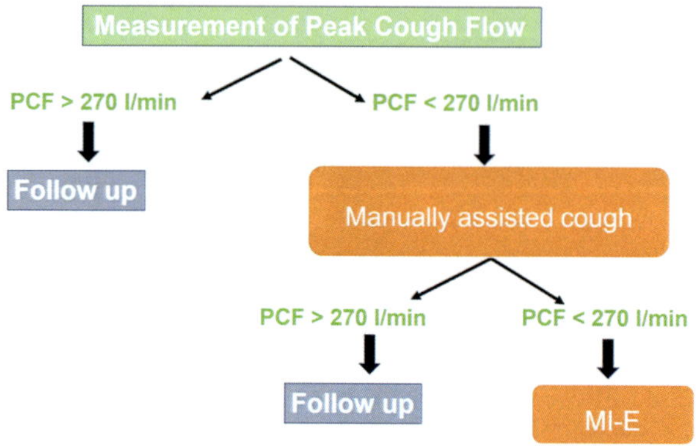

Fig. 9.3 Ineffective cough management. Legend: PCF peak cough flow, MI-E mechanical insufflation-exsufflation device

hypercapnia is detected [41, 50, 51]. Cough peak flow (PCF) is the most specific test to assess cough effectiveness. In adults and children older than 12 years old a PCF < 270 l/min is associated with a relevant risk of ARF due to accumulation of bronchial secretions in case of airway infections [3]. Manual cough-assist techniques are usually employed as the first-line approach. MI-E is indicated when manual techniques are ineffective. Figure 9.3 outlines the most commonly used protocol for managing ineffective cough in NMD patients.

In cases of ARF, the use of NIV in combination with MI-E and antibiotics constitutes the standard treatment for patients with NMDs, both at home [30, 35, 38, 40, 52] and during hospital admission [22, 43, 53]. Oxygen therapy alone should be avoided [21–23, 35, 38]. When oxygen supplementation together with NIV is required in the hospital setting, it is essential to monitor CO_2 levels [21, 22, 35, 38].

When NIV in combination with MI-E is insufficient, tracheal intubation is indicated and should not be delayed [21, 22, 53]. Moreover, in these patients the tracheal intubation maneuver may be challenging due to limited mouth opening, macroglossia, and anatomical airway alterations [54–56].

When the acute condition that required intubation has resolved, NMD patients should be extubated using a dedicated ventilator weaning protocol. This protocol includes the use of MI-E while the patient is still intubated to manage desaturations, and the use of NIV combined with MI-E after extubation [57, 58].

9.4 Pathophysiology During Pregnancy

During physiological pregnancy, maternal pulmonary function, respiratory pattern, and gas exchange are influenced both by hormonal changes induced by pregnancy itself and by the mechanical effects of uterine enlargement [59]. Hormonal modifications represent the main cause of respiratory function alterations observed during pregnancy. In particular, the increase in progesterone levels leads to a rise in oxygen consumption and basal metabolic rate (up to 21% and 14%, respectively), and consequently to an increased ventilatory demand. Moreover, progesterone enhances the sensitivity of the respiratory centers to CO_2. This leads to an increase in minute ventilation, primarily due to an increase in tidal volume [59]. The rise in respiratory drive can be assessed by measuring the increase of the tidal volume—inspiratory time ratio and the increase in the mouth occlusion pressure at 100 ms, known as P0.1 [60, 61]. During the first trimester of pregnancy, due to the increase in tidal volume, minute ventilation significantly rises, by up to 48%, whereas the respiratory rate remains unchanged. This ventilatory pattern remains stable throughout pregnancy [60, 61], resulting in a progressive decrease of pCO_2 levels until reaching a plateau between 27 and 32 mmHg.

As a result of hyperventilation and the reduction in arterial PCO_2 levels, arterial PO_2 increases, reaching values of 106–108 mmHg and 101–104 mmHg in the first and third trimesters of pregnancy, respectively [62]. Although arterial PO_2 rises, pregnant women are more prone to hypoxemia [59]. Indeed, during pregnancy, maternal respiratory reserve is reduced due to the decrease in functional residual capacity (FRC), caused by fetal growth that displaces the diaphragm upwards, and by the increased oxygen consumption [59]. Despite the reduction in PCO_2, blood pH remains almost constant (7.40–7.47) thanks to the concomitant renal compensation resulting from increased renal bicarbonate excretion [62, 63].

Progressive uterine enlargement is the main cause of the changes in lung volume and thoracic wall configuration observed during pregnancy, including diaphragm elevation and alteration of the thoracic cage configuration [59, 60]. The increased uterine size leads to higher intra-abdominal pressure and raises the diaphragm by approximately 5 cm. This results in a significant reduction in FRC and expiratory reserve volume (ERV). FRC decreases by 9.5–25%, while inspiratory capacity increases proportionally to maintain a stable total lung capacity (TLC) [62, 63]. The reduction in FRC is accompanied by thoracic cage widening, which compensates for the shortening of thoracic dimensions caused by the upward displacement of the diaphragm, thereby preserving TLC. During pregnancy, spirometry remains within normal limits, with forced vital capacity (FVC), forced expiratory volume in the first second (FEV_1), peak expiratory flow (PEF), and FEV_1/FVC ratio remaining unchanged [62–64].

During the third trimester, the further increase in abdominal contents reduces chest wall compliance, thereby increasing respiratory workload [59]. On the other hand, maximum inspiratory and expiratory airway pressures do not change during pregnancy or after childbirth, indicating that, despite alterations in chest wall geometry, respiratory muscle strength is preserved [63].

Dyspnea, or shortness of breath, occurring during normal daily activities is reported from the first trimester of pregnancy and is observed in approximately 70% of pregnant women. Such an early onset excludes a significant role of pregnancy-induced mechanical changes in the development of dyspnea [62]. It has been hypothesized that dyspnea during pregnancy may result from the sensation of physiological hyperventilation and/or from the increased respiratory drive associated with pregnancy itself.

9.5 Pulmonary Restrictive Diseases During Pregnancy

Pulmonary restrictive diseases are caused by interstitial alterations of the lung parenchyma, chest wall disorders, or NMDs. Since these are rare conditions, limited data are available regarding both the risks during pregnancy and their management [65].

Physiological decrease in tidal volume, the increase of ventilatory need and the respiratory workload, manifesting during pregnancy, expose women with a preexisting restrictive disease to the risk of respiratory complications [9]. Particularly women with severe restrictive disease (FVC < 1 liter) are at risk of hypoxemic-hypercapnic ARF in the peripartum [65, 66].

Restrictive lung disease can indeed limit the ability to increase minute ventilation as required during pregnancy due to the resulting increase in respiratory workload and oxygen consumption [65, 66]. Furthermore, in women with NMDs, progressive intrauterine fetal growth, by further increasing respiratory workload, worsens alveolar hypoventilation and reduces the ability to maintain an effective cough [4, 11]. Finally, in patients with kyphoscoliosis, pelvic abnormalities may be present, potentially limiting or even precluding normal vaginal delivery [65].

Given the potential for high maternal morbidity, some authors recommend discouraging pregnancy in women with restrictive lung disease who have an FVC below 1.0 L [66]. Nevertheless, others suggest that even women with severe restrictive lung disease can tolerate pregnancy and delivery well if managed throughout gestation with a multidisciplinary approach, including close monitoring of spirometry and gas exchange, as well as careful planning of labor and delivery [4, 11, 65, 67]. A review of 15 pregnancies in 12 women with severe restrictive lung disease due to kyphoscoliosis, NMDs or pulmonary disease showed that even a marked reduction in FVC can be tolerated during pregnancy with minimal maternal complications and favorable neonatal outcomes [65]. Half of the women included had an FVC below 1.0 L. It is also important to note that in the majority of cases reported in this study, deliveries were preterm (60% of cases), and cesarean section was performed in 10 instances. Furthermore, in six of these cases, severe spinal deformity precluded neuraxial anesthesia, necessitating the use of general anesthesia [65].

9.6 Management of NMD Patients Undergoing Delivery

9.6.1 Delivery in NMD Patients: Strategies to Consider

Vaginal delivery is not considered an absolute contraindication for women with NMDs, as the uterus is composed of smooth muscle under autonomic innervation and, therefore, its musculature is not affected in most NMDs. However, in myotonic dystrophy, some abnormalities of the uterine musculature have been reported [13, 68], and ineffective contractions have also been described in some women affected by spinal muscular atrophy [69, 70]. On the other hand, women with NMDs often exhibit weakness of the pelvic and abdominal muscles [8, 12, 67], and pelvic anatomical compromise may also be present [67, 71]. All these alterations can hinder normal labor and may necessitate assisted vaginal delivery or cesarean section [68–72].

The mode of delivery in women with NMDs should be determined using a multidisciplinary approach, taking into account the severity of scoliosis, respiratory compromise, and overall muscle strength [15, 68]. In a recent study of 94 pregnancies in women with NMDs, 77% underwent cesarean section. Among the remaining 22 women who delivered vaginally, vacuum-assisted delivery was required in five cases [15]. Vacuum assistance was indicated due to ineffective uterine contractions in four cases and cephalopelvic disproportion in one case. Furthermore, in five cases from this cohort, urgent cesarean section was performed due to failure to progress during labor [15].

9.6.2 Relevant Anesthesiological Considerations

Patients with NMDs often present respiratory and/or cardiovascular impairments that increase perioperative risk when undergoing surgical procedures requiring general anesthesia [16, 17]. In addition, certain anesthetic agents—such as volatile anesthetics and succinylcholine—may potentially trigger life-threatening complications, including malignant hyperthermia, rhabdomyolysis, and hyperkalemic cardiac arrest secondary to denervation [73–75]. For these reasons, people with NMDs are at higher risk of intra- and postoperative complications compared to the general population.

Ideally, surgical procedures in these patients should be performed in centers with professionals experienced in the management of these conditions [17]. When specialized centers are not available, or in case of emergency procedures, anesthesia may still be safely performed in non-specialized centers, provided that specific guidelines for anesthesia and perioperative management in patients with NMDs are strictly followed.

The preoperative assessment of respiratory function should include pulmonary function tests and an evaluation of cough effectiveness [16, 17]. Patients with an FVC below 30–50% of the predicted value or with a PCF below 270 L/min should be trained in the use of assisted cough techniques and NIV prior to surgery. In these cases, whenever general anesthesia is required, these patients should be extubated directly to NIV combined with MI-E [16, 17, 54, 76].

Patients with myopathies should also undergo a thorough evaluation of cardiac function and, when necessary, optimization of cardiac therapy in the preoperative period [17, 73, 77].

In these patients, the use of regional or local anesthesia offers a significant advantage in preventing and reducing intra- and postoperative complications. For these reasons, regional anesthesia is considered the first-line technique, especially in patients with NMDs complicated by impaired respiratory function [17, 54, 73, 77]. However, in these patients, neuraxial anesthesia may be technically challenging due to the presence of severe scoliosis [8]. In a recent study of pregnant women with

Table 9.4 Use of succinylcholine and inhaled anesthetics in patients with neuromuscular disorders

Disorders	Use of succinylcholine	Use of halogenated agents
Amyotrophic lateral sclerosis	Must be avoided	May be used
Spinal muscular atrophies	Must be avoided	May be used
Charcot-Marie-Tooth disease	Must be avoided	May be used
Myasthenia gravis	Must be avoided	May be used
Dystrophypathies	Must be avoided	Must be avoided
Myotonic dystrophy	Must be avoided	Must be avoided
Limb-girdle muscular dystrophy	Must be avoided	Must be avoided
Facioscapulohumeral muscular dystrophy	Must be avoided	Must be avoided
Congenital muscular dystrophy	Must be avoided	Must be avoided
Congenital myopathies	Must be avoided	Must be avoided
Glycogen storage myopathies	Must be avoided	Must be avoided
Mitochondrial encephalomyopathies	Must be avoided	May be used

NMDs, 72 patients underwent cesarean delivery; the majority (65 out of 72) were managed with regional anesthesia, while only seven required general anesthesia [15]. It should be noted, however, that only five patients in this cohort had severe scoliosis.

Regarding the choice of agents for general anesthesia, when regional anesthesia is not feasible, the use of succinylcholine should be strictly avoided in all patients with NMDs to prevent the potentially life-threatening complications already described in this review [17, 73] (Table 9.4). If rapid-sequence induction is indicated, succinylcholine should be replaced with a combination of rocuronium and sugammadex [17, 73]. Furthermore, in patients with myopathies, the administration of halogenated agents should be avoided, except for those with mitochondrial myopathies, in whom halogenated anesthesia should be preferred over total intravenous anesthesia with propofol (Table 9.4) [17, 73].

NMD patients also exhibit increased sensitivity to sedatives, inhaled anesthetics, and neuromuscular blocking agents. Therefore, ultra-short-acting drugs, as propofol and remifentanil, should be preferred, with careful monitoring of anesthesia depth and neuromuscular function to appropriately titrate dosing [17, 73]. Finally, at the end of the surgery, the effect of neuromuscular blocking agents should be fully reversed. For this reason, rocuronium should be used as it can be completely reversed with sugammadex [73].

Tracheal intubation can be challenging in patients with NMDs, and literature reports frequent use of fiber-optic–assisted endotracheal intubation [54–56]. Indeed, in these patients airway management may be complicated by one or more of the following conditions: mandibular ankylosis, atrophy of the masseter and/or other masticatory muscles, macroglossia, a narrow and high-arched hard palate, and limited cervical spine mobility [54–56]. In a recent study of pregnant women with NMDs, intubation difficulties were reported in five of the seven patients who underwent general anesthesia for cesarean delivery [15]. Specifically, three patients underwent awake fiber-optic intubation, and two were intubated using a videolaryngoscope.

For NMDs patients undergoing vaginal delivery, epidural analgesia should always be ensured. However, it should be noted that severe scoliosis may sometimes be present in these patients, making both neuraxial block placement and epidural analgesia technically challenging [8]. In a recent study, among the 22 patients who underwent vaginal delivery, 15 received epidural analgesia [15].

In the postoperative period, opioid infusion should be avoided in patients with NMDs, particularly in those with reduced respiratory function or documented obstructive sleep apnea syndrome [17].

Additionally, for all patients at risk of respiratory or cardiac complications, post-operative admission to an intensive care unit should be considered [17]. Specifically, patients with reduced respiratory muscle strength who have undergone intubation for general anesthesia require careful postoperative respiratory management, which includes clearing bronchial secretions using MI-E while the patient is still intubated, followed by early extubation with immediate transition to NIV combined with MI-E. Oxygen therapy alone should never be used without concurrent NIV [17].

9.6.3 Respiratory Protocol for the Management of Pregnant Women with NMDs

Since, during pregnancy, the progressive intrauterine growth of the fetus compromises the diaphragmatic function and increases the respiratory workload—further worsening alveolar hypoventilation and cough effectiveness in women with NMDs—a prepartum respiratory assessment is strongly recommended to identify patients who require specific management to prevent and, when necessary, treat PCs [4, 11].

The results of a recent prospective study [15] confirmed, in a large cohort, findings that had previously been described only through case reports. These retrospective studies, based on the description of individual cases of women with NMDs—particularly those affected by poliomyelitis, spinal muscular atrophy, limb-girdle muscular dystrophy, amyotrophic lateral sclerosis, and mitochondrial myopathies—had highlighted that: (i) different categories of NMDs share common complications, such as alveolar hypoventilation and impaired cough, and (ii) the use of NIV in the peripartum period prevents maternal PCs, allowing the birth of healthy neonates despite severe pre-pregnancy maternal respiratory impairment (very low FVC and cough peak flows, severe kyphoscoliosis, and pre-pregnancy noninvasive ventilatory support) [6, 11, 78–81]. It is also noteworthy that none of these studies reported the use of MI-E, either during pregnancy or labor.

A recent multicenter Italian study, including 94 patients with NMDs, reported that only 25% of pregnant women were at risk of developing respiratory complications [15]. The protocol included a preliminary respiratory assessment to evaluate cough effectiveness, gas exchange, and lung volumes between the 28th and 30th week of gestation [15]. The respiratory risk assessment also considered preexisting dependence on respiratory support (long-term NIV and home use of MI-E) as well as the presence of swallowing difficulties or scoliosis. Patients were classified as being at risk of respiratory complications if any of the following conditions were present: (i) oxygen saturation in room air <95%, (ii) daytime or nighttime hypercapnia, (iii) central or obstructive apneas, (iv) history of weak cough or recurrent respiratory illness, (v) long-term use of NIV, (vi) use of home cough-assisted techniques, (vii) FVC < 50% of predicted value, (viii) PCF < 270 L/min, (ix) presence of swallowing difficulties, and (x) scoliotic curve with a cobb angle ≥50° [15]. Women classified as being at risk of respiratory complications were therefore trained in the use of NIV and/or bronchial secretion clearance techniques prior to delivery. Training on the use of NIV and MI-E was conducted in an outpatient setting between 1 and 4 weeks before delivery. At the end of the training, patients were instructed to use NIV daily, for a minimum of 30 min and to perform at least one daily session of MI-E. Regarding anesthesiologic management in case of cesarean delivery, all patients were treated according to the Italian recommendations for anesthesia in patients with NMDs [17]. Specifically, patients at risk of PCs underwent spinal anesthesia and, when necessary, used NIV and MI-E both during cesarean section and in the postoperative period [15]. If endotracheal intubation was required to perform general anesthesia, NIV and MI-E were applied immediately after extubation in all patients who were already using these devices prior to pregnancy, as well as in women with preoperatory FVC < 30% of the predicted value and/or PCF < 270 L/min. Overall, 10 of the 94 women with NMDs included in the study developed respiratory complications [15]. Seventeen women required NIV after delivery, with ten of them also using MI-E [15]. Maternal and neonatal outcomes were favorable [15]. In particular, although 9 of the 24 women classified as at risk developed postpartum respiratory complications, none required re-intubation or tracheostomy. Only one patient without pulmonary risk factors developed a postpartum respiratory complication. The most frequent complication was bronchial secretion retention, which occurred in all ten affected patients. Furthermore, considering the entire study population, the mean neonatal birth weight and Apgar scores were within the normal range. It is also noteworthy that the authors [15] highlighted that the subgroup of patients with respiratory risk factors, compared with those without pulmonary risk factors, not only had a higher percentage of respiratory complications but also a higher rate of admission to intensive or sub-intensive care units, longer average hospital and intensive care units stays, lower Apgar scores, and lower neonatal birth weight [15]. This study was the first to document the use of MI-E during pregnancy [15]. Among the ten pregnant women with PCs who experienced secretion retention, nine used MI-E. No complications related to MI-E were reported in these patients either before or after delivery. Therefore, the analysis of these data suggests that MI-E can be safely used in combination with NIV in women with NMDs to prevent and treat secretion retention even during pregnancy [15].

9.7 Conclusions

In conclusion, pregnant women with NMDs, who are at high risk for complications during the peripartum period, should be managed within a multidisciplinary protocol that also includes screening for and prevention of respiratory insufficiency throughout pregnancy. Anesthetic management should be carefully planned, and the mode of delivery should be determined by a multidisciplinary team. Patients identified as being at risk for PCs should receive pre-delivery training in the use of MI-E and NIV. The combined use of NIV and MI-E during the peripartum period enables effective prevention and management of alveolar hypoventilation and airway secretion retention. Accordingly, all pregnant women with NMDs should be cared for in highly specialized centers.

References

1. Finkel RS, Sejersen T, Mercuri E. 218th ENMC International Workshop: revisiting the consensus on standards of care in SMA Naarden, The Netherlands, 19-21 February 2016. Neuromuscul Disord. 2017;27:596605.
2. Sansone VA, Gagnon C. Participants of the 207th ENMC Workshop. 207th ENMC Workshop on chronic respiratory insufficiency in myotonic dystrophies: management and implications for research, 27-29 June 2014, Naarden, The Netherlands. Neuromuscul Disord. 2015;25(5):43242.
3. Hull J, Aniapravan R, Chan E, Chatwin M, Forton J, Gallagher J, et al. British Thoracic Society guideline for respiratory management of children with neuromuscular weakness. Thorax. 2012;67(1):140.
4. Norwood F, Rudnik-Schoneborn S. 179th ENMC international workshop: pregnancy in women with neuromuscular disorders. Neuromuscul Disord. 2011;22(2):183–90.
5. Guidon AC, Massey EW. Neuromuscular disorders in pregnancy. Neurol Clin. 2012;30(3):889–911.
6. McLoughlin L, Bhagvat P. Anaesthesia for caesarean section in spinal muscular atrophy type III. Int J Obstetr Anesth. 2004;13:1925.
7. Flunt D, Andreadis N, Menadue C, Welsh AW. Clinical commentary: obstetric and respiratory management of pregnancy with severe spinal muscular atrophy. Obstet Gynecol Int. 2009;2009:942301.
8. Foster RN, Boothroyd KP. Caesarean section in a complicated case of central core disease. Anaesthesia. 2008;63:5447.
9. Elkus R, Popovich J Jr. Respiratory physiology in pregnancy. Clin Chest Med. 1992;13(4):55565.
10. LoMauro A, Aliverti A. Respiratory physiology of pregnancy. Breathe. 2015;11:297–301.
11. Bach JR. Successful pregnancies for ventilator users. Am J Phys Med Rehabil. 2003;82:226–9.
12. Awater C, Zerres K, Rudnik-Sch€oneborn S. Pregnancy course and outcome in women with hereditary neuromuscular disorders: comparison of obstetric risks in 178 patients. Eur J Obstet Gynecol Reprod Biol. 2012;162(2):153–9.
13. Johnson NE, Hung M, Nasser E, Johnson NE, Hung M, Nasser E, Hagerman KA, Chen W, Ciafaloni E, et al. The impact of pregnancy on myotonic dystrophy: a registry-based study. J Neuromuscul Dis. 2015;2(4):447–52.

14. Racca F, Longhitano Y, Zanza C, Draisci G, Stoia PA, Gollo E, Maio M, Grattarola C, Astuto M, Vaschetto R, Sansone VAM, Conti G, Gregoretti C. Peri-partum respiratory management in neuromuscular disorders (IT-NEUMA-Pregn study): a proposal by an Italian panel and a call for an international collaboration. Pulmonology. 2023:S2531-0437(23)00041-7.
15. Racca F, Longhitano Y, Zanza C, Balzanelli MG, Draisci G, Stoia PA, Gollo E, Maio M, Grattarola C, Astuto M, Ciccarelli A, Racca G, Romenskaya T, Giordano B, Serraino A, Sansone VAM, Gregoretti C, Conti G, Piccolella F, Vaschetto R. Peri-partum respiratory management of pregnant women with neuro-muscular disorders: a prospective observational study (IT-NEUMAPregn study). BMC Anesthesiol. 2023;23(1):342.
16. Birnkrant DJ, Panitch HB, Benditt JO, Boitano LJ, Carter ER, Cwik VA, et al. American College of Chest Physicians consensus statement on the respiratory and related management of patients with Duchenne muscular dystrophy undergoing anesthesia or sedation. Chest. 2007;132:1977–86.
17. Racca F, Mongini T, Wolfler A, Vianello A, Cutrera R, Del Sorbo L, et al. Recommendations for anesthesia and perioperative management of patients with neuromuscular disorders. Minerva Anestesiol. 2013;79:419–33.
18. Islander G. Anesthesia and spinal muscle atrophy. Paediatr Anaesth. 2013;23:804–16.
19. Bach JR, Sabharwal S. High pulmonary risk scoliosis surgery: role of noninvasive ventilation and related techniques. J Spinal Disord Tech. 2005;18:527–30.
20. Mehta S. Neuromuscular disease causing acute respiratory failure. Respir Care. 2006;51:1016–21.
21. Racca F, Vianello A, Mongini T, Ruggeri P, Versaci A, Vita GL, Vita G. Practical approach to respiratory emergencies in neurological diseases. Neurol Sci. 2020 Mar;41(3):497–508.
22. Racca F, Del Sorbo L, Mongini T, Vianello A, Ranieri VM. Respiratory management of acute respiratory failure in neuromuscular diseases. Minerva Anestesiol. 2010 Jan;76(1):51–62.
23. Sansone VA, Racca F, Ottonello G, Vianello A, Berardinelli A, Crescimanno G, Casiraghi JL, Italian SMA Family Association. 1st Italian SMA Family association consensus meeting: management and recommendations for respiratory involvement in spinal muscular atrophy (SMA) types I-III, Rome, Italy, 30-31 January 2015. Neuromuscul Disord. 2015;25:979–89.
24. Buu MC. Respiratory complications, management and treatments for neuromuscular disease in children. Curr Opin Pediatr. 2017;29:326–33.
25. Britton D, Karam C, Schindler JS. Swallowing and secretion management in neuromuscular disease. Clin Chest Med. 2018;39:449–57.
26. Knuijt S, Kalf JG, de Swart BJ, et al. Dysarthria and dysphagia are highly prevalent among various types of neuromuscular diseases. Disabil Rehabil. 2014;36:1285–9.
27. Pane M, Vasta I, Messina S, et al. Feeding problems and weight gain in Duchenne muscular dystrophy. Eur J Paediatr Neurol. 2006;10:231–6.
28. Waito AA, Valenzano TJ, Peladeau-Pigeon M, et al. Trends in research literature describing dysphagia in motor neuron diseases (MND): a scoping review. Dysphagia. 2017;32:734–47.
29. Baydur A, Gilgoff I, Prentice W, et al. Decline in respiratory function and experience with long-term assisted ventilation in advanced Duchenne's muscular dystrophy. Chest. 1990;97:884–9.
30. Finder JD, Birnkrant D, Carl J, et al. Respiratory care of the patient with Duchenne muscular dystrophy: ATS consensus statement. Am J Respir Crit Care Med. 2004;170:456–65.
31. Mayer OH. Scoliosis and the impact in neuromuscular disease. Paediatr Respir Rev. 2015;16:35–42.
32. Bach JR, Turcios NL, Wang L. Respiratory complications of pediatric neuromuscular diseases. Pediatr Clin N Am. 2021;68:177–91.
33. Poponick JM, Jacobs I, Supinski G, et al. Effect of upper respiratory tract infection in patients with neuromuscular disease. Am J Respir Crit Care Med. 1997;156(2 Pt 1):659–64.
34. Calvert LD, McKeever TM, Kinnear WJM, et al. Trends in survival from muscular dystrophy in England and Wales and impact on respiratory services. Respir Med. 2006;100:1058–63.

35. Tzeng AC, Bach JR. Prevention of pulmonary morbidity for patients with neuromuscular disease. Chest. 2000;118:1390–6.
36. Goodwin FC, Muntoni F. Cardiac involvement in muscular dystrophies: molecular mechanisms. Muscle Nerve. 2005;32:577–88.
37. Simonds AK, Muntoni F, Heather S, et al. Impact of nasal ventilation on survival in hypercapnic Duchenne muscular dystrophy. Thorax. 1998;53:949–52.
38. Bach JR, Ishikawa Y, Kim H. Prevention of pulmonary morbidity for patients with Duchenne muscular dystrophy. Chest. 1997;112:1024–8.
39. Trucco F, Pedemonte M, Racca F, et al. Tele-monitoring in paediatric and young home-ventilated neuromuscular patients: a multicentre case-control trial. J Telemed Telecare. 2019;25:414–24.
40. Vianello A, Savoia F, Pipitone E, et al. "Hospital at home" for neuromuscular disease patients with respiratory tract infection: a pilot study. Respir Care. 2013;58:2061–8.
41. Wang CH, Finkel RS, Bertini ES, et al. Consensus statement for standard of care in spinal muscular atrophy. J Child Neurol. 2007;22(8):1027–49.
42. Tzeng AC, Bach JR. Prevention of pulmonary morbidity for patients with neuromuscular disease. Chest. 2000;118(5):1390–6.
43. Chatwin M, Toussaint M, Gonçalves MR, Sheers N, Mellies U, Gonzales-Bermejo J, Sancho J, Fauroux B, Andersen T, Hov B, Nygren-Bonnier M, Lacombe M, Pernet K, Kampelmacher M, Devaux C, Kinnett K, Sheehan D, Rao F, Villanova M, Berlowitz D, Morrow BM. Airway clearance techniques in neuromuscular disorders: a state of the art review. Respir Med. 2018;136:98–110.
44. American Thoracic Society/European Respiratory Society ATS/ERS. Statement on respiratory muscle testing. Am J Respir Crit Care Med. 2002;166:518–624.
45. Toussaint M. The use of mechanical insufflation-exsufflation via artificial airways. Respir Care. 2011;56:1217–9.
46. Vianello A, Corrado A, Arcaro G, Gallan F, Ori C, Minuzzo M, Bevilacqua M. Mechanical insufflation-exsufflation improves outcomes for neuromuscular disease patients with respiratory tract infections. Am J Phys Med Rehabil. 2005;84:83–8.
47. Gregoretti C, Pisani L, Cortegiani A, Ranieri VM. Noninvasive ventilation in critically ill patients. Crit Care Clin. 2015;31:435–57.
48. Birnkrant DJ, Bushby K, Bann CM, Apkon SD, Blackwell A, Colvin MK, Cripe L, Herron AR, Kennedy A, Kinnett K, Naprawa J, Noritz G, Poysky J, Street N, Trout CJ, Weber DR, Ward LM, DMD Care Considerations Working Group. Diagnosis and management of Duchenne muscular dystrophy, part 3: primary care, emergency management, psychosocial care, and transitions of care across the lifespan. Lancet Neurol. 2018;17:445–55.
49. Birnkrant DJ, Bushby K, Bann CM, et al. DMD Care Considerations Working Group. Diagnosis and management of Duchenne muscular dystrophy, part 2: respiratory, cardiac, bone health, and orthopaedic management. Lancet Neurol. 2018;17:347–61.
50. Mercuri E, Bertini E, Iannaccone ST. Childhood spinal muscular atrophy: controversies and challenges. Lancet Neurol. 2012;11(5):443–52.
51. Mellies U, Dohna-Schwake C, Stehling F, Voit T. Sleep disordered breathing in spinal muscular atrophy. Neuromuscul Disord. 2004;14(12):797–803.
52. Sancho J, Servera E. Noninvasive ventilation for patients with neuromuscular disease and acute respiratory failure. Chest. 2008;133:314–5.
53. Vianello A, Bevilacqua M, Arcaro G, et al. Non-invasive ventilatory approach to treatment of acute respiratory failure in neuromuscular disorders. A comparison with endotracheal intubation. Intensive Care Med. 2000;26:384–90.
54. Racca F, Longhitano Y, Wolfler A, et al. Perioperative management of children with neuromuscular disorders based on a common protocol: a prospective, national study in Italy. Acta Anaesthesiol Scand. 2021;65:1195–204.

55. Graham RJ, Athiraman U, Laubach AE, et al. Anesthesia and perioperative medical management of children with spinal muscular atrophy. Paediatr Anaesth. 2009;19:1054–63.
56. Muenster T, Mueller C, Forst J, et al. Anaesthetic management in patients with Duchenne muscular dystrophy undergoing orthopaedic surgery: a review of 232 cases. Eur J Anaesthesiol. 2012;29:489–94.
57. Bach JR, Gonçalves MR, Hamdani I, et al. Extubation of patients with neuromuscular weakness: a new management paradigm. Chest. 2010;137:1033–9.
58. Vianello A, Arcaro G, Braccioni F, et al. Prevention of extubation failure in high-risk patients with neuromuscular disease. J Crit Care. 2011;26:517–24.
59. LoMauro A, Aliverti A. Respiratory physiology in pregnancy and assessment of pulmonary function. Best Pract Res Clin Obstet Gynaecol. 2022;85(Pt A):3–16. https://doi.org/10.1016/j.bpobgyn.2022.05.007. Epub 2022 Jun 27. PMID: 35868980.
60. Contreras G, Gutiérrez M, Beroíza T, et al. Ventilatory drive and respiratory muscle function in pregnancy. Am Rev Respir Dis. 1991;144:837–41.
61. Kolarzyk E, Szot WM, Lyszczarz J. Lung function and breathing regulation parameters during pregnancy. Arch Gynecol Obstet. 2005;272:53–8.
62. Weinberger SE, Weiss ST, Cohen WR, et al. Pregnancy and the lung. Am Rev Respir Dis. 1980;121:559–81.
63. Jensen D, Webb KA, Davies GA, et al. Mechanical ventilatory constraints during incremental cycle exercise in human pregnancy: implications for respiratory sensation. J Physiol. 2008;586:4735–50.
64. Grindheim G, Toska K, Estensen ME, et al. Changes in pulmonary function during pregnancy: a longitudinal cohort study. BJOG. 2012;119:94–101.
65. Lapinsky SE, Tram C, Mehta S, Maxwell CV. Restrictive lung disease in pregnancy. Chest. 2014;145(2):394–8. https://doi.org/10.1378/chest.13-0587. PMID: 24493511.
66. King TE Jr. Restrictive lung disease in pregnancy. Clin Chest Med. 1992;13(4):607–22.
67. Boggess KA, Easterling TR, Raghu G. Management and outcome of pregnant women with interstitial and restrictive lung disease. Am J Obstet Gynecol. 1995;173(4):1007–14.
68. Hopkins AN, Alshaeri T, Akst SA. Neurologic disease with pregnancy and considerations for the obstetric anesthesiologist. Semin Perinatol. 2014;38:359–69.
69. Elsheikh BH, Zhang X, Swoboda KJ, et al. Pregnancy and delivery in women with spinal muscular atrophy. Int J Neurosci. 2017;127(11):953–7.
70. Rudnik-Schoneborn S, Breuer C, Zerres K. Stable motor and lung function throughout pregnancy in a patient with infantile spinal muscular atrophy type II. Neuromuscul Disord. 2002;12:137–214.
71. Pugh CP, Healey SK, Crane JM, et al. Successful pregnancy and spinal muscular atrophy. Obstet Gynecol. 2000;95(6 Pt 2):1034.
72. Argov Z, de Visser M. What we do not know about pregnancy in hereditary neuromuscular disorders. Neuromuscul Disord. 2009;19:675–9.
73. Schmitt HJ, Muenster T. Anesthesia in patients with neuromuscular disorders. Minerva Anestesiol. 2009;75:632–7.
74. Veyckemans F. Can inhalation agents be used in the presence of a child with myopathy? Curr Opin Anaesthesiol. 2010;23:348–55.
75. Klingler W, Lehmann-Horn F, Jurkat-Rott K. Complications of anaesthesia in neuromuscular disorders. Neuromuscul Disord. 2005;15:195–206.
76. Khirani S, Bersanini C, Aubertin G, et al. Non-invasive positive pressure ventilation to facilitate the post-operative respiratory outcome of spine surgery in neuromuscular children. Eur Spine J. 2014;23(Suppl 4):S406–11.
77. Romero A, Joshi GP. Neuromuscular disease and anesthesia. Muscle Nerve. 2013;48:451–60.

78. Yim R, Kirschner K, Murphy E, et al. Successful pregnancy in a patient with spinal muscular atrophy and severe kyphoscoliosis. Am J Phys Med Rehabil. 2003;82:222–5.
79. Allen T, Maguire S. Anaesthetic management of a woman with autosomal recessive limb-girdle muscular dystrophy for emergency caesarean section. Int J Obstet Anesth. 2007;16(4):370–4.
80. Kock-Cordeiro DBM, Brusse E, van den Biggelaar RJM, Eggink AJ, et al. Combined spinal-epidural anesthesia with non-invasive ventilation during cesarean delivery of a woman with a recent diagnosis of amyotrophic lateral sclerosis. Int J Obstet Anesth. 2018;36:108–10. Yuan N, El-Sayed YY, Ruoss SJ, et al. Successful pregnancy and cesarean delivery via noninvasive ventilation in mitochondrial myopathy. J Perinatol. 2009;29(2):166–7.
81. Díaz-Lobato S, Gómez Mendieta MA, Moreno García MS, et al. Two full term pregnancies in a patient with mitochondrial myopathy and chronic ventilatory insufficiency. Respiration. 2005;72(6):654–6.

Patient Positioning for Surgical Procedures and Invasive Interventions: What the Anesthesiologist Needs to Know

10

Andrea De Gasperi, Stefania Colombo, and Laura Petrò

The role of patient posture or positioning on the surgical table has long been recognized as clinically relevant (Courington FW, Little DM Jr. The role of posture in anesthesia. Clin Anesth 1968; 3:24).

10.1 Introduction

In surgical practice, patient positioning refers to the position in which the patient is placed on the operating table with the aim of easing the procedure and, at least in principle, optimizing its outcome. Interventional procedures—not necessarily surgical in nature—also require specific positions tailored to the procedure requirements [1–4]. The choice of patient positioning on the operating table must take into account factors such as age, body weight and body size, comorbidities (with particular attention to cardiac or respiratory conditions), as well as the presence of anatomical or physiological alterations (including but not limited to mediastinal masses, severe kyphosis, malformations) and late-term pregnancy. Patient positioning for surgical or interventional procedures is a shared responsibility among the surgeon (or interventional physician), anesthesiologist, and operating room nursing staff. In most cases it results from a compromise between optimal surgical access and the position best tolerated by the patient [1–4]. General anesthesia, deep

A. De Gasperi (✉)
Former Director AR2, Ospedale Niguarda Ca' Granda, Milano, Italy
e-mail: dottdega@gmail.com

S. Colombo
AR 2 – ASST GOM Niguarda, Milan, Italy
e-mail: stefania.colombo@ospedaleniguarda.it

L. Petrò
Post-Transplant ICU, Ospedale Policlinico San Martino, Genoa, Italy
e-mail: petro.laura82@gmail.com

D. Chiumello, A. De Gasperi (eds.), *Practical Trends in Anesthesia and Intensive Care 2026*, https://doi.org/10.1007/978-3-032-25721-5_10

sedation, and central (or peripheral) nerve blocks may significantly modify or exacerbate the consequences of a position that would otherwise be poorly tolerated by a conscious patient [1, 2]. The selected position may therefore lead to (i) alterations in the cardiovascular and respiratory physiology and potentially metabolic changes; (ii) pressure-related injuries to the skin and soft tissues (including pressure injuries or ulcers); (iii) musculoskeletal damage; (iv) nerve injuries caused by compression or malpositioning resulting in peripheral neuropathies; and (v) compartment syndrome (particularly the lower limbs). Correct patient positioning on the surgical or procedural table is therefore a key component of perioperative risk management for the anesthesiologist and for the entire surgical team [3]. This underscores the importance of documenting both the "initial patient positioning (e.g., supine, prone, etc.) and its regular reassessment during surgery in the anesthetic record, especially during prolonged or high-risk procedures. The selected position should remain appropriate throughout the procedure and should not expose the patient to avoidable harm or complications [3, 4]. Correct patient positioning is thus fundamental to patient safety. Clear, shared protocols—recognized by all members of the surgical team—should be established, ideally with departmental, if not an institutional, endorsement [1, 3, 4]. Within the informed consent process, any specific risk associated with the planned position for the procedure (surgical or interventional) should be explicitly addressed [3]. In developing or updating internal protocols, both the (albeit dated) American standards from the Association of Surgical Technologists (AST) [4] and the more recent Canadian recommendations in the relevant section [3] may serve as valuable references.

In this update, we will discuss (i) the "basic" methods of positioning surgical or interventional patients; (ii) general issues related to injuries of the skin, soft tissues, and nervous structures; (iii) position-related changes in the physiological profile (cardiovascular, respiratory, neurological effects) associated with the most commonly used positions (*supine, Trendelenburg, reverseTrendelenburg, lithotomy, lateral decubitus, prone, sitting or "beach chair"*). Within each dedicated section, critical issues related to so-called "extreme" positions—frequently adopted in laparoscopic and robotic surgery—will be highlighted. For further details, interested readers are invited to refer to specific surgical literature (some of which is covered in this volume).

10.2 General Considerations

Operating Tables Although it may seem obvious, inappropriate/sudden movements of the operating table should be avoided during patient positioning: should it be required, the patient must be secured, with operating room staff on all sides of the table to prevent falls or shifts [2, 3]. To prevent serious accidents, the weight limits specified for the surgical table are to be respected. For example, tilting the table alters its load-bearing capacity, and the orientation of the table (head-to-foot) must also be respected, as weight limits are different (lower) if the patient is positioned in a reverse orientation [1–4]. This is particularly important in bariatric surgery.

Trial Positioning Although uncommon, certain morphological alterations (marked dorsal kyphosis, mediastinal masses, anatomical deformities due to disease, position tolerance related to comorbidities, term pregnancy) may require a sort of *positioning trial* to assess patient comfort. In fact, whenever possible, the intraoperative position should be well tolerated, if not comfortable, for a fully awake or consciously sedated patient. Limitations in limb movement (upper and lower) must be recognized and taken into account to avoid malpositioning, stretching, or compression that could lead to complications during the procedure, whether under deep sedation, general, or regional anesthesia. Specific positions achieved during surgery through particular movements of the operating table (generally corresponding to lateral tilts or Trendelenburg and anti-Trendelenburg positions, sometimes extremes) must ensure stability, safety, and tolerability ([1–4]).

Anesthesia Techniques, Positioning, and Changes in Physiological Profile It is well known that both general and neuraxial anesthesia can alter the mechanisms regulating cardiovascular stability (vasodilation and variable reduction in cardiac performance, sometimes associated with hypotension) as well as the adequacy of ventilation (hypoxemia due to alterations in the ventilation/perfusion ratio (Va/Q)). It is also important to note that all positions used during surgical procedures can cause cardiovascular changes as well as alterations in ventilation and gas exchange. Even the supine position—which humans assume for at least a quarter of their lives—can, under certain circumstances or conditions (including, but not limited to, obesity, anatomical deformities, mediastinal masses, heart failure, and women at the end of pregnancy), present challenges [1]. Perioperative compression of the skin and soft tissues (more susceptible to injury in frail, elderly, obese, diabetic, vasculopathic patients, or those with connective tissue disorders), as well as of vascular or neural structures—especially if prolonged—can result in injuries correlated with malpositioning or pressure. These may become the subject of medicolegal litigations and claims for temporary or permanent damage attributed to malpractice or negligence [1–4]. The following sections will address the general aspects of injuries involving the skin and soft tissues, and neural structures.

Tissue Injuries and Risk Factors Pressure-induced injuries are common among hospitalized patients in general, and surgical patients in particular. The incidence of these injuries in surgical patients varies widely depending on the clinical context, being reported in 10–37% of the cases during hospital stays [5–9]. Pressure ulcers are particularly significant, and without appropriate preventive measures, their incidence can reach up to 53% on the heels, 16% in the sacral area, and up to 25% on the upper limbs in patients placed in the prone position [7–9]. A number of risk factors contribute to the development of pressure injuries in the perioperative period, including (but not limited to) ASA class ≥ 3, frailty, high preoperative Braden scale score, extreme body mass index (BMI), advanced age, peripheral vascular disease, and diabetes. Depending on the case series, other factors may also be present (though not necessarily), such as prolonged surgical duration, hypotension, use of vasopressors and blood products, and intraoperative acidosis. All these factors highlight the complexity of the procedure and the challenges related to peripheral tissue perfusion [1, 2, 5–9]. In elderly patients undergoing central blocks or peripheral regional anesthesia, sensory and motor blocks may facilitate the development of pressure ulcers. Identification of high-risk areas (pressure points) and frequent checks to detect early signs of pressure-related injury are relevant in risk management [10]. Although rare, compartment syndrome of the lower limbs can occur in patients in the lithotomy position. Since risk factors for pressure injuries may overlap with those for intraoperative nerve injuries, strategies to reduce or even prevent such injuries are to be widely implemented [4]. If pressure reduction is the key factor, identifying the areas most prone to injury and ensuring their protection is essential. Tissue pressures are highest over bony prominences where skeletal support points come into contact with external surfaces (for example, heels, occiput, sacrum, iliac crests, ischial tuberosities). These contact points must be adequately protected with appropriate pressure-relieving materials or kept "free" (not in contact with surfaces). The risk is greater if these points are covered by surgical drapes and are not immediately visible or easily checked.

Pressure redistribution is the most important factor in preventing this type of injury [4, 11] and can be achieved by (i) using devices and surfaces that reduce pressure; (ii) frequent repositioning of the patient's head and limbs; and (iii) correct (re) positioning of the patient. Often overlooked [2], stopcocks, connectors, and plastic lines for intravenous therapy or cardiovascular monitoring may cause pressure injuries. Best available materials and tools for protection are available in dedicated texts. Textile materials should be avoided, as they are often responsible for abrasions due to their rigidity or roughness. Gel, "reactive foam," or *memory foam* is strongly recommended. Dressings such as *multilayer soft silicone foam dressing*, *Mepilex border sacral dressings*, and *Mölnlycke Health Care* are used in frail patients and can be highly effective in surgical settings to protect areas at risk for pressure injuries or pressure ulcers [2, 4, 11].

Peripheral Nerve Injuries Due to Positioning and Risk Factors Malpositioning and/or prolonged compression of peripheral neural structures can result in injuries to peripheral nerves, leading to temporary or permanent motor or sensory deficits, paresthesias, or prolonged pain syndromes, and may become the subject of medicolegal disputes. Although rare (<0.1%), nerve injuries unrelated to either surgery or anesthetic maneuvers are also possible, and likely attributable to malpositioning or compression [12–14]. Peripheral nerve injury is a complex phenomenon that can occur during any type of procedure (surgical or interventional) or anesthesia, including the NORA settings (outside the operating room). Awake patients or those under conscious sedation may be at lower risk of position-related nerve injuries (as they are "*able to move an uncomfortable limb or report paresthesia or pain*"); however, upper limb nerve injuries have been reported during neuraxial anesthesia and during MAC [1, 4, 12–14]. The mechanisms of perioperative nerve injury (still not fully understood) may involve local mechanical trauma related to (mal)positioning (compression and stretching), ischemia, or inflammatory stimuli: these factors must be carefully considered and, where possible, prevented (as already emphasized for skin injuries) in cases of preexisting subclinical neuropathy, diabetes mellitus, arterial hypertension, or dysmorphisms. Certain nerve structures/ peripheral nerves are particularly at risk of position-related injury due to a superficial course that is especially exposed to compression (e.g., common peroneal nerve at the fibular head, ulnar nerve in the ulnar groove at the elbow) [15] or due to potential stretching (e.g., brachial plexus with excessive head rotation). Risk factors for peripheral nerve injury not related to the surgical procedure include prolonged procedures, obesity, advanced age, smoking, hypertension, peripheral vascular disease, and diabetes [1, 4, 5, 13, 14]. Of particular importance in this context is the 2018 ASA document aimed at preventing perioperative peripheral neuropathies [13]. The recommendations, based on observational studies, case reports, and expert opinion, emphasize the importance of *protecting contact points* with suitable/appropriate materials and safe positioning in cases at risk due to the type of surgery and/or patient comorbidities. The "time" factor is certainly relevant, although precise intervals have not yet been well defined (a duration greater than 2 h is considered "*prolonged*," while in other cases "prolonged" refers to more than 4 h). Early diagnosis and a proactive approach are crucial, as most perioperative nerve injuries are potentially reversible [13, 14].

A summary of the 2018 ASA document has been presented both in UPTODATE 2025 [2] and by Hagan et al. [1]. "Routine" electrophysiological monitoring, which is present in highly specialized surgeries or in known, particularly high-risk situations (where it is mandatory, e.g., somatosensory evoked potentials, SSEPs, in spinal surgery), is logistically and technically not feasible as a risk reduction tool. There are, in fact, preliminary studies involving the use of a device for automated SSEPs during cardiac [16] and shoulder surgery [17]: for the electrophysiological monitoring as considered above, confirmation of benefits in terms of outcomes and, above all, their diagnostic accuracy requires, at least for now, further investigation [1, 2].

Treatment for this type of injury still lacks solid evidence: steroids, high-dose B vitamin complexes, and hyperbaric oxygen are proposed. A very recent review on the role of hyperbaric oxygen therapy documents positive effects in 88% of studies, with stimulation of peripheral nerve regenerative capacity, reduced healing times, and a substantial absence of major adverse events [18]]. Ozone therapy is not addressed in this review.

An uncommon but extremely complex problem with significant clinical and medicolegal impact concerns visual changes (up to blindness) in the postoperative period [1, 2]. The incidence varies widely (0.06–25.6%, with a reliable value around 3% according to ASA Closed Claims analysis reviews) depending on the type of injury, ranging from temporary minor damage to anatomical structures to true permanent blindness. While most are minor injuries (corneal abrasions, periorbital edema, subconjunctival hemorrhage among these) easily avoidable with well-known precautions and care (humidification, occlusion, protection), significant, rare but devastating problems may include vitreous loss, retinal detachment, central retinal artery thrombosis, temporary loss of visual acuity, and permanent loss of visual function (blindness) [1, 2]. Attention must also be paid to protective devices or practices (solutions, protective goggles, etc.): for further details on this issue, refer to the dated but still relevant ASA document. After spinal surgery in the prone position, postoperative visual loss has been associated with posterior ischemic optic neuropathy; however, it can also occur after other prolonged procedures, including those performed in the Trendelenburg position (e.g., gynecological and robotic urological procedures) [1, 2].

10.3 Surgical Positions: What Anesthesiologists Need to Know

10.3.1 Supine Position

In the supine position, the patient lies on their back; one or both arms may be abducted (*always at an angle less than 90°*), or adducted (0–10°), and should rest on supports always protected with pressure-relieving material. To prevent malpositioning—which is often a cause of lumbosacral pain and poor tolerance in the event of prolonged "fixed" positioning in awake patients—it is recommended to keep the hip and knee joints slightly flexed by placing a pressure-relieving support under the knees. There are operating tables that allow this configuration with appropriate supports. As previously mentioned, essential is to use pressure-relieving materials to protect the head (occiput), heels, and sacrum, especially in frail, elderly, diabetic, and vasculopathic patients. To be addressed is the particular vulnerability of the peroneal nerve to pressure injuries (e.g., from contact with support structures), with the risk of external popliteal sciatic nerve (EPSN) palsy, resulting in "foot drop" [1–3, 19, 20].

10.3.2 Effects on the Physiological Profile of the Supine Position (Table 10.1)

Cardiovascular Effects In the supine position, the *cardiovascular system* exhibits minimal gradients [1–3, 19, 20]. Heart rate (HR) and systemic vascular resistance (SVR) are generally lower in the supine position compared to those found in the sitting and prone positions. Elevating the lower limbs even by 20–30° increases venous return (VR) to the heart and, in a heart with normal pump function, cardiac output (CO) (leg raising effect); a similar effect can be achieved by tilting the operating table to the *head down* (Trendelenburg) position [1–3]. The most significant hemodynamic effects in the supine position are therefore those determined by the cardiovascular effects of drugs used in general anesthesia—both induction agents (usually intravenous, less commonly volatile) and maintenance agents (volatile or intravenous)—as well as the effects of central neuraxial blockade.

Table 10.1 Synoptic table with the effects of the supine position on the physiological profile

Modifications	Physiological effects	Clinical consequences/notes
Hemodynamic changes	↑ CBV ↓ HR ↓ MAP ↑ SVR ↑ SV /↑ CO	In uncompensated heart possible ↓ cardiac performance secondary to overload (rare) ↑ HR ↓ SV / CO ↓ MAP
Ventilatory changes	Cranial displacement of the diaphragm with ↓ FRC ↓ Cp Mismatch Va/Q Increased perfusion of pulmonary dependent zones with the same ventilation ↑ Basal atelectatic areas Closing volume reached earlier	Problems in the case of obese/COPD/elderly/frail subjects Use of protective ventilation during general anesthesia PEEP 5–10 cmH_2O TV 6–8 ml/kg Adequate RR to maintain minute ventilation

CBV central blood volume, *HR* heart rate, *MAP* mean arterial pressure, *SVR* systemic vascular resistance, *Cp* static pulmonary compliance, *SV* stroke volume, *CO* cardiac output, *FRC* functional residual capacity, *TV* tidal volume—see text for details

Respiratory Effects It has long been known that the supine position can significantly affect pulmonary physiology [21, 22]. The sitting or upright position is associated with better functional parameters than the supine position, both in healthy individuals and in patients with chronic heart failure (CHF), COPD, obesity, or neuromuscular diseases. Total lung capacity (TLC) and residual volume do not differ between the supine and upright positions in obese or healthy subjects [21–22]. Conversely, diffusing capacity for carbon monoxide (DLCO) in healthy individuals is better in the supine position. Forced vital capacity (FVC), instead, is reduced in the supine position in patients with CHF due to increased venous return, and in obese patients due to diaphragmatic elevation from increased abdominal pressure (cranial displacement of abdominal contents) [22]. Cranial displacement of the diaphragm is largely due to the upward shift of abdominal organs when moving from the upright to the supine position, reducing functional residual capacity (FRC) by 0.8–1 L (i.e., from about 3.5 L to 2.5 L); induction of anesthesia causes a further reduction in FRC of 0.4–0.5 L [19–22]. This may result in reduced lung compliance (C_p), earlier closing volume (CV), and the formation of atelectatic areas, especially at lung bases. Additionally, during mechanical ventilation, Va/Q mismatch may occur. *Perfusion* increases in dependent lung regions, while *ventilation* appears to be more even. These changes, generally well tolerated by healthy individuals, may be problematic in the elderly, obese, or COPD patients. Intraoperative ventilation, following well-defined protocols (protective ventilation), must be frequently (re)assessed during surgery. Of particular interest are recent studies conducted before and immediately after induction of anesthesia and during maintenance, using electrical impedance tomography (EIT), which, among others, allows (i) noninvasive definition of changes in respiratory mechanics [23], (ii) to individualize perioperative ventilation in both adult [23] and pediatric patients [24, 25]. EIT can therefore be used in preoperative assessment to prepare the patient for surgery, during anesthesia to guide and/or tailor the optimal ventilation strategy, and in the postoperative period for early diagnosis of respiratory complications (including atelectasis) [23–25]. A novel aspect of EIT monitoring, still under investigation, could be its application in noninvasive hemodynamic monitoring, tailoring, and personalizing the surgical positioning of the patient [23]. The supine position in advanced pregnancy or in patients with significant abdominal distension (for example, hepatorenal polycystic disease) may carry a risk of aortocaval compression and hypotension in the supine position: left lateral decubitus using an anti-decubitus wedged tool placed under the right hip usually resolves hypotension secondary to caval compression [19, 20].

Nerve Injuries Associated with the Supine Position The arms should be properly positioned to minimize the risk of brachial plexus and ulnar nerve injury: if abduction is necessary, it is recommended to keep it always less than 90° to avoid stretching the brachial plexus in the axilla. It should be noted that most perioperative nerve injuries occur despite optimal positioning: it is important to emphasize that the guidelines for arm positioning are mainly based on case reports and small studies [13]. Although it may seem redundant, it is worth repeating that the support surface must be adequately protected and should keep the upper arm at the same level as the operating table mattress: misalignments (“steps”) with the edge of the surgical bed mattress are to be avoided [2].

Ulnar Nerve Injuries The optimal position for the forearm with the arm abducted aims to eliminate or minimize pressure on the nerve in the ulnar groove at the elbow: based on an older study conducted in awake healthy volunteers [26], forearm should be neutral or supinated and slightly flexed to avoid hyperextension of the elbow. Ideally, the position should be individualized based on the patient’s anatomy, checking in the awake patient the “ideal” position [[13)]. The upper limbs in adduction (“alongside the patient’s body”) are usually in a neutral position, with the palm facing the patient. Similarly to positioning with the arms abducted, no specific forearm position has been shown to reduce nerve injury [2].

Radial Nerve Injuries The radial nerve is rarely injured due to positioning (instead, more frequently traumatized by repeated attempts during radial artery cannulation), but it is theoretically at risk of compression as it runs in the spiral groove of the humerus on the posterior aspect of the arm, between the heads of the triceps muscle. “Steps” between the anti-decubitus padding of the arm support and the operating table mattress should be avoided, as misalignment can compress the radial nerve [2].

Brachial Plexus Injuries Brachial plexus injuries are usually associated with stretching: a particular situation is related to sternotomy, especially after asymmetric sternal retraction (typical in cardiac surgery for internal mammary artery dissection). The literature on this topic is not very recent, but it remains an important issue to be aware of [27, 28].

Back Pain It may occur after procedures in the supine position (especially in elderly, frail, or predisposed patients, or those with preexisting conditions) and may be related to the loss of physiological lumbar lordosis associated with musculoskeletal relaxation during anesthesia (paravertebral musculature). Measures to alleviate postoperative back pain include placing appropriate supports under the lumbar spine to maintain the lordotic curve, slight flexion of the hip and knee joints to reduce tension on the thoracolumbar spine, and placing anti-decubitus padding under the knees (popliteal support, to avoid compression).

Hyperextension of the Head and Neck This is often required for thyroid and parathyroid surgery and other procedures on neck structures. It is important to assess the patient's ability to extend the neck before surgery. To facilitate surgical exposure the neck could be extended avoiding "extreme" positions (which can cause postoperative vertigo, headache, and nausea), and placing a roll (anti-decubitus material) or an inflatable cushion under the shoulders after intubation (pre-induction simulation is strongly recommended). The head should always be adequately supported under the occiput: "floating" of the head ("air under the head") should be avoided.

Supine Position and Pressure/Decubitus Injuries The bony prominences in contact with the operating table mattress, arm supports, and head supports can cause pressure-related skin injuries and must be adequately protected with specific anti-decubitus materials (gel pads, etc.). While prolonged pressure on the occiput can cause alopecia, the heels and sacrum are at risk for pressure ulcers, especially during lengthy procedures. Protective measures must include:

(i) Anti-decubitus supports under the lower legs to elevate the heels.
(ii) Special heel protectors (*padding*): It is important that the feet are supported without creating pressure on the Achilles tendon or hyperextension at the knee joint.
(iii) Positioning the head on a foam or gel "donut-shaped cushion" to eliminate pressure on the occiput. When possible, intermittent repositioning of the head during surgery can reduce pressure on specific occipital areas.

10.4 Trendelenburg Position

The Trendelenburg Position (named after the Berlin surgeon Friedrich Trendelenburg, 1844–1924, who demonstrated its importance and indications in abdominal surgery) is the position with the patient lying supine with the head of the operating table *tilted downward* (*head down*) by at least 15°: this position improves visceral exposure during abdominal and laparoscopic surgery and is now also recommended to facilitate central venous cannulation. Depending on the degree of downward tilt (*steep Trendelenburg*, with inclination up to 45° *head down,* as in robotic surgery) special devices are to be used to maintain the patient in a secured (and safe) position on the operating table: among these tools (but not limited to) are the use of anti-slip material on the operating bed, appropriate fixation at thoracic level, knee flexion, and supports (always protected and of appropriate material) for the shoulders. When the patient's arms are abducted, supports must be firmly secured and adequately protected with pressure-relieving material: the aim is to prevent movement, misalignment, or slipping during position changes. In robotic surgery, a *steep Trendelenburg* is usually required for abdominal procedures, while for abdominal wall surgery, the surgeon's preferences determine the degree of tilt. Vascular access and monitoring systems should be planned preoperatively and positioned in a way that the anesthesiologist can work independently of the surgical drapes and the position required for the procedure. Assessing the safety of the patient's position is particularly relevant in case of morbid obesity and when significant tilting is necessary. Some authors suggest evaluating the tilt and safety of the position before skin prep and draping: the goals are safety (preventing slippage) and ventilation quality (addressing changes in respiratory mechanics and gas exchange) [1–4].

10.4.1 Physiological Effects of the Trendelenburg Position (Table 10.2)

In young patients, the position is generally well tolerated, although it introduces significant cardiovascular, respiratory, and central nervous system changes compared to the supine position. Obese, elderly, or patients with chronic cardiorespiratory or neurological diseases may experience more pronounced alterations, potentially compromising their baseline compensation. In addition to the tilt required by the operator (often "significant" and generally between 15° and 45°), laparoscopic and robotic surgery also involve pneumoperitoneum, today managed with lower intra-abdominal pressures (and thus with a reduced physiological impact) compared to the early days of these techniques: however, significant cardiorespiratory, neurological, and metabolic effects may become evident. The Trendelenburg position may increase the risk of aspiration, and airway management during procedures in this position should prioritize maximum safety, favoring endotracheal intubation. For the use of supraglottic devices in laparoscopic surgery and the Trendelenburg position, please refer to an interesting *pro-con* discussion published by the APSF (Anesthesia Patient Safety Foundation) in 2023 [29, 30].

Cardiocirculatory Changes Transition from the supine to the Trendelenburg position increases venous return and central blood volume, increasing preload. In patients with normal cardiac function, cardiac output (CO) and mean arterial pressure (MAP) increase: filling pressures rise, variations depending on volemia and cardiac competence [31–33]. A somewhat dated study on the hemodynamic effects of laparoscopy in the Trendelenburg position during laparoscopic radical prostatectomy with an intra-abdominal pressure of 12 mmHg and a 45° Trendelenburg tilt [34] reported a two- to threefold increase in central venous pressure (CVP), mean

Table 10.2 Synoptic table of the effects of the Trendelenburg position on the physiological profile

Modifications	Physiological changes	Clinical consequences/notes
Hemodynamic changes	↑ CBV ↑ VR ↓ / ↔ HR ↑ MAP ↑ SV / ↑CO	In uncompensated heart possible ↓ cardiac performance secondary to overload (rare) ↑ HR ↓ SV/CO ↓ MAP Gradual positioning recommended to avoid critical cardiovascular changes
Ventilatory changes	1. Cranial displacement of the diaphragm with ↓FRC ↓ Cp Va/Q mismatch Increased perfusion of pulmonary dependent zones with the same ventilation ↑atelectatic areas Earlier closing volume	1. Issues in obese/COPD/elderly/frail patients 2. Increased mean airway pressure and risk of barotrauma 3. Use PEEP 5–10 cmH_2O 4. Protective ventilation TV 6–8 ml/kg RR to maintain adequate minute volume ventilation
Cerebral perfusion	↑ intracranial pressure ↑ intraocular pressure	Caution in patients with glaucoma and/or increased intracranial pressure

CBV central blood volume, *HR* heart rate, *MAP* mean arterial pressure, *SVR* systemic vascular resistance, *SV* stroke volume, *CO* cardiac output, *Cp* static pulmonary compliance, *FRC* functional residual capacity, *RR* respiratory rate, *TV* tidal volume—see text for explanations

pulmonary artery pressure (mPAP), and pulmonary artery wedge pressure (PAWP), as well as a 35% increase in MAP; notably, there were no changes in cardiac output/stroke volume or heart rate. These changes, usually well tolerated in patients with normal cardiac function, may lead to signs of overload or even acute cardiac decompensation in patients with impaired cardiac performance. Cerebral perfusion (cerebral blood flow) may be reduced in the *head down* position: despite increased carotid MAP, elevated venous pressure (hindered outflow) can reduce perfusion pressure due to increased intracranial pressure. Reported complications may include (i) ocular injury from increased intraocular pressure with venous thrombosis and retinal detachment, an issue to be addressed in patients with glaucoma; (ii) cases of visual loss after prolonged procedures in the Trendelenburg position, possibly due to posterior ischemic optic neuropathy. Potential solutions include the anticipation of the problem, less extreme *head down* positions, and maintaining lower mean airway pressures [1].

Changes in Respiratory Mechanics and Gas Exchange The Trendelenburg position causes alterations in respiratory mechanics and gas exchange [35]: cranial displacement of the abdominal viscera elevates the diaphragm, reduces functional residual capacity (FRC) and pulmonary compliance (C_p) (increasing resistance to insufflation), and may cause atelectasis. The work of breathing (WoB) increases in spontaneously ventilating patients [1]. Possible solutions include the use of protective ventilation during anesthesia with tidal volumes of 6–8 ml/kg of ideal body weight (some recommend 8 ml/kg), while avoiding volutrauma or barotrauma due to excessive increases in mean airway pressure, and the use of PEEP between 5 and 10 cm H_2O. In this context as well, EIT can provide an important contribution to personalizing the ventilation [36, 37]. In a recent trial conducted during robotic surgery for prostatectomy, the use of PEEP between 11 and 14 cm H_2O improved oxygenation and reduced the incidence of pulmonary infiltrates in the early postoperative period; however, the length of hospital stay was not affected [37]. It is important to emphasize, in such a context, the role of recruitment maneuvers in reducing the incidence of consolidations/atelectasis in the postoperative period. A problem often underestimated but to be carefully considered is the possible distal displacement of the endotracheal tube. Cranial displacement of the diaphragm and compression of the lung bases caused by the *head down position* can alter the position of the carina and result in selective bronchial intubation [1, 2]. Pneumoperitoneum can exacerbate this issue. If not carefully managed, fluid balance can also contribute to changes in respiratory mechanics due to increased chest wall stiffness, especially in patients with comorbidities. Since the goal is circulating volume optimization, both fluid overload and hypovolemia should be avoided with careful fluid management: monitoring of dynamic indices (Pulse Pressure Variations, PPV, and/or Stroke Volume Variations, SVV), now possible even with noninvasive devices, should be considered mandatory in patients with comorbidities [38]. Interventions in this regard aim to maintain adequate oxygen delivery (DO_2) both peripherally and at the cerebral level, where hypoperfusion has been observed: in this context, in selected patients, noninvasive monitoring of cerebral oxygenation (NIRS) might become crucial (see also the section on the Beach Chair position). Reports indicate, especially in cases of prolonged *head down* position, facial edema, and sometimes increased laryngeal swelling: here too, optimization of fluid balance can play an important role in reducing peri-extubation complications. Some authors recommend performing the *leak test* before extubation (deflating the endotracheal tube cuff and assessing for air leak) to detect possible laryngeal edema [1]. Extubation may even be performed using protected extubation techniques, utilizing dedicated devices with a nitinol guidewire [1, 19, 20]. For the effects of pneumoperitoneum and associated neuroendocrine changes, for ventilation strategies and hemodynamic monitoring, and for issues related to hypercapnia (including, but not limited to, reduced contractility, cardiac arrhythmias due to increased catecholamine sensitivity, systemic vasodilation with reflex sympathetic stimulation), particularly during robotic surgery and thus with even extreme Trendelenburg positions, refer to the comprehensive review by Chiumello and Duscio [35].

Nerve Injuries Associated with the Trendelenburg Position In addition to nerve injuries reported in the supine position, injuries to the brachial plexus can also occur in Trendelenburg position: shoulder supports or straps (an important risk factor for brachial plexus injury in the ASA Closed Claims [12]) can compress the roots of the brachial plexus. Furthermore, with abducted arms, brachial plexus injuries due to stretching around the head of the humerus may be observed: duration and tension are risk factors.

10.5 Reverse Trendelenburg [19, 20]

The *reverse Trendelenburg* position (also called *anti-Trendelenburg*) involves tilting the head of the operating table upward (*head up*). This position is commonly used for upper abdominal surgery to improve access to the organs during both open and laparoscopic abdominal procedures. For interventions requiring an extreme position (head-up tilt of 40–45°) (e.g., laparoscopic cholecystectomy, gastric bypass), special attention must be paid to how the patient is secured to the surgical table: transverse table straps may be insufficient to prevent the patient from sliding, and anti-slip and pressure-relief mattresses should be used. The arms may be abducted (with the same considerations above addressed regarding possible brachial plexus stretch injuries) or adducted and positioned alongside the patient's body.

10.5.1 Physiological Effects of the Reverse Trendelenburg Position (Table 10.3)

Cardiovascular Changes The *reverse Trendelenburg* position, with the head elevated above the heart, induces significant changes in central hemodynamics: reduction in central blood volume, increased blood pooling in the splanchnic circulation and lower limbs (venous pooling), decreased venous return, and consequently reduced cardiac filling, with lower SV and CO [39, 40]. In healthy subjects not under general anesthesia or central block, the increase in sympathetic tone in

Table 10.3 Synoptic table of the effects on the physiological profile of the anti-Trendelenburg position

Modifications	Physiological effects	Clinical consequences/suggestions
Hemodynamic changes	↑ Venous pooling in the lower limbs and splanchnic regions ↓VR ↓ / ↔/ ↑HR ↓MAP ↓ CO/SV	Reduced sympathetic compensation under general anesthesia/central neuraxial blocks Gradual positioning to avoid critical cardiovascular changes Fluid and vasopressor support with close monitoring
Ventilatory changes	Caudal displacement of the diaphragm with ↑FRC ↑C_p ↑ Tidal Volume (TV)	1. Increased mean airway pressure with risk of 1. Barotrauma 2. Volutrauma (potential) 2. PEEP 5–10 cm H_2O 3. Protective ventilation TV 6–8 ml/kg
Cerebral perfusion	↓ CPP ↓ intracranial pressure (ICP)	Attention to the hydrostatic gradient between MAP at the brain level and MAP at the measurement site to avoid cerebral hypoperfusion in cases of "extreme positions"

VR venous return, *HR* heart rate, *MAP* mean arterial pressure, *SVR* systemic vascular resistance, *SV* stroke volume, *CO* cardiac output, *FRC* functional residual capacity, *Cp* static pulmonary compliance, *CPP* cerebral perfusion pressure—see text for details response leads to increased SVR to maintain MAP and increased HR: these compensatory mechanisms may be significantly blunted under general anesthesia or in the presence of central blocks. In this context, the greater the degree of *tilting* (extreme head-up, 40–45°), the more pronounced the hemodynamic effects may be. The presence of comorbidities requires hemodynamic monitoring with invasive arterial pressure (now possible within certain limits also with noninvasive methods), focusing on dynamic indices (PPV/SVV) and tailoring the degree of tilting to the patient's cardiovascular responses. Constant communication with the surgeon is essential in this context to optimize surgical requirements with the patient's hemodynamic responses. Unfavorable cardiovascular responses (hypotension/tachycardia/oliguria), which become more evident with closer monitoring cardiorespiratory and metabolic, can be managed using a proactive approach rather than a merely reactive or, worse, symptomatic one [38] with (i) fluids (always with careful monitoring to avoid overload); (ii) low doses of vasoconstrictors (norepinephrine as the agent of choice) to centralize the circulating blood volume at the splanchnic and lower limb levels; (iii) progressive and gradual reverse Trendelenburg, especially when extreme positioning (45°) is required; (iv) use of mechanical compression devices for the lower limbs. With the combined and proactive use of these and other precautions (e.g., keeping the lower limbs parallel and not angled relative to the floor, to have lower limbs at the same height as the pelvis), CO can be favorably influenced even during the creation of pneumoperitoneum. The *maintenance of cerebral perfusion pressure* in the *head up* position (identical to the issue observed in the sitting or *beach chair* position, *see below*) deserves particular attention. Blood pressure measurement must consider the hydrostatic gradient between the measurement site (usually at the level of the heart) and the position of the brain, to avoid a "reassuring" MAP reading that is not actually effective in maintaining cerebral perfusion (*see below beach chair*). In these cases, the reference point for measurement should be the tragus (external auditory canal) and not the heart. The effects of extreme *head up* positioning on cerebral perfusion are discussed in the section dedicated to the beach chair position.

Respiratory Changes The head up position reduces the pressure of abdominal contents on the diaphragm and thorax and increases FRC and C_p, especially in obese patients.

10.6 Lithotomy Position [19, 20]

The lithotomy position is a supine position, with the lower limbs flexed at both the hip and knee joints, with the legs separated and abducted; it can also be limited to one limb only (hemi-lithotomy, in orthopedics). The degree of flexion varies, but is always aimed at avoiding stretching and malpositioning that could lead to injury of the skin and soft tissues (which may result in compartment syndromes [40–45]) or peripheral neuropathies [46–51]. The lithotomy position *standard* is commonly used for urological, gynecological, and certain rectal procedures and can be combined with a certain degree of Trendelenburg. In the standard ("high") lithotomy position, the hip and knee joints are flexed to about 90 degrees: although an old technique, the lithotomy position remains valid and the entire surgical team should be familiar with the classification of possible lithotomy positions (low, standard, high, hemi, exaggerated, and tilted) [40]. The type of surgery determines the choice of the degree of inclination, in accordance with the patient's compensation and tolerance. To support the legs in this position, appropriate supports padded with anti-decubitus material are used, avoiding compression of nerve structures (e.g., accidental pressure of the fibular head against the lateral support and resulting peroneal nerve palsy). The arms may be adducted or abducted (always at an angle less than 90°) and should always be placed on dedicated arm supports covered with protective and anti-decubitus material to prevent, as much as possible, pressure injuries to the skin and soft tissues, postoperative neuropathies, muscle trauma from excessive traction ("muscular strain"), and low back pain [1, 2, 4, 40, 47–50].

10.6.1 Physiological Effects of the Lithotomy Position (Table 10.4)

Cardiovascular Changes In the lithotomy position, venous return is usually increased compared to the supine position, although this may be a minor and transient effect. Abdominal pressure may increase in the lithotomy position to the point of impeding venous return to the heart and causing hypotension: this can be observed in patients with obesity, significant abdominal mass, or a gravid uterus. The lithotomy position combined with Trendelenburg (usually for surgical reasons) in patients with cardiac or respiratory comorbidities has led, in older reports, to problems with coronary or cerebral perfusion: hence the recommendation to use *head down* no greater than 10°, and in any case to provide individualized cardiovascular monitoring (and, if indicated, cerebral monitoring). A proactive anesthetic approach and ad hoc monitoring for both the patient and his/her comorbidities are paramount and to be tailored to the type of procedure and the consequences positioning may have for the individual patient. In these cases (as with the beach chair position), attention should be addressed to the heart-brain gradient to avoid problems of altered intracranial drainage or hypoperfusion in at-risk individuals (elderly, frail, diabetic, vasculopathic, or with significant cardiovascular comorbidities) [1, 2]. Peripheral hypoperfusion due to "local" pressure changes, which may cause skin and muscle injury from hypoperfusion (from pressure ulcers to ischemic necrosis in the case of excessive duration of the position), should also be considered.

Respiratory System Changes The diaphragm may be displaced cranially by the abdominal contents, resulting in reduced FRC, C_p, and increased airway pressure. These effects (which may lead to basal areas of atelectasis and potentially cause hypoxia) are more pronounced in the *head down* position, in obese patients, and in extreme lithotomy positions, where the risk of aspiration must be carefully considered (for example, in patients with impaired esophageal sphincter tone or those with gastroesophageal reflux).

Table 10.4 Synoptic table of the effects of the standard lithotomy position on the physiological profile

Changes	Physiological effects	Clinical consequences/notes
Hemodynamic changes	↓ venous blood volume in the lower limbs secondary to redistribution to the central and splanchnic compartments ↑VR ↓ / ↔/ ↑HR ↓ / ↔/ ↑MAP ↓ / ↔/ ↑CO / SV	Position may be poorly tolerated in patients with reduced cardiac function Potential fluid overload secondary to increased VR Gradual positioning to avoid cardiovascular instability/critical changes
Ventilatory changes	Upward displacement of the diaphragm Possible ↑ in intra-abdominal pressure in obese patients ↓FRC ↓Cp	Increased mean airway pressure in obese patients with risk of barotrauma potential volutrauma 1. Use PEEP (5–10 cm H_2O) 2. Protective ventilation TV 6–8 ml/kg RR to maintain adequate minute ventilation
Cerebral perfusion changes	↓CPP ↑ ICP	Attention to the hydrostatic gradient between MAP at the brain level and MAP at the measurement site to avoid cerebral hypoperfusion in the event of a "head down" lithotomy position
Skin/soft tissue effects	Lower limb compartment syndrome is rare but may complicate prolonged procedures	Risk factors Comorbidities Duration (> 2 h? > 4 h?) Degree of inclination Hypotension Hypovolemia Hypoperfusion/reduced pressure gradient

HR heart rate, *MAP* mean arterial pressure, *SVR* systemic vascular resistance, *SV* stroke volume, *CO* cardiac output, *FRC* functional residual capacity, *RR* respiratory rate, *Cp* static pulmonary compliance, *CPP* cerebral perfusion pressure, *ICP* intracranial pressure. See text for details

Skin and Soft Tissue Injuries Although now rare, the possibility of compartment syndromes affecting the lower limbs is underscored even in recent reviews and is reported rarely (see below) in cases where the lithotomy position is used [1, 2, 40–45]. Compartment syndrome can occur in any surgical position and affect both the lower and upper limbs: a large part of the cases reported after surgical procedures (and not necessarily to be associated with "anesthesia") involving a lower limb were in patients in the lithotomy position. A compartment syndrome could affect the "well" (nonoperated) limb (Well Leg compartment syndrome (WLCS) in patients in the hemilithotomy position (orthopedic procedures) [44]. An old but relevant review of 575,000 orthopedic procedures reported 13 cases of compartment syndrome in the lithotomy position (1/8700), compared to 1/92,441 in the supine position; even the lateral decubitus position is not exempt from this issue (1/10,000). Since the occurrence of compartment syndrome was associated with longer surgical procedures (> 2–3 h, most likely 3 h), critical are the "time" factor (prolonged exposure to pressure "trauma") and a proactive anesthetic and surgical management.

Responsibility of the anesthesiologist, once the patient has been positioned by the entire surgical team, is to maintain adequate perfusion pressure (adequate MAP), particularly if in the presence of potential external compression factors (malpositioning and elastic stocking, excessive pressure from supports). Possible mechanisms related to positioning injuries include the weight of the extremities on supports, reduced perfusion pressure with the limb elevated, and decreased capacitance of the affected compartment. Since a key role in the etiology of these injuries is played by increased (com)pression and the duration of excessive pressure and/or hypoperfusion, proactive measures (particularly for WLCS) include (i) to consider patient comorbidities (obesity, diabetes, peripheral vascular disease, well-known contributing factors); (ii) to avoid in general hypotension, hypoperfusion, and hypovolemia; (iii) to limit to 2–3 h at maximum the time the "healthy" limb is kept above the right atrium [44]; and (iv) to use leg or heel supports of appropriate material [2, 44]. In case of prolonged procedures (no universally accepted definition, but generally over 3 h) [44] it should be possible for the anesthesiologist to assess peripheral perfusion and detect any hypoperfusion conditions. WLCS can also develop in the early postoperative period via a mechanism similar to reperfusion syndrome: for the interested reader, the recent review by Nester and Borrelli on the pathogenesis, diagnosis, and treatment of WLCS is recommended [44].

Nerve Injuries Associated with the Lithotomy Position Along with injuries to the skin and soft tissues, injuries to peripheral nerve structures are rare but feared complications [41, 46–51]. Transient peripheral neuropathies are reported in approximately 1.5% of cases. Techniques, manipulations, or surgical instruments used in the lithotomy or even supine position may be responsible for these injuries. Among these (but not limited to), the following should be noted:

- *Injuries to the lateral femoral cutaneous nerve or the femoral nerve* during gynecological surgery: retractors may be responsible (and not regional anesthesia, often improperly cited as the cause).
- *The peroneal nerve* may be at risk of compression injury at the level of the fibular head: peripheral damage has been reported due to prolonged pressure of the fibular head against support structures. The lateral side of the leg should be left free or protected with pressure-relieving material when using lateral support devices. Consequences may include motor deficits ("foot drop" due to common peroneal nerve injury) or sensory neuropathy without motor deficit. The superficial peroneal nerve may also be stretched by excessive plantar flexion of the foot.
- The *saphenous nerve* runs superficially and horizontally across the medial femoral epicondyle. It may be compressed by contact with the medial leg support; should it be the case, protection and, if necessary, periodic checks during prolonged procedures are warranted (time and pressure are both important risk factors).
- *Lateral femoral cutaneous and obturator nerves*: Although the mechanism of injury to these sensory nerves is not fully understood, it is likely associated with hip flexion on the pelvis greater than 90° (the so-called "extreme" angle)—such

excessive flexion (as documented in cadaver studies) stretches the inguinal ligaments, through which the lateral femoral cutaneous and obturator nerves pass, and, especially if prolonged, should be avoided [2].

- The *sciatic nerve* may be stretched at the hip or knee joint, or compressed distally in the popliteal fossa (mind type of supports and degree of flexion). Before surgery, it is essential to (i) check, with the patient awake, the maximum tolerated flexion of the thigh on the pelvis, to be kept as the ideal position for surgery, and (ii) ensure that the popliteal fossa is not subjected to pressure.
- *Postoperative low back pain*: The lithotomy position, which can exacerbate radicular pain in patients with degenerative disc disease or (worse) herniated discs, has also been associated with low back pain in individuals without preexisting pathology: the possible cause is "excessive" straightening of the physiological lumbar lordosis. In patients with radicular pain, *the planned position for the procedure must be simulated with the patient awake*, to determine the most comfortable position for the patient during the procedure: unfortunately, this did not prevent radiculopathies.
- As is evident, the lithotomy position, although widely used, can cause significant postoperative complications involving the skin, soft tissues, and peripheral nerve structures and may be the subject of medico-legal disputes (especially those related to peripheral nerve injuries) [4, 49–51]. A document from American operating room technicians [4] highlights the importance of coordinated positioning: for example, the lower limbs should be positioned *simultaneously* on supports or stirrups and performed by two assistants, to avoid (among other issues) twisting of the lumbar spine and excessive extension of the hip joint. The same recommendation applies to returning the patient to the supine position at the end of the procedure. The "time" factor should also be emphasized: prolonged procedures are associated with more frequent problems involving cutaneous, muscular, and nervous structures.

10.7 Lateral Decubitus

The lateral decubitus position can be used for procedures involving the thorax, retroperitoneal structures, or the hip joint. In the classic lateral decubitus position [1–4], the patient is placed on his/her side with the back perpendicular to the surface of the table. The head is supported so that the cervical spine is properly aligned with the rest of the body, and a support device (axillary roll or thoracic cushion) is placed under the dependent rib cage just below the axilla to prevent compression and injury to the axillary neurovascular bundle. The dependent lower limb is flexed at the hip and knee joints. The nondependent lower limb is partially flexed at the hip and knee joints, so that the pelvis is stabilized and excessive anterior tilt of the trunk is avoided. Adequate pressure-relieving protection must be ensured to protect all pressure points on the operating table for the dependent side (from head to feet). Major issues to be considered are the following:

1. Between the thighs and/or at the level of the knee joint, cushions/supports made of pressure-relieving material and pressure-relieving devices for the most prominent bony prominences of the lower limbs should be used. The dependent arm is flexed and supported on an adequately protected support. Invasive monitoring of arterial pressure and pulse oximetry confirm adequate perfusion.
2. To check the invasive arterial pressure waveform: there should be no overdamping or slow upstroke (in case consider malposition).
3. The nondependent arm is slightly abducted and flexed at the shoulder and elbow joints, moving the scapula away from the thorax. If placed overhead when necessary, it must be supported by a series of specific supports and positioned to avoid stretching or malposition that could potentially injure the brachial plexus (a possible cause of peripheral nerve injury): a pulse oximeter is recommended to verify consistent peripheral perfusion.
4. To be avoided are traumatic or pressure injuries caused by anterior and posterior supports (depending on the type of surgery), whose main aim is to provide stability during the procedure. The supports must be covered (or made) with materials able to provide the best support and maximum safety, and prevent pressure or decubitus injuries.
5. The head should be in a neutral position, with pressure-relieving protection, to avoid malposition of the cervical region (stretching or rotation) and pressure injuries to the auricular cartilage ("*keep the ears flat to the head*") and the dependent eyeball [2].
6. The eyes must be hydrated, closed, and protected (as for the prone position).
7. All precautions regarding the limbs and head (except for the eyes) must be implemented both in patients who are awake under central or peripheral block, in deep sedation with spontaneous ventilation (for example, during complex endoscopic procedures such as ERCP), and under general anesthesia with intubation and muscle relaxation.

In non-thoracic surgery requiring the lateral decubitus position (orthopedics, retroperitoneal surgery), intubation with a reinforced cuffed endotracheal tube appropriately secured/taped is recommended: from the supine position, the patient is then placed in lateral decubitus always with maximum coordination among team members to avoid trauma/injury to the patient, accidental extubation with loss of airway control, loss of venous access (infusions/monitoring), arterial access (monitoring), or dislodgement of the urinary catheter (all items to be appropriately secured). In case of intubation for thoracic surgery or procedures requiring double-lumen tubes or bronchial blockers, verification of correct double-lumen tube placement with fiberoptic bronchoscopy, cuff maneuvers, and anesthetic management is mandatory but beyond the scope of this discussion (see the dedicated chapter by Federico Piccioni).

10.7.1 Physiological Effects of Lateral Decubitus Positioning (Table 10.5)

Cardiovascular Effects In lateral decubitus, peripheral blood pooling may occur in the dependent limb, leading to reduced venous return and hypotension. Older studies documented stasis at the level of the inferior vena cava due to partial obstruction caused by excessive (if present) flexion of the hip joints. The "jackknife" position, widely used in the past for nephrectomy (operating table "broken" at an angle of about 30° for better "surgical" exposure, and resulting in this specific patient body position), was associated with a significant hypotension, secondary to decreased venous return and relative hypovolemia (reduced cardiac output and decreased filling pressures) [1, 2, 4]. Data still to be validated, although recently published, suggest a worsening of the hemodynamic profile due to the use of self-retaining retractors (with a greater impact in the lateral than in the supine position), but with full recovery of the circulatory profile after their removal [52].

Respiratory Effects The lateral decubitus changes the ventilation/perfusion ratio. In anesthetized and mechanically ventilated patients, moving from the supine to the lateral decubitus position increases perfusion and decreases ventilation in the dependent lung, where FRC and C_p decrease. The opposite occurs in the nondependent lung, with increased ventilation and decreased perfusion. This can result in a Va/Q mismatch, a potential cause of hypoxemia in patients with reduced pulmonary reserve; higher FiO_2 may be required. It should also be noted that lateral decubitus is often used in the ICU to improve gas exchange by placing the "injured" lung in the *nondependent* (upper) position. EIT studies may provide important information both in "normal" subjects and in those with chronic respiratory disease or localized pulmonary pathology.

Table 10.5 Synoptic table of the effects of the lateral (standard) decubitus position on the physiological profile

Modifications	Physiological changes	Clinical consequences/notes
Hemodynamic changes	Possible venous pooling in the dependent lower limb Possible temporary effect of retractors [52] ↓VR ↓ MAP ↓SV / ↓CO	Attention to correct measurement of arterial pressure, both invasive and noninvasive
Ventilatory changes	Possible Va/Q mismatch during general anesthesia with possible hypoxemia 1. Upper lung ↑ ventilation /↓ perfusion 2. Dependent lung ↑ perfusion /↓ ventilation	Va/Q ratio 1. Normal in subjects not under general anesthesia 2. Altered during general anesthesia (a) FiO_2 may need to be increased to correct hypoxemia

MAP mean arterial pressure, *VR* venous return, *SV* stroke volume, *CO* cardiac output; see text for details

Nerve Injuries (and Vascular Problems) in the Lateral Decubitus Position [4, 46–51] The brachial plexus is at risk of injury if a cushion or chest roll is not properly positioned (see text above). According to Welch [2] the so-called "axillary roll" should be made of pressure-relieving material and should be placed *caudally to the axilla*, to avoid compression of axillary vascular and nerve structures: the upper edge of inflatable devices (*deflatable bean bag*) [2] should be below the level of the axilla. As emphasized above, monitoring the radial "pulse" of the dependent arm with a pulse oximeter is an excellent method for assessing perfusion and, indirectly, confirming the absence of brachial plexus compression. The brachial plexus and the nerve branches originating from the cervical nerve roots, which are at risk, can be stretched and injured if the neck is excessively rotated and/or laterally flexed. Hence, the importance during positioning maneuvers of supporting the head and orotracheal tube by the anesthesiologist, and, once positioned, maintaining head and the endotracheal tube in a neutral position on the operating table to prevent trauma or injury. As already mentioned, optimal positioning of the "dependent" arm is crucial: it should rest on a support, protected with pressure-relieving materials, abducted no more than 90° from the trunk to avoid stretching the brachial plexus. The nondependent arm, when supported by appropriate devices (thoracic surgery position), should ideally be parallel to the dependent arm and positioned to avoid stretching. The duration of the position is also relevant for the risk of vascular or nerve injury. The quality of peripheral perfusion in the nondependent arm should be monitored with dedicated devices: as noted above, next-generation pulse oximeters with software designed to assess perfusion signal quality are a valid option.

Lower Limbs As previously noted, a point of particular vulnerability is the passage of the *peroneal nerve* (*common peroneal nerve, branch of the sciatic nerve*) behind the head of the fibula: in the lateral decubitus position, special attention must be paid to protecting the dependent lower limb. Compressive injury is especially possible if the duration is prolonged: although there is no definitive evidence, the critical time may be over 2 h. "Foot drop" (inability to dorsiflex the foot) and steppage gait (deficit in ankle and foot extension, leading to significant walking difficulties and tripping) are the typical signs/symptoms of this injury. The *saphenous nerve*, running along the medial femoral condyle, is also at risk of pressure injury and must be protected (see also lithotomy position).

10.8 Prone Position

In the prone position, the patient lies with the face, trunk, and abdomen in a dependent position: the head, neck, and spine are in a neutral position, and the arms may be adducted or, if abducted, at an angle less than 90° at the acromioclavicular and elbow joints, with the palms facing downward. The prone position is used for posterior spinal surgery, certain craniotomies, rectal and gluteal procedures, superficial trunk surgeries, and procedures involving the posterior surface of the lower limbs (or vascular structures). Induction and intubation are usually performed in the supine position on the operating table (some sources also mention the possibility of using a stretcher for induction), and then, with appropriate precautions and a sufficient number of trained staff (3 or 4, in some cases up to 6, and with suitable equipment in cases of obesity) [1–4, 40, 53]. There are reports of intubation using supraglottic devices or laryngeal masks with the patient in the prone position (discectomy surgery) [54–57].

The patient is then placed in the prone position on the operating table. The eyes must be moistened, closed, and protected. For the correct technique for proning the patient and for the distribution of tasks among the operating room staff (a maneuver also common in the intensive care setting for prone ventilation), refer to the AST document [4]. During proning, there are risks of extubation (with loss of airway control), dislodgement, and loss of venous and arterial lines for infusion and/or monitoring, or dislodgement of the urinary catheter. Therefore, certain precautions must be taken before rotating the patient. The breathing circuit and monitoring lines should be disconnected just before rotation, always maintaining a pulse oximeter with active and alarmed sound. Pre-oxygenation with 100% oxygen for several minutes should precede rotation. During rotation, the patient's neck must be kept in a neutral position (endotracheal tube, being part of the anesthesiologist's responsibilities). The arm on the side to which the patient is rotated must be kept alongside the torso to prevent injury. The connection to the ventilator must include [57]

1. Immediate re-verification of power-on and parameter settings
2. Verification that ventilation mechanics (pressures, volumes) and/or gas exchange are unchanged
3. Verification that pressure, volume, and respiratory rate alarms are enabled and that no pressure or volume alarms are triggered.

In the prone position, the head must be rotated without stretching or excessive rotation and should rest on a foam or gel headrest with attention to the position of the ear cartilage to avoid trauma. Lateral rotation of the head and neck can stretch the roots of the cervical plexus: care must also be taken to avoid malpositions that could lead to potential compression of nerves and vessels between the clavicle and the first rib. The head should be positioned at the same level as the heart or even slightly above to prevent venous stasis in the face.

For neurosurgical procedures, the position may be maintained using cranial pins with the Mayfield apparatus or its variants: refer to specialized publications for further details.

The torso, depending on the type of surgery and technical-surgical requirements, may be supported by a dedicated device to support the entire chest or by placing supports or gel pads under the iliac spines to reduce possible abdominal compression, which can decrease pressure both due to the gel material and the surface area that dissipates pressure.

The arms may be positioned with shoulders and elbows flexed and "hands up" (the "prone Superman" or "surrender" position) or placed alongside the patient's torso. The hip and knee joints are flexed, with the lower leg supported to avoid pressure on the toes. Both pressure-relief and fixation/support devices are important at points prone to pressure injuries of the upper and lower limbs: particular attention must be paid to correct facial positioning, secure fixation of the endotracheal tube (preferably reinforced to prevent kinking or angulation and to allow intraoperative checks), and eye protection. There are specific supports for the head and endotracheal tube.

10.8.1 Physiological Effects of the Prone Position (Table 10.6)

In surgery, the prone position addresses specific surgical needs. Excluding neurosurgery, certain aspects still require attention to reduce potential negative cardiovascular and respiratory impacts, and should be the subject of dedicated studies in the near future [53, 59–61].

Cardiovascular Effects In the prone position, it is important to avoid: (i) excessive abdominal pressure causing caval compression, splanchnic stasis (particularly in the epidural venous plexus, with a potential increase in venous bleeding during spinal surgery), and consequently in the lower limbs; (ii) reduced diaphragmatic excursion with increased intrathoracic pressure and potential reduction in left ventricular function (decreased ventricular compliance due to increased intrathoracic

Table 10.6 Synoptic table of the effects of the prone position on the physiological profile

Modifications	Physiological effects	Clinical consequences/notes
Hemodynamic changes	↓ VR ↓MAP ↓ SV / ↓CO ↓ / ↔/ ↑HR	1. Intrathoracic pressure increase affecting intramediastinal pressure increase with effects on VR and SV/CO Preload-dependent patients at risk of cardiovascular complications (up to cardiac arrest)
Ventilatory changes	↑FRC (possible reduction in obese patients) ↑PaO_2 ↔ Lung and chest wall compliance	1. Better respiratory mechanics and respiratory exchanges if free downward movement of the diaphragm (“free abdomen”) 2. Increased pulmonary blood flow in dependent areas with better Va/Q matching 3. Possible worsening of Va/Q matching in obese patients 4. Consider the use of PEEP
Cerebral perfusion	Potential ↓ cerebral arterial blood flow and venous drainage even for moderate head rotations	In subjects at risk head to be kept in a neutral position both during positioning and during surgery possible monitoring with TCD

VR venous return, *MAP* mean arterial pressure, *SV* systolic volume, *CO* cardiac output, *HR* heart rate, *FRC* functional residual capacity, *TCD* transcranial Doppler—in-text explanations pressure): these changes are observed with the "flat" supine position. Therefore, the abdomen should be "free" with pressure-relief supports placed under the iliac spines and upper thoracic region. If not properly managed, increased abdominal pressure leads to reduced functional residual capacity, venous stasis, decreased cardiac output, hypotension, and compensatory (sympathetic) increase in heart rate [53, 58–60]. Dynamic indices (SVV/PPV) may play an important role in this context. The lower limbs, especially in the jackknife position, may develop stasis and contribute, as noted above, to hypotension due to peripheral "venous pooling." An important point to emphasize is the possible need for cardiac massage in the event of cardiac arrest [62]: it is recommended to initiate both chest compressions (hands on both scapulae) and, if necessary, defibrillation (posterolateral defibrillator pads) in the prone position [53]. In at-risk patients, it is advisable to place the defibrillator pads while still in the supine position.

Effects on Respiratory Mechanics and Gas Exchange In the absence of abdominal compression and with unimpeded diaphragmatic excursion hindered (the importance of supports on the iliac spines and/or lateral to the trunk to keep the abdomen "free"), the prone position under anesthesia can have beneficial effects on pulmonary function [53, 60, 61]. In fact, during surgery in the prone position, abdominal compression, if not properly managed, leads to elevation of the diaphragm, reduced thoracic and pulmonary compliance, and an increase in peak airway pressure. Some issues may therefore arise in obese patients. In these cases, PEEP and increased FiO_2 [53] should be used. In addition to the classic discussions by Lumb and Nunn, reference is made to recent reviews on the prone position both in spontaneous and mechanical ventilation (the subject of numerous studies for prone positioning in acute hypoxemic respiratory failure and later during COVID), which will not be covered in this lesson. A very recent summary by Gattinoni et al. reiterates that the prone position makes the lung parenchyma more homogeneous: a direct consequence is a more uniform distribution of ventilation with a reduction in risk factors for volutrauma (VILI) [61].

The patient's head should never be excessively rotated (< 60°) to avoid problems with cerebral blood flow and venous drainage [1, 2, 53]. A reduction in cerebral blood flow has been documented in healthy volunteers ventilated with PEEP using transcranial Doppler (TCD) [53]. An aspect not always adequately considered in clinical practice is the position of the patient's face. If the patient's head is below the level of the heart (supports placed under the clavicles and under the iliac spines can cause this), facial edema due to venous stasis may be observed, but more importantly, there may be an increase in intraocular pressure: this becomes particularly important as it is considered potentially responsible, when present, for vision-related complications (up to postoperative loss of vision). Although fortunately very rare (1:60,000/1:125,000), this issue is becoming a subject of medicolegal dispute in spinal surgery (reported as 1:30,000) [1, 2, 53, 63].

Main Issues to Consider Are the Following

1. The position of the head, which is usually rotated, should not be excessively rotated, to avoid stretching of the roots, vascular kinking, or nerve compression, with appropriate anti-decubitus and protective supports.
2. The brachial plexus can be stretched when the neck is rotated: ideally, the possibility of neck rotation and the optimal position should be determined with the patient awake, using suitable protective supports. The eyes should be closed and protected.
3. The prone position carries potential risks of injury to peripheral nerve structures, resulting in both sensory and motor deficits. Ideal should be to determine the best position prior to surgery with the patient conscious, to avoid positions during general anesthesia and muscle relaxation that may later prove traumatic. Upper limb perfusion should be visually monitored, but the use of pulse oximeters is preferable: in particular, compression and stretching should be avoided when placing supports in the clavicular area. Finally, the ulnar nerve at the elbow must be adequately protected or left free to prevent compression or stretch injuries.
4. Trunk and pelvis: Devices must provide adequate support while being covered with anti-decubitus material to prevent pressure injuries at the level of the chest (sternal and acromioclavicular regions) and iliac crests. The purpose of the supports is to minimize pressure on the abdomen and chest.
5. Lower limbs: Protection of bony prominences (iliac spines, knees, ankle joints) must be ensured. Particular attention (as with other positions) should be paid to the positioning of the limbs and joints: at the joint(s) level, to be addressed are "abnormal" angles and pressure points able to cause peripheral nerve injuries. Attention should also be paid to the height of the supports to avoid malpositioning (misalignment), stretching, and pressure sores. Finally, care must be taken with the breasts and genitals, as well as the position of the urinary catheter.

It is recommended [1–4] to document in the medical record both the method of surgical positioning and the protective measures used. According to literature and medicolegal issues, it is suggested as a risk management measure to draft a shared protocol including the type of position and the precautions taken, to serve as a reference and to avoid complex descriptions, while providing administrative and clinical validation. Intraoperative periodic checks reduce the likelihood that prolonged exposure to trauma will result in postoperative injuries.

10.9 Sitting Position (Beach Chair Position, BCP)

The sitting position is usually used for neurosurgical procedures involving the posterior fossa, for posterior cervical spine surgery (widely used in the 1980s and 1990s) [64–66] and today for shoulder surgery [67, 68]. The variant of the sitting position used for shoulder surgery is often called the "beach chair" position *(beach chair)* [67–77]. The head can be elevated above an ideal horizontal plane to varying degrees, depending on surgical requirements (20–45° up to 70°, in some cases even 80°). In neurosurgery (for specific positions, refer to specialized literature) [57, 64–66] the head is fixed with cranial pins, and the arms are supported by devices adequately protected with anti-decubitus material [2]. According to an authoritative and expert opinion, though not yet a recommendation of scientific societies, it is suggested to make somatosensory (SSEP) and motor (MEP) evoked potentials monitoring mandatory in the supine position and to reassess in the sitting position for any changes. If amplitude decreases or latency increases, the recommendation is to modify the position (unpublished data, Dario Caldiroli). The sitting position offers many advantages for surgical procedures [66]: the neurosurgeon's arguments, to a specific list of anesthesiological issues (among others "*cardiovascular instability, jugular venous obstruction, airway oedema, quadriplegia, displacements of catheters and the endotracheal tube, ulnar, sciatic and lateral peroneal nerve compression, venous air embolism, and tension pneumocephalus*"), include better exposure of the surgical field, reduced blood loss, and better preservation of cranial nerves. The conclusion of the article is therefore an invitation to do everything possible to make the sitting position as safe (and as usable) as possible (*"This argues strongly for teaching and use of the sitting position whenever surgically indicated"*) [66].

In orthopedic surgery, the advantages are better surgical/anatomical access to the shoulder region with improved joint mobility and less blood in the surgical field [1, 2, 67, 68]. The BCP, however, requires from an anesthesiological perspective extreme attention and specific precautions for monitoring. The surgical advantages, in fact, should match with significant challenges the anesthesiologist has to face [68, 74]: among them are relevant clinical and medicolegal issues related to cerebral oxygenation and perfusion: even if extremely rare, neurological complications including post-anoxic coma and vision loss) could be devastating [63, 69, 72, 73]. These aspects are of utmost clinical, medicolegal, and even administrative importance, as the number of shoulder procedures in Italy has increased significantly over the past 15 years (data from the Istituto Superiore di Sanità [ISS] and the Italian Arthroplasty Registry [RIA]). Shoulder procedures are currently considered safe surgical procedures in Italy. The definition of a "safe procedure" is supported by the very low incidence of complications and the substantial benefits reported in a recent very large case series from the UK [73]. A review of 288,250 shoulder arthroscopies performed on 261,248 adult patients between 2009 and 2017 (approximately 15,000/year) found that major complications (death, major cardiac events such as pulmonary embolism or myocardial infarction, stroke, infections) were very rare but not absent (1.2%, range 0.2–1.7%): specifically, mortality was 0.05% and major neurological events 0.07%. The most frequent complication was pneumonia (0.3%), and the incidence of pulmonary embolism was very low (0.1%). The authors concluded that, despite a significant increase in procedures in the UK, complications remained very limited, but since maximum safety during surgery should always be pursued, the highest level of anesthesiologic vigilance is warranted to contribute to the definition of "safe" procedures [68, 73, 74]. It is therefore mandatory to understand (i) the cardiovascular changes [73–75], (ii) the impact sitting position (BCP) has on cerebral perfusion, and (iii) the need for appropriate ad hoc monitoring, even for minor, extremely common but potentially dangerous procedures (shoulder surgery).

10.9.1 Physiological Effects of the Sitting Position (BCP) (Table 10.7)

Cardiovascular effects: These effects have the greatest impact on the physiological changes in the sitting position [74–77]. The drugs used for induction and maintenance of general anesthesia (volatile or intravenous agents) cause a modest depression of cardiac performance and vasodilation, which, together with lower limbs venous pooling amplified by the sitting position, are responsible for the hypotension that may occur in the early phases of general anesthesia [74]. In fact, the orthosympathetic response present in non-anesthetized subjects is blunted during general anesthesia: the relative hypovolemia induced by the BCP is associated with reduced preload, decreased SV/CO (10–15%), reduced MAP, and decreased peripheral perfusion pressure. BCP is therefore at risk (particularly) for cerebral hypoperfusion (reduction of cerebral perfusion pressure by about 15%) [1, 67–70, 74]. Correction can be achieved with fluids or moderate doses of vasoconstrictors (usually noradrenaline, sometimes phenylephrine) [67, 73–77]. Among "physical" measures able to reduce the hemodynamic impact of the position and its negative consequences (reduced cerebral perfusion) are slow sitting positioning, elevation of the lower limbs, maintenance of slight flexion at the hip joints, and the use of pneumatic

Table 10.7 —Synoptic table of the effects of the sitting position on the physiological profile

Modifications	Physiological effects	Clinical consequences/notes
Hemodynamic changes	↓VR ↓MAP ↓SV / ↓CO ↓ / ↔/ ↑HR	1. During general anesthesia, hemodynamic effects related to peripheral venous pooling and reduced sympathetic response Regional anesthesia: possible strategy to mitigate the hemodynamic impact of general anesthesia
Ventilatory changes	↑FRC ↑ VC Possible ↑ in physiological dead space (PDS)	ABG
Cerebral perfusion	↓Cerebral arterial flow ↓ Intracranial venous drainage (stasis) ↓ Cerebral oxygenation Cerebral oxygenation monitoring (NIRS) Brain monitoring (see text)	*Blood pressure measurement* 1. *Invasive blood pressure*: should be measured at the "brain" level—transducer zeroed at the level of the external acoustic meatus (tragus) 2. *Noninvasive blood pressure*: should be corrected for the pressure difference between the cuff and the brain. 1. For every 1 cm difference between the cuff and the external acoustic meatus, MAP is 0.75 mmHg *lower in the brain than the MAP measured by the cuff* usually at heart level (1 mmHg for every 1.25 cm) 3. Maintain MAP within 20% of preoperative baseline at rest and in any case ≥70 mmHg

VR venous return, *MAP* mean arterial pressure, *SV* systolic volume, *CO* cardiac output, *HR* heart rate, *FRC* functional residual capacity, *VC* vital capacity—explanations in the text devices on the lower limbs [2] (this latter measure without evidence) [67, 73–77]. The problem of cerebral hypoperfusion with BCP is significant and may be observed with other positions [64–69]. The most extensive documentation for BCP was provided by Aguirre et al., studying risk factors able to alter cerebral blood flow during BCP [71]. The proposed solution(s) of using regional anesthesia to reduce BCP complications is of great clinical and safety interest, but outside the scope of this review and addressed in specific discussions elsewhere [68, 74]. Numerous cases of cerebral ischemia have been reported, including post-anoxic coma, blindness, spinal cord injury, and death in patients undergoing shoulder surgery performed using BCP [67–73]. Even if major neurological events are indeed extremely rare (0.05–0.07%) [69–71, 73], when they occur, the clinical and human consequences are devastating (and arguments for significant medicolegal litigations). Peripheral nerve injuries may also occur and are always associated with clinical and medicolegal issues [1, 2].

Efforts to prevent neurological injuries in BCP have focused on maintaining cerebral perfusion and oxygenation, even though very recent trials have not demonstrated a mandatory association between cerebral desaturation (occurring in up to 30% of cases) and postoperative cognitive dysfunction [76, 77]. The use of locoregional techniques instead of general anesthesia is recommended to reduce this risk [68, 74]. The effects of the BCP on cerebral perfusion and oxygenation are complex and not yet fully understood. In the awake patient, cerebral perfusion in BCP relies on compensatory mechanisms based on the sympathetic response (cerebral autoregulation). Since general anesthesia significantly impairs these mechanisms, closely associated with the orthosympathetic activation, this may result in cerebral hypoperfusion [67, 68, 74–77]. Hypocapnia associated with mechanical ventilation causes cerebral vasoconstriction and may further reduce cerebral perfusion; however, it should be noted that a paradoxical effect (reduction in cerebral blood flow) can also be associated with $PaCO_2 > 50$ mmHg [71]. The mechanism of cerebral autoregulation, which is supposed to maintain constant cerebral blood flow with MAP between 50 and 150 mmHg, has long been questioned. There is, in fact, wide individual variability within this range: in particular, hypertensive and elderly patients may require MAP values not of 50 mmHg but at least of 70 mmHg to maintain autoregulation. Hence the clinical importance of maintaining MAP >70 mmHg to prevent cerebral ischemia when BCPO is used [1, 2, 67, 74]. In 1997, Drummond [78] proposed maintaining higher MAP values (between 70 and 80 mmHg), especially for procedures performed in the BCP under general anesthesia. Lanier's commentary [79] in 2009 in the *Anesthesia Patient Safety Foundation* dealing with cerebral perfusion followed Drummond's observation [78], suggesting a higher MAP value ("*our practices should err on the side of providing excessive blood pressure to non-critical tissues, and adequate blood pressure to critical tissues*" [79]), to maintain adequate perfusion pressure in tissues most sensitive to hypotension (in this case, the brain). "*This approach also has merit because experience tells us that small reductions from normal blood pressure are statistically more likely to produce long-term injury (e.g., from ischemia)*" [79]. In the absence of definitive guidelines,

MAP >70 mmHg is strongly recommended [2, 79]. Controlled hypotension, as per surgeon's request, should instead be carefully considered and planned on a case-by-case basis before surgery, assessing patient risk factors and including in the informed consent form the position, type of technique, risks, benefits, and the type of cardiovascular, respiratory, and cerebral monitoring to be used [2, 74] (of interest are the very recent experiences of Golz et al. [76] and Lee et al. [77]. In the BCP setting, the recommendations on how (and where) to measure (invasive or noninvasive) arterial blood pressure [2, 68, 74, 75] as reiterated by Welch [2] are the following:

1. *Invasive arterial pressure (IAP)*: IAP should be measured at the "cerebral" level—transducer zeroed at the level of the external auditory meatus (tragus).
2. *Noninvasive arterial pressure*: The value should be corrected for the pressure difference between the cuff and the brain. This means that *for every cm of difference between the cuff and the external auditory meatus, MAP is 0.75 mmHg lower at the cerebral level compared to that measured at the cuff, which is usually at heart level (1 mmHg for every 1.25 cm) (brachial pressure).*
   (a) In BCP, with the external auditory meatus on average 30 cm above the cuff, MAP could be less than 50 mmHg (47 mmHg) when cuff MAP is 70 mmHg.
3. Maintain MAP within 20% of the preoperative resting baseline and $\geq$ 70 mmHg.

Cerebral Oxygenation [76–84] Episodes of cerebral desaturation are (i) statistically more frequent in surgery performed in the sitting position; (ii) particularly common in shoulder surgery in BCP under general anesthesia compared to locoregional anesthesia; (iii) the lateral supine position with minimal elevation, not always favored by the surgeon, has a protective effect. Cerebral oxygenation monitoring can be "gauged" using devices for assessing depth of anesthesia (BIS, ENTROPY, NARCOTREND), as well as transcranial Doppler (TCD), EEG, and cerebral oximetry with NIRS (increasingly used), with new opportunities in development, such as MESPERE [80]. Further improvement can be achieved in patients under controlled ventilation by maintaining $ETCO_2$ between 35 and 40 mmHg and avoiding both hyperventilation and hypoventilation.

Respiratory Effects FRC, VC, and C_p improve in the sitting position compared to the lateral supine and prone positions, as the abdominal content is displaced downward [1, 2, 19, 20]. The final effect on oxygenation depends on CO, which tends to decrease in the sitting position and may reduce the beneficial effects of improved respiratory function [68, 74, 85]. Theoretically, an increase in physiological dead space is possible due to reduced perfusion in the nondependent regions of the lung during positive pressure ventilation. Blood gas analysis is essential to assess gas exchange and maintain metabolic control. The topic of gas embolism, its risks, prevention strategies, and dedicated monitoring falls outside the scope of this discussion and is addressed in dedicated literature [1, 58, 64, 65], as is for gas embolism during posterior cranial fossa surgery [2, 58, 64, 65].

Nerve and Vascular Injuries Associated with the Sitting Position Neck flexion used during neurosurgical procedures in the posterior fossa had been associated with rare cases of tetraplegia: a review of these cases, however, revealed the presence of anatomical abnormalities compatible with an increased risk of cervical spinal cord injury. Some authors also highlight the possibility of vascular obstruction involving venous or arterial vessels due to extreme flexion, highlighting the relevance of maintaining the correct positioning. Possible causes in the case of venous obstruction can be identified in altered intracranial venous drainage, with edema of the oropharyngeal structures and tongue [2]. The brachial plexus, as already underlined for other positions, may be at risk of stretching, if the arms are not adequately supported, and of pressure injuries if supports are not properly padded. The ulnar nerve may be compressed at the elbow and should therefore be protected with pressure-relief devices and by checking its position to avoid compression against the operating table. Hands have to stay on supports and should not be left "free" out of the supports. As with other positions, the positioning of the lower limbs requires attention: in the sitting position, in thin patients, pressure on the sciatic nerve exit area or pressure injuries to the ischial tuberosities are to be avoided. The hip joints should not be flexed more than 90°. The knee joints should be placed in slight flexion. The purpose of these precautions is always to avoid stretching injuries to the sciatic nerve.

The sitting position may also be associated with problems related to malpositioning or kinking of the orotracheal tube (which should be reinforced to reduce risks and properly secured): some suggest maintaining a 2–3 cm space between the mandible and sternum during positioning. The proposal by Mannava et al. regarding operating room organization, patient positioning, and monitoring appears extremely useful for summarizing organizational and clinical issues [85].

10.10 Conclusions

The main aim of patient positioning on the operating table is the optimization of surgical outcomes. Then, strict criteria must be set to ensure, together with the best exposure, maximum patient safety: hence the need for training of all team members (surgeon, anesthesiologist, nurse, healthcare staff) to achieve the best result. The choice of position is the responsibility of the surgeon and the anesthesiologist, while the correctness of positioning and protective measures is a team responsibility, with clearly defined roles and tasks that constitute a true risk management operation. The various positions result in changes to cardiovascular, respiratory, and even cerebral perfusion profiles: the physiological changes introduced by different positions must therefore be well understood to be properly managed. A proactive—and not a merely reactive—approach is mandatory for the anesthesiologist. Pressure injuries to the skin and soft tissues and/or peripheral nerve and vascular structures are the most frequent complications related to positioning on the surgical or interventional table. Therefore surgical positioning deserves awareness, widespread dissemination, comprehensive training, and (the role of the Institution) investment in protective and monitoring devices aimed at the mandatory prevention: a protocol with at least an interdepartmental value (better if coming from the Institution) is warranted and should be implemented to avoid defensive medicine and to encourage proactive attitudes at all levels (clinical, administrative, organizational, and logistical).

Acknowledgments To Dario Caldiroli, MD, for his patient and expert review and for his extremely valuable suggestions.

References

1. Hagan K, Gottomukkala V. Chapter 23: Surgical positioning: physiology and perioperative implications. In: Longenecker DE, Brown DL, Newman MF, Zapol W, editors. Anesthesiology. McGraw Hill; 2018. p. 465–75.
2. Welch MB. Patient positioning for surgery and anesthesia in adults. UPTODATE October 26, 2025. Literature review current through: Sep 2025. Section Editor: A Wahr JA; Deputy Editor: Crowley M. Wolters Kluvers.
3. Dobson G, et al. Guidelines to the practice of anesthesia – revised edition 2021. Can J Anesth. 2021;68:92–129.
4. Association of Surgical Technologists – AST Standards of Practice for Surgical Positioning- 2011.
5. Tschannen D, Bates O, Talsma A, Guo Y. Patient-specific and surgical characteristics in the development of pressure ulcers. Am J Crit Care. 2012;21:116.
6. Schoonhoven L, Defloor T, van der Tweel I, Buskens E, Grypdonk MHF. Risk indicators for pressure ulcers during surgery. Appl Nurs Res. 2002;15:163.
7. Choi S, Kim YJ, Oh H, Yuh WT, Lee CH, Kim CH, et al. Factors associated with perioperative hospital acquired pressure injury in patients undergoing spine surgery in the prone position: a prospective observational study. J Neurosurg Anesthesiol. 2024;36:45.
8. Black J, Scott S, Fawcett D. Top ten tips: preventing pressure ulcers in surgical patients. Wounds Int. 2014;5:14.
9. O'Brien DD, Shanks AM, Talsma A, Brenner PS, Ramachandran SK. Intraoperative risk factors associated with postoperative pressure ulcers in critically ill patients: a retrospective observational study. Crit Care Med. 2014;42:40.
10. Shah JL. Lesson of the week: postoperative pressure sores after epidural anesthesia. BMJ. 2000;321:941.
11. Santamaria N, Gerdtz M, Sage S, McCann J, Freeman A, Vassiliou T, et al. A randomized controlled trial of the effectiveness of soft silicone multi-layered foam dressings in the prevention of sacral and heel pressure ulcers in trauma and critically ill patients: the border trial. Int Wound J. 2015;12:302.
12. Chui J, Murkin JM, Posner KL, Domino KB. Perioperative peripheral nerve injury after general anesthesia: a qualitative systematic review. Anesth Analg. 2018;127:134.
13. American Society of Anesthesiologists Task Force on Prevention of Perioperative Peripheral Neuropathies. Practice Advisory for the Prevention of Perioperative Peripheral Neuropathies 2018: An updated report by the American Society of Anesthesiologists Task Force on prevention of perioperative peripheral neuropathies. Anesthesiology. 2018;128:11.
14. Radkowski P, Fedrowska-Szleper M, Podhorodecka K, Mieszkowsk M. Neurological complications of regional anesthesia: an updated review with clinical guidelines. Med Sci Monit. 2023;29:e940399.

15. Warner MA, Warner DO, Matsumoto JY, Harper CM, Schroeder DR, Maxson PM. Ulnar neuropathy in surgical patients. Anesthesiology. 1999;90:54.
16. Chui J, Murkin JM, Turkstra T, McKenzie N, Guo L, Quantz M. A novel automated somatosensory evoked potential (SSEP) monitoring device for detection of intraoperative peripheral nerve injury in cardiac surgery: a clinical feasibility study. J Cardiothorac Vasc Anesth. 2017;31:1174.
17. Chui J, Murkin JM, Drosdowech D. A pilot study of a novel automated somatosensory evoked potential (SSEP) monitoring device for detection and prevention of intraoperative peripheral nerve injury in Total shoulder arthroplasty surgery. J Neurosurg Anesthesiol. 2019;31:291.
18. Brenna CT, Khan S, Katznelson R, Brull R. The role of hyperbaric oxygen therapy in the management of perioperative peripheral nerve injury: a scoping review of the literature. Reg Anesth Pain Med. 2023;48:443.
19. Armstrong M, Moore RA. Anatomy, Patient Positioning [Updated 2022 Oct 31]. In: StatPearls. Treasure Island (FL): StatPearls Publishing; 2024. Available from: https://www.ncbi.nlm.nih.gov/books/NBK513320/.
20. Ravula N, Zagaynov C. Patient positioning: physiologic effects. Last updated: 07/18/2023. In: StatPearls [Internet]. Treasure Island (FL): StatPearls Publishing; 2024. Available from: https://www.ncbi.nlm.nih.gov/books/NBK513320/.
21. Wahba RW. Perioperative functional residual capacity. Can J Anaesth. 1991;38:384.
22. Katz S, Arish N, Rokach A, Zaltzman Y, Marcus EL. The effect of body position on pulmonary function: a systematic review. BMC Pulm Med. 2018;18:159.
23. Spinelli MT, Fogagnolo A, Scaramuzzo G, Rundo A, Grieco DL, et al. Electrical impedance tomography in perioperative medicine: careful respiratory monitoring for tailored interventions. BMC Anesthesiol. 2019;19:140.
24. Nascimento MS, Rebello CM, Costa ELV, Correa LC, Alcala GC, Rossi FS, et al. Effect of general anesthesia and controlled mechanical ventilation on pulmonary ventilation distribution assessed by electrical impedance tomography in healthy children. PLoS One. 2023;18:e0283039.
25. Clasen D, Winter I, Rietzler S, Wolf GK. Changes in ventilation distribution during general anesthesia measured with EIT in mechanically ventilated small children. BMC Anesthesiol. 2023;23:118.
26. Prielipp RC, Morell RC, Walker FO, Santos CC, Bennet JJ, Butterworth J. Ulnar nerve pressure: influence of arm position and relationship to somatosensory evoked potentials. Anesthesiology. 1999;91:345.
27. Unlü Y, Velioğlu Y, Koçak H, Becit N, Ceviz M. Brachial plexus injury following median sternotomy. Interact Cardiovasc Thorac Surg. 2007;6:235.
28. Roy RC, Stafford MA, Charlton JE. Nerve injury and musculoskeletal complaints after cardiac surgery: influence of internal mammary artery dissection and left arm position. Anesth Analg. 1988;67:277.
29. Schwartz S, Peng YG. PRO Supraglottic airway devices (SADs) and laparoscopic surgery. APSF Newsletter. 2023.
30. Omenyo S, Duggan LV CON: Supraglottic airway devices: safety concerns in laparoscopic surgery. APSF Newsletter 2023; 38 May.
31. Bundgaard-Nielsen M, Sørensen H, Dalsgaard M, Rasmussen P, Secher NH. Relationship between stroke volume, cardiac output, and heart filling during tilt. Acta Anaesthesiol Scand. 2009;53:1324.
32. Harms MPM, van Lieshout JJ, Jenstrup M, Secher NH. Postural effects on cardiac output and mixed venous oxygen saturation in humans. Exp Physiol. 2003;88:611.
33. Gannedahl P, Odeberg S, Brodin LA, Sollevi A. Effects of posture and pneumoperitoneum during anesthesia on indices of left ventricular filling. Acta Anaesthesiol Scand. 1996;40:160.
34. Lestar M, Gunnarsson L, Lagerstrand L, Wiklund P. Hemodynamic perturbations during robot-assisted laparoscopic radical prostatectomy in 45° Trendelenburg position. Anesth Analg. 2011;113:1069.

35. Chiumello DA, Duscio E. Chapter 7: Anesthesia in robotic surgery. In: Chiumello D, editor. Practical trends in anesthesia and intensive care 2022; 2024. p. 101–16. https://doi.org/10.1007/978-3-031-43891-2_7.
36. Girrbach F, Petroff D, Schulz S, Hempel G, Lange M, Klotz C, et al. Individualized positive end-expiratory pressure guided by electrical impedance tomography for robot-assisted laparoscopic radical prostatectomy: a prospective, randomized controlled clinical trial. Br J Anaesth. 2020;125:373.
37. Zhou J, Wang C, Lv R, Liu N, Huang Y, Wang W, Yu L, Xie J. Protective mechanical ventilation with optimal PEEP during RARP improves oxygenation and pulmonary indices. Trials. 2021;22:351.
38. Brienza N, Biancofiore G, Cavaliere F, Corcione A, De Gasperi A, De Rosa RC, et al. Clinical guidelines for perioperative hemodynamic management of non-cardiac surgical adult patients. Minerva Anestesiol. 2019;85:1315–33.
39. Banerjee A, Saini S, Lal J. Evaluation of hemodynamic changes during laparoscopic cholecystectomy by transthoracic echocardiography. J Anaesthesiol Clin Pharmacol. 2021;37:436–42.
40. Martin JT. Positioning in anesthesia and surgery. Philadelphia: WB Saunders; 1997.
41. Warner MA, Warner DO, Harper CM, Schroeder DR, Maxson PM. Lower extremity neuropathies associated with lithotomy positions. Anesthesiology. 2000;93:938.
42. Mathews PV, Perry JJ, Murray PC. Well leg compartment syndrome as a result of the hemilithotomy position: a report of two cases and literature review. J Orthop Trauma. 2001;15:580.
43. O'Connor D, Radcliffe J. Patient positioning in anesthesia. Anaesth Intensive Care Med. 2015;16:543–7.
44. Nester M, Borrelli J. Well leg compartment syndrome: pathophysiology, prevention, and treatment. J Clin Med. 2022;11(21):6448. https://doi.org/10.3390/jcm11216448.
45. Halvachizadeh S, Jensen KO, Pape HC. Chapter 12: Compartment syndrome due to patient positioning. In: Mauffrey C, Hak DJ, Martin III MP, editors. Compartment syndrome: a guide to diagnosis and management. Cham: Springer; 2019. p. 113–24. https://doi.org/10.1007/978-3-030-22331-1_12.
46. Litwiller JP, Wells RE Jr, Halliwill JR, Carmichael SW, Warner MA. Effect of lithotomy positions on strain of the obturator and lateral femoral cutaneous nerves. Clin Anat. 2004;17:45.
47. Cheney FW, Domino KB, Caplan RA, Posner KL. Nerve injury associated with anesthesia: a closed claims analysis. Anesthesiology. 1999;90:1062.
48. Welch MB, Brummet CM, Welch DT, Tremper KK, Shanks AM, Guglani P, Manshor GA. Perioperative peripheral nerve injuries: a retrospective study of 380,680 cases during a 10-year period at a single institution. Anesthesiology. 2009;111:490–7.
49. Hewson DW, Bedforth NM, Hardman JG. Peripheral nerve injury arising in anesthesia practice. Anaesthesia. 2018;73(Suppl. 1):51–60.
50. Chui J, Murkin JM, Posner KL, Domino KB. Perioperative peripheral nerve injury after general anesthesia: a qualitative systematic review. Anesth Analg. 2018;127:134–43.
51. Sonawane K, Rao P, Haripriya T, Mystry T, Sekar C. Shedding light on perioperative nerve injury: an investigation using the SHED (symptoms categorization-history taking-examination-diagnostic evaluations) approach. Cureus. 2024;16:e54133.
52. Ghanem MA, El-Hefnawy AS. Cardiopulmonary effects of prolonged surgical abdominal retractor application during general anesthesia: a prospective observational comparative study. Braz J Anesthesiol. 2023;73:291–300.
53. Feix B, Sturgess J. Anaesthesia in the prone position. Contin Educ Anaesth Crit Care Pain (BJA Education). 2014;14:291–7.
54. Alexander NA, Raitt DG, Smith G. Induction of anesthesia and insertion of a laryngeal mask airway in the prone position for minor surgery. Anesth Analg. 2002;94:1194–8.
55. Agrawal S, Sharma J, Jindal P, Sharma U, Rajan M. Airway management in the prone position with an intubating laryngeal mask airway. J Clin Anest. 2007;19:293–5.
56. Weksler N, Klein M, Rozentsveig V, Weksler D, Sidelnik C, Lottan M, Gurman GM. Laryngeal mask in the prone position: mere showmanship or a valid technique? Minerva Anestesiol. 2007;73:33–7.

57. DeGasperi A. Adverse events in anesthesiology: definitions, organizational implications, and clinical applications. Update 2023. ATI 14 Lecture – September 2023. www.ATI14.it.
58. Emamimeybodi M, Hajikarimloo B, Abbasi F, Tavanei R, Toudeshki KK, Koohi N, et al. Position-dependent hemodynamic changes in neurosurgery patients: a narrative review. Interdisc Neurosurg Adv Tech Case Manag. 2024;36:101886.
59. Park JH, Kwon JY, Lee SE, Kim HK, Kim SH. Sudden hemodynamic collapse after prone positioning on a Jackson spinal table for spinal surgery. Korean J Anesthesiol. 2020;73:71.
60. Carreon LY, Glassman S, Chappell D, Garvin S, Lavelle AM, Gum JL, et al. Impact of predictive hemodynamic monitoring on intra-operative hypotension and postoperative complications in multi-level spinal fusion surgery. Spine. 2024; https://doi.org/10.1097/BRS.0000000000005121.
61. Gattinoni L, Brusatori S, D'Albo R, Maj R, Velati M, Zinnato C, et al. Prone position: how understanding and clinical application of a technique progress with time. Anesthesiol Perioper Sci. 2023;1:3. https://doi.org/10.1007/s44254-022-00002-2.
62. Dhoon TQ, Tiwari A, Villaluz E, Morrison DE. Understanding the physiological connection: cardiac arrest following prone positioning. Cureus. 2024;16:e63050. https://doi.org/10.7759/cureus.63050.
63. Roth S. Peri-operative visual loss: what do we know, what can we do? Br J Anaesth. 2009;103(Suppl. I):i31–40.
64. Singh G. Chapter 10: Positioning in Neurosurgery. In: Essentials of neuroanesthesia. Academic; 2017. p. 183–205. https://doi.org/10.1016/B978-0-12-805299-0.00010-5.
65. Mavarez-Martinez A, Israelyan LA, Soghomonyan S, Fiorda Diaz J, Sandhu G, Shimasky VN, Ammirati M, Palettas M, Lubnin AY, Bergese SD. The effects of patient positioning on the outcome during posterior cranial fossa and pineal region surgery. Front Surg. 2020;13(7):9.
66. Charbel F, Kehrli P, Pain L. The sitting position in neurosurgery: the surgeon's perspective. Ann Fr Anesth Reanim. 1998;17:160.
67. Murphy GS, Greenberg SB, Szokol JW. Safety of beach chair position shoulder surgery: a review of the current literature. Anesth Analg. 2019;129:101–18.
68. Hewson DW, Oldman M, Bedforth NM. Regional anesthesia for shoulder surgery. BJA Educ. 2019;19:98–104.
69. Pohl A, Cullen DJ. Cerebral ischemia during shoulder surgery in the upright position: a case series. J Clin Anesth. 2005;17:463.
70. Friedman DJ, Parnes NZ, Zimmer Z, Higgins LD, Warner JPJ, et al. Prevalence of cerebrovascular events during shoulder surgery and association with patient position. Orthopedics. 2009;32:256.
71. Aguirre JA, Mohajeri MS, Rupnik B, Brada M, Rosskopf AB, Meyer DC, Eichenberger U, Borgeat A. Early recognition of a transient ischemic attack utilizing cerebral oxygenation monitoring during shoulder surgery in the beach chair position: a case report. Anesth Analg Pract. 2019;13:176–80.
72. Bhatti MT, Enneking FK. Visual loss and ophthalmoplegia after shoulder surgery. Anesth Analg. 2003;96:899.
73. Rees JL, Crain R, Navra N, Balwin M, Lane JCE, Price A, Beard DJ, Abram S, Judge A, Prieto Alhambra D, Furniss D, Carr AJ. Serious adverse event rates and reoperation after arthroscopic shoulder surgery: population based cohort study. BMJ. 2022;378:e0699012022.
74. Mojica J, Ocker A, Barrat J, Schwenk ES. Anesthesia for the patient undergoing shoulder surgery. Anesthesiol Clin. 2024;42:219–31.
75. Larsen SL, Lyngeraa TS, Maschmann CP, Van Lieshout JJ, Pott FC. Cardiovascular consequence of reclining vs. sitting beach-chair body position for induction of anesthesia. Front Physiol. 2014;5:187.
76. Golz GA, Davis WJ, Perry ME, Tonino PM, Garbis NG, Salazar DH. Improving the safety of shoulder arthroscopy in the beach chair position: a prospective randomized trial investigating the effect of compression stockings on cerebral desaturation events in obese patients. J Shoulder Elb Surg. 2020;29:2027–35.

77. Lee CT, Lin CP, Chan KC, Wu YL, Teng HC, Wu CY. Effects of goal-directed hemodynamic therapy using a noninvasive finger-cuff monitoring device on intraoperative cerebral oxygenation and early delayed neurocognitive recovery in patients undergoing beach chair position shoulder surgery: a randomized controlled trial. Anesth Analg. 2023;136:355–64.
78. Drummond JC. The lower limit of autoregulation: time to revise our thinking? Anesthesiology. 1997;86:1431–3.
79. Lanier W. Cerebral perfusion: err on the side of caution. APFS Newsl. 2009;24:45–8.
80. Lee L, Caplan R. APSF workshop: cerebral perfusion experts share views on management of head-up cases. APSF J. 2009–2010;24(4):45–68.
81. Papadonikolakis A, Wiesler ER, Olympio MA, Poehling GG. Avoiding catastrophic complications of stroke and death related to shoulder surgery in the sitting position. J Arthrosc Relat Surg. 2008;24:481–2.
82. Thanaboriboon C, Vanichvithya P, Jinaworn P. What is the risk of intraoperative cerebral oxygen desaturation in patients undergoing shoulder surgery in the beach chair position? Clin Orthop Relat Res. 2021;479:2677–87.
83. Salazar DH, Davis WJ, Ziroglu N, Garbis NG. Cerebral desaturation events during shoulder arthroscopy in the beach chair position. JAAOS Glob Res Rev. 2019;3:e007.
84. Boukhemis K, Perez M, Olness E, Hensley JL, Lindstrom J, Berry McDonough E, Bal GK. Prospective evaluation of cognitive outcomes after anesthesia for patients in the beach chair position. Orthopedics. 2020;43:27–30.
85. Mannava S, Jinnah AH, Plate JF, et al. Basic shoulder arthroscopy: beach chair patient positioning. Arthrosc Tech. 2016;5(4):731–5.

Suggested Readings

86. Lumb AB, Nunn JF. Respiratory function and ribcage contribution to ventilation in body positions commonly used during anesthesia. Anesth Analg. 1991;73:422.
87. American Society of Anesthesiologists. Practice advisory for perioperative visual loss associated with spine surgery: a report by the american society of anesthesiologists task force on perioperative blindness. Anesthesiology. 2006;104:1319–28.
88. O'Connor D, Radcliffe J. Patient positioning in anaesthesia. Anesth Intensive Care J. 2024;25:743–8.
89. Patterson H, Eady J, Sommerfield A, Sommerfield D, Hauser N, von Ungern-Sternberg BS. Patient positioning and its impact on perioperative outcomes in children: A narrative review. Paediatr Anaesth. 2024;34(6):507–518. 28.
90. Mojica JJ, Ocker A, Barrata J, Schwenk ES. Anesthesia for the Patient Undergoing Shoulder Surgery. Anesthesiol Clin. 2024;42(2):219–31.

Postoperative Delirium and Neurocognitive Decline

11

Stefano Romagnoli

11.1 Introduction and Definitions

Cognitive changes affecting patients after anesthesia and surgery, particularly in the elderly, have been recognized in various forms for many years. Many clinicians are familiar with the clinical syndrome of delirium, a constellation of fluctuating changes in attention, mental status, and level of consciousness, which often occurs after anesthesia and surgery or during hospitalization in the intensive care unit or on the general ward. In addition to delirium, a substantial body of research has investigated postoperative cognitive dysfunction (POCD) or decline after full recovery of consciousness, which persists well beyond the expected pharmacological and physiological effects of anesthetic agents.

It is important, first of all, to distinguish *delirium* (see definition below) from *delusion*. Although in English both syndromes derive from the word "delirium" (e.g., *postoperative delirium*, POD; *delirium as a serious change in mental abilities*), in Italian they refer to two profoundly different pathological conditions.

- Delusion is a chronic and persistent neuropsychiatric condition; it is a psychotic symptom characterized by the presence of false beliefs or ideas, not corresponding to reality, not shared by others, and persistent despite contrary evidence.
- Delirium, according to the *Diagnostic Manual of Mental Disorders* (DSM-5) and the *10th revision of the International Statistical Classification of Diseases*

S. Romagnoli (✉)
Department of Health Sciences, University of Florence, Florence, Italy

Division of Oncologic Anesthesia and Intensive Care, Department of Anesthesiology and Intensive Care, Careggi University Hospital, Florence, Italy
e-mail: stefano.romagnoli@unifi.it

D. Chiumello, A. De Gasperi (eds.), *Practical Trends in Anesthesia and Intensive Care 2026*, https://doi.org/10.1007/978-3-032-25721-5_11

and Related Health Problems (ICD-10), is a form of brain dysfunction (organ failure) characterized by: acute onset, fluctuating course, inattention, disorganized thinking, and altered level of consciousness. Thus, delirium is a multidimensional syndrome defined by five essential elements:
1. Acute change in mental status associated with inattention
2. Fluctuating mental state
3. Disorganized thinking
4. Altered level of consciousness
5. May include hallucinations and illusions

Although this chapter addresses the topic of postoperative delirium (POD), the general features of this serious syndrome are entirely consistent with those characterizing delirium associated with hospitalization, with or without surgery. Some specific aspects (e.g., anesthesia, type and depth, open vs. minimally invasive surgery) will nonetheless be considered in relation to the postoperative form.

11.2 A Brief History

Awareness of the term delirium dates back to the time of *Celsus* in the early centuries before Christ. Celsus described his patients as suffering from mental disturbances when they presented with fever or head trauma. *Hippocrates* likewise recognized delirium as a "*bad omen.*" Hippocrates also used numerous different terms to refer to the clinical syndrome we now call delirium.

The word delirium derives from Latin (deliro—delirare; de-lira; to go out of the furrow). Thus, in Latin, delirium means to lose the right path, to go mad, to lose one's mind, etc.

In 1887, the surgeon *George H. Savage* in an article entitled "Insanity Following the Use of Anaesthetics in Operations" described one of his patients as "in weak condition, both mentally and physically. He would not stay still, was incoherent, and repeated meaningless words. He had entirely the appearance of a half-drunken man."

In 1995, an article by *P.D. Bedford* was published in *The Lancet*, now considered a milestone: "Adverse Cerebral Effects of Anaesthesia on Old People." In this important article, the author emphasized that patients over 65 years of age had an incidence of 7% (18 out of 251) of dementia (a condition of chronic and progressive dysfunction of brain functions leading to a decline in cognitive abilities) following general anesthesia. The significance of this scientific contribution lies in having highlighted, many years ago, the occurrence of *neurocognitive decline* in patients undergoing anesthesia. If anything was missing from Bedford's article, it was the relationship between neurocognitive decline and a set of factors that include anesthesia but cannot exclude hospitalization, surgery, and comorbidities.

Of great importance, however, was the emphasis on age as a significant risk factor. In this regard, as Anglo-Saxon authors say, in elderly patients, worsening neurocognitive function can represent *"the straw that breaks the camel's back"* or, as we would say, "the drop that makes the cup overflow."

This means that elderly patients who are admitted to hospital after living independently may return home in a state of dependency. In light of these considerations, utmost attention must be paid to preventing one of the most serious and frequent complications of hospitalization and surgery, namely, delirium and its close causal relationship with neurocognitive decline.

A lasting complication of delirium affecting patients discharged after one or more episodes (generally those admitted to intensive care) is profound cognitive deterioration, manifesting as loss of short- and long-term memory, executive dysfunction (i.e., the ability to plan, focus attention, remember instructions, and manage multiple tasks), as well as attention, visuospatial, and language disturbances.

11.3 Risk Factors, Clinical Features, Incidence, and Prevention

The exact mechanism underlying delirium remains unclear, and many hypotheses are currently under discussion. The most widely accepted, though still debated, hypothesis is that central neurotransmission is altered, with reduced cholinergic activity and hyperactivation of dopaminergic activity. It is also hypothesized that other central neurotransmitters, such as serotonin and gamma-aminobutyric acid (GABA), play a role in the onset of delirium.

All organs and systems possess a certain level of reserve functional. These reserves are well known and measurable for the cardiovascular system, kidneys, lungs, etc. The brain is no different from other organs and systems. Its functional reserve can be defined as neurocognitive reserve.

It is of fundamental importance to adequately stratify the risk of delirium using the tools currently available. In general, a preexisting deficit in neurocognitive functions represents a significant risk factor, along with age, malnutrition, polypharmacy, major surgery, sleep disturbances, anxiety, dehydration, etc. The presence of one or more of these risk factors at the time of hospitalization identifies what we can call individual cerebral vulnerability.

As a result, there will be patients with a strong neurocognitive reserve in whom delirium will only develop following profound alterations in multiorgan homeostasis (cardiovascular disturbances, fever, release of inflammatory mediators, tissue trauma, etc.), and extremely frail patients (low neurocognitive reserve) who may develop delirium and an increased risk of neurocognitive decline even after minimal perturbations (hospitalization and uncomplicated surgery).

Delirium should be considered the most common form of brain dysfunction occurring in intensive care. It must be regarded as a true organ failure, no different from respiratory, renal, or cardiovascular failure.

Delirium has three fundamental characteristics:

1. Severe
2. Frequent
3. Preventable in many cases

The incidence of delirium in hospitalized populations ranges from 10% to over 80% when considering patients admitted to intensive care and undergoing mechanical ventilation. The consequences of delirium are particularly severe and include: increased neurocognitive decline, high mortality, prolonged length of stay in intensive care and in hospital, increased duration of mechanical ventilation, functional decline at discharge, and higher costs.

Mortality associated with delirium is very high. In particular, at 1 and 6 months it can reach 14% and 22%, respectively—about twice the incidence compared to patients who did not develop delirium. Moreover, signs of delirium may persist even 12 months or more after hospitalization, especially in patients with dementia. According to some studies, only one-third of patients return to independent living after discharge back into the community. Following cardiac surgery, administration of a well-known cognitive test, the Mini-Mental State Examination (MMSE), showed that 6 months after surgery, scores were significantly lower in those who had experienced delirium.

A key aspect is that delirium can be prevented in up to 50% of cases. A meta-analysis demonstrated a 53% reduction in the incidence of delirium (*odds ratio* 0.47) through the implementation of non-pharmacological strategies based on a defined package known as the *Hospital Elder Life Program* (HELP), which included several core interventions:

- Orientation
- Cognitive stimulation
- Improvement of sleep quality
- Mobilization
- Correction of visual (glasses) and hearing (hearing aids) deficits
- Optimization of fluid intake (prevention of dehydration) and nutrition

And a series of additional interventions (hand hygiene, prevention of aspiration, management of pain and hypoxia, etc.).

In recent years, great attention has been devoted to the prevention and treatment of delirium by major scientific societies and international organizations, including the *Perioperative Brain Health Initiative*, the UK NICE guidelines, the *American College of Surgeons*, the *American Geriatric Society*, and, of course, the European Society of Anaesthesiology and Intensive Care (ESAIC), which has recently published guidelines on the prevention of postoperative delirium (see below).

Clinically, delirium can present in three forms, known as *motor subtypes*:

(a) *Hyperactive or hyperkinetic*: the most overt, aggressive, and dangerous for both the patient and healthcare staff.
(b) *Hypoactive or hypokinetic*: characterized by drowsiness, inattention, and *disengagement*. It is also the most hidden but also the most severe (because it is often unrecognized) and more frequent.
(c) *Mixed*.

According to a recent review published in 2022 [8], which included 131 studies and 13,902 patients, hypoactive delirium was present in 50.3% of cases, while both hyperactive and mixed forms accounted for 22.7% each. The hypoactive form was the most frequent, especially among patient populations over 65 years of age.

Delirium that develops during hospitalization is sometimes referred to as the "canary in the coal mine." In other words, delirium can be a prodromal symptom of disturbances in homeostatic balance.

Sometimes, for example, it may be an early manifestation of an infectious process. The fact that the incidence of delirium increased during the COVID-19 pandemic correlates closely with both predisposing and preventive factors: separation from family members was a predisposing factor, and the lack of a preventive factor (so-called *family engagement*). At the same time, the need for deep sedation in patients admitted to intensive care and the use of benzodiazepines have once again proven to be powerful predisposing factors.

Major international initiatives, such as the one promoted by the Society of Critical Care Medicine, the *ICU Liberation* campaign, emphasize the critical importance, in the A, B, C, D (Delirium), E, F sequence, of understanding delirium and its risk factors, knowledge of diagnostic tools, the importance of frequent assessments, and strategies for prevention and treatment (iculiberation@sccm.org).

In the 1990s, a famous advertisement stated: ***prevention is better than cure***. The advertisement referred to a well-known toothpaste and the prevention of cavities, but the underlying concept was that in many conditions, prevention is by far the most effective tool for managing a problem, whereas treatment can be very complex and less effective. The same applies to delirium: prevention is possible, treatment is very difficult! An extremely important aspect is that rarely in medicine does a single intervention suffice to resolve a major and complex problem. What generally proves most effective is the use of multiple interventions that target different areas and, when combined, significantly increase the probability of success. This is the concept of the *bundle*. As the Latins said, "E Pluribus Unum" (the phrase comes from the Moretum, a poem attributed to Virgil), meaning "Out of many, one." The most well-known use of this phrase is as the national motto of the United States of America: it can be found on the state seal, inscribed on a golden ribbon held in the beak of the bald eagle at the center of the shield, as well as on other government-issued items bearing the same symbol (for example, on coins).

The key concept of bundles is that the combination of interventions leads to the highest probability of success. To think, for example, that avoiding electroencephalographic (EEG) suppression during anesthesia for surgery could be the solution to postoperative delirium (POD) is rather utopian, even though, as we will see later, some studies have nonetheless achieved their goal by modulating general anesthesia based on EEG traces alone.

Especially in more complex clinical situations, such as delirium, it is the combination of interventions that increases the likelihood of success.

The main starting point is *risk stratification*. Identifying high-risk patients is the first step in prevention. Delirium is a multifactorial syndrome resulting from the complex interaction between an individual's baseline vulnerability (predisposing factors) and factors related to hospitalization (precipitating factors).

Table 11.1 lists the main risk factors, divided into three categories: patient, acute illness, and iatrogenic and environmental aspects.

There are also electronic tools that can help predict the development of delirium (e.g., *Prediction of Delirium in ICU Patients (Pre-deliric) model; Early (E) Pre-deliric*).

Delirium is a clinical condition and, as such, must be diagnosed using dedicated tools. Among the most commonly used are:

- *Richmond Agitation Sedation Scale* (first step before proceeding with the CAM-ICU) (Table 11.2).
- *Confusion Assessment Method for the ICU* (CAM-ICU); there are also smartphone applications available. In cases of deep sedation (RASS = −4 or −5), the CAM-ICU scale is not administered and the patient is described as "not assessable." With lighter levels of sedation (RASS ≥ −3), the second phase can be performed.

Table 11.1 Risk factors

Patient	Acute illness and treatments	Iatrogenic and environmental aspects
Age (> 65 years)	Acidosis	Immobilization
Male sex	Anemia	Medications (e.g., opioids, benzodiazepines)
Alcoholism	Fever	Anticholinergic drugs
Dementia and baseline cognitive impairment	Infection	Sleep disorders
Previous history of delirium	Sepsis	Isolation
Apolipoprotein E4 polymorphism	Acid-base and fluid-electrolyte imbalances	Lack of visits
Depression	Respiratory distress	Physical restraints
Hypertension	Poor pain control	Deep sedation (vs. light)
Smoking	Mechanical ventilation	Surgery
Visual and/or hearing impairment		EEG suppression during anesthesia
Frailty		

Table 11.2 RASS Scale

Score	Definition	Description	What to do
4	Combative	Clearly combative, violent, immediate danger to self and staff	Patient observation
3	Very agitated	Aggressive, immediate risk of removing catheters and tubes	
2	Agitated	Frequent purposeless movements, poor adaptation to mechanical ventilation	
1	Restless	Anxious but without aggressive or vigorous movements	
0	Alert and calm	Includes periods of physiological sleep	
-1	Drowsy	Not fully alert, opens eyes to verbal stimulus, maintains eye contact >10 sec	Verbal stimulation
−2	Lightly sedated	Brief awakening with verbal stimulus, eye contact <10 sec	
−3	Moderately sedated	Movement or eye opening to verbal stimulus (but without eye contact)	
−4	Deep sedation	No response to verbal stimulus, movement or eye opening to physical stimulation	Physical stimulation (tactile and/or painful)
−5	Unarousable	No response to tactile or painful stimulation	

- 4 AT; *Assessment Method.*
- *Intensive Care Delirium Screening Checklist (ICDSC).*

As previously mentioned, prevention is the most effective weapon against delirium. Albert Einstein once said, "*The clever person solves the problem, but the wise person prevents it.*" To prevent delirium, we must consider a multidisciplinary team in which each professional contributes according to their role: physicians (anesthesiologists, surgeons, internists, geriatricians, psychiatrists, etc.), nurses, physiotherapists, pharmacists, psychologists, dietitians, and healthcare assistants.

Within the context of POD, interventions should be implemented at every stage of the care pathway:

1. Preoperative:
   (a) Identification of patients at risk
   (b) Implementation of *Enhanced Recovery After Surgery* programs
   (c) Development of a dedicated pathway that includes active participation of family members
   (d) *Education*
   (e) Adjustment of polypharmacy
   (f) Assessment and management of cognitive disorders
   (g) Initiation of multimodal prehabilitation programs
   (h) Involvement of the geriatrician
   (i) Others
2. Intraoperative
   (a) Implementation of *Enhanced Recovery After Surgery* programs
   (b) Avoid hypothermia
   (c) Avoid EEG suppression (NO burst-suppression)
   (d) Multimodal and polypharmacological analgesia
   (e) *Opioid-sparing* and *opioid-free* strategies
   (f) Avoid hypoglycemia
   (g) Ensure hemodynamic stability
   (h) Promote minimally invasive surgery (laparoscopic and robotic)
   (i) Maximum attention in high-risk surgeries (cardiac, vascular, urological, general)
   (j) Others
3. Postoperative
   (a) Implementation of *Enhanced Recovery After Surgery* programs
   (b) Early resumption of feeding
   (c) Early mobilization
   (d) Involvement of family members
   (e) Use of glasses and hearing aids
   (f) Sleep hygiene
   (g) If admitted to ICU, promote light sedation
   (h) Early removal of devices (urinary catheter, nasogastric tube, drainage tubes)
   (i) others

As early as 1999, Prof. Inouye demonstrated that the implementation of a series of non-pharmacological interventions targeting six main aspects (cognitive stimulation, sleep hygiene, mobilization, visual aids, hearing aids, hydration) was sufficient to reduce the incidence of delirium in medical wards from 15% to 9% [6].

Some pharmacological interventions have proven useful in the context of anesthesia and intensive care to reduce the incidence of POD:

- According to the "*Best Practices for Postoperative Brain Health: Recommendations from the Fifth International Perioperative Neurotoxicity Working Group*" (Anesthesia & Analgesia 2018), the use of EEG is recommended to tailor the level of anesthesia to the actual needs of the patient.
- Numerous systematic reviews and meta-analyses have shown that avoiding burst-suppression during anesthesia significantly reduces the incidence of POD.
- The guidelines of the European Society of Anaesthesiology and Intensive Care suggest the use of *processed* EEG during anesthesia and recommend avoiding suppression states.
- In the case of intensive care admission, light sedation has been shown to be protective compared to deep sedation in patients on mechanical ventilation.

Table 11.3 summarizes the main strategies for delirium prevention.

Table 11.3 Non-pharmacological and pharmacological strategies for delirium prevention

Non-pharmacological strategies	Pharmacological strategies
Identification of at-risk patients (risk stratification)	Light vs. deep sedation
Patient orientation	Avoid burst-suppression during anesthesia and in intensive care
Noise management (reduction)	Dexmedetomidine for sedation in intensive care and to promote the sleep-wake cycle
Sleep hygiene (reduce noise and nighttime light)	
Patient mobilization	
Glasses	
Hearing aids	
Family involvement	
Natural feeding	
Management of malnutrition and preoperative fasting	
Preoperative prehabilitation pathways	
Minimally invasive surgery	
ERAS programs	
Avoid use of restraints	
Remove unnecessary devices	

11.4 Treatment of Delirium

As previously mentioned, the treatment of delirium is truly complex and much less effective than prevention.

First of all, all strategies that are part of prevention (Table 11.3) should be applied. If these fail, the most dangerous conditions (hyperactive delirium) can be managed with the use of specific agents.

Pharmacological treatment of delirium should be administered in cases of agitation that is dangerous for the patient and healthcare staff, for the shortest possible duration, and with frequent reassessment. Any psychoactive drug can worsen mental confusion, and to date, there is no ideal medication.

Among the most commonly used and currently indicated drugs are Neuroleptics (typical and atypical). Neuroleptics block post-synaptic dopaminergic receptors. Among these, the primary agent indicated is haloperidol.

- Haloperidol
  - Represents the first-line drug of choice
  - Initial dose 0.5–1 mg, repeat as needed after 30 minutes
  - Maintenance 0.1–1 mg 1–3 times/day
  - Risk of parkinsonism (especially if therapy lasts more than 7 days)
  - Rare but severe neuroleptic malignant syndrome
  - 2 mg/ml oral drops (1 drop = 0.1 mg): 3–5 drops twice daily; 2 mg/ml injectable solution: 1 ampoule intramuscularly or subcutaneously, repeat every hour until adequate symptom control is achieved, up to a maximum of 20 mg/day
- Atypical antipsychotics:
  - Quetiapine: 25–100 mg twice daily
  - Olanzapine: 2.5–10 mg daily (also sublingual and intramuscular)
  - Risperidone: 0.5–1 mg twice daily
  - Aripiprazole: 5–15 mg (also intramuscular)
- Benzodiazepines have been shown to be pro-delirogenic, but in cases of uncontrolled agitation they may be considered:
  - May be used as a second-line option when antipsychotics are ineffective or when anxiety predominates
  - Lorazepam 0.5–1 mg intramuscularly or orally
  - Midazolam 1 mg intramuscularly or intravenously (rapid sedation, very short half-life), repeatable
  - Long-acting benzodiazepines are not recommended (no diazepam!)
- In critical care settings, with monitored patients, dexmedetomidine has demonstrated useful preventive and therapeutic effects.

11.5 Relationship Between Delirium and Neurocognitive Decline

Neurocognitive decline involves one or more cognitive domains (learning and memory, language, executive function, complex attention, perceptual-motor function, social cognition). In the perioperative setting, to use correct and shared nomenclature, it is advisable to refer to a recent publication by Lisbeth Evered and colleagues [4].

According to the article by Evered and colleagues, a series of terminological recommendations have been presented.

- Recommendations for perioperative neurocognitive disorders

  They recommend using the term *perioperative neurocognitive disorders* as a general term for cognitive deterioration or change identified in the preoperative or postoperative period. This includes cognitive disorders diagnosed before surgery (described below as *neurocognitive disorders*, NCD); any form of acute event (such as delirium); and cognitive decline diagnosed up to 30 days after surgery (described below as delayed neurocognitive recovery) and up to 12 months (described below as NCD).
- Recommendations for preexisting cognitive impairment

  Preexisting cognitive impairment is the term used to indicate patients with subtle, objectively measurable cognitive impairment at baseline. As a preoperative assessment, this measure of impairment cannot be related to the imminence of anesthesia and surgery and should be considered in terms of cognitive decline that could be incidentally identified in the community as mild NCD (*mild cognitive impairment*, MCI) or major NCD (dementia).
- Recommendations for delirium

  Postoperative delirium (POD) should be recognized as a specific category, in line with DSM-5 terminology (see section on definitions), with appropriate specifications (substance intoxication, substance withdrawal, medication-induced, delirium due to other medical conditions, and delirium due to multiple etiologies), once other specific causes have been excluded and the patient is in the immediate postoperative period.

  POD refers to that which occurs in the hospital *up to one week after surgery* or *until discharge* (whichever comes first) and meets the DSM-5 diagnostic criteria.
- Recommendations for *postoperative cognitive dysfunction* (POCD)

  Objectively measurable decline in cognitive function at variable intervals after anesthesia and surgery. The criteria for POCD have been limited to research settings and have generally been based on an objective decline in cognition measured by neuropsychological tests, usually administered as a battery of multiple tests.

  Delirium significantly increases the risk of postoperative neurocognitive dysfunction and decline.

An article published in the *Wall Street Journal* describes several paradigmatic cases that closely link an episode of POD with cognitive decline.

- One is the story told by William Borten, husband of Judith Sue Borten. William did not imagine that his wife's colorectal surgery could affect her mind. But the day after the operation, Judith Sue Borten could not remember her birthday or who the President of the United States was. She exhibited symptoms of delirium, a confusional state common in elderly patients after surgery or during intensive care stays. The delirium resolved after a few days. However, Mrs. Borten's already compromised cognitive abilities declined rapidly.
- A recent study published in 2023 [7] demonstrated that delirium is associated with a *40% increase in the acceleration of cognitive decline after elective surgery*. In particular, the study's findings suggest that delirium is the most common postoperative complication in older adults and is associated with adverse outcomes, including long-term cognitive decline and incident dementia. The study assessed cognitive decline for up to 72 months (6 years) in a cohort of older adults followed after an episode of delirium following major elective surgery. This was a prospective observational cohort study with long-term follow-up that included 560 community-dwelling older adults (aged over 70 years). Delirium was assessed daily during hospitalization using the CAM method. Cognitive performance, using a comprehensive battery of neuropsychological tests, was evaluated before surgery and at multiple time points after surgery up to 72 months of follow-up. Longitudinal cognitive change was assessed using a composite measure of neuropsychological performance called general cognitive performance (GCP). Retest effects were adjusted using cognitive test results from a nonsurgical comparison group. The 560 participants (326 women [58%]; mean age [SD] 76.7 [5.2] years) provided a total of 2637 person-years of follow-up. One hundred thirty-four participants (24%) developed postoperative delirium. Cognitive change after surgery was complex: the authors found that participants with delirium showed a significantly faster long-term cognitive change, with an increase of −0.4 GCP units (95% CI, −0.1 to −0.7) or −1.4 units per year (about 0.14 population SD units per year). The study found that delirium is associated with *a 40% acceleration in the slope of cognitive decline up to 72 months after major elective surgery*.
- Another study evaluating *covert strokes* (clinically silent strokes identified by MRI) published in 2019 (Neurovision Investigators; Lancet 2019) observed that, in 12 centers enrolling 1114 participants aged >65 years, 78 (7%) had a *covert stroke* and that cognitive decline at 1 year was diagnosed in 42% of patients with a *covert stroke* and only in 29% of those who had not experienced one. The etiopathogenesis of these ischemic events shows substantial overlap with that of delirium.

Delirium and cognitive decline (e.g., dementia, Alzheimer's disease) find numerous common elements, and recent studies have shown that delirium and dementia share common pathophysiological features. For example, neuroinflammation has long been recognized in Alzheimer's disease. Studies on delirium have also demonstrated increased secretion of inflammatory markers by microglia (interleukin-1β, tumor necrosis factor, nitric oxide, and reactive oxygen species) and astrocytes (chemokines). Higher levels of amyloid-β and tau protein in the cerebrospinal fluid are associated with Alzheimer's disease pathology and have also been reported in patients with delirium. On the other hand, systemic inflammation is strongly associated with delirium, and in this context, major surgery may play a role, while minimally invasive approaches may be protective compared to traditional open surgery. Disruption of the blood-brain barrier integrity allows inflammatory cytokines to reach the brain, a phenomenon also observed in patients with dementia. Higher levels of plasma markers of neuronal injury, such as S100B and neuron-specific enolase, have also been described in patients with delirium and dementia. Furthermore, patients with long-term cognitive decline secondary to delirium exhibit atrophy of the prefrontal cortex, hippocampus, and alterations in white matter; these structural changes are also found in patients with dementia. These changes observed in neuroimaging are associated with worse cognitive scores up to 12 months after discharge.

11.6 ESAIC Guidelines on Postoperative Delirium

Recently, the European Society of Anaesthesiology and Intensive Care (ESAIC) published an important document, "*Update of the European Society of Anaesthesiology and Intensive Care Medicine evidence-based and consensus-based guideline on postoperative delirium in adult patients*" [1].

We summarize below some key elements of the document but recommend reading the full text given its relevance and scientific importance.

- *Risk factors*:

  It is recommended to assess the following preoperative risk factors for POD: (1) advanced age, (2) American Society of Anesthesiology physical status score > 2, (3) Charlson comorbidity index >2, and (4) Mini Mental State Examination score below 25 points.
- *Preventive measures* I: Effects of drugs on POD prevention

  In surgical patients, we do not suggest the use of any medication as a prophylactic measure to reduce the incidence of POD.

  When dexmedetomidine is used intraoperatively or postoperatively for the purpose of preventing POD, it is recommended to balance the expected benefits with the most significant side effects (bradycardia and hypotension).

  In surgical patients, we do not suggest any specific type of intervention or anesthesia to reduce the incidence of POD.
- Which *multicomponent or single non-pharmacological interventions* can be recommended to prevent POD?

  We recommend that preoperative anesthesiology consultation in elderly patients include screening for POD risk factors and address patient needs to optimize their preoperative status.

It is recommended that the results of POD risk factor screening be shared with the care team and that prevention strategies be discussed and documented in the medical record.

We recommend multicomponent, non-pharmacological interventions for all patients at risk of POD.

- Does *processed EEG monitoring* during anesthesia reduce POD?

  We suggest guidance of anesthetic depth monitoring based on EEG index to reduce the risk of POD.

  We suggest intraoperative multiparametric EEG monitoring (burst suppression, density spectral array, DSA) during anesthesia to reduce the risk of POD.
- Should *antipsychotics* be used for the treatment of POD?

  The use of low-dose haloperidol is suggested for the treatment of POD if non-pharmacological measures fail. Short-term, symptom-oriented therapy is recommended. Administration should be by bolus and at the lowest possible dose. Antipsychotic drugs should be used with caution or avoided altogether in individuals with preexisting neurological conditions, such as Parkinson's disease or Lewy body dementia.
- Should *benzodiazepines* be used for the treatment of POD?

  The use of benzodiazepines for the treatment of delirium in postoperative patients is not recommended. This recommendation should not be confused with delirium in the context of alcohol withdrawal, where benzodiazepines are recommended as the first-line drug (administered in bolus doses, at the lowest possible dose).
- Should *alpha-2 agonists* be used for the treatment of POD?

  We suggest the use of dexmedetomidine for the treatment of postoperative delirium in cardiac surgery.

11.7 Conclusions

Life expectancy continues to rise, and a 65-year-old European can expect to live approximately 20 more years. The need for surgical interventions (and consequently, anesthesia) increases with age. As a result, in the coming decades, complications related to surgery and anesthesia such as POD will increase in absolute numbers. To reduce the individual and societal burden of POD and its long-term sequelae, preventive strategies are necessary. This requires knowledge, understanding, training, and commitment from the entire perioperative and postoperative team. The implementation of dedicated pathways for the prevention, screening, and possible treatment of POD in routine clinical practice is urgently warranted. Prevention of POD is a fundamental component of the perioperative care pathway for at-risk patients and requires multicomponent strategies, delivered by multidisciplinary teams and ideally initiated before elective surgery. No two elderly patients undergoing scheduled (or unscheduled) surgery have the same risk profile, and therefore, cannot derive the same benefit from a standardized prevention plan. Nevertheless, such standardized strategies are necessary to enable a common, evidence-based approach. Necessary implementations include the assessment of preoperative risk factors, the use of prophylactic medications, biomarkers, type of surgical procedure or anesthesia, and the adoption of non-pharmacological interventions. Neuromonitoring plays a key role in the prevention of POD. If POD is unavoidable and non-pharmacological measures fail, pharmacological treatment options are available. Postoperative delirium and postoperative cognitive dysfunction are neurocognitive complications with negative consequences that may extend well beyond surgical recovery. Postoperative delirium significantly increases the risk of postoperative cognitive dysfunction. Postoperative delirium and postoperative cognitive dysfunction may be distinct manifestations of neurocognitive deficits, triggered by interactions between surgery, anesthesia, and one or more preoperative vulnerabilities (e.g., inflammation, preclinical Alzheimer's neuropathology, blood-brain barrier dysfunction). The nature of the relationship between postoperative delirium and postoperative cognitive dysfunction is not well characterized and is extremely complex. Delirium is associated with long-term cognitive decline, an observation that has been used to suggest a putative role for postoperative delirium in the pathogenesis of postoperative cognitive dysfunction.

More than 40% of delirium cases can be prevented. Consequently, interventions aimed at preventing delirium may also help reduce the risk of postoperative cognitive dysfunction. Research on POD has intensified significantly over the past decade, and discoveries regarding the underlying pathophysiological mechanisms will continue to emerge in the coming decade, refining or revising current knowledge. Finally, future research should investigate the effects of postoperative delirium, postoperative cognitive dysfunction, and their concurrence on functional decline, dementia, and mortality, to better understand the long-term course of the disease.

Suggested Readings

1. Aldecoa C, Bettelli G, Bilotta F, Sanders RD, Aceto P, Audisio R, Cherubini A, Cunningham C, Dabrowski W, Forookhi A, Gitti N, Immonen K, Kehlet H, Koch S, Kotfis K, Latronico N, MacLullich AMJ, Mevorach L, Mueller A, Neuner B, Piva S, Radtke F, Blaser AR, Renzi S, Romagnoli S, Schubert M, Slooter AJC, Tommasino C, Vasiljewa L, Weiss B, Yuerek F, Spies CD. Update of the European Society of Anaesthesiology and Intensive Care Medicine evidence-based and consensus-based guideline on postoperative delirium in adult patients. Eur J Anaesthesiol. 2024;41(2):81–108. https://doi.org/10.1097/EJA.0000000000001876. Epub 2023 Aug 30.
2. Bilotta F, Russo G, Verrengia M, Sportelli A, Foti L, Villa G, Romagnoli S. Systematic review of clinical evidence on postoperative delirium: literature search of original studies based on validated diagnostic scales. J Anesth Analg Crit Care. 2021;1(1):18. https://doi.org/10.1186/s44158-021-00021-8.
3. Daiello LA, Racine AM, Yun Gou R, et al.; SAGES Study Group. Postoperative delirium and postoperative cognitive dysfunction: overlap and divergence. Anesthesiology. 2019;131(3):477–91. https://doi.org/10.1097/ALN.0000000000002729. PMID: 31166241.
4. Evered L, Silbert B, Knopman DS, Scott DA, DeKosky ST, Rasmussen LS, Oh ES, Crosby G, Berger M, Eckenhoff RG. Nomenclature Consensus Working Group. Recommendations for the nomenclature of cognitive change associated with anaesthesia and surgery-2018. Br J

Anaesth. 2018;121(5):1005–12. https://doi.org/10.1016/j.bja.2017.11.087. Epub 2018 Jun 15. PMID: 30336844.

5. Evered LA, Chan MTV, Han R, Chu MHM, Cheng BP, Scott DA, Pryor KO, Sessler DI, Veselis R, Frampton C, Sumner M, Ayeni A, Myles PS, Campbell D, Leslie K, Short TG. Anaesthetic depth and delirium after major surgery: a randomised clinical trial. Br J Anaesth. 2021;127(5):704–12. https://doi.org/10.1016/j.bja.2021.07.021. Epub 2021 Aug 28. PMID: 34465469.
6. Inouye SK, Westendorp RG, Saczynski JS. Delirium in elderly people. Lancet 2014;383(9920):911–22. https://doi.org/10.1016/S0140-6736(13)60688-1. Epub 2013 Aug 28. PMID: 23992774.
7. Kunicki ZJ, Ngo LH, Marcantonio ER, Tommet D, Feng Y, Fong TG, Schmitt EM, Travison TG, Jones RN, Inouye SK. Six-year cognitive trajectory in older adults following major surgery and delirium. JAMA Intern Med. 2023;183(5):442–50. https://doi.org/10.1001/jamainternmed.2023.0144. PMID: 36939716.
8. la Cour KN, Andersen-Ranberg NC, Weihe S, Poulsen LM, Mortensen CB, Kjer CKW, Collet MO, Estrup S, Mathiesen O. Distribution of delirium motor subtypes in the intensive care unit: a systematic scoping review. Crit Care. 2022;26(1):53. https://doi.org/10.1186/s13054-022-03931-3. PMID: 35241132.
9. Mevorach L, Forookhi A, Farcomeni A, Romagnoli S, Bilotta F. Perioperative risk factors associated with increased incidence of postoperative delirium: systematic review, meta-analysis, and Grading of Recommendations Assessment, Development, and Evaluation system report of clinical literature. Br J Anaesth. 2023;130(2):e254–62. https://doi.org/10.1016/j.bja.2022.05.032. Epub 2022 Jul 7.
10. Nassar AP, Ely EW, Fiest KM. Long-term outcomes of intensive care unit delirium. Intensive Care Med. 2023;49(6):677–80. https://doi.org/10.1007/s00134-023-07029-4. Epub 2023 Mar 24. PMID: 36964214.
11. Needam MJ, Webb CE, Bryden DC. Postoperative cognitive dysfunction and dementia: what we need to know and do. Br J Anaesth. 2017;119(suppl_1):i115–25. https://doi.org/10.1093/bja/aex354. PMID: 29161395.
12. Sumner M, Deng C, Evered L, Frampton C, Leslie K, Short T, Campbell D. Processed electroencephalography-guided general anaesthesia to reduce postoperative delirium: a systematic review and meta-analysis. Br J Anaesth. 2023;130(2):e243–53. https://doi.org/10.1016/j.bja.2022.01.006. Epub 2022 Feb 17. PMID: 35183345.
13. Veronese N, Solimando L, Bolzetta F, Maggi S, Fiedorowicz JG, Gupta A, Fabiano N, Wong S, Boyer L, Fond G, Dragioti E, Dominguez LJ, Barbagallo M, Romagnoli S, Bellelli G, Solmi M. Interventions to prevent and treat delirium: an umbrella review of randomized controlled trials. Ageing Res Rev. 2024;97:102313. https://doi.org/10.1016/j.arr.2024.102313. Epub 2024 Apr 26.

Airway Management and One-Lung Ventilation: Current Techniques and Scientific Evidence

12

Federico Piccioni and Fabio Piccirillo

One-lung ventilation techniques are used in a variety of settings: pulmonary, mediastinal, esophageal, cardiac, vascular, and spinal surgery. The goal is to provide optimal exposure of the surgical field by avoiding ventilation of one lung or part of it. Sometimes, one-lung ventilation is required due to the presence of bronchopleural fistulas or for performing bronchoalveolar lavage. In any situation where one-lung ventilation is planned, it is crucial to define the objectives to be achieved, which depend on the planned surgical procedure, as well as to consider the anatomical and physiological aspects to be managed, the devices and tools available to the clinician, and the clinician's experience with these devices in order to determine the best operative strategy.

Airway anatomy is of utmost importance in this context and guides the technical choice, which today can rely on a wide range of devices available on the market. Two levels of assessment can be defined: that of the upper airways and that of the lower airways. The first is part of the routine preoperative evaluation and is necessary to anticipate cases of difficult ventilation or intubation. These specific aspects are beyond the scope of this discussion, although they will be briefly addressed in a dedicated section. The second level, the assessment of tracheobronchial anatomy, is a mandatory step as it helps determine the most appropriate device for each specific case. The importance of radiological imaging review by the anesthesiologist is therefore emphasized, especially computed tomography (CT), which allows for assessment of the caliber and course of the trachea and bronchi, the actual anatomy of the structures, and, particularly in thoracic surgery, the complexity of the surgical procedure.

F. Piccioni (✉) · F. Piccirillo
Anesthesia and Perioperative Medicine Unit, IRCCS Humanitas Research Hospital, Rozzano, Rozzano, Italy
e-mail: federico.piccioni@humanitas.it; fabio.piccirillo@humanitas.it

D. Chiumello, A. De Gasperi (eds.), *Practical Trends in Anesthesia and Intensive Care 2026*, https://doi.org/10.1007/978-3-032-25721-5_12

12.1 Lung Isolation and Separation: Definitions and Historical Overview

Technically, a distinction is made between lung isolation and lung separation. In the first case, the goal is to avoid ventilation of one lung (or a portion of it), while in the second, an additional objective is to prevent possible contamination of the ventilated, healthy lung by secretions, purulent material, or blood. Further indications for lung separation include situations where independent ventilation of both lungs may be necessary (large bronchopleural fistulas, pulmonary contusion, giant bullae). Lung isolation is achieved with bronchial blockers (BB), while lung separation is obtained using double-lumen tubes (DLT—Fig. 12.1). The indications for lung isolation or separation are summarized in Table 12.1. Historically, the possibility of achieving one-lung ventilation was first realized in 1931, three years after the introduction of the endotracheal tube, by advancing the tube into the bronchus of the lung to be ventilated (endobronchial intubation) [1]. In 1935, Archibald instead described the use of a cuffed rubber catheter positioned under radiological guidance to exclude ventilation of one of the two lungs [2]. This was the first description of a BB that was placed externally to the orotracheal tube. Other authors also described the use of BBs in subsequent years, but at that time, the use of such devices was complex because it relied solely on rigid bronchoscopes and radiological control to verify correct placement. For the anesthesiologist, managing BBs was very challenging without the aid of flexible bronchoscopy, which was introduced only 40 years later, and due to the frequent movements of patients during procedures, facilitated by the lack of muscle relaxants. In 1936, the use of a single-lumen bronchial tube equipped with two cuffs, one tracheal and one bronchial, was described [3]. This type of device, still commercially available today, allows, after positioning its distal end in the left main bronchus, for left single-lung ventilation when both cuffs are inflated. However, it was not until 1949 that the first DLT was introduced, developed by the Swedish physiologist Eric Carlens with the aim of performing separate spirometries [4]. This innovation radically changed the management of single-lung ventilation, improving not only anesthetic techniques but also surgical

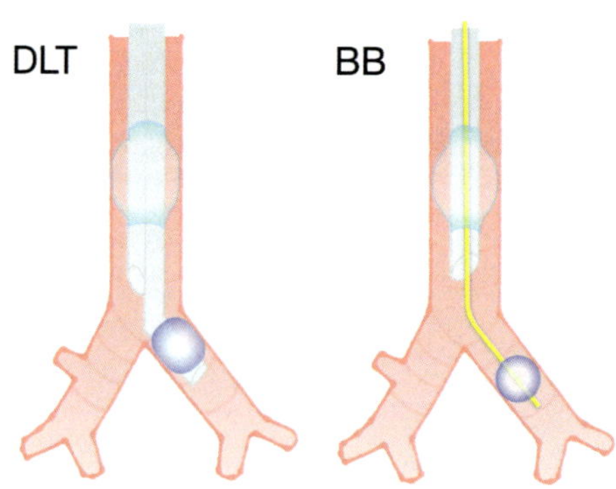

Fig. 12.1 Schematic representation of a left double-lumen tube (DLT) and a bronchial blocker (BB)

Table 12.1 Indications and objectives of one-lung ventilation with suggested optimal device

Indication	Objective	Device
Unilateral lung abscess	Protection of the contralateral lung	DLT
Massive bleeding/hemoptysis		DLT
Alveolar lavage for proteinosis		DLT
Bronchopleural fistula	Ensure gas exchange and airway safety	DLT
Severe unilateral disease (e.g., giant emphysematous bulla)	Separate lung ventilation	DLT
Lung transplantation	Separate lung ventilation and airway safety	DLT
Pneumonectomy, main bronchus sleeve resection	Surgical exposure	DLT
Tumors involving the main bronchus		DLT
Thoracic aneurysm		DLT
Lobectomy and minor resections		DLT / BB
Thymectomy		DLT / BB
Pleural surgery		DLT / BB
Thoracectomy		DLT / BB
Sympathectomy		DLT / BB
Esophagectomy		DLT / BB
Spinal surgery		DLT / BB
Minimally invasive cardiac surgery		DLT / BB

DLT double-lumen tube; *BB* bronchial blocker

possibilities. Since then, both BBs and DLTs have undergone significant development, allowing anesthesiologists today to have a wide range of devices to address different clinical situations.

12.2 Bronchial Blockers

As mentioned in the previous section, BBs function by preventing gas flow to the isolated portion of the lung. The cuff, when properly inflated, acts as a "plug," blocking ventilation distal to it (Fig. 12.2). While the operating principle is the same, many devices not specifically designed for this purpose have been used in the past: Fogarty embolectomy catheters, Swan-Ganz pulmonary artery catheters, and even Foley urinary catheters [1]. Since the 1980s, numerous BBs have been developed and are currently available on the market, with different characteristics and suitable for both adult and pediatric patients. It is worth recalling the introduction in 1984 of the Univent tube, a single-lumen endotracheal tube equipped with a channel in which a BB can be inserted and positioned, as needed, in either the right or left main bronchus [5]. This tube allows removal of the BB at the end of the procedure if the patient needs to remain intubated. Available in various sizes, the Univent has not gained widespread use among anesthesiologists because of its large diameter and, above all, because it is much stiffer than a standard single-lumen tube.

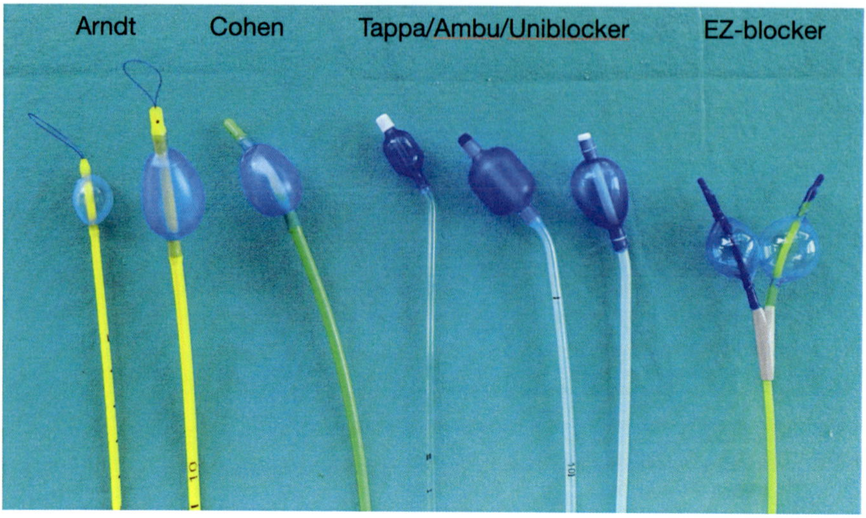

Fig. 12.2 Distal portion of the main types of bronchial blockers in various sizes. Note that the cuffs may be spherical or more elongated in shape. Refer to the text for a description of each model

Table 12.2 Characteristics of the main devices used for lung isolation

Device	Size	Length	Cuff	Cuff volume	Channel diameter
Fogarty	Pediatric 2–5 Fr	80 cm	HP spherical	0.2–3 mL	No channel
	Adult 6–8 Fr				
Univent	Pediatric ETT 3.5–4.5	ETT	HP spherical	1–3 mL	No channel
	Adult ETT 6–9			4–8 mL	2 mm
Uniblocker	5–9 Fr	66.5 cm	LP spherical	1–3 mL	2 mm
Arndt	Pediatric 5 Fr	65 cm	LP spherical	1–3 mL	0.7 mm
	Adult 7–9 Fr	65–78 cm	LP spherical/ elliptical	6–8 / 12 mL	1.4 mm
Cohen	9 Fr	65 cm	LP spherical	5–8 mL	1.6 mm
EZ-blocker	7 Fr	75 cm	HP spherical	4–12 mL	1.4 mm

HP high pressure; *LP* low pressure

The general characteristics of the main BBs and the Univent tube are summarized in Table 12.2.

All BBs are equipped with a channel that, although small in caliber, can be used for both suction and oxygen delivery. Suction through this lumen can facilitate collapse of the isolated lung, although it is rarely effective for removing secretions and blood. All BBs come with a dedicated connector for connection between the orotracheal tube and the ventilation circuit and are equipped with an access port for the

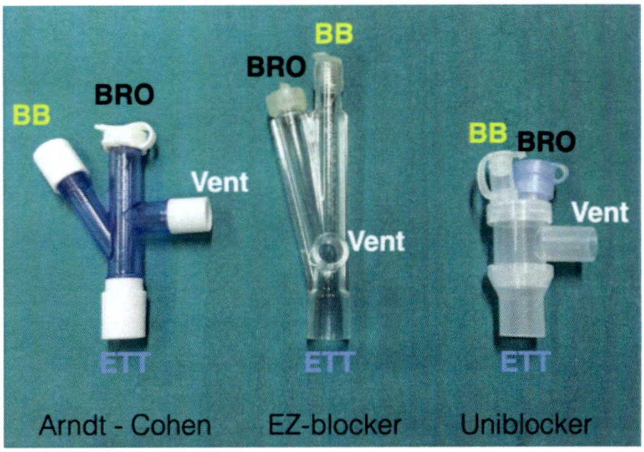

Fig. 12.3 Three types of connectors for bronchial blockers. Each connector is equipped with access ports for the blocker (BB), for the bronchoscope (BRO), and connectors for the ventilation circuit (Vent) and the endotracheal tube (ETT)

blocker itself and a suction port through which a video-bronchoscope can be introduced (Fig. 12.3).

The Arndt BB is the prototype of these devices and is available for adults (sizes 7 and 9 Fr) and pediatric patients (size 5 Fr) [6]. It is the only blocker that must be "guided" into the desired bronchus using a video-bronchoscope. This maneuver is possible by using the loop with which it is equipped, which, protruding from the distal channel, allows it to be anchored to the video-bronchoscope. Once the video-bronchoscope is introduced into the desired bronchus, the loop is loosened by advancing the BB, and the video-bronchoscope is withdrawn to the tracheal level to visualize the carina and optimize the BB's position. Other types of BBs, on the other hand, can be positioned under direct vision by keeping the tip of the video-bronchoscope at the exit of the endotracheal tube, allowing visualization of the tracheal carina, bronchi, and the blocker itself during placement. The Cohen BB is characterized by a flexible tip that, via a wheel at the proximal end of the device, allows the tip to be flexed to facilitate positioning [7]. This flexion of the distal tip is similar to that of a bronchoscope but is possible in only one direction (the side of the tip that can be flexed is indicated on the blocker with a black arrow). This blocker is available only in the 9 Fr size. Another type of BB, produced by various companies, features a distal tip bent at an angle between 20 and 30° [8]. By rotating the BB after it exits the tube, the tip can be directed into the desired bronchus. This blocker is essentially the same as the one incorporated in the Univent tube and is available in various sizes for adults (7 and 9 Fr) as well as for pediatric patients (5 Fr). Some models are available with a self-inflating cuff system, that is, they are equipped with a device connected to the cuff inflation channel which, similar to a small elastomeric pump, can be filled with air before the start of the positioning maneuver to inflate the cuff at the appropriate time with one hand and without the use of a syringe (Fig. 12.4). The most recent type of BB introduced to the market is the EZ-blocker, characterized by a Y-shaped distal portion with two ends equipped with cuffs that are to be positioned in both main bronchi [8]. This BB is available only in the 7 Fr size and, once positioned, is particularly stable because it is placed "straddling" the tracheal carina. To facilitate its placement, it is essential to initially maintain a

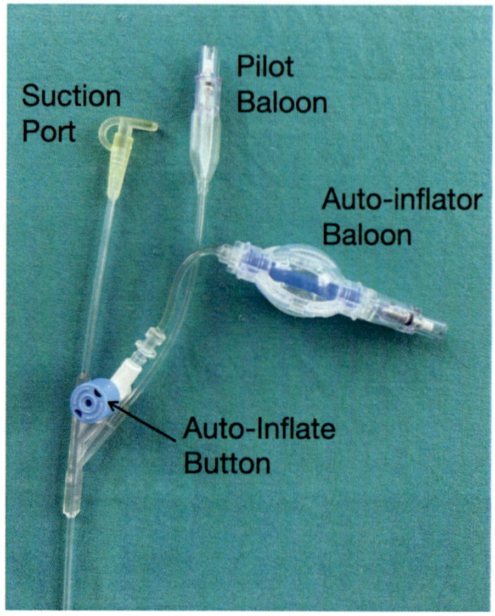

Fig. 12.4 Proximal portion of a bronchial blocker with a self-inflating cuff system. The blocker is equipped with a suction port for access to the device lumen, an inflation connector for manual cuff inflation using a syringe, and a self-inflating balloon that can be filled with air before starting the positioning procedure. Once the blocker is inserted into the desired bronchus, the cuff can be inflated by pressing the inflation button

distance of about 5 cm between the tip of the orotracheal tube and the carina so that the two Y-shaped ends can separate and be introduced into the two main bronchi (the opening angle of the ends is about 30°). Once the BB is properly positioned, if necessary, the tube can be advanced closer to the carina.

Few comparative studies between different BB models have demonstrated superiority of one model over the others. A randomized study found no differences among three blockers in terms of positioning time and quality of lung isolation [9]. However, in that study, the Arndt BB required more frequent repositioning compared to the Cohen BB and the Uniblocker. A comparative study between the EZ-blocker and the Cohen blocker reported shorter positioning times and a lower incidence of intraoperative repositioning for the former [10]. Another study reported a higher frequency of intraoperative repositioning with the Uniblocker compared to the EZ-blocker, although the latter required more repositioning interventions when isolating the right lung [11]. Inflation of the BB cuff and the small caliber of the internal channel hinder the collapse of the isolated lung regardless of the BB model used. To facilitate lung deflation, it is useful to perform an apnea during which the ventilation circuit is disconnected for 30 seconds, then inflate the BB cuff, reconnect, and finally restore mechanical ventilation. An interesting development of this strategy, when using the EZ-blocker, is the possibility of inflating the cuff of the dependent lung—that is, the lung to be ventilated—before the apnea phase, with the aim of counteracting alveolar derecruitment that occurs with disconnection of the ventilation circuit [12]. This cuff is then deflated upon resumption of one-lung ventilation. Finally, connecting a suction system to the BB lumen can further facilitate lung collapse.

When choosing which BB to use, it is extremely important to consider its size in relation to the single-lumen tube to be used and the size of the available video-bronchoscope. It should be noted that the size of blockers is expressed in French, which describes the circumference. To determine the diameter in millimeters, simply divide the size by 3 (for example: a 9 Fr BB has a diameter of 9/3 = 3 mm). This measurement should be considered together with the external diameter of the video-bronchoscope, which in this context is typically 3.8–4.0 mm, and the internal diameter of the endotracheal tube, which for 7 and 9 Fr BBs should not be less than 7.5 mm to ensure mechanical ventilation during positioning maneuvers or airway checks.

At present, it is not possible to recommend one type of BB over the others; rather, it is useful to consider the different types based on their specific characteristics, which may indicate their use according to individual circumstances. Each anesthesiologist should ideally have access to multiple BB models and acquire the technical skills to use them interchangeably according to the clinical context.

12.3 Double-Lumen Tube (DLT)

The double-lumen tube is currently the most widely used device for one-lung ventilation. According to several surveys, the DLT is the first choice for anesthesiologists in 89–100% of cases [13–17], because, once positioned, it ensures device stability and complete control of both pulmonary systems, both in terms of ventilation and the possibility of suction and video-bronchoscopic inspection. There are two versions of the double-lumen tube, left and right, which are shaped to fit the corresponding bronchial anatomy. Both versions have two ventilation lumens: one longer, called the bronchial lumen, which is placed in the desired main bronchus, and a shorter, tracheal lumen, whose opening remains above the carina. Both ends are equipped with cuffs, one tracheal and one bronchial, which serve to isolate the trachea and bronchus, allowing independent ventilation of the two lungs. As previously mentioned, the introduction of this device, in the left-sided version only, dates back to 1949 (Carlens tube) [4]. Subsequently, in 1960, the right-sided version was introduced—the White tube—which, equipped with a hole at the level of the bronchial cuff, allowed ventilation of the right upper lobe (Fig. 12.5) [18]. The described tubes were made of rubber, reusable, with circular-section ventilation lumens, equipped with high-pressure cuffs, and featured a hook between the bronchial cuff and the tracheal lumen opening designed to anchor the device to the carina and ensure stability during surgery. The next evolution of double-lumen tubes occurred in 1962 with the introduction of the Robertshaw tube, without a hook and with larger ventilation lumens and a "D"-shaped cross-section, which reduced resistance to gas flow [19]. The advent of plastics allowed, two decades later, the introduction of the devices currently used in operating rooms. Today's tubes are made of PVC or silicone; are single-use, equipped with high-volume, low-pressure cuffs; and have thinner walls that, for the same total diameter, provide larger ventilation lumens with minimal resistance to airflow and easier introduction of suction catheters and video-bronchoscopes. An in vitro study found that modern DLTs offer greater flow resistance compared to single-lumen tubes, but this difference is clinically

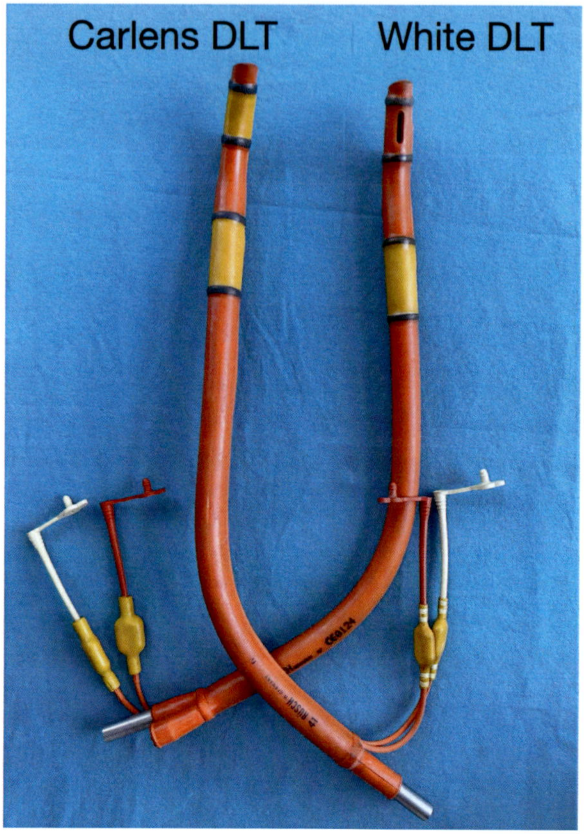

Fig. 12.5 Left (Carlens DLT) and right (White DLT) rubber double-lumen tubes. Note the slit-shaped distal opening of the bronchial portion of the right DLT, which is useful for ventilating the right upper lung lobe

negligible [20]. An observational study instead investigated the contribution of expiratory flow resistance of the DLT to autoPEEP [21]. The authors found that DLT resistance accounts for 30% of autoPEEP generation, but this effect does not differ when using different DLT sizes (35, 37, and 39 Fr). The debate over the choice of a double-lumen tube with or without a hook remains unresolved. Although the hook may provide greater tube stability during surgery, it potentially increases the risk of injury to the upper and lower airways and may interfere with correct device placement if it bends toward the proximal portion of the tube or enters the bronchus along with the bronchial lumen. A recent randomized study of 184 patients showed no difference between the use of the device with or without a hook in terms of benefits or complications [22], but nowadays, most anesthesiologists and the authors themselves prefer the hookless version (Fig. 12.6).

The available double-lumen tube sizes range from 26 to 41 Fr to accommodate both adult and pediatric patients. Choosing the appropriate size of the double-lumen tube is crucial to ensure correct and stable device placement during surgery. It should be emphasized that surgical maneuvers can easily cause displacement of these devices if the initial placement is not adequate. Several authors have proposed methods to facilitate the selection of the correct DLT size based on patient

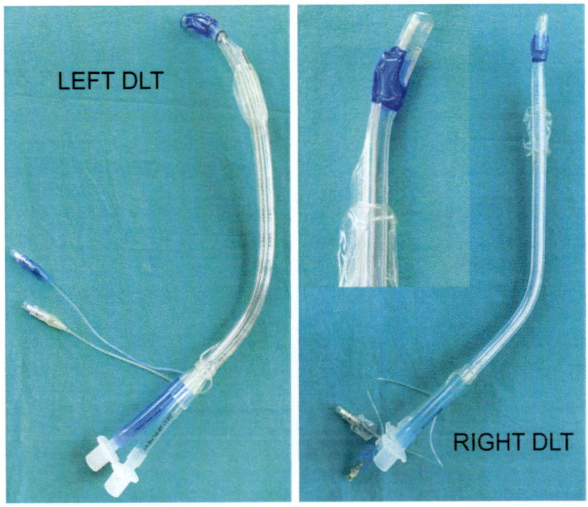

Fig. 12.6 Right and left PVC double-lumen tubes. In the inset, the bronchial end of the right DLT with the asymmetric cuff and the lateral opening for ventilation of the right upper lung lobe

characteristics. The simplest method is based on the patient's height and gender, while other approaches rely on the tracheal diameter measured on chest X-ray or the size of the left main bronchus obtained from computed tomography [23]. All these methods refer to the selection of the left-sided double-lumen tube. One study evaluated the selection of the right-sided DLT by considering the distance between the tracheal carina and the right upper lobe bronchus, but the results are not well suited to the European population, as they are based on a sample of Asian patients with different anthropometric characteristics [24]. In the authors' experience, chest CT analysis is well suited for selecting the left-sided tube in male patients, whereas in female patients it often leads to the selection of tubes that are too large and may be difficult to introduce, especially when passing the glottic plane. It is important to note that double-lumen tubes have large external diameters; for example, a 41 Fr tube is comparable to a size 12.5 single-lumen tube. For this reason, intubation with a DLT is always more difficult than with a single-lumen tube and must be managed with great care, avoiding forceful maneuvers if there is difficulty passing the glottic plane or advancing the device at the bronchial level, due to the risk of airway injury.

There are two techniques for positioning the DLT. The most common involves blind placement of the tube, followed by confirmation through auscultation, observation of airway pressure curves and capnometry, and finally with the aid of a video-bronchoscope introduced into the tracheal lumen. The second technique involves intubation with advancement of the first portion of the tube (the bronchial lumen) past the glottic plane, through which the video-bronchoscope is introduced and advanced into the desired bronchus, then serving as a guide for further advancement of the tube. In both cases, correct tube placement is confirmed by visualization and identification of anatomical structures and verification of the correct depth of the bronchial lumen in the target bronchus (relative to the tracheal carina, a small portion of the bronchial cuff should be visible without herniation). If video-bronchoscopic inspection is unclear, with uncertain identification of anatomical structures and consequent doubt about correct device placement, it is recommended to position the tip of the video-bronchoscope at the distal opening of the bronchial lumen and slowly withdraw the tube until the tracheal carina is clearly identified, then proceed with repositioning the tube. It should be noted that distinguishing the tracheal carina from the lower bronchial branches is often challenging. Therefore, DLT withdrawal should be performed without hesitation if there is any uncertainty in identifying the structures. Video-bronchoscopic control should be performed during DLT placement, after surgical positioning of the patient, and whenever necessary during one-lung ventilation, as surgical maneuvers can displace the device during the procedure. The use of the right-sided DLT is associated with greater difficulty in placement because it is necessary to identify the correct device depth so that the opening for ventilation of the right upper lobe bronchus is aligned with its origin, and the bronchial cuff does not protrude into the trachea beyond the carina. The greater complexity of positioning the right-sided DLT is the main reason why, in most cases, anesthesiologists preferentially use the left-sided version [13, 16].

The use of video-bronchoscopy has not yet become standard practice in thoracic anesthesia. According to an international survey conducted in 2017, the video-bronchoscope is routinely used in 82% of cases in Northern European countries, 57% in Southern European countries, and 21% in Eastern Europe [16]. The latter figure is related to the limited availability of bronchoscopes in operating rooms. In 2019, a prospective multicenter observational study involving 2217 Italian patients found that DLT placement was followed by bronchoscopic confirmation in only 54% of cases (100% when a BB was used) [24]. It is noteworthy that in this study, bronchoscopic confirmation of DLT placement was associated with a reduction in hypoxic events during one-lung ventilation. Today, the availability and use of video-bronchoscopes in the operating room are strongly recommended [25], and anesthesiologists must possess the technical skills required to use them.

While the most widely used double-lumen tubes today are made of polyvinyl chloride (PVC), silicone models are also available, characterized by greater softness and flexibility. In particular, this type of tube has a more flexible bronchial segment, allowing better adaptation to the bronchial tree, especially in cases of more pronounced anatomical curvature due to parenchymal traction, deviation from mass effect, or previous surgical procedures (a typical clinical scenario is upward torsion of the left main bronchus in patients who have undergone previous left upper lobectomy).

In addition to the double-lumen tubes described above, other devices with specific features are available. The Vivasight 2 DLT double-lumen tube is equipped with an integrated video camera at the end of the tracheal lumen, allowing visualization of the bronchial portion of the tube and the surrounding anatomical structures [26]. This device, combined with a dedicated display, enables real-time visual monitoring of correct positioning during surgery. Since the camera view may be compromised by secretions or blood, it can be cleaned by injecting air or saline through an accessory channel with a terminal opening at the camera itself. The Vivasight 2 DLT is available only in the left-sided version in sizes 35, 37, 39, and 41 Fr. The use of this device reduces the need for video-bronchoscopy and, according to some studies, may lower costs compared to a standard DLT combined with a reusable bronchoscope, although the comparison with single-use bronchoscopes is less clear [27–30]. The reduction in the need for video-bronchoscopy with the Vivasight 2 DLT has also been demonstrated in a recent meta-analysis, which also reported shorter DLT placement times compared to conventional methods. Overall, the literature has demonstrated the superiority of the Vivasight 2 DLT in other aspects, such as device displacement during surgery, quality of lung collapse, and postoperative hoarseness [31].

In 2023, a new double-lumen tube, the sOLVe Tube, was introduced, designed as a single size (35 Fr) and suitable for placement in either the right or left main bronchus [32]. The device was developed after analyzing radiological images from 195 patients, is made of silicone, features a trapezoidal-shaped bronchial cuff, and has a flexible septum dividing the two lumens to facilitate passage of the video-bronchoscope. This device is still in the testing phase and not yet commercially available, but it has already met Food and Drug Administration (FDA) safety standards for manufacturing, biocompatibility, and clinical use.

Of particular interest is the ECOM DLT, a left-sided tube available in sizes 35, 37, and 39 Fr, equipped with electrodes integrated into the tracheal cuff that, using a bioimpedance system, allow noninvasive hemodynamic monitoring of cardiac output and stroke volume variation [33].

12.4 Bronchial Blocker Versus Double-Lumen Tube

As previously mentioned, the DLT is the first choice for one-lung ventilation management for the vast majority of anesthesiologists [13–17, 24]. A 2015 meta-analysis of 13 randomized studies compared DLTs and BBs in terms of efficacy and adverse events [34]. DLTs were found to be positioned more quickly and accurately than BBs. It should be noted, however, that only 2 of the 13 studies used the right-sided DLT, which is more challenging to position. No significant difference was found between the two devices regarding the time to lung collapse or the quality of collapse. BBs, which are positioned through a single-lumen tube, were associated with a lower incidence of airway injury, sore throat, and hoarseness after extubation.

BBs, compared to DLTs, offer the possibility of selective isolation of a lobe in cases where it is difficult or impossible to ensure normoxemia during one-lung ventilation. The use of this strategy, which involves positioning the blocker cuff in a distal bronchus to isolate only a portion of the lung undergoing surgery, has been successfully described by several authors [35–38]. A randomized study conducted on 61 patients demonstrated that, during minimally invasive cardiac surgery, isolation at the level of the right intermediate bronchus allows for better oxygenation compared to exclusion of the entire right lung with a DLT [39]. For completeness, it should be noted that selective isolation has also been described by advancing a right or left DLT more distally, so that the bronchial cuff occludes the upper lobar bronchus [35].

There are no guidelines for training in airway management for one-lung ventilation. The anesthesiologist must be proficient in the use of the video-bronchoscope,

Table 12.3 Advantages and disadvantages of double-lumen tubes and bronchial blockers

	Double-lumen tube	Bronchial blockers
Advantages	Ensures lung separation Large lumens facilitate ventilation and suction Simple and rapid switch from double- to single-lung ventilation Both lungs can be examined by bronchoscopy during single-lung ventilation Allows independent lung ventilation Less expensive	After intubation, easier identification of anatomical structures during bronchoscopy Best choice for difficult intubation No need to replace the endotracheal tube if mechanical ventilation must continue after surgery Allow selective lobar blockade Can be used in already intubated patients Can be used in pediatric patients (< 8 years)
Disadvantages	Greater difficulty in selecting the appropriate device size More difficult intubation Higher risk of cuff rupture during intubation Higher risk of airway injury	Very small suction channels Higher risk of dislodgement during surgery More complex transition from double-lung to single-lung ventilation More expensive

which is an essential tool in this context, and have thorough knowledge of the devices to be used. Campos suggests participating in at least 20 cases in which bronchoscopy is performed in the operating room by an anesthesiologist or thoracic surgeon [40]. Slinger reports that the training program at the University of Toronto includes 22 DLT placements, and the guidelines of the Canadian Association of University Departments of Anesthesia recommend 38 [41]. Rispoli identified 15 cases as the number required to acquire adequate skills for correct placement of the EZ-blocker [42]. There are no data regarding the number of procedures to be performed annually to maintain competence, while participation in practical training courses and the use of simulators are considered useful, and increasingly accessible, for developing both basic and advanced skills in the management of these devices [41, 43]. Table 12.3 summarizes the main advantages and disadvantages of DLTs and BBs.

12.5 Difficult Airways and Lung Ventilation

Intubation with a double-lumen tube is a more challenging procedure than with a single-lumen tube because the DLT is a stiffer and larger device, not only in relation to the airways but also due to the obstruction it causes in visualizing anatomical structures during laryngoscopy. The aforementioned Italian multicenter observational study conducted on 2217 patients found an incidence of unexpected difficult intubation in 5.2% of cases [24]. In another retrospective observational Italian study, a rate of unexpected difficult intubation was reported in 13.6% of cases, most of which were managed using a video-laryngoscope [44]. From this perspective, the widespread adoption of video-laryngoscopy has made intubation with a double-lumen tube easier. A meta-analysis published in 2018, which analyzed comparative studies between video-laryngoscopy and direct laryngoscopy for DLT intubation, demonstrated a higher first-attempt success rate and a reduction in airway injuries with the former technique [45]. Another literature review from 2020, based on the results of 23 studies, confirmed that first-attempt intubation success is higher with video-laryngoscopy compared to standard laryngoscopy, but also noted that the procedure takes longer and is associated with a higher frequency of incorrect DLT placement [46]. While the video-laryngoscope is a highly useful tool that has profoundly changed the approach to unexpected or borderline difficult airways, it is always recommended to opt for awake intubation with a video-bronchoscope when difficulty is anticipated. These principles also apply in the context of thoracic anesthesia, and this approach therefore involves the use of a single-lumen tube combined with a BB. This strategy is also safer during extubation and does not require replacement of the double-lumen tube at the end of the procedure if the patient is expected to remain intubated. Although there are no specific guidelines for airway management in thoracic anesthesia, several algorithms have been proposed and suggest resorting to the use of a DLT only when there is an absolute indication [23, 47, 48]. In such cases, replacement of the single-lumen tube with a double-lumen tube must be performed by experienced personnel, as it is a maneuver with a high failure rate. The combined use of a video-laryngoscope and an airway exchange catheter represents the safest strategy in what must always be considered a potentially complex and risky procedure. In this regard, it is worth mentioning a retrospective observational study that reported a failure rate of 13.8% for orotracheal tube exchanges using an airway exchange catheter in 527 patients [49]. In this cohort, the failure rate was very high when replacing a single-lumen tube with a DLT (39.9% – 43/110), while no failures occurred when performing the reverse procedure. The same study emphasized also the risk of airway injury during such maneuvers, including cases of pneumothorax. To minimize the risk of procedural difficulties, the tube exchanger must therefore be carefully selected before starting the maneuver, ensuring its compatibility with the DLT in terms of both external diameter and length. The latter should be 65–70 cm, considering the sum of the length of the double-lumen tube (usually about 40–42 cm) and the distance from the teeth to the glottic plane (about 20 cm).

12.6 Special Clinical Contexts

12.6.1 Patients with Tracheostomy

In airway management of patients with tracheostomy, both double-lumen tubes and bronchial blockers can be used. In the first case, the Tracheopart tube can be employed, which has the same design as conventional DLTs but is shorter and curved between the intratracheal and extratracheal portions. This device is equipped with an adjustable flange and collar to stabilize the tube after insertion, similar to standard tracheostomy cannulas. When positioning this DLT, the tracheal lumen must always be oriented toward the dorsal wall of the trachea, and the use of a video-bronchoscope is mandatory. This device corresponds to a 39 Fr, is available in both right and left versions, and comes in three sizes based on the intratracheal length of the double-lumen segment: 75 mm for patients up to 165 cm in height, 85 mm (height 165–175 cm), and 95 mm (height over 180 cm). To facilitate tube size selection, tracheal length can be estimated by performing a chest X-ray in inspiration. The distance between the center of the first thoracic vertebra and the carina usually corresponds to the distance between the tracheostomy and the carina. In the Tracheopart, this distance corresponds to the length from the apex of the curvature to the cranial edge of the cuff: this length is 105 mm for the 75 mm model, 115 mm for the 85 mm model, and 125 mm for the 95 mm model.

In this type of patient, it is also possible to replace the tracheostomy cannula with a single-lumen tube, which can be positioned in the left main bronchus if isolation of the right bronchus is required, or alternatively, a BB can be used [50, 51]. Each of these strategies requires familiarity with the devices and the use of a video-bronchoscope, as the space between the stoma and the tracheal carina is limited.

12.6.2 Pneumonectomy with Resection of the Tracheobronchial Angle

Pulmonary tumors involving the carina or tracheobronchial angle are rare and complex to manage. In such cases, surgery involves extended pneumonectomy with resection of the bronchus, carina, and trachea, necessitating reconstruction by direct tracheobronchial anastomosis (tracheal-sleeve pneumonectomy). In these cases, intubation with a DLT under careful video-bronchoscopic guidance is generally preferred, but during the resection of the carina and reconstruction phases, it is necessary to withdraw the DLT into the trachea and continue ventilation with a single-lumen tube inserted directly from the surgical field for the time required to suture the anastomosis (this technique requires periods of apnea during placement and removal of the endobronchial tube). Another approach involves the use of small-diameter endobronchial single-lumen tubes positioned via the trachea. For this purpose, the Wrett tube is noteworthy—a 40 cm long device with a shorter cuff to better adapt to bronchial placement (available sizes: 5.5, 6.5, and 7.5). Other authors have reported experience with high-frequency jet ventilation for this type of procedure, also using the BB of the Univent tube [52–54]. Recently, the authors have also successfully described the use of veno-venous extracorporeal membrane oxygenation (ECMO v-v), which allows management of the carinal resection and reconstruction phases without the need for pulmonary ventilation, leaving the surgical field unobstructed for the surgeon, which is particularly advantageous during tracheobronchial anastomosis suturing [55, 56].

12.6.3 Pediatric Patients

Although this text refers to airway management in adults, it is useful to provide some essential information regarding pediatric patients, in whom the small size of the airways is a significant limitation in device selection. In general, DLTs in sizes 26, 28, and 32 Fr can be used in patients aged 8 years and older [57, 58]. These devices are more challenging to manage because, being smaller, they have ventilation lumens of small diameter, requiring the use of small-diameter video-bronchoscopes (external diameter 2–2.5 mm), which are not available in all centers, are delicate to use, and are unable to aspirate secretions or blood that may impair adequate visualization of the structures. It should be noted that, in general, the ratio between the external diameter of the video-bronchoscope (OD_B) and the internal diameter of the tube lumen (ID_{TT}) should be less than 0.9 to allow passage of the instrument through the tube, but to avoid high airflow resistance values that could impede ventilation, the OD_B/ID_{TT} must be less than 0.7. For patients younger than 8 years and down to 6 years of age, the Univent tube (sizes 3.5 and 4.0) may be considered. Bronchial blockers (BBs), on the other hand, represent the most flexible solution for pediatric patients. Orotracheal intubation is facilitated by the ability to use a single-lumen tube as in other anesthetic settings. Various sizes of BBs, including the pediatric 5 Fr size (and a 3 Fr size currently being marketed by a manufacturer), can be used in conjunction with this tube. The authors have direct experience with the placement of the EZ-blocker via the extra-luminal (also called *parallel*) approach, that is, outside the single-lumen tube [59]. Similarly, other authors have described the extra-luminal use of the Arndt blocker [60, 61]. This approach makes device placement more complex but, by leaving the ventilation lumen unobstructed, is highly advantageous for the use of a video-bronchoscope and for reducing inspiratory flow resistance. Finally, especially in smaller patients, endobronchial placement of the single-lumen tube is possible, although this may increase the risk of lumen obstruction by secretions or blood [57].

12.6.4 Non-intubated Thoracic Surgery (NITS)

In the past 10 years, several groups have proposed the management of pulmonary surgical procedures without resorting to orotracheal intubation. This approach is the subject of considerable debate within the scientific community, as it pits the potential advantage of reduced invasiveness in airway management and mechanical ventilation against the increased complexity of management, particularly if intubation becomes necessary after the surgical procedure has begun. The term NITS actually encompasses various approaches that always involve the use of regional anesthesia techniques combined with sedation and spontaneous breathing using a Venturi mask, high-flow oxygen therapy cannulas, noninvasive ventilation, and even the use of a laryngeal mask, sometimes in combination with a BB. These techniques have been proposed for both low-complexity procedures, such as diagnostic pleural biopsies or for interstitial lung diseases, and major resective procedures such as lobectomy. A survey of Italian thoracic surgery centers found that 78% of centers perform NITS procedures, but predominantly for minor diagnostic procedures and in patients with significant comorbidities to reduce the perioperative impact of general anesthesia [62]. A literature review indicated that the laryngeal mask is the most commonly used device for airway management during these procedures, with a conversion rate to tracheal intubation of 3% [63]. When considering patients for NITS, preoperative airway assessment is crucial to ensure the highest level of safety during the procedure, as the possibility of requiring urgent intubation must always be considered. Interest in this approach is steadily increasing for pulmonary resective surgery, especially in Asia, which accounts for the majority of publications on the topic.

12.7 Conclusions

Airway management for one-lung ventilation is complex and requires expertise in the use of the video-bronchoscope, the many specific devices now available, and their techniques of use. Double-lumen tubes and bronchial blockers can be used with different indications depending on the clinical context, that is, the patient's characteristics and the type of planned procedure. Appropriate expertise and careful planning of the anesthetic strategy are essential to ensure optimal outcomes and patient safety. Although the scientific literature provides extensive information on devices and management techniques, further studies are needed to define the most effective solutions for many clinical scenarios.

References

1. Brodsky JB, Lemmens HJM. The history of anesthesia for thoracic surgery. Minerva Anestesiol. 2007;73:513–24.
2. Archibald E. A consideration of the dangers of lobectomy. J Thorac Surg. 1935;4:335–51.
3. Rovenstine EA. Anaesthesia for intrathoracic surgery: the endotracheal and endobronchial techniques. Surg Gynecol Obstet. 1936;63:325–30.
4. Carlens E. A new flexible double-lumen catheter for bronchospirometry. J Thorac Surg. 1949;18:742–6.
5. Inoue H, Shohtsu A, Ogawa J, et al. Endotracheal tube with movable blocker to prevent aspiration of intratracheal bleeding. Ann Thorac Surg. 1984;37:497–9.
6. Arndt GA, Buchika S, Kranner PW, et al. Wire-guided endobronchial blockade in a patient with a limited mouth opening. Can J Anaesth. 1999;46:87–9.
7. Cohen E. The Cohen flexitip endobronchial blocker: an alternative to a double lumen tube. Anesth Analg. 2005;101:1877–9.
8. Licker M, Le Guena M, Diapera J, et al. Isolation of the lung: double-lumen tubes and endobronchial blockers. Trends Anaesth Crit Care. 2014;47:e54.
9. Narayanaswamy M, McRae MK, Slinger P, et al. Choosing a lung isolation device for thoracic surgery: a randomized trial of three bronchial blockers versus double-lumen tubes. Anesth Analg. 2009;108:1097–101.
10. Kus A, Hosten T, Gurkan Y, et al. A comparison of the EZ-blocker with a cohen flex-tip blocker for one-lung ventilation. J Cardiothorac Vasc Anesth. 2014;28:896–9.

11. Shum S, Garijo JM, Tomlinson G, et al. A clinical comparison of 2 bronchial blockers versus double-lumen tubes for one-lung ventilation. J Cardiothorac Vasc Anesth. 2023;37:2577–83.
12. Rispoli M, Nespoli MR, Ferrara M, et al. A practical guide for using the EZ-blocker endobronchial blocker: tips and tricks after 10 years of experience. J Cardiothorac Vasc Anesth. 2023;37:1884–93.
13. Shelley B, Macfie A, Kinsella J. Anesthesia for thoracic surgery: a survey of UK practice. J Cardiothorac Vasc Anesth. 2011;25:1014–7.
14. Eldawlatly A, Turkistani A, Shelley B, et al. Anesthesia for thoracic surgery: a survey of Middle Eastern practice. Saudi J Anaesth. 2012;6:192–6.
15. Della Rocca G, Langiano N, Baroselli A, et al. Survey of thoracic anesthetic practice in Italy. J Cardiothorac Vasc Anesth. 2013;27:1321–9.
16. Defosse J, Schieren M, Loop T, et al. Current practice of thoracic anaesthesia in Europe—a survey by the European Society of Anaesthesiology Part I—airway management and regional anaesthesia techniques. BMC Anesthesiol. 2021;21:266.
17. Wang YC, Chang CH, Wang YT, et al. A survey of one-lung ventilation devices in lung resection surgeries in Taiwan: a population-based nationwide cohort study. J Formosan Med Assoc. 2020;119:449e454.
18. White GMJ. A new double lumen tube. Br J Anaesth. 1960;32:232–4.
19. Robertshaw FL. Low resistance double-lumen endobronchial tubes. Br J Anaesth. 1962;34:576–9.
20. Slinger P, Lesiuk L. Flow resistances of disposable double-lumen, single-lumen, and Univent tubes. J Cardiothorac Vasc Anesth. 1998;12:142–4.
21. Spaeth J, Ott M, Karzai W, et al. Double-lumen tubes and auto-PEEP during one-lung ventilation. Br J Anaesth. 2016;116:122–33.
22. Dumans-Nizard V, Parquin JF, Moyer JD. Left double-lumen tube with or without a carinal hook. A randomised controlled trial. Eur J Anaesthesiol. 2015;32:1–7.
23. Merli G, Guarino A, Della Rocca G, et al. Recommendations for airway control and difficult airway management in thoracic anesthesia and lung separation procedures. Minerva Anestesiol. 2009;75:59–96.
24. Langiano N, Fiorelli S, Deana C, et al. Airway management in anesthesia for thoracic surgery: a "real life" observational study. J Thorac Dis. 2019;11:3257–69.
25. Piccioni F, Droghetti A, Bertani A et al. Recommendations from the Italian intersociety consensus on Perioperative Anesthesia Care in Thoracic surgery (PACTS) part 2: intraoperative and postoperative care. Perioper Med. 2020;9:31.
26. Schuepbach R, Grande B, Camen G, et al. Intubation with VivaSight or conventional left-sided double-lumen tubes: a randomized trial. Can J Anesth. 2015;62:762–9.
27. Onifade A, Lemon-Riggs D, Smith A, et al. Comparing the rate of fiberoptic bronchoscopy use with a video double lumen tube versus a conventional double lumen tube—a randomized controlled trial. J Thorac Dis. 2020;12:6533–41.
28. Larsen S, Højberg Holm J, Nørgaard Sauer T, et al. A cost-effectiveness analysis comparing the VivaSight double-lumen tube and a conventional double-lumen tube in adult patients undergoing thoracic surgery involving one-lung ventilation. Pharmacoecon Open. 2020;4:159–69.
29. Granell M, Petrini G, Kot P, et al. Intubation with VivaSight double-lumen tube versus conventional double-lumen tube in adult patients undergoing lung resection: a retrospective analysis. Ann Card Anaesth. 2022;25:279–85.
30. Singh Heir J, Guo SL, Purugganan R, et al. A randomized controlled study of the use of video double-lumen endobronchial tubes versus double-lumen endobronchial tubes in thoracic surgery. J Cardiothorac Vasc Anesth. 2018;32:267–74.
31. Sharapi M, El-Samahy M, Rizk MA, et al. VivaSight double-lumen tube versus conventional double-lumen tube for one-lung ventilation: a systematic review and meta-analysis of randomized controlled trials. Asian J Anesthesiol. 2023;61:46–60.

32. Nwajuaku P, Barjaktarevic I, Hoftman N. Research and development of the sOLVe Tube™ dual lumen endobronchial tube: from concept to construct. Front Med Technol. 2023;5:1158154.
33. https://ecommedical.com/
34. Clayton-Smith A, Bennett K, Alston RP, et al. A comparison of the efficacy and adverse effects of double-lumen endobronchial tubes and bronchial blockers in thoracic surgery: a systematic review and meta-analysis of randomized controlled trials. J Cardiothorac Vasc Anesth. 2015;29:955–66.
35. Morikawa T, Sugiura H, Kaji M, et al. Feasibility of lobe-selective bronchial blockade for video-assisted thoracic surgery. Surg Endosc. 2002;16:327–30.
36. Campos JH. Update on selective lobar blockade during pulmonary resections. Curr Opin Anaesthesiol. 2009;22:18–22.
37. Morales J, Granell M, Biosca E, et al. Right lobar isolation by different methods in two patients with previous left lung resection. J Cardiothorac Vasc Anesth. 2017;31:S53.
38. Cedrone M, Rosboch GL, Ceraolo E, et al. Selective lobar exclusion in robot-assisted thoracic surgery using EZ Blocker. J Cardiothoracic Vasc Anesth. 2022;36:3221–3.
39. Ren Y, Lyu Y, Yu Y, et al. Selective right middle and lower lobar blockade for minimally invasive cardiac surgery: a prospective, single-center, randomized controlled study. Ann Transl Med. 2021;9:254.
40. Campos JH. Update on tracheobronchial anatomy and flexible fiberoptic bronchoscopy in thoracic anesthesia. Curr Opin Anaesthesiol. 2009;22:4–10.
41. Slinger P. Acquisition of competence in lung isolation: simulate one, do one, teach…repeat PRN. J Cardiothorac Vasc Anesth. 2014;28:873–6.
42. Rispoli M, Zani G, Bizzarri F, et al. Bronchial blocker positioning: learning curve and confidence in its use. Minerva Anestesiol. 2018;84:1254–60.
43. Solidoro P, Corbetta L, Patrucco F, et al. Competencies in bronchoscopy for intensive care unit, anesthesiology, thoracic surgery, and lung transplantation. Panminerva Med. 2019;61:367–85.
44. Corso RM, De Fazio C, Nigotti E, et al. Incidence of difficult airway in thoracic anesthesia practice. Minerva Anestesiol. 2018;84:1421–2.
45. Liu TT, Li L, Wan L, et al. Videolaryngoscopy vs. Macintosh laryngoscopy for double-lumen tube intubation in thoracic surgery: a systematic review and meta-analysis. Anaesthesia. 2018;73:997–1007.
46. Kim YS, Song J, Lim BG, et al. Different classes of videoscopes and direct laryngoscopes for double-lumen tube intubation in thoracic surgery: a systematic review and network meta-analysis. PLoS One. 2020;15(8):e0238060.
47. Campos JH. Lung isolation techniques for patients with difficult airway. Curr Opin Anaesthesiol. 2010;23:12–7.
48. Granell M, Parra MJ, Jiménez MJ, et al. Review of difficult airway management in thoracic surgery. Rev Esp Anestesiol Reanim. 2018;65:31–40.
49. McLean S, Lanam CR, Benedict W, et al. Airway exchange failure and complications with the use of the cook airway exchange catheter®: a single center cohort study of 1177 patients. Anesth Analg. 2013;117:1325–7.
50. Rispoli M, Nespoli MR, Salvi R, et al. One-lung ventilation in tracheostomized patients: our experience with EZ-Blocker. J Clin Anesth. 2016;31:288–90.
51. Campos JH, Musselman ED, Hanada S, et al. Lung isolation techniques in patients with early-stage or long-term tracheostomy: a case series report of 70 cases and recommendations. J Cardiothorac Vasc Anesth. 2019;33:433–9.
52. Williams H, Gothard J. Jet ventilation via a Univent tube for sleeve pneumonectomy. Eur J Anaesthesiol. 2001;18:407–9.
53. Rea F, Marulli G, Schiavon M, et al. Tracheal sleeve pneumonectomy for non-small cell lung cancer (NSCLC): short and long-term results in a single institution. Lung Cancer. 2008;61:202–8.
54. Chin JH, Lee EH, Choi DK, et al. High frequency jet ventilation of one lung using a bronchial blocker of Univent during carinal resection. J Korean Med Sci. 2010;25:1083–5.

55. Spaggiari L, Sedda G, Petrella F, et al. Preliminary results of extracorporeal membrane oxygenation assisted tracheal sleeve pneumonectomy for cancer. Thorac Cardiovasc Surg. 2021;69:240–5.
56. Marziali V, Mangiameli G, Crepaldi A, et al. Right tracheal sleeve pneumonectomy with VV-ECMO support for non-small cell lung cancer via anterior thoracotomy: a single center experience. Front Surg. 2023;10:1238462.
57. Templeton TW, Piccioni F, Chatterjee D. An update on one-lung ventilation in children. Anesth Analg. 2021;132:1389–99.
58. Letal M, Theam M. Pediatric lung isolation. BJA Educ. 2017;17:57–62.
59. Piccioni F, Vecchi I, Spinelli E, et al. Extraluminal EZ-blocker placement for one-lung ventilation in pediatric thoracic surgery. J Cardiothorac Vasc Anesth. 2015;29:e71–3.
60. Stephenson LL, Seefelder C. Routine extraluminal use of the 5F Arndt Endobronchial Blocker for one-lung ventilation in children up to 24 months of age. J Cardiothorac Vasc Anesth. 2011;25:683–6.
61. Templeton TW, Downard MG, Simpson CR, et al. Bending the rules: a novel approach to placement and retrospective experience with the 5 French Arndt endobronchial blocker in children <2 years. Paediatr Anaesth. 2016;26:512–20.
62. Rosboch GL, Giunta F, Ceraolo E, et al. Italian survey on non-intubated thoracic surgery: results from the INFINITY group. BMC Anesthesiol. 2022;22:2.
63. Rosboch GL, Lyberis P, Ceraolo E, et al. The anesthesiologist's perspective regarding non-intubated thoracic surgery: a scoping review. Front Surg. 2022;9:868287.

Neuraxial and Fascial Plane Blocks in Pediatric Age

13

Giovanna Chidini and Giuliana Anna Porro

Abbreviations

ADARPEF	Association des Anesthésistes Réanimateurs Pédiatriques d'Expression Française
CYP	Cytochrome P450
EA	Esophageal atresia
EMLA	Eutectic mixture of local anesthetics
ERAS	Enhanced Recovery After Surgery
ESPB	Erector Spinae Plane Block
GA	General anesthesia
LA	Local anesthetic
LOR	Loss of resistance
MH	Malignant hyperthermia
NMDA	N-methyl-D-aspartate
PA	Posterior arch
PCA	Post-conceptual age
SA	Spinal anesthesia
TAP	Transversus abdominis plane

G. Chidini (✉)
Department of Emergency and Critical Care, Pediatric Intensive Care, Fondazione IRCCS Cà Granda Ospedale Maggiore Policlinico, Milan, Italy
e-mail: giovanna.chidini@policlinico.mi.it

G. A. Porro
Department of Emergency and Critical Care, Pediatric Anesthesia, Fondazione IRCCS Cà Granda Ospedale Maggiore Policlinico, Milan, Italy
e-mail: giuliana.porro@policlinico.mi.it

D. Chiumello, A. De Gasperi (eds.), *Practical Trends in Anesthesia and Intensive Care 2026*, https://doi.org/10.1007/978-3-032-25721-5_13

TEF	Tracheoesophageal fistula
US	Ultrasound
VACTERL	Vertebral anomalies, Anorectal malformations, Cardiovascular anomalies, Tracheoesophageal fistula, Esophageal atresia, Renal anomalies, Limb defects

13.1 Introduction

Neuraxial anesthesia and analgesia are becoming increasingly common practices in the perioperative care of pediatric patients. For many children undergoing surgery, the use of a neuraxial technique can provide excellent postoperative analgesia, significantly reducing the need for general anesthetics (GA) and opioids, and in some cases eliminating the need for GA altogether. As early as 1909, Lord Tyrell Gray reported his experience with spinal anesthesia (SA) in 100 patients [1].

Gray became an advocate of SA, stating that the disadvantages encountered were "relatively negligible compared to general anesthesia administered under the same conditions." He concluded that "the enormous advantages derived from the use of spinal anesthesia have so impressed me that I am convinced it will have a prominent role in the pediatric surgery of the future."

With improvements in the safety of GA over the twentieth century, SA and other pediatric neuraxial techniques gradually lost ground. Only in the twenty-first century, thanks to a carefully controlled international multicenter study focused on comparing GA and regional anesthesia in neonates, were the benefits of neuraxial anesthesia confirmed. This study, originally conducted to assess possible neurodevelopmental harm related to GA exposure, also revealed several notable advantages of regional anesthesia. Neonates who underwent regional anesthesia experienced less hypotension and early apnea compared to those exposed to GA. Furthermore, they had a lower likelihood of significant postoperative desaturation episodes, slightly shorter times to first feeding, and lower postoperative pain scores [2–4]. The ability to perform many surgeries in neonates and infants without the need for GA or sedatives is particularly important in contemporary pediatric anesthesia practice, given the attention to the potential neurotoxic effects of anesthetic and sedative drugs. This concern was first raised in 1999 when Ikonomidou and colleagues discovered that antagonism of N-methyl-D-aspartate receptors was associated with widespread neurodegeneration in the brains of young rats. As this field developed, the finding of increased neuroapoptosis was replicated in numerous species and with most commonly used anesthetics and sedatives. Although recent clinical studies in healthy children have provided reassuring results, uncertainty regarding the neurological effects of anesthesia on brain development continues to make reducing the need for GA more attractive [13–16].

Neuraxial anesthesia and analgesia are now an integral part of pediatric perioperative care, and consequently, a thorough understanding of their implications is essential for all professionals involved in neonatal care. Effective postoperative pain relief achieved through epidural analgesia offers numerous advantages, including early mobilization, weaning from mechanical ventilation in patients with chronic respiratory insufficiency (such as bronchopulmonary dysplasia or patients on chronic home ventilation), reducing the time spent in a catabolic state, and lowering circulating levels of surgical stress hormones. Although a comprehensive discussion of the risks of anesthesia in neonates is beyond the scope of this review, we cannot discuss the benefits of neuraxial anesthesia in neonates without briefly outlining the risks of general anesthesia in this population. In recent years, more and more institutions have introduced policies requiring that all children under 3 years of age be cared for by a specialized pediatric anesthesiologist. The American College of Surgeons standards recommend that every child under 2 years of age be managed by a pediatric anesthesiologist. These regulatory changes have arisen from several large database studies demonstrating that perioperative risk in children increases inversely with age [5]. Of particular concern is the risk of GA in patients with a history of congenital heart disease. In many cases, the adverse events described in these studies are directly associated with failures in some of the core elements of GA, including airway management, opioid-based pain control, and the effects of GA on neonatal physiology [6–8].

The risks associated with opioid therapy in neonates deserve specific mention. In all patients, opioids lead to various adverse effects, including respiratory depression up to apnea, sedation, pruritus, constipation, bradycardia/hypotension. When these adverse events are combined with the residual effects of GA after surgery, they can result in significant morbidity and even mortality. Finally, opioid withdrawal is well documented in neonates and infants and can occur after only a few days of therapy. Based on these findings and ongoing concerns about the risks of GA in young patients, interest in neuraxial techniques continues to grow [9–24].

The aim of this chapter is therefore to review the indications and established procedures in the literature regarding the practice of epidural anesthesia (caudal, thoracic, and lumbar), subarachnoid anesthesia, postoperative epidural analgesia, and the use of peripheral nerve blocks in infants and children.

13.2 Anatomical Features Related to Pediatric Age

There are significant anatomical differences in children compared to adults that must be considered when using neuraxial anesthesia. For example, in neonates and young children, the conus medullaris is located lower in the vertebral column (L3) than in adults, where it is at L1. This is the result of the discrepancy in growth rates between the spinal cord and the vertebral column in neonates. However, by about 1 year of age, the conus medullaris reaches the L1 level, similar to that of an adult.

The sacrum in children is also flatter and narrower than in the adult population. At birth, the sacral lamina, formed by five sacral vertebrae, is not completely ossified and continues to fuse until about 8 years of age (although it may take up to 21 years). There is a 6% incidence of sacral atresia. Incomplete fusion of the sacral vertebral arch forms the sacral hiatus. The caudal epidural space can be easily accessed in neonates and children through the sacral hiatus. Due to the ongoing development of the sacral canal roof, there is considerable variation in the sacral hiatus. In young children, the sacral hiatus is located more cranially than in older children, and the dural sac may terminate more caudally: at S4 in neonates under 1 year of age and at S2 in older children. Therefore, due to the higher risk of accidental dural puncture, caution is required when performing caudal blocks in neonates. The amount of cerebrospinal fluid per body weight is greater in neonates and children (4 mL/kg) than in adults (2 mL/kg), and the CSF is mainly located in the spinal canal. Furthermore, in neonates the spinal cord is still unmyelinated, which means that lower concentrations of local anesthetic can be used effectively. Since children have a higher cardiac output compared to adults, the systemic absorption of local anesthetic occurs more rapidly. This can lead to toxic plasma levels and a shorter duration of the block. The presence of vertebral canal fusion malformations or ossification anomalies contraindicates the use of epidural techniques unless preceded by radiological assessment (MRI). The VACTERL syndrome defines the most common malformative association that contraindicates the use of neuraxial block techniques.

The VACTERL association (also known as VACTERL association or syndrome) describes a set of congenital defects that frequently occur together. The acronym stands for the following anomalies:

- V: Vertebral anomalies
- A: Anorectal malformations
- C: Cardiovascular anomalies
- T: Tracheoesophageal fistula (TEF)
- E: Esophageal atresia (EA)
- R: Renal anomalies
- L: Limb defects, including radial anomalies

These anomalies involve structures derived from the embryonic mesoderm. In addition to the primary anomalies listed, patients with VACTERL association may also present with other congenital abnormalities: hypoplastic, dysplastic, absent, or supernumerary vertebrae; hemivertebrae; wedge vertebrae; vertebral clefts and fusions; caudal regression; tethered cord; sacral agenesis, dysplastic sacral vertebrae, scoliosis or kyphoscoliosis secondary to costovertebral anomalies; C5-C6 dislocation and severe stenosis with spinal cord compression [25–28].

13.3 Techniques for Identifying the Epidural/Caudal Space

Various techniques have been developed to safely and accurately locate and access the epidural space. The traditional landmark-based approach relies on identifying anatomical features, such as the spinous processes, interspinous spaces, and the midline, to guide epidural needle insertion [29]. In addition, the loss-of-resistance technique is commonly used to confirm the position of the epidural space. This involves perceiving resistance to gentle injection of air or saline with the epidural needle when it is not in the epidural space, and a sudden loss of resistance when the space is entered [29, 30].

The caudal epidural block is a specific technique involving the administration of local anesthetic agents into the caudal epidural space located at the sacral apex. This technique is often used in pediatric anesthesia and in specific procedures involving the lower limbs and perineum in adults. The most common shape of the sacral hiatus is a U-inversion, seen in both males and females. The length from the apex of the sacral hiatus to the first sacral spine is slightly greater in females than in males; however, the width of the sacral cornua is similar in both sexes. Understanding these morphometric parameters is crucial for successful epidural anesthesia procedures. The sacral canal is formed by the union of the pedicle and lamina of the five sacral vertebrae and contains important structures such as the cauda equina and sacral nerves [30]. Correct needle placement can only be achieved by identifying anatomical landmarks (e.g., sacral cornua, lateral sacral crests, and the apex of the sacral hiatus). Even with anatomical landmark identification, clinicians fail to correctly place a caudal epidural block 30% of the time due to anatomical variations; ultrasound is often used to guide placement [8]. Therefore, clinicians must have a thorough understanding of the anatomy of the sacral region to have any chance of successfully administering a caudal epidural block [31].

Ultrasound-guided epidural block is an advanced procedure that incorporates ultrasound imaging to facilitate correct epidural needle placement during epidural anesthesia. In neonates, spinal cord fibers, cerebrospinal fluid, and the dura mater are easily identified using high-frequency linear ultrasound probes. It has also been suggested that epidural fat is less densely packed in children than in adults. Loosely packed epidural fat may facilitate the spread of local anesthetic and contribute to a more rapid onset of block. In the pediatric context, it is important to know the depth at which the needle encounters the epidural space. Table 13.1 summarizes some formulas for calculating this depth in children.

Table 13.1 Commonly reported clinical models for estimating skin-to-epidural distance in pediatric patients

Predictive variable	Estimation model	Population	Clinical use
Body weight (simple approximation)	≈ 1 mm per kg body weight	Infants and young children	Rapid bedside estimate
Age-based relationship	Depth (cm) = 1 + (0.15 × age in years)	Older pediatric patients	Alternative when weight is unavailable
Weight-based regression model	Depth (cm) = 0.8 + (0.05 × weight in kg)	Broad pediatric range	More refined estimate derived from regression analysis
Ultrasound assessment	Direct pre-procedural measurement	Neonates to adolescents	Most accurate individualized assessment

In the pediatric setting, where anatomical variations are more pronounced, ultrasound-guided epidural block can be particularly advantageous for improving accuracy and reducing associated risks. Where available, ultrasound allows real-time identification of anatomical landmarks and a much more precise estimation of epidural space depth. It is highly recommended to examine the anatomy with ultrasonography in all children before performing the block, especially in difficult cases such as patients with scoliosis or sacral dimples. Ultrasound also allows visualization of the needle in the epidural space in neonates. In smaller children, ultrasound can detect the advancement of the epidural catheter, either directly or indirectly by observing the injection of fluid [32].

Here are some common landmarks used during ultrasound-guided pediatric epidural block:

1. Dura Mater:
    - The dura mater appears as a thin hyperechoic line on ultrasound. It is important to clearly identify the dura mater to avoid accidental perforation during epidural needle insertion.
2. Epidural Space:
    - The epidural space is the area between the dura mater and the surrounding structures. During ultrasound, the operator looks for an epidural space free of echogenic signals that could indicate the presence of vascular or bony structures. As a general rule, the epidural space in children weighing more than 10 kg is found at a depth of 1 mm/kg of body weight. However, pre-procedural ultrasound imaging is useful for determining the depth of the epidural space.
3. Spinal Denticulation:
    - Spinal denticulation is an indentation in the dura mater caused by the spinal processes. It can be identified as a notch along the dura mater line and may help confirm the correct location of the epidural space.
4. Posterior Arch (PA):
    - The posterior arch is the posterior bony surface of the vertebrae. It can be visualized as an echogenic structure adjacent to the dura mater. The operator uses the posterior arch as a reference for needle orientation and depth.
5. Spinous Processes:
    - The spinous processes are the bony prominences along the midline of the back. They can be used as landmarks to identify different vertebrae and guide the operator during needle insertion.
6. Paravertebral Muscles:
    - The paravertebral muscles surround the epidural space and can be visualized as hyperechoic structures. The operator considers these muscles to assess the suitability of the needle position.
7. Vascular Structures:
    - During ultrasound, the operator monitors for the presence of vascular structures, such as epidural arteries, to avoid accidental puncture and reduce the risk of bleeding.

Anthropometric formulas provide approximate guidance based on age or body weight; however, interindividual variability may limit accuracy. However, pre-procedural ultrasound assessment allows individualized measurement and is considered the preferred method when available. Common clinical models for estimating skin to epidural distance in pediatrics are reported in Table 13.1.

Integrated clinical and instrumental approaches for confirming epidural catheter position in pediatric patients during intraoperative and postoperative phases are reported in Table 13.2. Instrumental methods provide direct anatomical confirmation when available, while clinical indicators should be interpreted cautiously and in conjunction with continuous monitoring.

Table 13.2 Clinical and instrumental confirmation of epidural catheter position in pediatric patients

Timing	Category	Method	Assessment strategy	Indicative findings
Intraoperative (under general anesthesia)	Instrumental	Ultrasound	Visualization of local anesthetic spread at or adjacent to the catheter tip within the epidural space	Imaging evidence of epidural distribution at expected segmental levels
	Clinical/ procedural	Aspiration and incremental dosing	Careful aspiration followed by slow, fractionated injection of small aliquots	Hemodynamic stability and absence of clinical signs suggestive of intrathecal or intravascular injection
	Clinical	Ventilatory pattern	Maintenance of spontaneous ventilation when clinically appropriate	May assist in indirect detection of excessive cephalad spread or unintended high neuraxial block
	Instrumental	Radiography with contrast	Contrast medium outlining catheter trajectory and epidural space	Radiological confirmation of catheter location
Postoperative (awake patient)	Instrumental	Ultrasound	Bedside assessment of catheter position and spread of local anesthetic	Non-invasive confirmation of epidural placement in the recovery setting
	Clinical/ pharmacologic	Lidocaine test dose (if ultrasound unavailable)	Incremental administration of 2% lidocaine solution with monitoring	Sensory changes consistent with the intended dermatomal distribution

(continued)

Table 13.2 (continued)

Timing	Category	Method	Assessment strategy	Indicative findings
Postoperative (awake patient)	Clinical-level assessment	Lumbar catheter tip	Neurological examination	Bilateral lower limb sensory changes with variable motor involvement; warming of plantar surfaces
	Clinical-level assessment	Lower thoracic catheter tip	Neurological and autonomic assessment	Decreased hip flexion strength; attenuation of abdominal cutaneous reflexes; possible mild reductions in heart rate and arterial pressure
	Clinical-level assessment	Upper thoracic catheter tip	Neurological and autonomic assessment	Reduction in heart rate and arterial pressure; warming of palmar surfaces; unilateral or bilateral Horner syndrome

13.4 Pharmacology of Local Anesthetic Agents in Neonates and Infants

Since most pediatric patients receive epidural analgesia in conjunction with general anesthesia, the primary purpose of the epidural catheter is to deliver a sufficient amount of local anesthetic solution to ensure both intraoperative and postoperative analgesia. As in adult epidural anesthesia, the concentration and volume of the local anesthetic are important factors in determining the density and level of the block. However, in pediatric patients, knowledge of the total drug dose is equally important to avoid local anesthetic toxicity and must take into account pharmacodynamic and pharmacokinetic factors (related to the development and maturation of hepatic cytochromes), as well as the different physiology of cerebrospinal fluid clearance.

There are several considerations to keep in mind when evaluating epidural analgesia in children [33–35]

- The larger volume of distribution of local anesthetics in children reduces peak plasma concentrations after a single dose.
- Hepatic and renal functions are immature until 3 months of age.
- Drug metabolism and clearance are reduced during this period. The infusion rate in neonates should be decreased after 24 h to prevent accumulation.
- The relatively high cardiac output in children increases the absorption of local anesthetic agents from neuraxial compartments, resulting in higher initial plasma concentrations and a shorter duration of action.

- Lower plasma protein concentrations for drug binding in neonates, particularly alpha-1-acid glycoprotein, increase the amount of free local anesthetic available for potential toxicity.
- The blood-brain barrier is more permeable to local anesthetics in neonates.

Local anesthetics are metabolized by cytochrome P450 (CYP). The main CYP isoforms involved are CYP3A4 for lidocaine and bupivacaine and CYP1A2 for ropivacaine. At birth, the CYP3A4 system is not fully mature but is partially replaced by CYP3A7. At 1 month of age, the intrinsic clearance of bupivacaine is only one-third that of adults and two-thirds at 6 months. CYP1A2 does not reach full maturity before 3 years of age. In fact, the clearance of ropivacaine does not reach its maximum until 8 years of age. The volumes of distribution of local anesthetics in neonates and children are larger than in adults, thus reducing the risk of high serum drug concentrations after a single injection, but not after multiple injections. The greater volume of distribution of local anesthetics in children reduces peak plasma concentrations after a single bolus dose. However, it increases the risk of drug accumulation after continuous infusion or multiple injections.

Alpha-1-acid glycoprotein is the main protein binding local anesthetics. The concentration of alpha-1-acid glycoprotein is very low at birth and increases progressively during the first year of life. This is why neonates and young infants have a much higher free fraction of local anesthetics compared to adults. Alpha-1-acid glycoprotein is an acute phase protein, and its concentration rises rapidly in inflammatory states. High cardiac output in children tends to accelerate the vascular absorption of drugs from tissues, resulting in higher initial plasma concentrations and a shorter duration of action, with a potential increased systemic toxicity of local anesthetics [36, 37].

The dosage of local anesthetics in children under 2 years of age should be reduced due to their higher baseline heart rate, which increases vulnerability to cardiac toxicity from local anesthetics. In children under 1 year, the risk of systemic toxicity is further heightened by higher free concentrations of local anesthetics associated with persistently low serum protein levels. This risk is even greater before 6 months of age, when the liver is immature, especially when continuous infusions or repeated bolus doses are used.

The physiology of cerebrospinal fluid circulation of anesthetics also influences the duration of neuraxial block. The duration of spinal block is shorter in neonates compared to adults, likely due to the larger volume of cerebrospinal fluid. Indeed, a relationship between the duration of motor block and age has been reported. Additionally, there is a proportionally greater blood flow to the spinal cord, resulting in more rapid absorption of drugs from the subarachnoid space. These phenomena are more pronounced in preterm neonates than in term neonates [37].

Bupivacaine, ropivacaine, and levobupivacaine are the most commonly used local anesthetics for neuraxial epidural anesthesia in children. High concentrations of local anesthetics, such as 0.5% bupivacaine or 0.5% ropivacaine, are not recommended in the pediatric population. Since myelination is incomplete, lower concentrations of amino-amide local anesthetics are effective (e.g., 0.125%

levobupivacaine). Instead, larger volumes of more diluted local anesthetic are commonly used to cover multiple dermatomes. Body weight is usually a better predictor than patient age for estimating the spread of local anesthetic after a caudal block. Dosage ranges reflect commonly reported clinical practice and should be individualized according to age, weight, surgical indication, and institutional protocols. Continuous clinical monitoring is essential, particularly in neonates. Dosing strategies are based on commonly described pediatric regional anesthesia practice standards (Table 13.3) [38].

Table 13.3 Practical dosing considerations for caudal, lumbar, and thoracic epidural techniques in pediatric patients

Technique	Local anesthetic	Concentration	Initial volume	Maximum single dose	Infusion rate (if applicable)
Caudal block—single injection	Ropivacaine	0.2% (range 0.1–0.375%)	0.5 mL/kg (sacral) 1 mL/kg (lumbar) 1.25 mL/kg (lower thoracic)	2 mg/kg	–
	Bupivacaine/Levobupivacaine	0.125–0.25%	Same dermatomal guidance as above	2.5 mg/kg	–
Lumbar epidural—bolus technique	Ropivacaine	0.2%	0.5 mL/kg (initial loading)	≤1.7 mg/kg	–
	Bupivacaine/Levobupivacaine	0.125–0.25%	0.5 mL/kg (initial loading)	≤1.7 mg/kg	–
Thoracic epidural—bolus technique	Ropivacaine	0.2%	0.3 mL/kg (initial loading)	≤1.7 mg/kg	–
	Bupivacaine/Levobupivacaine	0.125–0.25%	0.3 mL/kg (initial loading)	≤1.7 mg/kg	–
Continuous epidural infusion	Bupivacaine	0.125%	–	–	Neonates: 0.2 mg/kg/h; Older children: 0.4 mg/kg/h
	Ropivacaine	0.1%	–	–	Neonates: 0.2 mg/kg/h; Older children: 0.4 mg/kg/h

13.5 Caveats and Practical Considerations in Neonates and Children

Although ropivacaine has been associated with a lower incidence of early motor block compared with bupivacaine, drug selection should always consider the clinical context, expected duration of analgesia, and institutional experience. Bupivacaine and levobupivacaine remain widely used and well-established agents in pediatric epidural practice. Dose and volume must be tailored to the surgical level, patient age, and overall clinical condition. Incremental administration with careful aspiration between aliquots is advised in order to reduce the risk of inadvertent intravascular or intrathecal injection. Thoracic epidural techniques require particular attention to hemodynamic stability, and enhanced monitoring is recommended during and after block placement. For continuous epidural infusion, strict clinical and neurological surveillance is essential, especially in neonates and young infants, in whom reduced hepatic clearance may increase the risk of local anesthetic accumulation. In routine practice, infusion duration is commonly limited to approximately 48 h, although this should be individualized according to clinical response and institutional protocols.

13.6 Adjuvants for Neuraxial and Peripheral Blocks

With the exception of clonidine and preservative-free morphine, no other adjuvant agent mentioned in the ESRA guidelines is approved for spinal/epidural administration or for peripheral blocks.

Even long-acting local anesthetics have a limited duration (typically 4–12 h) to ensure analgesic coverage for the postoperative period following intermediate or major surgery (24–72 h). This issue can be managed by combining a single-shot injection with the placement of an epidural catheter to allow repeated administration or continuous infusion of local anesthetics. However, most pediatric surgical procedures do not justify the use of these more complex and resource-intensive options for postoperative analgesia. Therefore, an alternative to prolong the nerve block from a single injection is to use adjuvant drugs mixed with local anesthetics to increase the duration of nerve block.

The advantages associated with the use of adjuvant drugs include:

1. Prolongation of the duration of the block and the analgesic effect.
2. Reduction in the requirement for general anesthetics.
3. Allowing a smooth emergence from anesthesia and a relaxed stay in the recovery room.
4. Reduction in the incidence of postoperative delirium and shivering.

Key requirements for adjuvant drugs include:

1. There should be sufficient understanding of the adjuvant's mechanism of action.
2. The side effect profile must be tolerable compared to the use of pure local anesthetics.
3. The adjuvant must be available as a preservative-free preparation.

In conclusion:

- Clonidine (1–2 μg/kg) and morphine (10–30 μg/kg) can be administered intrathecally to prolong the duration of spinal block in children. Data on toxicity in children are very limited; the dose used should be the minimum necessary to achieve the desired benefits and minimize potential adverse effects.
- Racemic ketamine (0.5 mg/kg) and S-ketamine have been used as neuraxial adjuvants in children. However, ketamine is not recommended for intrathecal use in neonates and children due to the potential risk of neuronal apoptosis. Data on toxicity in children are very limited; the dose used should be the minimum necessary to achieve the benefits and minimize potential adverse effects [39–42].
- Dexmedetomidine has been used to prolong postoperative analgesia when used as an adjuvant in neuraxial blocks (e.g., caudal block).
- Magnesium acts as a voltage-dependent calcium channel blocker and is also a non-competitive antagonist of NMDA receptors. A comprehensive review, compiling data from animal and human studies, concluded that magnesium is useful in reducing postoperative pain by enhancing opioid analgesia [43]. While systemic magnesium has demonstrated efficacy in reducing postoperative pain in adults [44], the same effect has not been consistently observed in pediatric patients [45], and the reason for this difference remains unclear. Neuraxial administration of magnesium is thought to be more potent than systemic administration, primarily because magnesium does not easily cross the blood-brain barrier [46]. Studies in adults have shown that epidural administration of magnesium can prolong the time to first analgesic request by approximately 109 min without causing delays in sensory block regression [47]. However, in pediatric patients undergoing surgery, the analgesic effect of caudal administration of magnesium appears to be inconsistent.

13.7 Technique and Materials

Among the various epidural analgesia techniques, the most common include caudal analgesia (see previous section), which is the most widely used regional technique in children, as well as lumbar and thoracic epidural analgesia [48–50].

13.7.1 Caudal Epidural Analgesia: Single-Shot Technique (Fig. 13.1)

The single-shot caudal epidural block is widely used to provide adequate perioperative analgesia in children undergoing urological, general, and orthopedic surgery involving the lower abdomen and lower limbs. It should be noted that, as a single-injection technique, it may not be suitable for all cases due to its limited segmental spread [51].

Contraindications to caudal anesthesia in children include: local infection at the site, pilonidal cyst, or spinal dysraphism such as tethered cord syndrome. In the presence of other spinal or meningeal anomalies, we recommend preoperative anatomical assessment by ultrasound or magnetic resonance imaging [52, 53].

The use of ultrasound compared to the traditional landmark-based method in caudal anesthesia offers clear advantages. While the conventional approach can achieve a convincing success rate, it is subject to significant complications and may result in inadequate analgesia [54–56]. On the other hand, the use of ultrasound provides two main benefits: it assists in identifying small anatomical structures and allows visualization of local anesthetic spread [57, 58]. Furthermore, ultrasound guidance does not require specific patient positioning or additional aseptic technique. However, it is essential to perform sterile preparation of the ultrasound probe [58–60]. In all children, it is essential to ensure adequate prevention of heat loss during the procedure. In neonates, it is recommended to prevent heat loss with a sterile, transparent drape, which also allows for visualization of the patient's breathing.

The patient is positioned laterally with the neck flexed and the knees drawn up toward the chest. After proper positioning, the landmarks for caudal epidural block are easily identified in children: the coccyx is first located, and by palpating along the midline in a cephalad direction, the sacral cornua can be felt on either side of the midline, approximately 1 cm apart. The sacral hiatus is perceived as a depression between the two bony prominences of the sacral cornua. Under sterile conditions, the needle is inserted and advanced into the sacral hiatus at an angle of about 70° to the skin until a distinct "pop" is felt as the sacrococcygeal ligament is pierced. After this puncture, the needle angle should be reduced to approximately 20–30° as the needle is advanced 2–4 mm into the caudal canal (Table 13.4).

13.7.2 Needle Selection for Caudal/Epidural Analgesia

There are several types of needles used for single-shot caudal epidural block. The size or type of needle does not appear to affect either the success rate or the incidence of complications of the caudal block. Tuohy or Crawford needles with a short bevel (5 cm in length), accompanied by a stylet, provide better tactile feedback when piercing the sacrococcygeal ligament. For children 1 year of age or older, a 22-gauge needle is preferred, while for those younger than 1 year, a 25-gauge needle may be used. Using a needle with a stylet can reduce the risk of introducing a

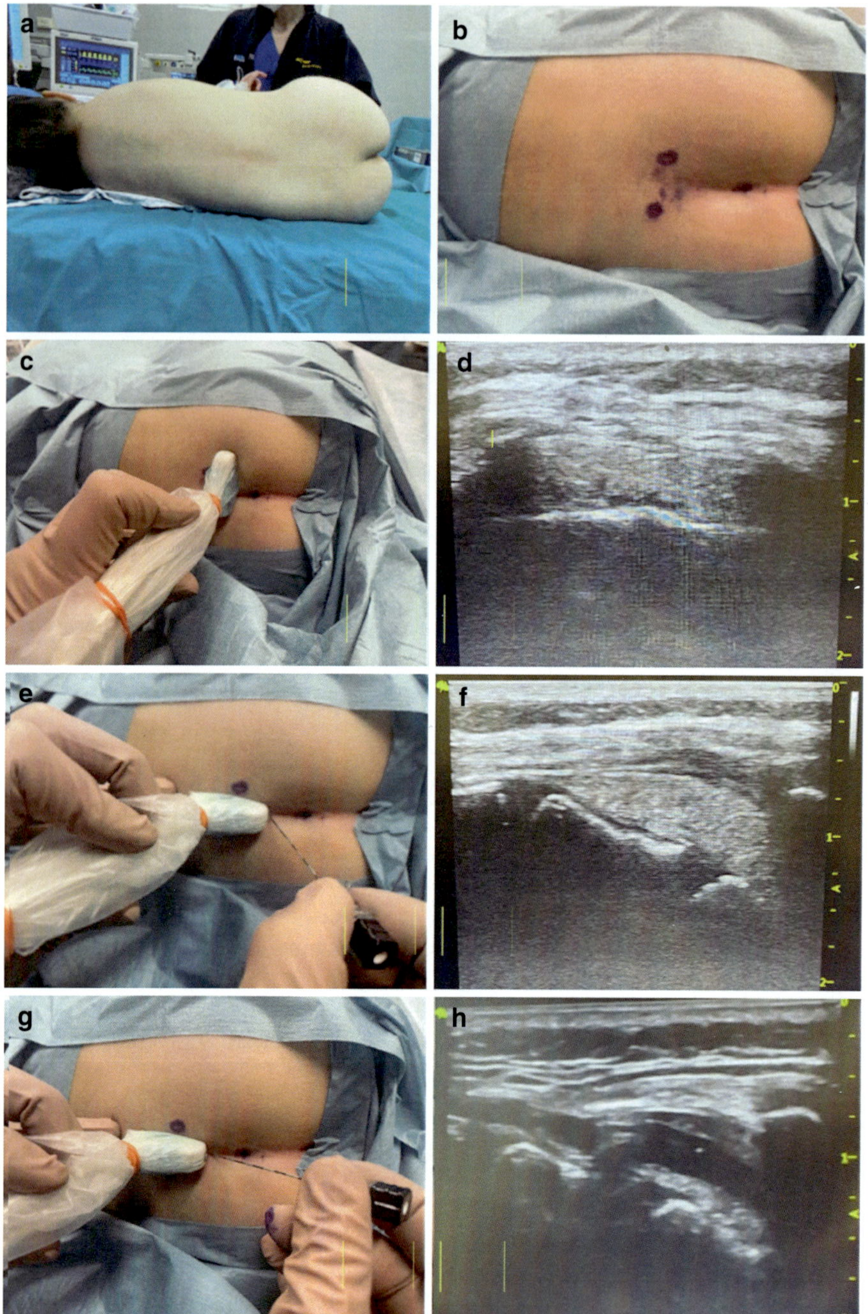

Fig. 13.1 Caudal anesthesia. (**a**) Lateral patient positioning. (**b**) Identification of anatomical landmarks. (**c**) Probe positioning in short-axis view. (**d**) Short-axis ultrasound view. (**e**) Probe positioning in long-axis view, initiation of needle insertion perpendicular to the skin. (**f**) Long-axis ultrasound view. (**g**) Advancement of the needle after adjusting the angle to approximately 45°. (**h**) Ultrasound view showing caudal dural displacement following infusion of local anesthetic into the caudal space

Table 13.4 Procedure for caudal epidural anesthesia

Patient and probe positioning:
Patient in lateral position with knees flexed toward the chest
Ultrasound machine positioned in front of the operator
Sterile high-frequency ultrasound probe (linear or joystick)
Probe placed transversely over the sacrum for short-axis (SA) view
Rotated 90° to a central sagittal position for long-axis (LA) view
Anatomical assessment:
Precise identification of the sacral cornua and sacrococcygeal membrane
Sacrococcygeal membrane centered in the long-axis view
Clear identification of the dural sac and layers of the sacral bone
Needle insertion procedure:
Introduction of the needle into the sacral groove with the probe in SA or LA view
Out-of-plane technique in SA view
In-plane technique in LA view
Documentation of the needle insertion angle
Confirmation of optimal positioning:
Advancement of the needle 2–4 mm into the caudal space
Removal of the stylet
Administration of a small amount of saline or local anesthetic under ultrasound guidance
Probe positioned cephalad to visualize the dural sac on the display
Injection monitoring:
Observation of ventral displacement of the dura during injection
Monitoring the spread of local anesthetic by moving the probe cephalad

skin plug into the caudal space. Some authors suggest the use of a 22-gauge angiocath catheter, as it facilitates detection of intravascular or intraosseous placement. This catheter is intended only for single-shot caudal epidural block and is withdrawn after administration of the dose, avoiding continuous injections.

13.7.3 Choice of Local Anesthetic

For caudal block in children, commonly used drugs include:

- (Levo)bupivacaine: 0.125–0.25%
- Ropivacaine: 0.1–0.375%

These agents are used at a volume of 0.5–1.5 mL/kg, depending on the desired dermatomal level. Current guidelines recommend not exceeding doses of 2 mg/mL for ropivacaine and 2.5 mg/mL for bupivacaine. The recommended volumes are 0.5 mL/kg for sacral dermatomes, 1.0 mL/kg for lumbar dermatomes, or 1.25 mL/kg for lower thoracic dermatomes [61]. See Table 13.3.

13.7.4 Lumbar and Thoracic Epidural Block

Lumbar epidural anesthesia is a well-established practice, frequently employed for continuous infusion and rarely used as a single-shot technique. Direct access to the lumbar region is primarily indicated for pain control during and after major abdominal or orthopedic surgery. Placement of the lumbar epidural catheter is performed after induction of general anesthesia.

Placement of the lumbar epidural needle is performed via a midline approach. Identification of the epidural space is commonly achieved by loss of resistance (LOR) to saline. It is essential to avoid LOR with air, due to the associated risk of air embolism, especially in neonates and infants [58–61].

Children should be positioned in the lateral decubitus position for direct lumbar epidural placement. Typically, in individuals older than 2 years, an 18-gauge Tuohy needle, 5 cm in length with 0.5 cm markings, is used together with a 20-gauge epidural catheter. For children under 1 year of age, a 20-gauge Tuohy needle, 5 cm in length with 0.5 cm markings, may be considered, accompanied by a 22-gauge catheter. However, it should be noted that these thinner catheters are more prone to kinking, occlusion, and leakage. Although identification of the intervertebral space and ligamentum flavum is generally straightforward in most pediatric patients, it is important to recognize that the ligamentum flavum may be less tense in children, resulting in a less distinct perception of loss of resistance. Additionally, the distance from the skin surface to the epidural space may be extremely shallow. While formulas have been proposed to estimate the distance from the skin to the epidural space, it is crucial to recognize that these formulas serve only as guidelines and vary according to the angle of epidural needle insertion. Currently, the most reliable method for assessing epidural depth is ultrasound (US) imaging. Using a probe placed in an oblique paramedian sagittal plane, the distance from the skin to the ligamentum flavum is measured. This measurement provides an accurate estimate of the depth at which loss of resistance will be encountered. Advancement of catheters from the lumbar and caudal epidural spaces to the thoracic level is feasible only in children up to 1 year of age. However, such advancement becomes progressively more difficult with increasing age due to the development of lumbar curvature.

13.7.5 Lumbar-to-Thoracic Epidural Approach

Catheters placed via the lumbar approach can be progressively advanced to thoracic vertebral levels. Similar to the difficulties encountered in advancing catheters through the caudal space in older children, advancing lumbar epidural catheters to thoracic levels is hindered by significant resistance [19–22].

13.7.6 Thoracic Epidural Analgesia

There remains controversy regarding the safety of thoracic epidural placement under deep sedation or general anesthesia, as unconscious patients are unable to report symptoms that might alert the anesthesiologist to potential neurological complications. Although direct needle trauma to the spinal cord during epidural insertion is rare, it can result in devastating complications. Cases of direct needle trauma to the spinal cord have been documented during epidural placement in both awake patients and those under general anesthesia.

The pharmacological approach is similar to caudal anesthesia, with common use of ropivacaine 0.2% or levobupivacaine/bupivacaine 0.25%, with a recommended dose of 0.5 mL/kg for the initial lumbar epidural bolus, 0.3 mL/kg for the thoracic epidural bolus, and 0.25 mL/kg for subsequent top-ups.

13.7.7 Postoperative Epidural Analgesia

To ensure effective and safe epidural analgesia, it is advisable to adopt a systematic, protocol-based approach to patient care. A dedicated pediatric acute pain team, consisting of anesthesiologists and nurses, is essential for standardized pain assessments, close patient monitoring, and appropriate management of adverse effects. The average duration of epidural infusion is approximately 72 h, but longer infusion periods may be necessary, especially in children with complex medical histories or prolonged analgesic requirements. In neonates, the duration of epidural infusion should be limited to 48 h due to the risk of systemic toxicity [33, 34].

For postoperative pain control, the use of 0.125% bupivacaine or 0.1–0.2% ropivacaine, with or without fentanyl 1–2 mcg/mL, is recommended at the following dosages:

- Age < 3 months: 0.2 mg/kg/h
- Age > 3 months: 0.4 mg/kg/h
- Age > 6 years or thoracic epidural: max 6–7 ml/h

13.8 Subarachnoid Anesthesia (SA)

Spinal anesthesia is considered the "gold standard" technique for abdominal or lower limb surgical procedures lasting less than 60 min in preterm neonates with a post-conceptual age (PCA) of less than 60 weeks. These neonates, especially those with a PCA below 48 weeks, have an increased incidence of apnea, further exacerbated by factors such as bronchopulmonary dysplasia, intracranial hemorrhage, and anemia. SA has demonstrated benefits in reducing the incidence of apnea, bradycardia, desaturation, and the need for postoperative ventilation. In some cases, spinal anesthesia may be combined with caudal or epidural anesthesia to prolong analgesia [62–64].

Some advantages of SA include:

1. Avoiding tracheal intubation and the respiratory effects of general anesthesia (GA) and intravenous opioids in high-risk patients (with subglottic stenosis, laryngotracheomalacia, respiratory distress, muscular dystrophy, hyperreactive airways, epidermolysis bullosa).
2. Greater efficacy compared to GA or epidural block in attenuating the neuroendocrine stress response and adverse reactions to surgery.
3. Preferred choice in children at risk of developing malignant hyperthermia (MH), as aminoamide anesthetics can be safely used in patients susceptible to MH. Additionally, it is an alternative technique in patients with medical and respiratory conditions who would otherwise be at high risk under GA [65–70].

13.8.1 Preparation of the Child for SA

The application of a local anesthetic cream (EMLA or LMX) may precede the procedure, taking into account the risk of methemoglobinemia in very small preterm infants. The operating room should be pre-warmed before the patient enters, with warm blankets and radiant heat lamps to mitigate heat loss in neonates. In older children, the room should be quiet and, if possible, surgical instruments should be covered to reduce patient anxiety. Midazolam, atropine, and ketamine, alone or in combination, have been used via various routes (oral/rectal/IM) to provide sedation and anxiolysis. Standard monitoring (pulse oximetry, electrocardiogram, and blood pressure cuff) is required before the block. The use of concomitant intravenous sedation or inhalational general anesthesia should be planned according to the patient's medical condition, age, and the nature and expected duration of the procedure.

13.8.2 Patient Positioning

Spinal anesthesia is traditionally administered in the lateral or sitting position in children. The lateral position requires the patient to be placed at the edge of the operating table and stabilized by an assistant. Alternatively, the patient may be positioned in the center of the table on multiple blankets to allow adequate hand positioning for the anesthesiologist during the block. The sitting position requires particular attention in neonates to avoid neck flexion that could cause airway obstruction. Careful monitoring of oxygen saturation in neonates during the procedure is essential, and neck flexion is not necessary and may be avoided in smaller children [66, 71–75].

13.8.3 Technique

In neonates, it is recommended to identify the L4-L5 or L5-S1 interspace; for older children, the L3-L4 space is appropriate, possibly using ultrasound guidance [76, 77].

The specific dose of spinal local anesthetic should be calculated and prepared before dural puncture to ensure precise administration. Given the small amount of local anesthetic required in neonates, it is crucial to carefully measure the volume corresponding to the needle hub and include it in the total anesthetic dose. A short 22- or 25-gauge spinal needle is often preferred, and a midline approach is recommended over a paramedian one. The ligamentum flavum in children is less resistant, and the characteristic "pop" may be less perceptible during dural penetration. The drug should be administered slowly once clear cerebrospinal fluid flow from the needle is confirmed. The barbotage technique is not recommended, as it can cause unacceptably high levels of motor block and carries the risk of total spinal block. Elevating the lower limbs c to place the return electrode use of the electrosurgical pad on the back can result in a total spinal block. To prolong surgical anesthesia in the case of bilateral hernia repair, spinal anesthesia can be supplemented with a caudal block.

Types of local anesthetics and dosages are provided in Table 13.5.

13.8.4 Block Assessment

Assessing the level of the block can be challenging in neonates and young children, especially in patients who have received sedation or in those in whom the block is performed under general anesthesia. In neonates, techniques such as stimulation with a fine needle or response to cold stimuli (e.g., an alcohol swab), along with observation of respiratory rate and pattern, can be used. In children over 2 years of age, the Bromage scale is commonly employed. After administration of the block, it is essential to avoid placing the patient in the Trendelenburg position or elevating

Table 13.5 Recommended doses for spinal anesthesia (SA) with local anesthetics (LA) in neonates and children

Type of LA	<5 kg	5–15 kg	>15 kg
0.5% Hyperbaric bupivacaine	0.5–0.6 mg/kg (0.1–0.12 ml/kg)	0.4 mg/kg (0.08 ml/kg)	0.3 mg/kg (0.06 ml/kg)
0.5% Hyperbaric tetracaine	0.5–0.6 mg/kg (0.1–0.12 ml/kg)	0.4 mg/kg (0.08 ml/kg)	0.3 mg/kg (0.06 ml/kg)
0.5% Isobaric ropivacaine	0.5–1 mg/kg (0.1–0.2 ml/kg)	0.5 mg/kg (0.1 ml/kg)	0.5 mg/kg (0.1 ml/kg)

Note: Dosages are expressed in milligrams per kilogram (mg/kg) and milliliters per kilogram (ml/kg). Duration is indicated in minutes, with the range in parentheses and the mean the lower limbs, for example, to place an electrosurgical pad on the neonate's back. In the event of a rapid increase in block level, the patient may be placed in the reverse Trendelenburg position.

13.8.5 Complications

Complications of spinal and epidural anesthesia in children are generally minor and infrequent. The prospective ADARPEF study conducted in patients from prematurity to adolescence reported a single complication out of 506 SA cases (intravenous injection) [78, 79].

Some of the complications that may occur include:

- Cardiorespiratory insufficiency: Hypotension and desaturation are rare in children. If they occur, they are usually due to a high block or the use of sedatives. One report describes the occurrence of bronchospasm with a higher block [13].
- Back pain: (5–10%), but a causal relationship has not been established.
- High or total spinal anesthesia: (0.6%) may occur if the child's legs are elevated after drug injection or with overdose and barbotage. Limited thoracic kyphosis facilitates cephalad spread, causing apnea and requiring assisted ventilation [80].
- Transient neurological symptoms: (3–4%) are described as the onset of pain and dysesthesia in the gluteal region radiating to the lower limbs [17]. In most cases, symptoms are mild. Neurological examinations and imaging studies are usually negative. No transient neurological symptoms were observed in 307 patients undergoing surgery with SA using 0.5% bupivacaine or 2% lidocaine.
- Infection: Only anecdotal reports of septic meningitis with SA in children have been described, with no proven causal relationship [81].

13.9 Fascial Plane Blocks

Analgesia is a crucial aspect of the recovery phase in pediatric surgery, and the introduction of regional anesthesia has had a particularly significant impact. Regional techniques have been associated with a reduction in general anesthesia requirements, resulting in fewer side effects and the prospect of a faster and smoother awakening, decreased need for opioids, quicker recovery of bowel function, and a reduction in the hormonal stress response. These advantages can be especially relevant for lower abdominal surgeries, which are commonly performed and often associated with a notable incidence of chronic postoperative pain. Both types of blocks—neuraxial (caudal, epidural) and fascial plane blocks—have been shown to be successfully applicable in this context, but there is currently a lack of data, particularly regarding the duration and quality of analgesia in these specific situations. The introduction of ultrasound-guided techniques into anesthetic practice has made it possible to extend postoperative analgesia using fascial plane blocks to the pediatric population as an alternative to classic neuraxial blocks (caudal, lumbar, and thoracic epidural).

Currently, it is unclear whether the implementation of fascial plane blocks is advantageous compared to more traditional techniques. The combined results of a recent meta-analysis [91] showed a longer duration of analgesia (approximately 1.76 h more) when using the transversus abdominis plane (TAP) block compared to isolated caudal block. This trend was associated with a significant reduction in the number of rescue analgesic doses in the first 24 h after surgery with the TAP block, but there was no overall difference in the total amount of acetaminophen administered in the first 24 h.

The recent introduction of the erector spinae plane block has also made it possible to extend this type of analgesia to patients undergoing thoracic surgery and for the management of postoperative pain following, for example, the placement of a chest drain.

13.9.1 Erector Spinae Plane Block (ESPB) (Fig. 13.2)

The erector spinae plane block (ESPB), originally described by Forero in 2016 for the treatment of thoracic neuropathic pain, has been applied in the management of postoperative pain in pediatric patients since 2017. Interest in this technique has rapidly spread in the pediatric population, not only in the context of perioperative analgesia but also in the management of pain unrelated to surgical procedures [81]. However, the location, timing, and pharmacological approach of ESPBs vary considerably among practitioners, and there are currently no standardized protocols. The level of evidence remains limited, and there is no general consensus on these aspects. ESPBs have been proposed for a wide range of possible applications, especially as part of a multimodal perioperative analgesia regimen to promote enhanced recovery after surgery (ERAS) in numerous types of procedures, ranging from thoracic and abdominal surgeries to inguinal and lower limb procedures. In fact, analgesia can be achieved in a wide range of anatomical areas depending on the vertebral level of local anesthetic injection, with extensive craniocaudal spread providing anesthetic coverage to multiple dermatomes [82, 83]. Notably, evidence has emerged supporting the non-inferiority of ESPBs compared to quadratus lumborum block in pediatric lower abdominal surgeries [84–86]. Further evidence indicates that ESPBs may provide more effective and longer-lasting postoperative analgesia than ilioinguinal/iliohypogastric blocks in unilateral inguinal hernia repairs [87]. The pharmacological approach described in the current literature is heterogeneous, as the procedure has multiple applications and the specific pharmacological approach varies according to the clinical context. Bupivacaine, ropivacaine, and levobupivacaine at different concentrations and volumes have been most commonly used in ESPBs in pediatric patients, with no significant differences in postoperative pain management among them. Most pediatric ESPBs currently described in the literature are performed with 0.25% bupivacaine, with volumes ranging from 0.3 to 0.6 ml/kg

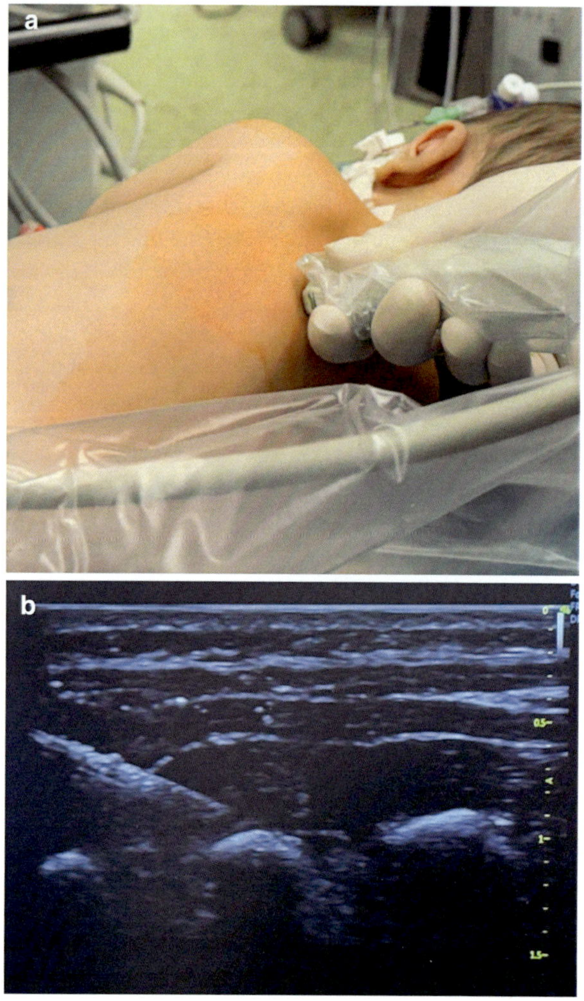

Fig. 13.2 Erector spinae plane block (ESP block). (**a**) Patient and ultrasound probe positioning. (**b**) Ultrasound view during needle insertion, with the needle tip located between the erector spinae muscle and the transverse process of the vertebra

[89, 90]. The ESP block is most commonly performed at the T5-T7 paravertebral levels, but can also be performed at lower levels. Proper ultrasound visualization is achieved with a linear probe positioned in a cephalocaudal direction over the midline of the back at the desired level. The probe should then be slowly moved laterally until the transverse process is visible. After identifying the transverse process, the trapezius muscle, the rhomboid major muscle (if performed at T5 or above), and the erector spinae muscle superficial to the transverse process should be identified (in-plane technique). The tip of the Tuohy needle should be directed posteriorly and inferiorly, advancing under ultrasound guidance through the trapezius, rhomboid major, and erector spinae muscles toward the transverse process; once the needle tip is beneath the erector spinae muscle, a small bolus of local anesthetic should be administered through the Tuohy needle. The erector spinae muscle should be

visualized separating from the transverse process. This separation from the transverse process confirms correct needle placement [88]. In conclusion, ESPBs represent a promising prospect in perioperative pain management, but further research is needed to thoroughly assess their efficacy and safety compared to other common techniques such as caudal epidural analgesia [85–87].

13.9.2 Transversus Abdominis Plane (TAP) Block (Fig. 13.3)

The transversus abdominis plane (TAP) block is an interfascial block technique in which a local anesthetic is deposited between the internal oblique muscle and the transversus abdominis muscle under ultrasound guidance. Several approaches to this block have been described, but all involve depositing the anesthetic in this interfascial plane and can provide analgesia from dermatomes T10 to L1 [91, 92]. The technique and related fascial plane blocks are becoming increasingly popular with

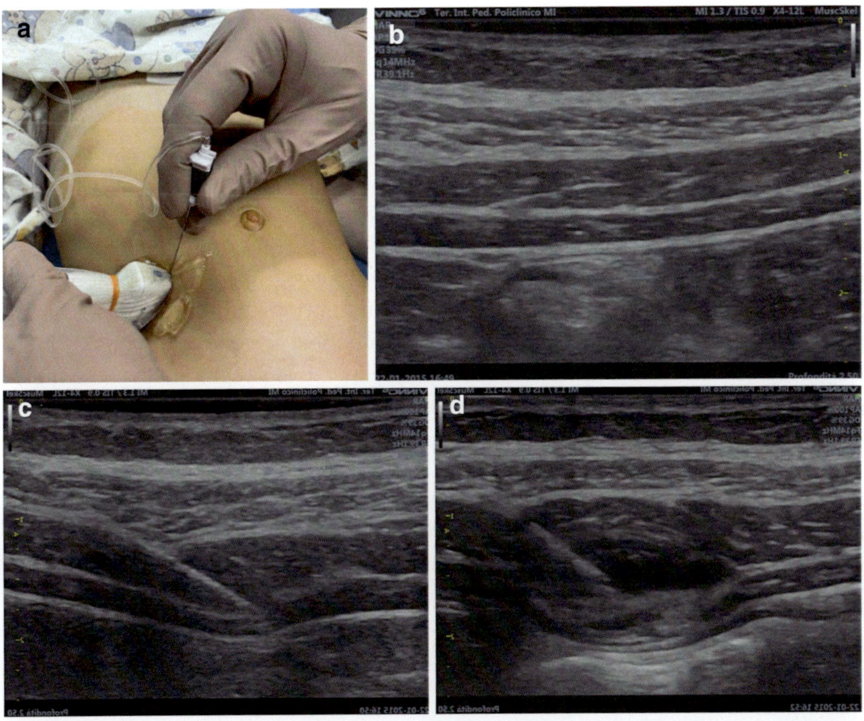

Fig. 13.3 Transversus abdominis plane (TAP) block. (**a**) Patient and ultrasound probe positioning. (**b**) Ultrasound view of the three abdominal muscle layers, from superficial to deep: external oblique, internal oblique, and transversus abdominis muscles. (**c**) Insertion of the hyperechoic needle, with the tip positioned within the fascial plane between the internal oblique and transversus abdominis muscles. (**d**) Infusion of local anesthetic, with ultrasound visualization of fascial plane separation

the widespread adoption of ultrasound technology in pediatric practice. Complications from the TAP block are rare, but there is a potential risk of systemic local anesthetic toxicity, and cases of hepatic injury and intestinal hematoma have been reported when the block is performed without ultrasound guidance [92]. Analgesia from the TAP block can last up to 18 h. This presumed prolonged duration may be attributed to a more sustained depot of local anesthetic at the injection site, in contrast to the highly vascularized epidural space, which has been shown to decrease the duration of epidural analgesia [93–96].

The block is performed under ultrasound guidance, using a microconvex or linear probe, in-plane.

The needle is inserted parallel to the ultrasound beam (in a direction parallel to the ultrasound beam) from the posterolateral side of the probe and advanced medially and anteriorly. To obtain a clear image of the needle, it is preferable to introduce it 1–2 cm away from the probe to avoid a steep acute angle that is unfavorable for ultrasound beam reflection. The needle is advanced through the various layers with a tactile "pop" sensation as each fascial layer is traversed. A gentle tap on the needle can help identify the advancing tip under ultrasound. Alternatively, the correct plane can be confirmed by injecting a few milliliters of saline or local anesthetic (hydrolocalization). The correct position is identified by the solution separating the internal oblique muscle superficially from the deeper transversus abdominis muscle. Pharmacological safety data in pediatric patients indicate that the use of levobupivacaine 0.4 $mg \cdot kg^{-1}$ administered either as a high-volume, low-concentration, or low-volume, high-concentration regimen provides good block duration and is not associated with a risk of systemic local anesthetic toxicity [97]. A similar study using different concentrations of ropivacaine and TAP block after unilateral pediatric inguinal hernia repair reported that administration of ropivacaine 0.2% (0.4 ml/kg) is safe and effective for postoperative pain control [98]. Catheter placement offers the advantage of prolonging the analgesic effect beyond the duration of the block and can also be used in patients with preoperative coagulopathy, which precludes neuraxial block. The procedure uses the same technique as previously described for the block. However, instead of a 22 G blunt needle, a Tuohy needle is used, and the space between the two muscles is dissected with 3–5 ml of saline, followed by insertion of a catheter approximately 2–4 cm beyond the needle tip. Some authors have described surgical placement of the catheter under direct vision and the use of an infusion device during the procedure.

13.10 Conclusion

In conclusion, the use of pediatric epidural and spinal anesthesia has emerged as a fundamental and well-established practice in perioperative care for children. Its effectiveness in providing adequate postoperative pain relief translates into numerous benefits, including early mobilization, reduced dependence on general anesthetics and opioids, and overall improvement in the well-being of pediatric patients. The most recent peripheral block techniques have expanded the therapeutic arsenal, offering valid alternatives, but epidural anesthesia retains its importance by allowing targeted pain control with lower doses of local anesthetics and greater precision in block management. Although scientific evidence is limited in some areas, it supports the adoption of pediatric epidural anesthesia as a safe and effective strategy. However, ongoing research is essential to broaden our understanding of long-term effects and refine clinical practices, ensuring optimal pain management in children undergoing surgical procedures.

Conflicts of Interest The authors declare no conflicts of interest related to this presentation.

The authors declare that they have no financial or non-financial conflicts of interest related to this chapter.

This work did not receive any specific grant from funding agencies in the public, commercial, or not-for-profit sectors.

References

1. Gray HT. A study of spinal anesthesia in children and infants: from a series of 200 cases. Lancet. 1909;174:913–7.
2. Abajian JC, Mellish RW, Browne AF, et al. Spinal anesthesia for surgery in the high-risk infant. Anesth Analg. 1984;63:359–62.
3. McCann ME, de Graaff JC, Dorris L, et al. Neurodevelopmental outcome at 5 years of age after general anaesthesia or awake-regional anaesthesia in infancy (GAS): an international, multicentre, randomised, controlled equivalence trial [published correction appears in Lancet. 2019 Aug 24;394(10199):638]. Lancet. 2019;393(10172):664–77.
4. Davidson AJ, Disma N, de Graaff JC, et al. Neurodevelopmental outcome at 2 years of age after general anesthesia and awake-regional anesthesia in infancy (GAS): an international multicenter, randomized controlled trial. Lancet. 2016;3870:239–50.
5. American College of Surgeons. Optimal resources for children's surgical care v.1 2019.
6. Morray JP, Geiduschek JM, Ramamoorthy C, et al. Anesthesia-related cardiac arrest in children: initial findings of the pediatric perioperative cardiac arrest (POCA) registry. Anesthesiology. 2000;93:6–14.
7. Nunnally ME, O'Connor MF, Kordylewski H, et al. The incidence and risk factors for perioperative cardiac arrest observed in the national anesthesia clinical outcomes registry. Anesth Analg. 2015;120:364–70.
8. Ramamoorthy C, Haberkern CM, Bhananker SM, et al. Anesthesia-related cardiac arrest in children with heart disease: data from the Pediatric Perioperative Cardiac Arrest (POCA) registry. Anesth Analg. 2010;110(5):1376–82.
9. Dahan A, Aarts L, Smith TW. Incidence, reversal, and prevention of opioid-induced respiratory depression. Anesthesiology. 2010;112:226–38.
10. Morton NS, Errera A. APA national audit of pediatric opioid infusions. Paediatr Anaesth. 2010;20:119–25.
11. Carbajal R, Eriksson M, Courtois E, et al. Sedation and analgesia practices in neonatal intensive care units (EUROPAIN): results from a prospective cohort study. Lancet Respir Med. 2015;3:796–812.
12. Lewis T, Erfe BL, Ezell T, et al. Pharmacoepidemiology of opiate use in the neonatal ICU: increasing cumulative doses and iatrogenic opiate withdrawal. J Opioid Manag. 2015;11:305–12.
13. Ikonomidou C, Bosch F, Miksa M, et al. Blockade of NMDA receptors and apoptotic neurodegeneration in the developing brain. Science. 1999;283:70–4.

14. Zou X, Liu F, Zhang X, et al. Inhalation anesthetic-induced neuronal damage in the developing rhesus monkey. Neurotoxicol Teratol. 2011;33:592–7.
15. Young C, Jevtovic-Todorovic V, Qin YQ, et al. Potential of ketamine and midazolam, individually or in combination, to induce apoptotic neurodegeneration in the infant mouse brain. Br J Pharmacol. 2005;146:189–97.
16. Pearn ML, Hu Y, Niesman IR, et al. Propofol neurotoxicity is mediated by p75 neurotrophin receptor activation. Anesthesiology. 2012;116:352–61.
17. Warschkow R, Steffen T, Lüthi A, et al. Epidural analgesia in open resection of colorectal cancer: is there a clinical benefit? A retrospective study on 1,470 patients. J Gastrointest Surg. 2011;15:1386–93.
18. Rigg JR, Jamrozik K, Myles PS, et al. Epidural anesthesia and analgesia and outcome of major surgery: a randomized trial. Lancet. 2002;359:1276–82.
19. Choi DH, Kim JA, Chung IS. Epidural depth in infants and children: correlation with age and body weight. Anesth Analg. 1999;88:617–20.
20. Rapp HJ, Folger A, Grau T. Ultrasound-guided epidural catheter insertion in children. Anesth Analg. 2005;101:333–9.
21. Nishimori M, Ballantyne JC, James HS. Epidural pain relief versus systemic opioid-based pain relief for abdominal aortic surgery. Available at: http://www.thecochranelibrary.com/view/0/index.html.
22. Jørgensen H, Wetterslev J, Møiniche S, et al. Epidural local anesthetics versus opioid-based analgesic regimens for postoperative gastrointestinal paralysis, PONV and pain after abdominal surgery. Available at: http://www.thecochranelibrary.com/view/0/index.html.
23. Taqi A, Hong X, Mistraletti G, et al. Thoracic epidural analgesia facilitates the restoration of bowel function and dietary intake in patients undergoing laparoscopic colon resection using a traditional, non-accelerated, perioperative care program. Surg Endosc. 2007;21:247–52.
24. Zingg U, Miskovic D, Hamel CT, et al. Influence of thoracic epidural analgesia on postoperative pain relief and ileus after laparoscopic colorectal resection: benefit with epidural analgesia. Surg Endosc. 2009;23:276–82.
25. Solomon BD. VACTERL/VATER association. Orphanet. 2011;6:1–12.
26. Yıldız TŞ, Özcan D, Solak M, Toker K. VACTERL syndrome and anesthesia. J Anesth. 2012;20:174–5.
27. Luce V, Mercier FJ, Benhamou D. Anesthetic management for a parturient affected by the VACTERL association. Anesth Analg. 2004;98:870–8.
28. Khatavkar SS, Jagtap SR. Anaesthetic management of cataract surgery in VACTERL syndrome case report. Indian J Anaesth. 2009;53:94–7.
29. Brogly N, Guasch Arévalo E, Kollmann Camaiora A, Alsina Marcos E, García García C, Gilsanz RF. Modern approach to an old technique: narrative review of techniques used to locate the epidural space. Rev Esp Anestesiol Reanim. 2017;64:460–6.
30. Punja R, Sumalatha S, Afrah F, Hosapatna M. Clinically relevant morphometry of sacral hiatus and morphology of sacrum. Turk Neurosurg. 2023;33:373–8.
31. Yan TT, Yang XL, Wang S, et al. Application of continuous sacral block guided by ultrasound after comprehensive sacral canal scanning in children undergoing laparoscopic surgery: a prospective, randomized, double-blind study. J Pain Res. 2023;16:83–92. Published 2023 Jan 10. https://doi.org/10.2147/JPR.S39150131.
32. Chawathe MS, Jones RM, Gildersleve CD, et al. Detection of epidural catheters with ultrasound in children. Paediatr Anaesth. 2003;13:681–4.
33. Bosenberg AT, Cronje L, Thomas J, et al. Ropivacaine plasma levels and postoperative analgesia in neonates and infants during 48–72 hr continuous epidural infusion following major surgery. Paediatr Anaesth. 2003;13:851–22.
34. Lerman J, Nolan J, Eyres R, et al. Efficacy, safety, and pharmacokinetics of levobupivacaine with and without fentanyl after continuous epidural infusion in children: a multicenter trial. Anesthesiology. 2003;99:1166–74.

35. Ivani G, DeNegri P, Conio A, et al. Comparison of racemic bupivacaine, ropivacaine, and levo-bupivacaine for pediatric caudal anesthesia: effects on postoperative analgesia and motor block. Reg Anesth Pain Med. 2002;27:157–61.
36. Joshi G, Gandhi K, Shah N, Gadsden J, Corman SL. Peripheral nerve blocks in the management of postoperative pain: challenges and opportunities. J Clin Anesth. 2016;35:524–9.
37. Desgranges FP, Desebbe O, de Souza P, Neto E, Raphael D, Chassard D. Respiratory variation in aortic blood flow peak velocity to predict fluid responsiveness in mechanically ventilated children: a systematic review and meta-analysis. Paediatr Anaesth. 2016;26:37–47.
38. Ivani G, Suresh S, Ecoffey C, et al. The European Society of Regional Anaesthesia and Pain Therapy and the American Society of Regional Anesthesia and Pain Medicine joint committee practice advisory on controversial topics in pediatric regional anesthesia. Reg Anesth Pain Med. 2015;40:526–32.
39. Woolf CJ, Thompson SW. The induction and maintenance of central sensitization is dependent on N-methyl-D-aspartic acid receptor activation; implications for the treatment of post-injury pain hypersensitivity states. Pain. 1991;44:293–9.
40. McCartney CJL, Sinha A, Katz J. A qualitative systematic review of the role of N-methyl-D-aspartate receptor antagonists in preventive analgesia. Anesth Analg. 2004;98:1385–400.
41. Schnabel A, Poepping DM, Kranke P, Zahn PK, Pogatzki-Zahn EM. Efficacy and adverse effects of ketamine as an additive for pediatric caudal anesthesia: a quantitative systematic review of randomized controlled trials. Br J Anaesth. 2011;107:601–11. https://doi.org/10.1093/bja/aer258.
42. Walker SM, Westin BD, Deumens R, Grafe M, Yaksh TL. Effects of intrathecal ketamine in the neonatal rat. Anesthesiology. 2010;113:147–59. https://doi.org/10.1097/ALN.0b013e3181dcd71c.
43. Bujalska-Zadrożny M, Tatarkiewicz J, Kulik K, Filip M, Naruszewicz M. Magnesium enhances opioid-induced analgesia–what have we learned in the past decades? Eur J Pharm Sci. 2017;99:113–27.
44. Guo B-L, Lin Y, Hu W, Zhen C-X, Bao-Cheng Z, Wu H-H, et al. Effects of systemic magnesium on postoperative analgesia: is the current evidence strong enough? Pain Physician. 2015;18:405–18.
45. Min X, Xiang-Kui LI, Yu P. Magnesium sulfate for postoperative complications in children undergoing tonsillectomies: a systematic review and meta-analysis. J Evid Based Med. 2017;10:16–25.
46. Thurnau GR, Kemp DB, Jarvis A. Cerebrospinal fluid levels of magnesium in patients with preeclampsia after treatment with intravenous magnesium sulfate: a preliminary report. Am J Obstet Gynecol. 1987;157:1435–8.
47. Albrecht E, Kirkham KR, Liu SS, Brull R. The analgesic efficacy and safety of neuraxial magnesium sulfate: a quantitative review. Anaesthesia. 2013;68:190–202.
48. Campbell MF. Caudal anesthesia in children. J Urol. 1933;30:245e50.
49. Veyckemans F, Van Obbergh LJ, Gouverneur JM. Lessons from 1100 pediatric caudal blocks in a teaching hospital. Reg Anesth. 1992;17:119e25.
50. Ecoffey C, Lacroix F, Giaufre E, Orliaguet G, Courr eges P. Association des Anesthesistes Reanimateurs P ediatriques d'Expression Franc¸aise (ADARPEF). Epidemiology and morbidity of regional anesthesia in children: a follow-up one-year prospective survey of the French-Language Society of Paediatric Anaesthesiologists (ADARPEF). Paediatr Anaesth. 2010;20:1061e9.
51. Johr M, Berger T. Caudal blocks. Paediatr Anaesth. 2012;22:44e50.
52. Flandin-Blety C, Barrier G. Accidents following extradural analgesia in children. The results of a retrospective study. Paediatr Anaesth. 1995;5:41e6.
53. Polaner DM, Taenzer AH, Walker BJ, et al. Paediatric Regional Anesthesia Network (PRAN): a multi-institutional study of the use and incidence of complications of pediatric regional anesthesia. Anesth Analg. 2012;115:1353e64.

54. Mirjalili SA, Taghavi K, Frawley G, Craw S. Should we abandon landmark-based technique for caudal anesthesia in neonates and infants. Paediatr Anaesth. 2015;25:511e6.
55. Lonnqvist PA. Is ultrasound guidance mandatory when performing pediatric regional anesthesia? Curr Opin Anaesthesiol. 2010;23:337–41.
56. Liu JZ, Wu XQ, Li R, Zhang YJ. A comparison of ultrasonography versus the traditional approach for caudal block in children. Zhonghua Yi Xue Za Zhi. 2012;92:882–5.
57. Lundblad M, Lonnqvist PA, Eksborg S, Marhofer P. Segmental distribution of high-volume caudal anesthesia in neonates, infants, and toddlers as assessed by ultrasonography. Paediatr Anesth. 2011;21:121–7.
58. Lundblad M, Eksborg S, Lonnqvist PA. Secondary spread of caudal block as assessed by ultrasonography. Br J Anaesth. 2012;108:675–81.
59. Marhofer P, Lonnqvist PA. The use of ultrasound-guided regional anesthetic techniques in neonates and young infants. Acta Anaesthesiol Scand. 2014;58:1049–60.
60. Mirjalili SA, Taghavi K, Frawley G, Craw S. Should we abandon the landmark-based technique for caudal anesthesia in neonates and infants? Paediatr Anaesth. 2015;25:511–6.
61. Suresh S, Ecoffey C, Bosenberg A, et al. The European Society of Regional Anaesthesia and Pain Therapy/American Society of Regional Anesthesia and Pain Medicine recommendations on local anesthetics and adjuvant dosage in pediatric regional anesthesia. Reg Anesth Pain Med. 2018;43:211–6.
62. Krane EJ, Harberkern CM, Jacobson LE. Postoperative apnea, bradycardia, and oxygen desaturation in formerly premature infants: prospective comparison of spinal and general anesthesia. Anesth Analg. 1995;80:7–13.
63. Williams RK, Adams DC, Aladjem EV, Kreutz JM, Sartorelli KH, Vane DW, et al. The safety and efficacy of spinal anesthesia for surgery in infants: the Vermont Infant Spinal Registry. Anesth Analg. 2006;102:67–71.
64. Lönnqvist PA. Spinal anesthesia in children: a narrative review. Best Pract Res Clin Anaesthesiol. 2023;37(2):133–8. https://doi.org/10.1016/j.bpa.2023.01.002. Epub 2023 Feb 7. PMID: 37321762.
65. Kokki H. Spinal blocks. Paediatr Anaesth. 2012;22:56–64.
66. Nickel US, Meyer RR, Brambrink AM. Spinal anesthesia in an extremely low birth weight infant. Paediatr Anaesth. 2005;15:58–62.
67. Williams RK, McBride WJ, Abajian JC. Combined spinal and epidural anesthesia for major abdominal surgery in infants. Can J Anaesth. 1997;44:511–4.
68. O'Higashi T, Shirakami G, Sasai S, Shinomura T, Kato S, Tomoda K. Spinal anesthesia for patients with progressive muscular dystrophy. [Article in Japanese]. Masui. 1995;44:723–8.
69. Gingrich BK. Spinal anesthesia for a former preterm infant undergoing upper abdominal surgery. Anesthesiology. 1993;79:189–90.
70. Arora MK, Nagaraja G, Lakhe ST. Combined spinal-epidural anesthesia for a child with Freeman-Sheldon syndrome and a difficult airway. Anesth Analg. 2006;103:1624.
71. Walker SM, Yaksh TL. Neuraxial analgesia in neonates and infants: a review of clinical and preclinical strategies for the development of safety and efficacy data. Anesth Analg. 2012;115:638–62.
72. Singh R, Batra YK, Bharti N, Panda NB. Comparison of propofol versus propofol-ketamine combination for sedation during spinal anesthesia in children: randomized clinical trial of efficacy and safety. Paediatr Anaesth. 2010;20:439–44.
73. Hermanns H, Stevens MF, Werdehausen R, Braun S, Lipfert P, Jetzek-Zader M. Sedation during spinal anesthesia in infants. Br J Anaesth. 2006;97:308–4.
74. Gleason CA, Martin RJ, Anderson JV, Carlo WA, Sanniti KJ, Fanaroff AA. Optimal position for a spinal tap in preterm infants. Pediatrics. 1983;71:31–5.
75. López T, Sánchez FJ, Garzón JC, Muriel C. Spinal anesthesia in pediatric patients. Minerva Anestesiol. 2012;78:78–87.
76. Arthrus OJ, Murray M, Zubier M, Tooley J, Kelsall W. Ultrasonographic determination of neonatal spinal canal depth. Arch Dis Child Fetal Neonatal Ed. 2008;93:F451–4.

77. Wright TE, Orr RJ, Haberkern CM, Walbergh EJ. Complications during spinal anesthesia in infants: high spinal blockade. Anesthesiology. 1990;73:1290–2.
78. Ecoffey C, Lacroix F, Giaufré E, Orliaguet G, Courrèges P. Association des Anesthésistes Réanimateurs Pédiatriques d'Expression Française (ADARPEF). Epidemiology and morbidity of regional anesthesia in children: a one-year prospective follow-up survey by the French-Language Society of Pediatric Anesthesiologists (ADARPEF). Paediatr Anaesth. 2010;20:1061–9.
79. Imbelloni LE, Vieira EM, Sperni F, Guizellini RH, Tolentino AP. Spinal anesthesia in children with isobaric local anesthetics: report on 307 patients under 13 years of age. Pediatr Anaesth. 2006;16:43–8.
80. Dohi S, Seino H. Spinal anesthesia in premature infants: dosage and effects of sympathectomy. Anesthesiology. 1986;65:559–61.
81. Wright TE, Orr RJ, Haberkern CM, Walbergh EJ. Complications during spinal anesthesia in infants: High spinal blockade. Anesthesiology. 1990;73:1290–2. 86. Forero M, Adhikary SD, Lopez H, Tsui C, Chin KJ. The erector spinae plane block: a novel analgesic technique in thoracic neuropathic pain. Reg Anesth Pain Med. 2016;41:621–9.
82. Muñoz F, Cubillos J, Bonilla AJ, Chin KJ. Erector spinae plane block for postoperative analgesia in pediatric oncological thoracic surgery. Can J Anaesth. 2017;64:880–2.
83. Adhikary SD, Bernard S, Lopez H, Chin KJ. Erector spinae plane block versus retrolaminar block: a magnetic resonance imaging and anatomical study. Reg Anesth Pain Med. 2018;43:756–62.
84. Mostafa SF, Abdelghany MS, Abdelraheem TM, Abu Elyazed MM. Ultrasound-guided erector spinae plane block for postoperative analgesia in pediatric patients undergoing splenectomy: a prospective randomized controlled trial. Aksu C, Şen MC, Akay MA, Baydemir C, Gürkan Y. Erector spinae plane block vs quadratus lumborum block for pediatric low. Paediatr Anaesth. 2019;29:1201–7.
85. Singh S, Jha RK, Sharma M. The analgesic effect of bilateral ultrasound-guided erector spinae plane block in pediatric lower abdominal surgeries: a randomized, prospective trial. Indian J Anaesth. 2020;64:762–7.
86. El-Emam EM, El Motlb EAA. Ultrasound-guided erector spinae versus ilioinguinal/iliohypogastric block for postoperative analgesia in children undergoing inguinal surgeries. Anesth Essays Res. 2019;13:274–9.
87. Villalobos MA, Veneziano G, Miller R, Beltran RJ, Krishna S, Tumin D, et al. Evaluation of postoperative analgesia in pediatric patients after hip surgery: lumbar plexus versus caudal epidural analgesia. J Pain Res 2019; 12: 997-1001. 12. Jöhr M, Berger TM. Caudal blocks. Paediatr Anaesth. 2012;22:44–50.
88. Lucente M, Ragonesi G, Sanguigni M, et al. Erector spinae plane block in children: a narrative review. Korean J Anesthesiol. 2022;75:473–86.
89. Nardiello MA, Herlitz M. Bilateral single shot erector spinae plane block for pectus excavatum and pectus carinatum surgery in 2 pediatric patients. Rev Esp Anestesiol Reanim (Engl Ed). 2018;65:530–3.
90. Çiftçi B, Ekinci M. Ultrasound-guided single shot preemptive erector spinae plane block for thoracic surgery in a pediatric patient. Analgesic efficacy of preemptive erector spinae plane block after thoracic surgery in a pediatric patient. Agri. 2020;32:58–9.
91. Hafeman M, Greenspan S, Rakhamimova E, Jin Z, Moore RP, Al Bizri E. Caudal block vs. transversus abdominis plane block for pediatric surgery: a systematic review and meta-analysis. Front Pediatr. 2023;11:1173700. Published 2023 May 30. https://doi.org/10.3389/fped.2023.1173700.
92. Dontukurthy S, Mofidi R. The role of interfascial plane blocks in pediatric regional anesthesia: a narrative review of current perspectives and updates. Anesthesiol Res Pract. https://doi.org/10.1155/2020/8892537.
93. Taylor R Jr, Pergolizzi JV, Sinclair A, Raffa RB, Aldington D, Plavin S, et al. Transversus abdominis block: clinical uses, side effects, and future perspectives. Pain Pract. 2013;13:332–44.

94. Frigon C, Mai R, Valois-Gomez T, Desparmet J. Bowel hematoma following an iliohypogastric-ilioinguinal nerve block. Paediatr Anaesth. 2006;16:993–6.
95. Carney J, Finnerty O, Rauf J, Curley G, McDonnell JG, Laffey JG. Ipsilateral transversus abdominis plane block provides effective analgesia after appendectomy in children: a randomized controlled trial. Anesth Analg. 2010;111:998–1003.
96. Latzke D, Marhofer P, Kettner SC, Koppatz K, Turnheim K, Lackner E, et al. Pharmacokinetics of the local anesthetic ropivacaine after transversus abdominis plane block in healthy volunteers. Eur J Clin Pharmacol. 2012;68:419–25.
97. Sola C, Menacé C, Bringuier S, Saour AC, Raux O, Capdevila X, Dadure C. Transversus abdominal plane block in children: efficacy and safety: a randomized clinical study and pharmacokinetic profile. Anesth Analg. 2019;128:1234–41.
98. Lee H, Chung J, Lee M, Yang S, Lee H. Comparison between post-operative analgesic efficacy of low-concentration high-volume and high-concentration low-volume combinations of Ropivacaine for transverse abdominis plane block in pediatric open inguinal hernia repair. J Clin Med. 2019;8:1133. https://doi.org/10.3390/jcm8081133. PMID: 31366079; PMCID: PMC6723931.

Intraoperative Mechanical Ventilation

14

Marina Roger Coscojuela, Miguel Linares Torras,
Jordi Vallverdú Martínez, and Carlos Ferrando Ortolá

14.1 Introduction

Globally, an estimated 310–313 million major surgical procedures requiring general anesthesia and mechanical ventilation are performed each year. The primary objective of mechanical ventilation is to replace the respiratory system's function in gas exchange [1]. However, inadequate adjustment of ventilatory parameters can promote lung injury and, consequently, the development of respiratory complications during the postoperative period, known as postoperative pulmonary

M. Roger Coscojuela (✉) · M. Linares Torras
Hospital Clínic de Barcelona, Department of Anesthesiology and Critical Care,
Barcelona, Spain
e-mail: mroger@clinic.cat; milinares@clinic.cat

J. Vallverdú Martínez
Hospital Clínic de Barcelona, Department of Anesthesiology and Critical Care,
Barcelona, Spain

Institut d'Investigacions Biomèdiques August Pi i Sunyer (FRCB-IDIBAPS), Fundació de
Recerca Clínic Barcelona, Barcelona, Spain
e-mail: vallverdu@clinic.cat

C. Ferrando Ortolá
Hospital Clínic de Barcelona, Department of Anesthesiology and Critical Care,
Barcelona, Spain

Institut d'Investigacions Biomèdiques August Pi i Sunyer (FRCB-IDIBAPS), Fundació de
Recerca Clínic Barcelona, Barcelona, Spain

Centro de Investigación Biomédica en Red Enfermedades Respiratorias (CIBERES),
Madrid, Spain
e-mail: cmferrando@clinic.cat

D. Chiumello, A. De Gasperi (eds.), *Practical Trends in Anesthesia and Intensive Care 2026*, https://doi.org/10.1007/978-3-032-25721-5_14

complications. Postoperative pulmonary complications (PPCs) are adverse events in the respiratory system following anesthesia and surgery. The prevalence is widely heterogeneous ranging from 1% to almost 50% [2–4], depending, among other factors, on the definition used or the number of PPCs reported. PPCs are contributors to the overall risk of surgery with a significant association with postoperative morbidity and mortality. The risk of mortality can increase up to five times in patients presenting PPCs [2, 6, 7]. PPCs also impose a considerable financial burden on healthcare systems, mainly due to an associated increase in length of stay and use of resources [8].

PPCs range from mild transient hypoxemia to severe life-threatening acute respiratory distress syndrome (ARDS). Despite significant variability in the definition of PPCs used in the literature, current European guidelines provide standardized definitions for both: the overall group of PPCs and each individual complication [4, 5, 9]. PPCs usually occur during the first postoperative days, although they are considered as such until 30 days after surgery. Their etiology is complex and influenced by modifiable and non-modifiable factors. Known influential factors can also be distinguished as patient-related (i.e., age, American Society of Anesthesiologists [ASA] status, comorbidities, smoking, preexisting pulmonary diseases, nutritional status, obesity) or procedure-related (duration of surgery, surgical approach, emergency surgery, anesthesia, mechanical ventilation [MV], and fluids, among others) [2–10].

Given the clinical relevance of PPCs and their multifactorial etiology, we consider it especially important for anesthesiologists to have a thorough understanding of respiratory physiology and the changes associated with general anesthesia and neuromuscular relaxation, and to understand the different techniques and methods of respiratory support, as well as respiratory monitoring. Last but not least, an anesthesiologist should understand the pathophysiology of PPCs and the different lung-protective ventilation strategies.

14.2 Basic Physiology Relevant to Intraoperative Ventilation

14.2.1 Respiratory Mechanics Under Anesthesia

The induction of general anesthesia induces profound changes in respiratory mechanics that differ significantly from those observed in the awake state. The *functional residual capacity (FRC)* decreases within minutes of anesthetic induction, primarily due to the loss of diaphragmatic and intercostal muscle tone [11]. This loss of tonic activity allows the diaphragm to be displaced cephalad by abdominal contents, reducing lung volume at end-expiration. The magnitude of this reduction varies but is generally reported to be 15–20% in healthy adults, with more pronounced decreases in obese patients, pregnant patients, and those undergoing abdominal or thoracic procedures [12].

The compliance of the respiratory system decreases during anesthesia, reflecting changes in both the lung parenchyma and chest wall. Static compliance typically falls by 10–40%, largely due to reduced lung volumes and an increased tendency toward airway closure. Dynamic compliance may be further compromised by increased airway resistance, which can result from reduced upper airway tone, endotracheal intubation, or increased bronchial reactivity in susceptible individuals. These changes mean that higher airway pressures are required to deliver equivalent tidal volumes compared to the awake state [11, 13–15]. The *airway resistance* itself can rise under anesthesia. Although endotracheal intubation bypasses upper airway structures, the artificial airway imposes its own resistance, and turbulent flow through smaller-caliber tubes can increase the work of breathing [13, 14]. Additionally, inhaled anesthetics may variably influence airway smooth muscle tone: agents such as sevoflurane exert bronchodilatory effects, while desflurane may initially provoke airway irritation and transient bronchoconstriction. The distribution of ventilation becomes less uniform under anesthesia. Reduced diaphragmatic excursion and changes in chest wall mechanics preferentially limit ventilation in dependent lung regions. As a result, ventilation is redistributed toward nondependent zones, which are less well perfused, contributing to ventilation-perfusion (V/Q) inequality [11, 16].

14.2.2 Gas Exchange and Anesthetic-Induced Changes

Gas exchange during anesthesia is altered through several mechanisms. The decrease in FRC reduces the buffer volume between tidal ventilation and residual volume, predisposing to airway closure during tidal breathing. Closure of small airways increases the degree of intrapulmonary shunt and worsens V/Q mismatch [11, 13, 16]. Oxygenation typically declines after induction, necessitating higher fractions of inspired oxygen (FiO_2) to maintain adequate arterial oxygen tension. Anesthetic agents also influence pulmonary physiology at the vascular level. Volatile anesthetics impair hypoxic pulmonary vasoconstriction (HPV) [17], a physiologic mechanism that diverts blood flow away from poorly ventilated regions of the lung. Inhibition of HPV accentuates shunt physiology, particularly in conditions where alveolar collapse or one-lung ventilation is present. Intravenous anesthetics tend to preserve HPV more effectively, which may be clinically relevant in thoracic surgery. Carbon dioxide homeostasis is also affected. Most anesthetics blunt the central chemoreceptor response to hypercapnia, rendering patients unable to maintain adequate minute ventilation spontaneously. Controlled mechanical ventilation is therefore required in most general anesthetics to avoid progressive hypercapnia and respiratory acidosis. During controlled ventilation, the increased dead space fraction observed under anesthesia—due to factors such as decreased pulmonary blood flow, airway instrumentation, and positive pressure ventilation—must be compensated for by adjusting tidal volume and respiratory rate [13].

14.2.3 Effects of Positioning, Neuromuscular Blockade, and Pneumoperitoneum

Beyond the intrinsic effects of anesthesia, intraoperative physiology is further influenced by surgical positioning, neuromuscular blockade, and pneumoperitoneum. Patient positioning has marked effects on pulmonary mechanics. The *supine position*, commonly adopted for induction and many surgeries, reduces FRC by approximately 0.8–1.0 L compared to the upright position [18]. *Trendelenburg positioning*, frequently employed in pelvic and robotic surgery, exaggerates cephalad displacement of the diaphragm, reducing compliance and increasing plateau pressure, and therefore, proportionally, peak inspiratory pressures. Conversely, the *reverse Trendelenburg position* can improve diaphragmatic mechanics and oxygenation, although venous return may be compromised [19]. In the *lateral decubitus position*, ventilation and perfusion distribution become markedly asymmetric. Gravity increases perfusion to the dependent lung, but diaphragmatic movement and ribcage mechanics favor ventilation of the nondependent lung [20]. In awake, spontaneously breathing individuals, this effect is mitigated by greater diaphragmatic excursion of the dependent lung. Under anesthesia with neuromuscular blockade, however, this advantage is lost, and the dependent lung tends to be underventilated relative to its perfusion, worsening gas exchange. These principles are particularly important during thoracic surgery and one-lung ventilation [18, 20].

Neuromuscular blockade eliminates spontaneous breathing and stabilizes the surgical field, but it also abolishes the beneficial diaphragmatic contractions that preferentially ventilate dependent regions [21]. This promotes uniformity of tidal ventilation at the expense of dependent lung aeration. Paralysis also increases chest wall compliance, further predisposing to reductions in FRC. The degree of impairment correlates with the depth of blockade and the duration of paralysis [15].

Pneumoperitoneum, used during laparoscopic and robotic surgery, introduces substantial mechanical and gas exchange challenges. Insufflation of carbon dioxide elevates intra-abdominal pressure, which displaces the diaphragm cephalad, reduces thoracic compliance, and increases peak and plateau airway pressures [13, 19]. Lung volumes decline, particularly in the basal regions, and V/Q mismatch worsens. In addition, absorption of insufflated CO_2 into the systemic circulation can increase arterial CO_2 tension ($PaCO_2$), requiring adjustments in minute ventilation to maintain normocapnia. The hemodynamic effects of pneumoperitoneum—such as reduced venous return and altered pulmonary blood flow—further contribute to changes in ventilation-perfusion relationships. Moreover, during thoracic procedures such as robotic-assisted surgery, the development of a capnothorax from continuous CO_2 insufflation can further impair respiratory mechanics, markedly reducing lung compliance and increasing driving pressure, necessitating higher individualized PEEP to maintain alveolar recruitment [23].

The interplay of positioning, paralysis, and pneumoperitoneum frequently requires individualized ventilatory adjustments. For example, low tidal volume strategies combined with appropriate levels of positive end-expiratory pressure (PEEP) may mitigate compliance reduction and oxygenation impairment, though optimal parameters vary depending on surgical and patient-specific factors.

14.3 Atelectasis

14.3.1 Physiopathology of Atelectasis

Perioperative pulmonary atelectasis is the most frequent respiratory complication during anesthesia and surgery. It is classically defined as the collapse of functional lung tissue, leading to a reduction in pulmonary volume and impaired gas exchange. The principal consequences are the development of intrapulmonary shunt and an increase in dead space, both of which contribute to hypoxemia. From a mechanistic standpoint, atelectasis may arise either from airway obstruction, as in obstructive atelectasis, or from impaired lung expansion, producing compressive atelectasis. In the perioperative setting, the latter mechanism predominates, although resorptive mechanisms also play a significant role when high fraction of inspired oxygen (FiO_2) is used [24].

The induction of general anesthesia constitutes a pivotal moment for the development of atelectasis. Loss of consciousness reduces respiratory drive and leads to apnea [25], which is accompanied by a cephalad displacement of the diaphragm due to abdominal pressure. This diaphragmatic shift compresses dependent lung zones, initiating collapse that can be detected within minutes of induction. Imaging studies, including computed tomography and electrical impedance tomography, demonstrate that up to 90% of patients develop atelectatic regions after induction of anesthesia [24, 26]. In addition to diaphragmatic mechanics, anesthesia also reduces functional residual capacity (FRC) and promotes airway closure, creating the conditions for progressive loss of aeration. Several physiological mechanisms converge in the formation of intraoperative atelectasis. First, resorptive atelectasis occurs when oxygen replaces nitrogen in the alveoli. High FiO_2 accelerates the resorption of alveolar gas into the blood, leaving alveoli prone to collapse if they are not periodically reinflated. Second, compressive atelectasis results from the reduction in lung volumes below the closing capacity, often triggered by diaphragm displacement, supine positioning, pneumoperitoneum during laparoscopy, or obesity. Third, obstructive atelectasis arises when small airways are blocked by secretions or mucus plugs, a less common but relevant mechanism in surgical patients [24].

The physiological consequences of atelectasis extend beyond simple collapse. The immediate effect is a reduction in FRC, which redistributes tidal ventilation to the non-collapsed lung. This may favor regional overdistension and increased pulmonary strain, conditions that predispose to ventilator-induced lung injury (VILI) [27]. At the same time, perfusion persists in collapsed areas, giving rise to intrapulmonary shunt. Normally, HPV serves to divert blood flow away from poorly ventilated regions, but this protective reflex is attenuated by volatile anesthetics, thereby worsening shunt-induced hypoxemia. As a result, even relatively small areas of atelectasis can lead to clinically significant desaturation. Furthermore, the redistribution of perfusion toward dependent, atelectatic zones aggravates the mismatch between ventilation and perfusion, reinforcing hypoxemia during anesthesia [17]. Patient characteristics and surgical conditions may amplify these processes. Obese individuals are particularly vulnerable, as increased abdominal pressure and reduced chest wall compliance exacerbate diaphragmatic elevation and airway closure [28]. Similarly, laparoscopic surgery [22] with pneumoperitoneum markedly reduces compliance and promotes further lung collapse. Pediatric patients, because of their smaller closing volumes and the frequent use of high FiO_2 during induction, are also at increased risk.

In summary, intraoperative atelectasis arises from a multifactorial interplay of mechanical, physiological, and pharmacological factors. It is characterized by alveolar collapse due to loss of FRC, airway closure, oxygen absorption, and diaphragmatic displacement. The consequences are reduced lung compliance, increased pulmonary strain, impaired gas exchange through shunt, and heightened risk of VILI. Recognizing this pathophysiology is essential, as it underscores the need for protective ventilation strategies aimed at preventing or minimizing collapse and its deleterious effects during anesthesia.

14.3.2 Diagnosis of Atelectasis

The accurate detection of pulmonary atelectasis during anesthesia is crucial for optimizing ventilation strategies and preventing postoperative pulmonary complications. Although computed tomography (CT) remains the gold standard for identifying and quantifying collapsed lung tissue, it is impractical [29]. Consequently, several bedside and functional methods have been developed to assess atelectasis dynamically and noninvasively in the perioperative setting. Among these, the Air-Test, lung ultrasound, and electrical impedance tomography represent the most relevant tools for real-time evaluation of lung aeration during surgery.

14.3.2.1 The Air-Test

The Air-Test is a simple, noninvasive bedside method for identifying atelectasis based on changes in arterial oxygenation after transient withdrawal of supplemental oxygen. In this approach, the patient breathes room air for a short period while oxygen saturation is continuously monitored. When alveolar units are collapsed, the resulting intrapulmonary shunt leads to a reduction in peripheral oxygen saturation despite normal ventilation and perfusion elsewhere in the lung. A fall in SpO_2 after switching to room air suggests a significant degree of atelectasis. The Air-Test has been validated to detect atelectasis in the postoperative period [29–31], comparing its results with chest CT findings. These make the Air-Test a practical, inexpensive, and repeatable diagnostic tool. Although it was developed for postoperative assessment, its underlying physiological principle is equally applicable in the intraoperative setting. During anesthesia, short reductions in inspired oxygen fraction may help confirm the presence of lung collapse when hypoxemia occurs, provided patient stability and monitoring allow safe execution [32].

14.3.2.2 Lung Ultrasound

Lung ultrasound (LUS) has emerged as the most versatile and widely applicable bedside technique for the morphological diagnosis of pulmonary atelectasis [29, 33]. The method relies on the fact that air strongly reflects ultrasound beams, producing distinctive patterns when lung aeration is lost. Collapsed or fluid-filled regions appear as tissue-like or "hepatized" structures, frequently with visible static air bronchograms. When aeration loss is partial, the presence of multiple or coalescent B-lines indicates interstitial fluid or incomplete collapse. LUS has been validated as a highly sensitive tool for the detection of atelectasis both in adults and children. In cardiac surgery, recent evidence confirms that lung ultrasound provides greater diagnostic accuracy than chest radiography and correlates with the extent of collapse seen on CT imaging [34]. These findings support its integration into perioperative monitoring, where ultrasound can be used to localize atelectatic regions, assess the effectiveness of recruitment, and guide individualized positive end-expiratory pressure settings. In practice, LUS can be rapidly performed at the bedside using standard probes, with the thorax divided into predefined scanning zones [35]. Each zone is evaluated for signs of aeration loss, producing a semiquantitative score that reflects the overall degree of lung collapse. Although interpretation requires training [33], the technique is radiation-free, repeatable, and suitable for continuous evaluation throughout the surgical procedure. Its main limitations include restricted acoustic windows in obese patients or in the presence of dressings and pneumoperitoneum, as well as the difficulty in distinguishing between atelectasis and consolidation when dynamic air bronchograms are absent. In such cases, transesophageal or Doppler ultrasound can provide complementary information about deeper or poorly accessible regions and regional perfusion patterns.

14.3.2.3 Other Bedside and Functional Techniques

Electrical impedance tomography (EIT) is another emerging tool for bedside assessment of ventilation distribution and lung aeration. The technique uses low-amplitude electrical currents applied through thoracic electrodes to generate real-time images of regional impedance changes [29], which correspond to local ventilation. Because air has high electrical resistance, areas of collapse exhibit a marked reduction in impedance. EIT allows continuous monitoring of aeration changes during anesthesia and has been used to evaluate the regional effects of PEEP and recruitment maneuvers. Although it provides valuable functional data, EIT does not offer direct anatomical visualization and should be interpreted in combination with other clinical findings.

Traditional monitoring of respiratory mechanics also remains useful for indirect detection of atelectasis. A progressive decrease in respiratory system compliance or an increase in driving pressure during constant-volume ventilation may suggest loss of aerated lung tissue. While not specific, these changes can serve as early warning signs of collapse, prompting the use of recruitment strategies or imaging confirmation. Similarly, continuous monitoring of oxygenation and the ratio between oxygen saturation and FiO_2 may provide additional information about the presence of shunt and impaired gas exchange.

14.4 Ventilation-Induced Lung Injury

Mechanical ventilation, while indispensable for supporting gas exchange during anesthesia and critical illness, is not free from risks. In certain conditions, the very intervention designed to sustain life can aggravate preexisting pulmonary injury or even initiate de novo damage, a phenomenon known as ventilator-induced lung injury (VILI). Both experimental and clinical studies have consistently shown that positive-pressure ventilation may exert deleterious effects on lung structure and function, and it is now clear that VILI represents a major pathophysiological mechanism underlying PPCs [36] and poor outcomes in acute respiratory distress syndrome (ARDS).

Several distinct but overlapping mechanisms have been described to explain how ventilation becomes injurious. *Volutrauma* refers to the overdistension of alveoli resulting from the delivery of high tidal volumes, producing stretch injury of alveolar walls, while *barotrauma* arises from excessive airway pressures and may manifest as complications such as pneumothorax or interstitial emphysema [37]. *Atelectrauma* occurs through the repetitive collapse and reopening of unstable alveolar units, which generates shear forces at the interfaces between collapsed and aerated regions [37, 38]. Beyond these mechanical processes, the concept of *biotrauma* underscores the inflammatory dimension of VILI [39]: mechanical stretch activates mechanotransduction pathways that lead to the release of cytokines (including TNF-α, IL-1β, and IL-6), recruitment of neutrophils, and oxidative stress, initiating an inflammatory response that may extend beyond the lung and contribute to multi-organ dysfunction. Together, these conditions generate abnormal stress and strain that disrupt the epithelial and endothelial compartments of the alveolo-capillary membrane, compromise the extracellular matrix (ECM), and amplify inflammatory signaling. The ECM—composed of collagen, elastin, proteoglycans, and hyaluronic acid—plays a key role in maintaining the lung's mechanical stability, yet exposure to high tidal volumes and heterogeneous stress gradients leads to ECM injury, interstitial edema, and activation of matrix metalloproteinases. The resulting fragmentation of ECM components, particularly low-molecular-weight hyaluronans, not only weakens lung architecture but also acts as a potent stimulus for local and systemic inflammatory cascades, further aggravating the cycle of ventilator-induced lung injury.

In addition to these classical concepts, more recent research has emphasized the role of *mechanical power* as a unifying framework to understand VILI. This concept will be better explained in the following sections.

Clinically, VILI is highly relevant, as even patients with previously healthy lungs undergoing surgery can develop postoperative complications secondary to intraoperative ventilatory strategies [36, 40]. Mild forms may manifest as transient hypoxemia or atelectasis, while more severe cases may progress to pneumonia, acute lung injury, or respiratory failure. Lung-protective ventilation strategies (which will be explained in the following sections), initially developed in the context of ARDS, have been translated to the operating room and perioperative care. At present, optimization of ventilator settings according to lung-protective principles remains the most effective and evidence-based strategy to mitigate VILI and its clinical consequences.

14.5 Ventilation Modes

Modern anesthesia ventilators have evolved to incorporate functions once exclusive to intensive care unit (ICU) devices, offering a wide range of ventilation modes that can be tailored to the physiological needs of the patient and the requirements of surgery. Although terminology is not always standardized across manufacturers, the main categories of ventilation modes available in the operating room include volume-controlled ventilation (VCV), pressure-controlled ventilation (PCV), dual-controlled ventilation, and assisted ventilation modes such as pressure support ventilation (PSV). The choice among these modes should be individualized according to patient factors, surgical procedure, and available technology.

14.5.1 Controlled Ventilation Modes

14.5.1.1 Volume-Controlled Ventilation (VCV)

Volume-controlled ventilation remains the most widely employed mode in the operating room. In this mode, also referred to as volume-cycled or volume-limited ventilation, the clinician sets a desired tidal volume and respiratory rate, thereby ensuring a predetermined minute ventilation [41]. The ventilator delivers the set volume with a constant inspiratory flow, producing a square flow waveform and a linear increase in tidal volume until the target is reached. An important advantage of VCV is the guarantee of stable minute ventilation, which is especially valuable during general anesthesia when maintaining adequate carbon dioxide elimination is essential. For this reason, many anesthesiologists still consider VCV the first-line mode for routine cases. However, this mode does not limit inspiratory pressure: if lung compliance decreases or airway resistance increases, the same set tidal volume may require higher airway pressures, potentially predisposing the patient to barotrauma or volutrauma. Modern anesthesia machines mitigate these risks by incorporating compliance compensation systems and pressure limits that trigger alarms when thresholds are exceeded.

14.5.1.2 Pressure-Controlled Ventilation (PCV)

Pressure-controlled ventilation, in contrast, is a pressure-targeted mode. Here, the clinician sets the inspiratory pressure, respiratory rate, and inspiratory time, while tidal volume becomes a dependent variable, influenced by compliance and resistance of the respiratory system [41]. During PCV, inspiratory flow is initially high and then decelerates as alveolar pressure equilibrates with the set inspiratory pressure. The absence of guaranteed tidal volume can be problematic in the intraoperative setting, where compliance may change rapidly due to factors such as pneumoperitoneum during laparoscopy, patient positioning, or depth of neuromuscular blockade. In such circumstances, PCV requires vigilant monitoring and frequent adjustments to maintain adequate ventilation.

14.5.1.3 Dual-Controlled Ventilation (DCV)

With the aim of taking advantage of the benefits of both VCV and PCV, newer ventilators increasingly offer dual-controlled ventilation modes. Although different manufacturers use different terms—such as autoflow, pressure-controlled ventilation with volume guarantee (PCV-VG), or pressure-regulated volume control (PRVC)—these modes share a common principle: they aim to combine the stability of tidal volume control with the benefits of lower peak pressures obtained through a decelerating flow pattern [41, 42]. In practice, the ventilator continuously assesses respiratory system compliance and adapts the inspiratory pressure on a breath-by-breath basis to deliver the target tidal volume at the lowest possible pressure. Such hybrid modes are particularly useful in situations where compliance is dynamic, such as laparoscopic or thoracic surgery, or in obese patients where intra-abdominal pressure varies significantly. Recent evidence demonstrates that DCV significantly reduces peak airway pressures and increases dynamic compliance compared to VCV, especially during challenging scenarios such as one-lung ventilation [42, 43], laparoscopic surgery with pneumoperitoneum and steep Trendelenburg positioning [42]. These improvements in airway mechanics may theoretically reduce the risk of barotrauma and ventilator-induced lung injury. However, current evidence does not show a consistent reduction in postoperative pulmonary complications or hypoxemia with DCV compared to controlled ventilation modes [44, 45].

14.5.1.4 Flow Control Ventilation

Flow-controlled ventilation (FCV) is an emerging mode of mechanical ventilation that allows precise control of both inspiratory and expiratory flow. Unlike conventional modes, FCV operates with an actively managed inspiration and expiration, typically using an I:E ratio close to 1:1 and eliminating pauses throughout the respiratory cycle [46]. This continuous, bidirectional flow results in a linear pressure curve, avoiding the abrupt rises and falls in intrathoracic pressure characteristic of traditional ventilation patterns. As a consequence, lung tissue strain may be reduced, gas flow is sustained longer within the alveoli, and sudden alveolar collapse is minimized. Clinically, FCV has been primarily applied in laryngeal surgery through the use of the Tritube® [47], a narrow-bore endotracheal tube with an external diameter of only 4.4 mm, which enables efficient ventilation and effective CO_2 clearance even in the presence of a small airway lumen. Beyond the operating room, preclinical studies have shown that FCV may improve lung recruitment and enhance gas exchange in models of severe acute respiratory distress [48], suggesting potential benefits in protective ventilation strategies.

14.5.2 Assisted Ventilation Modes

14.5.2.1 Pressure Support Ventilation (PSV)

Pressure support ventilation is a purely assisted mode, triggered by the patient's spontaneous inspiratory effort. Once an effort is detected, the ventilator delivers a preset inspiratory pressure, which then decreases as inspiratory flow decays, producing variable tidal volumes depending on lung mechanics [41, 49]. PSV is often employed in patients undergoing minor procedures, during sedation with regional anesthesia, or in the emergence phase from general anesthesia, when it can reduce the work of breathing, lower anesthetic drug consumption, and shorten recovery time. Its use is particularly attractive with supraglottic airways, as it can decrease air leaks and gastric insufflation, provided that inspiratory pressures are kept within a safe range [41].

In addition, several parameters can be adjusted to optimize patient–ventilator interaction. The trigger determines how sensitive the ventilator is to the patient's inspiratory effort, allowing synchronization between spontaneous and mechanical breaths. The rise time, or ramp, controls how quickly the target inspiratory pressure is reached [49]. Finally, the inspiratory-to-expiratory (I:E) ratio defines the relative duration of each phase of the respiratory cycle, shaping gas exchange efficiency and mean airway pressure.

14.5.3 Monitoring Intraoperative Ventilation

14.5.3.1 Basic Monitoring: Tidal Volume, Pressures, and Compliance

Intraoperative mechanical ventilation requires continuous monitoring of key ventilatory parameters to ensure adequate gas exchange, lung protection, and identification of derangements in respiratory mechanics. At the most basic level, three parameters are indispensable: tidal volume (VT), airway pressures, and respiratory system compliance (Crs) [50, 51].

- Tidal volume (VT): Contemporary evidence shows that 6–8 mL/kg predicted body weight (PBW) *VT* has the lowest incidence of PPC and VILI. Monitoring delivered *VT* (via ventilator display or flow sensors), ensuring that set and actual volumes match (accounting for circuit compliance and fresh-gas flow), is essential in the anesthesia work-station environment.
- Airway pressures: Two pressures are routinely monitored: peak inspiratory pressure (Ppeak) and plateau pressure (Pplat) during volume-controlled ventilation or maximal set inspiratory pressure during pressure-controlled modes. Pplat, measured during an end-inspiratory pause, reflects the pressure required to distend the respiratory system (lung and chest wall) at zero flow. Elevated Pplat (>30 cmH_2O) signals potential overdistension risk; consistently high Ppeak sug-

gests increased resistance or low compliance. Monitoring these pressures allows assessment of mechanical load and potential risk of VILI.

- Respiratory system compliance (Crs): Compliance is calculated as Crs = VT / (Pplat – PEEP). A decline in Crs intraoperatively often indicates worsening lung mechanics due to atelectasis, pulmonary edema, surgical positioning, pneumoperitoneum, or intra-abdominal pressure changes. Since Crs integrates both lung and chest-wall compliance, changes in compliance alert the anesthesiologist to evolving pathophysiology.

14.5.3.2 Advanced Monitoring: Driving Pressure, Transpulmonary Pressure, Mechanical Power, Flow–Volume Loops

Beyond basic parameters, more refined monitoring techniques enable deeper assessment of lung stress and strain, offering the potential for individualized intraoperative ventilation. Key advanced metrics include driving pressure (ΔP), transpulmonary pressure (Ptp), and analyses of flow–volume loops [51, 52].

- Driving pressure (ΔP): Defined as ΔP = Pplat – PEEP in volume-controlled ventilation (or equivalently VT/Crs), driving pressure has emerged as a powerful prognostic and monitoring tool. Lower ΔP is associated with reduced VILI and PPCs. It also correlates with better oxygenation and improved compliance. In practice, a $\Delta P \leq 15$ cmH_2O is generally considered a safe threshold [53].
- Transpulmonary pressure (Ttp): Transpulmonary pressure represents the pressure difference between alveolar pressure (approximated by airway pressure when flow is zero) and pleural pressure: Ttp = Paw – Ppl [52]. Because pleural pressure cannot be directly measured easily, an esophageal balloon catheter is usually used as a surrogate. Measurement of Ttp enables differentiation between chest-wall and lung contributions to mechanical load, improving ventilator titration in patients with altered chest-wall mechanics. Safety targets typically include keeping end-inspiratory Ttp below 20–25 cmH_2O and avoiding negative end-expiratory values [54].
- Mechanical power: Mechanical power reflects the total energy delivered to the respiratory system per unit time, combining volume, pressure, flow, and respiratory rate. Experimental data suggest that exceeding an energy threshold of roughly 12 J/min promotes lung injury [55], emphasizing that VILI risk depends on the cumulative energy load rather than any single parameter. As lung heterogeneity increases, higher pressures and flows further elevate mechanical power, perpetuating injury [36, 37]. Although exact clinical limits remain uncertain, reducing mechanical power—by avoiding high tidal volumes, excessive pressures, and unnecessarily high respiratory rates—is a key principle of protective ventilation.
- Flow–volume loops and waveform monitoring: Continuous inspection of ventilator waveforms such as flow–volume and pressure–time curves provides real-time insight into respiratory mechanics and evolving intraoperative challenges [41, 51], including secretion accumulation, bronchospasm, or changes in compliance due to surgical conditions. These tools often allow earlier detection of abnormalities than intermittent static measurements alone [56].

14.6 Protective Ventilation Strategies

Intraoperative ventilation strategy should aim to maintain adequate gas exchange while minimizing VILI and the formation or propagation of atelectasis. Over the last decade, a body of randomized trials and mechanistic studies has refined perioperative practice: tidal volume is now chosen on the basis of PBW rather than actual weight [57–59]; positive end-expiratory pressure (PEEP) is used to prevent end-expiratory collapse but requires titration to balance recruitment and overdistension [60]; recruitment maneuvers can reopen collapsed units but must be combined with adequate PEEP and performed cautiously; and avoidance of unnecessary hyperoxia minimizes the risk of absorption (resorption) atelectasis. The following sections review the evidence and practical approaches for each component.

14.6.1 Tidal-Volume Selection (Based on Predicted Body Weight)

Tidal volume should be set relative to predicted (ideal) body weight because lung size correlates with height rather than with total body mass. Contemporary practice and the major trials have converged on a protective intraoperative tidal-volume target in the range of roughly 6–8 mL/kg [57]. The physiologic rationale is to limit cyclic lung strain and tidal overdistension, which are central mechanisms of VILI. Early trials that combined low tidal volumes with PEEP and recruitment maneuvers suggested improved physiologic endpoints, but larger pragmatic trials comparing low versus more conventional tidal volumes with similar background PEEP have not uniformly demonstrated robust reductions in short-term postoperative pulmonary complications. This suggests that tidal volume is one element of a ventilatory bundle (including PEEP and avoidance of injurious pressures) and that the net effect on clinical outcomes depends on the whole strategy rather than on tidal volume alone [59–61]. For daily practice, targeting 6–8 mL/kg PBW is reasonable, avoiding tidal volumes above 10 mL/kg PBW when there is no specific indication to do otherwise, and watching for excessive driving pressure as a marker of injurious strain.

14.6.2 Use of PEEP: Benefits, Risks, and Individualized Titration

PEEP prevents end-expiratory alveolar collapse and thereby reduces intrapulmonary shunt, improves oxygenation, and attenuates cyclic opening and closing of unstable lung units. Physiologically, appropriate PEEP increases end-expiratory transpulmonary pressure and maintains alveolar patency; clinically, modest levels of PEEP (e.g., 5–8 cmH_2O) are frequently sufficient in nonobese patients under general anesthesia to improve oxygenation and respiratory mechanics [60, 62, 63]. Randomized trials that attempted to define a universally superior PEEP level have produced mixed results; higher PEEP has been associated with more hemodynamic instability [64]. PEEP should be individualized, and the "one-size-fits-all" high-PEEP prescription is not supported by results. Individualized PEEP titration aims to select a level that maintains recruitment without producing significant overdistension or adverse hemodynamics. Several physiologic targets and bedside methods have been proposed and tested:

- Driving-pressure minimization: selecting PEEP producing the lowest driving pressure for a given tidal volume has been associated with improved physiological surrogates [65] and is attractive because driving pressure correlates with lung strain. It must be taken into account that, using this method, the best PEEP depends on the tidal volume (TV) used, and lower TV usually requires higher PEEP levels [61].
- Transpulmonary-pressure (esophageal-balloon) guidance: using esophageal pressure to estimate pleural pressure allows selection of PEEP that secures a positive end-expiratory transpulmonary pressure; this approach has rationale from physiological studies [66], but clinical trials in critically ill patients have had mixed results, and the technique requires experience and careful interpretation [67].
- Electrical impedance tomography (EIT): EIT provides continuous, regional, bedside information about ventilation distribution and end-expiratory impedance; EIT-guided PEEP titration can identify the level at which dependent derecruitment is minimized without excessive nondependent overdistension [68].
- Incremental/decremental PEEP after recruitment with best compliance: the classical open-lung approach applies a recruitment maneuver followed by decremental PEEP steps to identify the PEEP with best respiratory compliance [69]; it is widely used but may lead to transient hemodynamic effects if pressures are high [64].

Each method has strengths and limitations. Esophageal-pressure guidance estimates pleural pressure but can be affected by positioning and chest-wall mechanics; EIT is noninvasive and continuous but provides cross-sectional rather than volumetric images and requires equipment and interpretation; driving-pressure optimization is simple but not specific to regional overdistension. Current evidence therefore favors individualized PEEP selection guided by physiologic measurements (driving pressure, compliance, or imaging when available) rather than routine application of very high PEEP for all patients.

14.6.3 Recruitment Maneuvers: Types and Techniques

Recruitment maneuvers (RMs) are transient applications of increased end-inspiratory transpulmonary pressure intended to reopen collapsed alveoli. Several techniques are used in the operating room and around anesthesia induction or pneumoperitoneum: sustained inflation (a single prolonged inflation at a moderate–high airway pressure for 20–40 s), stepwise increases of tidal volume or of PEEP/airway pressure (progressive increments for a few breaths), as seen in Fig. 14.1, and "sigh" maneuvers consisting of one or a few larger breaths [69, 70]. RMs reliably improve

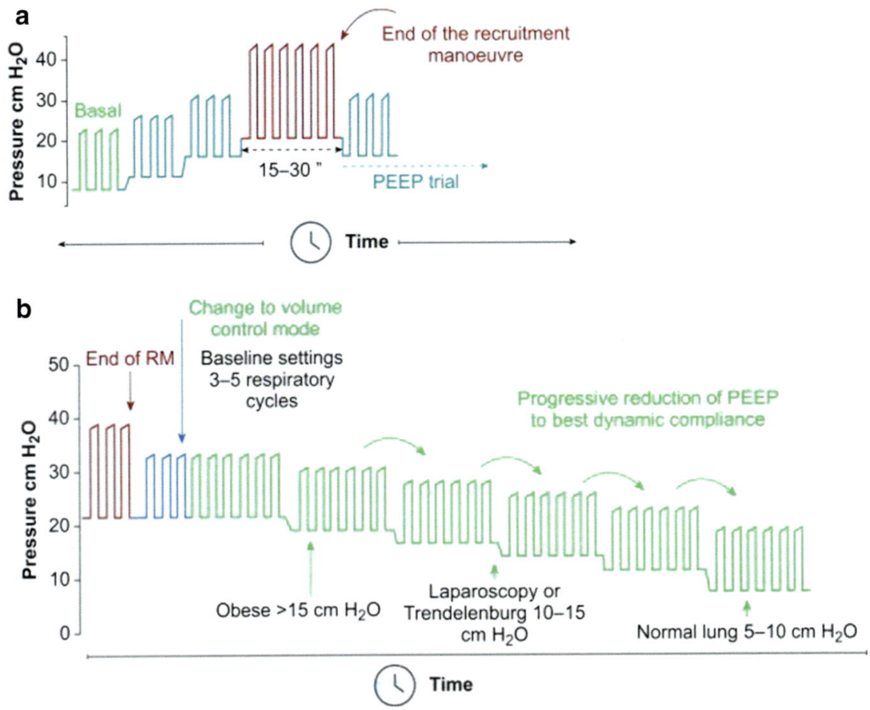

Fig. 14.1 Stepwise recruitment maneuver using pressure-controlled ventilation, followed by a PEEP titration trial. PEEP is gradually increased to an opening pressure of ~40 cmH$_2$O, held briefly, then reduced in 2 cmH$_2$O steps while monitoring compliance to identify the individualized optimal PEEP (iPEEP)

oxygenation and lung compliance in the short term and reduce radiographic atelectasis when combined with appropriate PEEP; their positive effects are most likely when applied in patients with significant collapse (e.g., obesity, pneumoperitoneum, or prolonged anesthesia) and when a maintenance PEEP sufficient to prevent re-collapse is used.

However, recruitment maneuvers are not benign. They can reduce venous return and cardiac output, provoke transient barotrauma if pressures are excessive, and their beneficial effect may be transient if PEEP is not optimized afterwards. Large pragmatic trials that bundled higher PEEP plus repeated RMs did not show consistent reductions in postoperative pulmonary complications and showed increases in intraoperative hemodynamic interventions in several cohorts [63, 71]. Consequently, recruitment maneuvers should be reserved for selected patients with clinical or imaging evidence of collapse, performed with the lowest effective pressures and the shortest necessary duration, and always followed by individualized PEEP to maintain the gains. Whenever possible, RMs should be performed under continuous hemodynamic monitoring [64] and in a controlled manner using ventilator-delivered maneuvers rather than manual bagging.

14.6.4 Avoiding Hyperoxia and Resorption (Absorption) Atelectasis

Administration of very high inspired oxygen fractions (FiO_2), particularly 100% O_2 during preoxygenation, induction, or just before extubation, accelerates absorption (resorption) atelectasis [72] in regions with low ventilation or transient airway closure. Oxygen replaces nitrogen in alveoli; because O_2 is rapidly absorbed into the blood, alveoli that are not replenished by ventilation may collapse. Classic physiologic and CT studies demonstrated that induction with 1.0 FiO_2 produces larger early atelectatic areas than lower FiO_2, and more recent randomized data confirm that higher perioperative FiO_2 increases the amount of atelectasis compared with lower FiO_2 in abdominal surgery [73, 74]. There is a balance to be struck, because preoxygenation with high FiO_2 is still employed to extend the time to desaturation during apnea or difficult airway management; practical strategies therefore include limiting 1.0 FiO_2 to periods when it is clinically needed (rapid-sequence induction or expected prolonged apnea), minimizing the duration of 1.0 FiO_2, and using the lowest FiO_2 that ensures safe oxygen reserves after induction or before extubation. When feasible, moderate FiO_2 (e.g., 0.3–0.6) during maintenance [72, 75] and avoidance of unnecessary use of 1.0 FiO_2 will reduce the risk of absorption atelectasis without compromising patient safety.

References

1. Weiser TG, Haynes AB, Molina G, Lipsitz SR, Esquivel MM, Uribe-Leitz T, et al. Size and distribution of the global volume of surgery in 2012. Bull World Health Organ. 2016;94(3):201–9F.
2. Fernández-Bustamante A, Frendl G, Sprung J, et al. Postoperative pulmonary complications, early mortality, and hospital stay following noncardiothoracic surgery: a multicenter study. JAMA Surg. 2017;152(2):157–66.
3. Neto AS, da Costa LGV, Hemmes SNT, Canet J, Hedenstierna G, Jaber S, et al. The LAS VEGAS risk score for prediction of postoperative pulmonary complications: An observational study. Eur J Anaesthesiol. 2018;35(9):691–701.
4. Canet J, Gallart L, Gomar C, Paluzie G, Vallès J, Castillo J, et al. Prediction of postoperative pulmonary complications in a population-based surgical cohort. Anesthesiology. 2010;113(6):1338–50.
5. Miskovic A, Lumb AB. Postoperative pulmonary complications. Br J Anaesth. 2017;118(3):317–34.
6. Jogiat U, Mocanu V, Birch DW, Switzer NJ, Turner SR, Karmali S. Pulmonary complications are a strong independent predictor of 30-day mortality following elective bariatric surgery. Obes Surg. 2022;32(3):696–703.
7. Ghaferi AA, Birkmeyer JD, Dimick JB. Variation in hospital mortality associated with inpatient surgery. N Engl J Med. 2009;361(14):1368–75.
8. Linde-Zwirble WL, Bloom JD, Mecca RS, Hansell DM. Postoperative pulmonary complications in adult elective surgery patients in the US: severity, outcomes and resources use. Crit Care. 2010;14(1):P210.
9. Jammer I, Wickboldt N, Sander M, et al. Standards for definitions and use of outcome measures for clinical-effectiveness research in perioperative medicine: European Perioperative Clinical Outcome (EPCO) definitions: a statement from the ESA-ESICM joint taskforce on perioperative outcome measures. Eur J Anaesthesiol. 2015;32(1):88–105.

10. Smetana GW, Lawrence VA, Cornell JE. Preoperative pulmonary risk stratification for noncardiothoracic surgery. Ann Intern Med. 2006;144(8):581–95.
11. Hedenstierna G, Edmark L. Effects of anesthesia on the respiratory system. Best Pract Res Clin Anaesthesiol. 2015;29(3):273–84.
12. Ma Z, Qvist T, Jakobsen JC, et al. Effects of general anesthesia on functional residual capacity: An updated review. Anesth Analg. 2021;132(5):1234–46.
13. Pelosi P, Gregoretti C. Perioperative lung mechanics and ventilation strategies. Curr Opin Crit Care. 2010;16(4):352–8.
14. Norlander O, Herzog P, Nordén I, Hossli G, Schaer H, Gattiker R. Compliance and airway resistance during anaesthesia with controlled ventilation. Acta Anaesthesiol Scand. 1968;12(2):135–41.
15. Brismar B, Hedenstierna G. Alveolar collapse and compliance changes during anesthesia. Acta Anaesthesiol Scand. 1989;33:121–5.
16. Hedenstierna G. Oxygen and anesthesia: what lung do we deliver to the post-operative ward? Acta Anaesthesiol Scand. 2012;56(6):675–85.
17. Lumb AB, Slinger P. Hypoxic pulmonary vasoconstriction: physiology and anesthetic implications. Anesthesiology. 2015;122(4):932–46.
18. Lumb AB, Nunn JF. Respiratory function and ribcage contribution to ventilation in body positions commonly used during anesthesia. Anesth Analg. 1991;73:422–6. https://doi.org/10.1213/00000539-199110000-00010.
19. Fahy BG, Barnas GM, Nagle SE, Flowers JL, Njoku MJ, Agarwal M. Effects of Trendelenburg and reverse Trendelenburg postures on lung and chest wall mechanics. J Clin Anesth. 1996;8(3):236–44.
20. Vidal Melo MF, Musch G, Kaczka DW. Pulmonary pathophysiology and lung mechanics in anesthesiology: a case-based overview. Anesthesiol Clin. 2012;30(4):759–84.
21. Hedenstierna G, Edmark L. Effects of anesthesia and muscle paralysis on the respiratory system. Best Pract Res Clin Anaesthesiol. 2010;24(2):157–69.
22. Atkinson TM, Giraud GD, Togioka BM, Jones DB, Cigarroa JE. Cardiovascular and ventilatory consequences of laparoscopic surgery. Circulation. 2017;135(7):700–10.
23. Buñuel Á, Navarro-Ripoll R, Italiano S, López-Baamonde M, Barbeta E, Gatherer R, Ferrando C. Effect of tension capnothorax on respiratory mechanics and individualized PEEP during robotic-assisted thoracic surgery: a prospective pilot observational study. Minerva Anestesiol. 2025;91(5):404–12.
24. Zeng C, Lagier D, Lee JW, Vidal Melo MF. Perioperative pulmonary atelectasis: part I. Biology and mechanisms. Anesthesiology. 2022;136(1):181–205.
25. Teppema LJ, Baby S. Anesthetics and control of breathing. Respir Physiol Neurobiol. 2011;177(2):80–92.
26. Lundquist H, Hedenstierna G, Strandberg A, Tokics L, Brismar B. CT-assessment of dependent lung densities in man during general anaesthesia. Acta Radiol. 1995;36(6):626–32.
27. Hubmayr RD, Kallet RH. Understanding pulmonary stress-strain relationships in severe ARDS and its implications for designing a safer approach to setting the ventilator. Respir Care. 2018;63(2):219–26.
28. Zhu C, Yao JW, An LX, Bai YF, Li WJ. Effects of intraoperative individualized PEEP on postoperative atelectasis in obese patients: study protocol for a prospective randomized controlled trial. Trials. 2020;21(1):618.
29. Lagier D, Zeng C, Fernandez-Bustamante A, Vidal Melo MF. Perioperative pulmonary atelectasis: part II. Clinical implications. Anesthesiology. 2022;136(1):206–36.
30. Ferrando C, Romero C, Tusman G, et al. The accuracy of postoperative, non-invasive Air-Test to diagnose atelectasis in healthy patients after surgery: a prospective, diagnostic pilot study. BMJ Open. 2017;7(5):e015560.
31. Ferrando C, Suárez-Sipmann F, Librero J, Pozo N, Soro M, Unzueta C, et al. A noninvasive postoperative clinical score to identify patients at risk for postoperative pulmonary complications: the Air-Test Score. Minerva Anestesiol. 2020;86(4):404–15.

32. Ferrando C, Tusman G, Suarez-Sipmann F, León I, Pozo N, Carbonell J, et al. Individualized lung recruitment maneuver guided by pulse-oximetry in anesthetized patients undergoing laparoscopy: a feasibility study. Acta Anaesthesiol Scand. 2018;62(5):608–19.
33. Rouby JJ, Arbelot C, Gao Y, Zhang M, Lv J, An Y, et al. Training for lung ultrasound score measurement in critically ill patients. Am J Respir Crit Care Med. 2018;198(3):398–401.
34. Huang D, Li Z, Zhao J, Li H, Wang W, Fu S. Lung ultrasound as a diagnostic tool for pulmonary consolidation and atelectasis after cardiac surgery. J Thorac Dis. 2025;17(7):4794–802.
35. Wu L, Yang Y, Yin Y, Yang L, Sun X, Zhang J. Lung ultrasound for evaluating perioperative atelectasis and aeration in the post-anesthesia care unit. J Clin Monit Comput. 2023;37(5):1295–302.
36. Slutsky AS, Ranieri VM. Ventilator-induced lung injury. N Engl J Med. 2013;369(22):2126–36.
37. Gattinoni L, Protti A, Caironi P, Carlesso E. Ventilator-induced lung injury: the anatomical and physiological framework. Crit Care Med. 2010;38(10 Suppl):S539–48.
38. Güldner A, Braune A, Ball L, Silva PL, Samary C, Insorsi A, et al. Comparative effects of volutrauma and atelectrauma on lung inflammation in experimental acute respiratory distress syndrome. Crit Care Med. 2016;44(9):e854–65.
39. Curley GF, Laffey JG, Zhang H, Slutsky AS. Biotrauma and ventilator-induced lung injury: clinical implications. Chest. 2016;150(5):1109–17.
40. Thornton LT, Marini JJ. Optimized ventilation power to avoid VILI. J Intensive Care. 2023;11(1):57.
41. Ball L, Dameri M, Pelosi P. Modes of mechanical ventilation for the operating room. Best Pract Res Clin Anaesthesiol. 2015;29:285–99.
42. Park JH, Park IK, Choi SH, Eum D, Kim MS. Volume-controlled versus dual-controlled ventilation during robot-assisted laparoscopic prostatectomy with steep trendelenburg position: a randomized-controlled trial. J Clin Med. 2019;8(12):2032.
43. Schick V, Dusse F, Eckardt R, Kerkhoff S, Commotio S, Hinkelbein J, Mathes A. Comparison of volume-guaranteed or -targeted, pressure-controlled ventilation with volume-controlled ventilation during elective surgery: a systematic review and meta-analysis. J Clin Med. 2021;10(6):1276.
44. Liu Z, Liu W, Zhao P, Ma Z, Li Y. Effect of pressure-controlled ventilation-volume guaranteed mode on intraoperative respiratory mechanics, oxygenation and postoperative pulmonary complications: a systematic review and network meta-analysis. Ann Med. 2025;57(1):2579790.
45. Li XF, Mao WJ, Jiang RJ, Yu H, Zhang MQ, Yu H. Effect of mechanical ventilation mode type on postoperative pulmonary complications after cardiac surgery: a randomized controlled trial. J Cardiothorac Vasc Anesth. 2024;38(2):437–44.
46. Bialka S, Palaczynski P, Szuldrzynski K, et al. Flow-controlled ventilation - a new and promising method of ventilation presented with a review of the literature. Anaesthesiol Intensive Ther. 2022;54(1):62–70.
47. Schmidt J, Günther F, Weber J, et al. Flow-controlled ventilation during ear, nose and throat surgery: a prospective observational study. Eur J Anaesthesiol. 2019;36(5):327–34.
48. Schmidt J, Wenzel C, Spassov S, et al. Flow-controlled ventilation attenuates lung injury in a porcine model of acute respiratory distress syndrome: a preclinical randomized controlled study. Crit Care Med. 2020;48(3):e241–8.
49. MacIntyre NR. Patient-ventilator interactions: optimizing conventional ventilation modes. Respir Care. 2011;56(1):73–84.
50. Placenti A, Fratebianchi F. Interpretation and use of intraoperative protective ventilation parameters: a scoping review. Anaesthesiol Intensive Ther. 2022;54(4):320–33.
51. Ball L, Costantino F, Orefice G, Chandrapatham K, Pelosi P. Intraoperative mechanical ventilation: state of the art. Minerva Anestesiol. 2017;83(10):1075–88.
52. Jimenez-Santana JD, Spadaro S, Argente Navarro MP, Mazzinari G. Advanced respiratory monitoring in the perioperative setting. Curr Anesthesiol Rep. 2024;14(4):551–66.

53. Urner M, Jüni P, Rojas-Saunero LP, et al. Limiting dynamic driving pressure in patients requiring mechanical ventilation. Crit Care Med. 2023;51(7):861–71.
54. Grieco DL, Chen L, Brochard L. Transpulmonary pressure: importance and limits. Ann Transl Med. 2017;5(14):285.
55. Cressoni M, Gotti M, Chiurazzi C, et al. Mechanical power and development of ventilator-induced lung injury. Anesthesiology. 2016;124(5):1100–8.
56. Dhand R. Ventilator graphics and respiratory mechanics in the patient with obstructive lung disease. Respir Care. 2005;50(2):246–61.
57. Brower RG, Matthay MA, Morris A, Schoenfeld D, Thompson BT, Wheeler A, et al. Ventilation with lower tidal volumes as compared with traditional tidal volumes for acute lung injury and the acute respiratory distress syndrome. N Engl J Med. 2000;342(18):1301–8.
58. Young CC, Harris EM, Vacchiano C, Bodnar S, Bukowy B, Elliott RRD, et al. Lung-protective ventilation for the surgical patient: international expert panel-based consensus recommendations. Br J Anaesth. 2019;123(6):898–913.
59. Serpa Neto A, Hemmes SN, Barbas CS, Beiderlinden M, Biehl M, Binnekade JM, et al. Protective versus conventional ventilation for surgery: a systematic review and individual patient data meta-analysis. Anesthesiology. 2015;123(1):66–78.
60. Turan A, Esa WAS, Rivas E, Wang J, Bakal O, Stamper S, et al. Tidal volume and positive end-expiratory pressure and postoperative hypoxemia during general anesthesia: a single-center multiple crossover factorial cluster trial. Anesthesiology. 2022;137(4):406–17.
61. Yang D, Grant MC, Stone A, Wu CL, Wick EC. A meta-analysis of intraoperative ventilation strategies to prevent pulmonary complications: is low tidal volume alone sufficient to protect healthy lungs? Ann Surg. 2016;263(5):881–7.
62. Severgnini P, Selmo G, Lanza C, Chiesa A, Frigerio A, Bacuzzi A, et al. Protective mechanical ventilation during general anesthesia for open abdominal surgery improves postoperative pulmonary function. Anesthesiology. 2013;118(6):1307–21.
63. Hemmes SN, Gama de Abreu M, Pelosi P, Schultz MJ. High versus low positive end-expiratory pressure during general anaesthesia for open abdominal surgery (PROVHILO trial): a multicentre randomised controlled trial. Lancet. 2014;384(9942):495–503.
64. Cavalcanti AB, Suzumura ÉA, et al. Effect of lung recruitment and titrated positive end-expiratory pressure (PEEP) vs low PEEP on mortality in patients with acute respiratory distress syndrome: a randomized clinical trial. JAMA. 2017;318(14):1335–45.
65. Zhang C, Xu F, Li W, et al. Driving pressure-guided individualized positive end-expiratory pressure in abdominal surgery: a randomized controlled trial. Anesth Analg. 2021;133(5):1197–205.
66. Talmor D, Sarge T, Malhotra A, et al. Mechanical ventilation guided by esophageal pressure in acute lung injury. N Engl J Med. 2008;359(20):2095–104.
67. Beitler JR, Sarge T, Banner-Goodspeed VM, et al. Effect of titrating positive end-expiratory pressure (PEEP) with an esophageal pressure-guided strategy vs an empirical high PEEP-Fio2 strategy on death and days free from mechanical ventilation among patients with acute respiratory distress syndrome: a randomized clinical trial. JAMA. 2019;321(9):846–57.
68. Pereira SM, Tucci MR, Morais CCA, et al. Individual positive end-expiratory pressure settings optimize intraoperative mechanical ventilation and reduce postoperative atelectasis. Anesthesiology. 2018;129(6):1070–81.
69. Ferrando C, Vallverdú J, Zattera L, Tusman G, Suárez-Sipmann F. Improving lung protective mechanical ventilation: the individualised intraoperative open-lung approach. Br J Anaesth. 2025;134(2):281–7.
70. Hartland BL, Newell TJ, Damico N. Alveolar recruitment maneuvers under general anesthesia: a systematic review of the literature. Respir Care. 2015;60(4):609–20.
71. Ferrando C, Soro M, Unzueta C, et al. Individualised perioperative open-lung approach versus standard protective ventilation in abdominal surgery (iPROVE): a randomised controlled trial. Lancet Respir Med. 2018;6(3):193–203.

72. Nimmagadda U, Salem MR, Crystal GJ. Preoxygenation: physiologic basis, benefits, and potential risks. Anesth Analg. 2017;124(2):507–17.
73. Park M, Jung K, Sim WS, et al. Perioperative high inspired oxygen fraction induces atelectasis in patients undergoing abdominal surgery: a randomized controlled trial. J Clin Anesth. 2021;72:110285.
74. Meyhoff CS, Wetterslev J, Jorgensen LN, et al. Effect of high perioperative oxygen fraction on surgical site infection and pulmonary complications after abdominal surgery: the PROXI randomized clinical trial. JAMA. 2009;302(14):1543–50.
75. Hol L, Nijbroek SGLH, Schultz MJ. Perioperative lung protection: clinical implications. Anesth Analg. 2020;131(6):1721–9.

Actions to Make Sustainable the Impact of Clinical Practice in Anesthesia and Intensive Care

15

Edoardo De Robertis, Rachele Simonte, and Giulia Masuzzo

15.1 Introduction

In 2019, the healthcare sector accounted for a total of 5.2% of global greenhouse gas emissions (compared to 4.9% in 2018), with Europe ranking third as an emitter after the USA and China.

Inhalational anesthetic agents play a key role, accounting for 2% of total healthcare system emissions (data from England), while waste management is also highly significant, with operating rooms generating up to 20% of all hospital waste.

This situation calls for targeted interventions to reduce the environmental impact of the sector, with anesthesiologists and intensivists acting as active contributors to the development of a more sustainable healthcare system (especially with a view to the future), with particular attention to the appropriate use of drugs and the management of waste generated during surgical procedures.

Despite growing awareness of climate change, the last decade has seen an increase in greenhouse gas emissions. Given the urgency of the issue, the European Society of Anaesthesiology and Intensive Care (ESAIC) published the "Glasgow Declaration" in July 2023, followed by Guidelines in 2024, aimed at providing recommendations specifically for the fields of anesthesiology, perioperative medicine, and intensive care that can help European countries move increasingly toward sustainable healthcare. This document is inspired by the European Green Deal, which aims to achieve climate neutrality by 2050 and reduce emissions by 55% by 2030 compared to 1990 levels.

E. De Robertis (✉) · R. Simonte · G. Masuzzo
Section of Anesthesia, Intensive Care, Critical Care and Pain Management – Department of Medicine and Surgery, University of Perugia, Perugia, Italy
e-mail: edoardo.derobertis@unipg.it; rachele.simonte@unipg.it; giulia.masuzzo95@gmail.com; giulia.masuzzo@specializzandi.unipg.it

D. Chiumello, A. De Gasperi (eds.), *Practical Trends in Anesthesia and Intensive Care 2026*, https://doi.org/10.1007/978-3-032-25721-5_15

The key points of the declaration, outlined through the recommendations of the ESAIC, are as follows:

- In the field of inhalational anesthesia, given the global warming potential of inhaled anesthetics, judicious use according to precise clinical indications and optimization of their administration, with a preference for low-flow techniques and, where possible, the use of intravenous anesthesia.
- Proper use of energy and its application in the ventilation and heating systems of operating rooms, use of LED devices, and generation of electricity from environmentally sustainable technologies such as photovoltaic systems.
- Proper management of hospital waste, particularly that generated by anesthesiology clinical practice, and its disposal.

Similarly, the European Society of Intensive Care Medicine (ESICM) has recently published a document that, by examining the significant environmental impact of intensive care units and their correlation with climate change, sets objectives aimed at fostering positive change shared by healthcare professionals.

15.2 Environmental Sustainability: Why it Is Important to Understand and Support It

When discussing environmental sustainability, it is essential to understand its fundamental aspects in order to implement actions that raise awareness and prevent even more severe effects on the planet, some of which we are already witnessing. This issue becomes even more significant when the audience is broad and the context for applying appropriate preventive measures, in this case perioperative and emergency medicine, plays a direct active role in the issue of pollution.

15.2.1 The Greenhouse Effect

The greenhouse effect and ozone layer depletion are distinct phenomena, although they are closely linked and, in part, share the same anthropogenic causes.

Specifically, the greenhouse effect is a natural process necessary to maintain temperatures on Earth compatible with life. In fact, the most abundant naturally occurring gases in the atmosphere—such as carbon dioxide, methane, and nitrous oxide—can absorb heat from solar radiation and retain it, preventing its dissipation into space.

However, this effect has progressively intensified due to the accumulation in the atmosphere of additional gases with similar effects, originating from industrial activities and the combustion of fossil fuels.

As a result, the amplification of the greenhouse effect represents one of the main causes of climate change, which in turn leads to rising global temperatures and increasingly frequent adverse weather events. Some examples of these anthropogenic gases include fluorinated gases, such as hydrofluorocarbons (HFCs), which are of particular concern because, compared to CO_2 (the reference parameter), they have a much higher global warming potential (GWP). In relation to our clinical practice, fluorinated inhalational anesthetics also fall into this category, with desflurane—whose use has been declared banned from 2026 by the Council of the European Union due to its high Global Warming Potential (GWP).

15.2.2 Ozone Layer Depletion

The ozone layer, normally present in the stratosphere, is essential for shielding the Earth's surface from harmful ultraviolet (UV-B) radiation, acting as a filter. In fact, if the ozone layer thins, a greater proportion of ultraviolet rays reaches the surface, which is undesirable as it causes harmful effects not only on human health but also on ecosystems. The discovery that the ozone layer over the Arctic and Antarctic is subject to depletion, resulting in thinning—the so-called ozone hole first identified over Antarctica—is relatively recent, dating back to the 1970s, when it was hypothesized that chlorine contained in chlorofluorocarbons could reach the stratosphere and cause its deterioration. The mechanism was identified as the catalytic destruction by chlorine and bromine, especially under certain cold conditions, leading to the signing of the Montreal Protocol (1987): an international agreement aimed at reducing the production of ozone-depleting substances containing chlorine and bromine.

Not only chlorofluorocarbons but also hydrochlorofluorocarbons and hydrofluorocarbons contain chlorine and have ozone-depleting properties (albeit to a lesser extent than the former). Among anesthetic agents, nitrous oxide plays a central role in the current issue of environmental pollution: in addition to being a highly significant greenhouse gas, due to its ability to persist in the atmosphere for an estimated 114 years, it is considered a primary agent in the destruction of atmospheric ozone.

15.3 Drugs Used in Anesthesia and Their Impact on Direct Greenhouse Gas Emissions

Inhalational anesthetics are potent greenhouse gases that contribute significantly to global warming. At a time when environmental sustainability is becoming an integral part of our clinical practice, it is important that anesthesiology is also aware of and trained in their proper use, thereby contributing to the achievement of emission reduction targets.

15.3.1 Inhalational Anesthetics

All inhalational anesthetic agents are potent greenhouse gases (Table 15.1) that exert their effect at the level of the troposphere; the goal is to align with the European

Table 15.1 Impact of the main inhalational anesthetics used in clinical practice, referenced to CO_2, using Global Warming Potential

	GWP 100	GWP20
CO_2	1	
Sevoflurane	144	508
Desflurane	2540	6810
Isoflurane	510	1800

From: European Society of Anaesthesiology and Intensive Care consensus document on sustainability, Patricio Gonzalez-Pizarro et al. [7]

Commission's target of becoming a net-zero emissions continent by 2050, in accordance with the European Climate Law.

Volatile anesthetic agents are inert molecules that are only minimally metabolized and, as a result, once used for intraoperative administration or as sedative agents in intensive care units, are released into the atmosphere as gases that are almost entirely unchanged. This pharmacological class includes nitrous oxide (N_2O) and the halogenated agents: sevoflurane, desflurane, isoflurane, enflurane, and halothane. Modern halogenated agents contain fluorine atoms, which makes them thermostable and reduces their risk of flammability.

Special mention should be made of sevoflurane and desflurane, which, since their introduction to the market in the mid-1990s, have shown a steadily increasing use in clinical practice, and consequently, their concentrations measured in the atmosphere (including in remote global areas such as Antarctica) have also progressively risen.

European anesthetists predominantly use sevoflurane (85%) for inhalational anesthesia, followed by desflurane (10%) and isoflurane (3%). Globally, these three inhalational anesthetics contribute 0.02–0.1% to greenhouse gas emissions, with desflurane alone estimated to account for 80% of this impact compared to the others.

In general, the effect a substance has on climate warming is defined by its "Global Warming Potential" (GWP), referring to a 100-year time horizon (GWP100), which is determined by its atmospheric lifetime and the range of atmospheric reflection of infrared radiation. Compared to CO_2, which has a GWP100 of 1, inhalational anesthetics have much higher values for their greenhouse gas effect: sevoflurane 144, nitrous oxide 298, isoflurane 510, and desflurane 2540.

It should also be noted that molecules such as nitrous oxide and isoflurane possess ozone-depleting properties and are therefore potentially capable of destroying ozone molecules, leading to thinning of the atmospheric layer.

However, these same inhalational anesthetics have a much shorter average atmospheric lifetime compared to the most prevalent greenhouse gases, N_2O and methane, which is why experts consider it more appropriate to measure GWP over a 20-year time frame (GWP20), which is: 508 for sevoflurane, 1800 for isoflurane, and 6810 for desflurane.

In addition, there is a close correlation with the effect exerted through the fresh gas flow (FGF): depending on the concentration at which these agents are administered to achieve the desired depth of anesthesia, the final contribution to environmental emissions of inhalational anesthetics—and thus directly to greenhouse gas emissions—will vary. Hence the need to implement and adopt low-flow ventilation strategies (Low Flow Anesthesia, LFA) that can help reduce the consumption of inhalational anesthetics and fresh gas flows by utilizing the recirculation of patient-expired gases through the ventilator's rotary circuit with a CO_2 absorber.

Nitrous oxide (N_2O) is widely used in clinical settings, not only in operating rooms but also in other areas such as maternity wards and dental offices, as well as in the industrial and agricultural sectors. Its extensive use is a key factor in the problem of ozone depletion: the global contribution from perioperative use of nitrous oxide is estimated to be between 1% and 3%, with some regions of the world (including the Middle East and Africa) where the impact from anesthetic practice reaches up to 5%. It is important to closely monitor its use, limiting it to situations where it is truly necessary.

In recent years, awareness of the contribution of fluorinated gases to global warming has increased significantly, to the extent that amendments (the "Kigali Amendment" to the Montreal Protocol, adopted in 2016) have banned the use of these substances in industrial products such as solvents, foams, and spray cans starting in 2030. Only medicinal substances, including inhaled anesthetics, are exempt from these restrictions. However, in 2022 the European Commission proposed an update to the regulation of fluorinated gases, banning the use of desflurane in Europe from 2026 due to its significant impact on global warming. It should be noted that this is the only inhaled anesthetic that exceeds the GPW100 threshold of 2500, and therefore, if the proposal is approved, desflurane will no longer be permitted for inhalational anesthesia except in cases with specific clinical indications.

What Can We Do?

- Use inhaled anesthetics according to appropriate clinical indications, opting for agents with lower environmental impact whenever possible, taking their GWP into account.
- Use low-flow ventilator circuits and, where possible, reduce FGF to minimal flow (<0.5 L/min).
- Consider the use of capture systems; canisters that retain halogenated molecules exhaled by the patient, allowing for safe storage and preventing their release into the atmosphere through a scavenging system.
- Provide clinicians with reports on annual inhaled anesthetic consumption and sedation hours, to raise awareness about appropriate usage.
- Where possible and indicated, prefer regional anesthesia techniques and intravenous anesthesia.

15.3.2 Propofol

Propofol is the most widely used hypnotic-induction agent in anesthesia, as well as a general anesthetic for TIVA/TCI intravenous anesthesia approaches. Compared to inhaled agents, its pharmacokinetic properties result in a lower impact on direct greenhouse gas emissions, since its metabolic byproducts are not released into the air but rather into aquatic ecosystems (being excreted in urine as 88% inactive metabolites and 1% unchanged drug). The direct effect of propofol on greenhouse gas emissions is therefore related to the use of electronic devices such as infusion pumps for intravenous administration, as well as the predominantly plastic waste generated by single-use infusion sets and the incineration processes required for disposal of unused product.

Propofol is toxic to aquatic organisms, and traces have been detected in both drinking water and fish, although it is considered a low environmental pollutant on a risk scale. However, further studies on wastewater analysis and proper disposal processes are needed, as current data indicate that less than half of the product is correctly disposed of as waste and thus incinerated.

There are also no clear guidelines regarding the use of the different concentrations available on the market, 2% (20 mg/ml dilution) versus 1% (10 mg/ml), as there are no trials to determine whether these have different environmental impacts, even though there are no differences in terms of use or efficacy.

What does change is the blood lipid concentration measured in patients receiving propofol at 2% concentration, which is lower than with the other concentration. This seems to suggest that using a higher dosage at the same infusion rate may result in a lower total amount of drug required and therefore, in terms of environmental sustainability, less energy consumption and "waste" in infusion devices.

What Can We Do?

- Prevent waste by drawing up and drawing up medications from vials only when necessary, and reusing, where possible, devices that do not come into direct contact with patient fluids (e.g., changing the infusion set while retaining the syringe pumps).
- Monitor the patient's depth of cerebral anesthesia (e.g., continuous EEG) to adjust the infused dose and avoid overdosing.

In reality, all the drugs we use, all the devices, and all the techniques we employ have an environmental impact. It is too simplistic to single out a particular drug or technique as more or less polluting. The reality is that sustainability is a complex issue that requires a comprehensive analysis, considering the Life Cycle Assessment of each intervention or drug. For example, a recent study on a small cohort showed that even the use of a locoregional technique (subarachnoid) is not necessarily less impactful from an environmental perspective than inhalational or combined anesthesia, once factors such as the use of sterile materials, electricity consumption, oxygen use, and other resources are taken into account.

15.4 Indirect Emissions Related to Energy Use

Energy consumption is one of the main contributors to the environmental impact of the hospital setting, especially in high-intensity areas such as operating rooms and intensive care units. The high use of resources for sterilization processes, the operation of advanced equipment, and the control of vital functions through machinery all require careful and sustainable energy management. To this end, the concept of the "energy triad" has been introduced, aiming to reduce overall energy consumption through three key principles: minimizing energy use, promoting renewable sources, and preventing waste.

15.4.1 Energy Consumption, Renewable Sources, and Water Management

Perioperative medicine requires significant expenditure of resources and materials, which are used across both surgical and anesthesiological fields. This includes, among others, the management and maintenance of mechanical ventilators, machines for supporting vital functions and patient monitoring, air conditioning and exhaust gas disposal systems, surgical instruments, as well as the management of resources needed for sterilization processes and the supply of energy, oxygen, and medical gases. For this reason, the so-called energy triad has been coined, based on three actions aimed at promoting the reduction of energy consumption: minimizing energy use, shifting toward renewable energy sources, and preventing energy waste.

One key area to focus on is the management of heating and air conditioning systems, which are present throughout the hospital and are fundamental to the proper functioning of operating room ventilation systems and beyond.

Another important aspect is water management. In a healthcare setting, where water is used for multiple purposes, proper consumption can make a significant difference in terms of environmental sustainability.

Hospitals should also be equipped with renewable energy systems (such as photovoltaic panels), and the use of windows and natural light should be encouraged to reduce reliance on artificial lighting powered by electricity.

What Can We Do?

- Reduce energy consumption: Optimize heating and air conditioning systems with high-efficiency technologies and automatic controls. Use renewable energy sources and heat recovery systems to lower energy use.
- Maintain correct temperature and humidity: Set optimal ranges in the operating room using precision sensors and automatic controls to avoid unnecessary thermal energy waste.
- Use LED lighting: Replace conventional lights with LEDs to significantly reduce electricity consumption and increase the lifespan of indoor lighting.
- Efficient sterilization procedures: Implement low-consumption technologies for material sterilization and ensure accurate management of sterile kits for perioperative use, avoiding waste and unnecessary use.
- Conductive heating methods: Use conductive devices to warm patients in the operating room, which are more efficient and perform better than conventional methods due to reduced heat loss.

- Switch off unused devices: At night and on weekends, turn off scavenger systems, computers, Wi-Fi networks, and other unused devices to reduce standby energy consumption.
- Use rechargeable batteries: Implement rechargeable batteries, thereby reducing hazardous waste; in the case of non-rechargeable batteries, ensure their proper disposal in accordance with environmental regulations.
- Avoid water waste: Install motion sensors at surgical washing stations and prefer the use of purified water where it is not intended for human use (e.g., drains and sewage systems).
- Renewable energy sources: Equip hospital facilities with renewable energy systems.

15.5 Production of Healthcare Waste, Management of Medications, and Their Proper Disposal

Waste management, including the proper handling of available resources, in the healthcare sector represents a crucial challenge for making clinical practice more sustainable. Hospitals are responsible for a significant portion of the waste produced nationally and contribute substantially to global greenhouse gas emissions. However, a large amount of this waste (especially from operating rooms) should be managed differently and subjected to appropriate recycling processes.

15.5.1 Waste Production

Waste production and its proper recycling are of utmost importance for making our clinical practice sustainable. Hospitals are responsible for producing up to 4.2% of the total solid waste generated by a country, and their impact on greenhouse gas emissions is estimated at 2.1% annually.

The vast majority of hospital waste produced is considered nonhazardous and therefore can be sorted: this means that most of the waste generated in a surgical/operating context is nonhazardous and can be disposed of similarly to household waste (e.g., plastic and cardboard packaging, bags, and uncontaminated materials that do not come into direct contact with the patient). Operating rooms produce about one-third of all hospital waste (half of which is recyclable), and of the total, anesthesiology practice alone accounts for 25%.

In this context, another significant issue is that, in preparation for surgery, a large amount of waste is generated due to the preemptive opening of sterile kits, surgical instruments, and other materials that might be needed during surgery or anesthetic procedures. Often, if these items are not used, their packaging must also be disposed of, and, where possible, new sterilization cycles are required (e.g., for surgical instruments and reusable devices that must remain sterile), resulting in additional energy and water consumption.

What Can We Do?

- Educate staff on the importance of waste sorting, especially for materials such as plastic and paper that have not been visibly contaminated with patient fluids.
- Increase the availability of waste bins, prioritizing the disposal of operating room waste in those designated for uncontaminated materials.
- Be conscientious when opening instruments and/or sterile kits that might go unused; prefer reusable devices (specifically, laryngoscope blades, fabric surgical gowns, procedure carts and trays, sharps disposal containers, etc.).
- Properly dispose of all items that are not normally separated into plastic waste, according to institutional protocols.

It is very important that hospital staff are well-trained in sorting and recycling procedures, particularly regarding materials that can potentially be separated and require proper disposal. Common examples include aluminum bottles containing inhaled anesthetics or the batteries of devices such as temporary cardiac pacemakers, which are often not properly disposed of due to the lack of adequate separation stations.

15.5.2 Medication Preparation

Especially in emergency settings, it is common practice to prepare and dilute medications for urgent use, which, however, often remain unused in about half of cases.

A specific mention should be made of propofol, which, particularly in the operating room, is frequently drawn up in advance and prepared in syringes without actually being administered to the patient (it is estimated that this occurs in more than one-third of cases). Proper disposal requires collecting unused medication in dedicated containers that must be incinerated in authorized facilities: it is important that it is not discarded with general waste or, worse, into the water system, as it ultimately ends up in the sewage due to its known toxicity to aquatic systems.

What Can We Do?

- Prepare medications by aspirating them only when truly necessary and, if available, use pre-filled saline syringes for dilution. This approach helps reduce the consumption of disposable materials and also prevents potential errors by the administering staff.
- Avoid the wastage of unused propofol, dispose of it properly, and reserve the aspiration of large quantities of the drug only when required for use in TCI/TIVA infusion syringes.

15.5.3 Use of Plastics in the Healthcare Industry and Medical Devices

In the healthcare industry, polymers are widely used for the production of disposable materials and beyond, due to their resistance to high temperatures.

Today, PVC (polyvinyl chloride) has been largely replaced by "polypropylene" (together, these are the two most widely used polymers) because PVC production requires higher energy consumption, resulting in increased fossil CO_2 emissions. Nevertheless, many devices used in anesthesiology practice are still made of PVC (e.g., laryngeal masks, face masks, etc.) or are supplemented with DEHP (di-2-ethylhexyl phthalate), a phthalate used to make plastic devices such as infusion sets and endotracheal tubes more flexible. The latter is of particular concern, as it has been classified by the United States Environmental Protection Agency as a potential carcinogen and an endocrine disruptor in humans.

What Can We Do?

- Prefer the use of reusable devices, ideally made from materials such as silicone or polypropylene (to be favored over those containing PVC and DEHP).
- Avoid the use of disposable instruments, especially when not truly necessary for patient care, and in nonemergency settings, consider using equipment according to a model that respects and avoids the expiration of materials.

15.6 Promoting Health, Psychological and Physical Well-Being of Staff, and Transportation

The psychological and physical well-being of healthcare personnel, particularly physicians working as anesthesiologists and intensivists, is essential to ensure the quality and safety of care provided to patients, especially in emergency and urgent care settings. Studies conducted in various European countries have shown that fatigue, stress, and a high burden of night work negatively affect the performance of medical staff, increasing the risk of errors and compromising not only patient safety but also the safety of the healthcare providers themselves.

15.6.1 Psychological and Physical Well-Being and Care of Staff

The psychological and physical well-being, rest, and care of healthcare professionals working as anesthesiologists and intensivists are fundamental to ensure the clarity and concentration required to care for patients, especially in care settings such as emergencies and urgent care, where the ability to respond to critical and unforeseen situations becomes even more crucial.

According to multiple studies conducted in various European countries, staff (including both residents and consultants) report fatigue and stress as predominant work-related feelings, mainly caused by shift work, particularly at night. There is increasing awareness that perioperative outcomes of emergency surgeries performed at night are worse compared to those performed during other shifts. While this is partly due to the condition of the patients (who are certainly more severe and unstable than those undergoing elective procedures), it is also important to consider the fatigue experienced by staff, which exposes them to a higher risk of errors in medical decision-making and anesthetic management.

In addition to the direct effects on patients, there is also an indirect link to the personal safety of the staff themselves: supporting this, the most significant statistics regarding accidents or near-misses are reported at the end of night shifts, with a percentage ranging from 37% to 45% among all medical personnel.

Other important issues that emerge among staff relate to the fact that, in addition to sleep deprivation (which, as already mentioned, increases the risk of improper patient management), there is a lack of training on strategies that could be implemented to improve night-time performance (such as sleep management during work hours, use of checklists to reduce risk, proper shift rotation and scheduling and rest periods), and above all, additional stress due to the inability to obtain a second opinion or assistance from colleagues during night shifts, should the need arise.

Another significant aspect concerns the mental health of staff, as surveys administered to anesthesiologists have revealed a high incidence of suicidal ideation (ranging from 3% to 25%) among those working in operating rooms and intensive care units, and that the prevalence of mental health issues affects up to 41% of individuals.

Not only mental health but also physical health is correlated with shift work conditions, which appear to negatively impact the cardiovascular health of Anesthesiologists and Intensive Care Physicians. It is estimated that these professionals have an increased risk of developing diseases and experiencing adverse events compared to other workers (with a risk increase of up to 40%).

What Can We Do?

- Provide rest areas that are accessible during and at the end of night shifts.
- Ensure the availability of assistance or consultation from another colleague when needed.
- Allow access to healthy food and beverages during work shifts.
- Offer psychological support: this is strategically important to ensure workers have the psychological well-being necessary to perform at their best.

15.6.2 Transport of Healthcare Personnel and Patients

The carbon footprint of the healthcare system is not limited to resource use, waste production, and energy consumption, but also revolves around how staff and patients physically reach healthcare facilities. The use of cars and the resulting road traffic increase air pollution, noise pollution, and the rate of accidents: all of which negatively impact the environment by increasing fossil fuel consumption.

These factors, together with the increasingly relevant issue of sedentary lifestyles (which is itself associated with conditions such as obesity, increased metabolic disorders, and cardiovascular diseases), are themselves causes of disease.

What Can We Do?

- Promote telemedicine to reduce patient travel, and also try to schedule multiple appointments for patients on the same day and at the same healthcare facilities.
- Prioritize the use of electric vehicles by providing adequate charging stations and, where possible, encourage "green" transportation for both healthcare workers and patients (bike sharing, pedestrian pathways).

15.7 Intensive Care Units: A Strategic Role in Clinical Sustainability

As highlighted in the recent document published by ESICM, it is important that, in addition to all previously mentioned actions aimed at implementing daily practices for environmental sustainability (involving both anesthesiology and intensive care and requiring practical, concrete measures), both staff and external users accessing intensive care units (ICUs) are actively involved and, above all, educated on the importance of this issue. The complexity of critically ill patients admitted to these units requires significant use of resources such as electricity, water, and medical supplies to meet the needs of advanced medical support and intensive monitoring of vital functions. Available data indicate that greenhouse gas emissions associated with a single day of ICU hospitalization are double those of other acute care wards; it is estimated that supporting fragile and complex patients, such as transplant recipients, results in an energy expenditure of 1.5 kW/h/day, equivalent to the consumption of an average European household.

There is not only a one-way relationship between pollution generated by clinical practice and climate change but also the reverse: environmental disasters that we increasingly witness as a consequence of the climate crisis (e.g., floods, hurricanes, wildfires) and health problems related to high temperatures also lead to increased admissions to high-intensity care units.

Moreover, climate change is also responsible for the resistance and adaptive mechanisms developed by microorganisms, making the problem of infections caused by multidrug-resistant organisms even more significant. For example, fungi have become more virulent due to thermotolerance developed as an adaptation to higher temperatures, and some pathogenic bacteria found in food tend to cause more illnesses during the summer months, suggesting a close correlation with the intensification of hot climates.

In this context, migratory flows driven by the need to move to more economically stable areas also contribute to the spread of pathogens or the emergence of new infections (concrete examples include dengue fever and tuberculosis), which inevitably increase the burden of healthcare services.

For these reasons, staff working in these critical settings, with such significant environmental impacts, must be adequately trained and informed about practical ways to act more sustainably in their daily activities.

What Can We Do?

- Review current company policies on waste disposal, improving proper recycling practices.
- Identify a multidisciplinary team and leadership to promote correct habits among staff.
- Engage patients and their families by proposing environmentally sustainable actions (waste separation, use of alternative means of transportation to reach the hospital).

15.8 Conclusion

Environmental sustainability is today not only a concern for individuals and international policies, but rotation also relies on the awareness that medical practice can play an active role in its prevention. It is therefore essential to adequately train staff so that they are aware and equipped with the necessary tools to implement actions that make the clinical environment sustainable.

The environmental effects of anesthesiology practice manifest through well-known mechanisms such as the greenhouse gas effect and ozone layer depletion, necessitating the adoption of anesthetic techniques that minimize environmental impact. In this regard, recommendations and regulations have been adopted at the European level to reconsider the use of inhalational anesthetics, the most significant of which is the ban on desflurane, whose use will be prohibited in Europe starting in 2026 due to its substantial greenhouse gas effect. Not only desflurane but also other agents such as nitrous oxide require judicious clinical use, and all are recommended to be administered with low-flow ventilation strategies, aiming to reduce the amount of inhalational anesthetics in the patient's exhaled gases that contribute to the greenhouse effect and ozone depletion.

Special attention should also be given to the use of propofol, which, according to recent studies, although it does not directly contribute to greenhouse gas emissions, is nonetheless a significant pollutant of aquatic systems and therefore requires separate disposal from other waste and elimination through incineration processes. This is particularly significant because it is one of the most widely used drugs by anesthesiologists and intensivists, yet a large portion remains aspirated and unused. Hence the need for its proper management.

A key area for improving the sustainability of our clinical practice is waste management, with operating rooms representing, on a national scale, some of the largest producers of waste within the healthcare system. It is important not only to reduce waste production but, above all, to apply proper collection and separation methods, allowing different materials to be disposed of appropriately. To ensure this, it is necessary to act conscientiously, paying attention to the actual need for equipment that is often prepared but not used, enabling the use of reusable devices, and providing adequate collection points.

Proper energy use, management of alternative sources, water conservation, and appropriate drug preparation are required to ensure optimal use of available resources. It is important that hospital facilities, particularly operating rooms and intensive care units where the most critical care is provided, are equipped with efficient air conditioning and heating systems to prevent heat and humidity loss (especially in operating suites). For the same purpose, LED devices should be preferred for electronic equipment, and motion sensors for surgical wash stations, among others. Resource management also depends on individual actions, such as turning off lights and systems during periods of nonuse and making thoughtful decisions about preparing and diluting drugs, opening sterile materials, and applying patient monitoring only when truly necessary to avoid waste.

The use of materials in the medical industry, particularly plastics used in clinical devices, is also considered, as it is not free from environmental impact or health risks.

Finally, the issue of the physical and psychological well-being of those working in anesthesiology and emergency settings is at the center of recommendations aimed at highlighting the central role that stress, fatigue, and excessive workload can have on the skills and abilities required for emergency work. It is important not to overlook that shift work, especially night shifts, is the leading cause of stress and negatively affects patient outcomes, as decisions are often made under conditions of insufficient rest and clarity, and in urgent or emergency situations without the support of another colleague.

In conclusion, we can state that there are many and diverse areas in which action can be taken to reduce the environmental impact of clinical practice in anesthesia and intensive care. It is important that awareness of this highly relevant issue is shared by everyone, so that every future action in the medical field becomes increasingly sustainable.

Suggested Readings

1. Lenzen M, Malik A, Li M, Fry J, Weisz H, Pichler P-P, Chaves LSM, Capon A, Pencheon D. The environmental footprint of health care: a global assessment. Lancet Planet Health. 2020;4:e271–9.
2. Romanello M, McGushin A, Di Napoli C, et al. The 2021 report of the lancet countdown on health and climate change: code red for a healthy future. Lancet. 2021;398:1619–62.
3. Romanello M, Di Napoli C, Drummond P, et al. The 2022 report of the lancet countdown on health and climate change: health at the mercy of fossil fuels. Lancet. 2022;400:1619–54.
4. Tennison I, Roschnik S, Ashby B, et al. Health care's response to climate change: a carbon footprint assessment of the NHS in England. Lancet Planet Health. 2021;5:e84–92.
5. Gonzalez-Pizarro P, Koch S, Muret J, et al. Environmental sustainability in the operating room: a worldwide survey among anaesthesiologists. Eur J Anaesthesiol. Intensive Care Med. 2023;2:4(e0025).
6. Buhre W, De Robertis E, Gonzalez-Pizarro P. The Glasgow declaration on sustainability in Anaesthesiology and intensive care. Eur J Anaesthesiol. 2023;40:461–4.

7. Gonzalez-Pizarro P, Brazzi L, Koch S, Trinks A, Muret J, Weiland NS, Jovanovic G, Cortegiani A, Fernandes TD, Kranke P, Malisiova A, McConnell P, Misquita L, Romero CS, Bilotta F, De Robertis E, Buhre W, on behalf of the Sustainability National Representatives. European Society of Anaesthesiology and Intensive Care consensus document on sustainability: four scopes to achieve more sustainable practice. Eur J Anaesthesiol. 2024;41:260–77.
8. Gonzalez-Pizarro P, Muret J, Brazzi L. The green anaesthesia dilemma: to what extent is it important to preserve as many drugs as possible. Curr Opin Anesthesiol. 2023;36:196–201.
9. Struys MMRF, Eckelman MJ. Environmental footprint of anesthesia: more than inhaled anesthetics! Anesthesiology. 2021;135:937–9.
10. McGain F, Sheridan N, Wickramarachchi K, et al. Carbon footprint of general, regional, and combined anesthesia for Total knee replacements. Anesthesiology. 2021;135:976–91.
11. De Waele JJ, Hunfeld N, Baid H, Ferrer R, Iliopoulou K, Ioan A-M, Leone M, Ostermann M, Scaramuzzo G, Theodorakopoulou M, Touw H, Citerio G, Derde LPG, Donadello K, Jufermans NP, Galarza L, Grasselli G, Maggiore SM, Martin-Loeches I, Alexandre J, Cecconi M, Azoulay E. Environmental sustainability in intensive care: the path forward. An ESICM Green Paper. Intensive Care Med. 50:1729–39.
12. The environment in Europe: Second assessment Chapter 3. Destruction of stratospheric ozone, European Environment Agency.
13. The Environmental Impact of Inhaled Anesthetics, ASA Committee on Environmental Health, date of last update: January 29, 2024.
14. REGULATION (EU) 2024/573 OF THE EUROPEAN PARLIAMENT AND OF THE COUNCIL of 7 February 2024 on fluorinated greenhouse gases.
15. Chipperfield MP, et al. Quantifying the ozone and ultraviolet benefits already achieved by the Montreal protocol. Nat Commun. 2015;6:7233. https://doi.org/10.1038/ncomms8233.

Part II

Care of the Critically Ill Patient

The Human Factor in Airway Management

16

Luigi La Via, Daniele Salvatore Paternò, and Massimiliano Sorbello

The technological, pharmacological, and cultural evolution of Medicine—and particularly of anesthesia and intensive care—has seen exponential growth in recent years, resulting in ever greater availability of patient monitoring systems, new techniques, and new devices that expand the horizons of airway management.

Today, increasingly precise and bedside-appropriate monitoring tools are available and sustainable, from capnography to tissue perfusion monitoring, from hemoglobin measurement to oxygenation indices. Ultrasound technology is becoming ever more sophisticated, incorporating templates and tutorials, and the ongoing refinement and miniaturization of video sensors has enabled the development of increasingly advanced videolaryngoscopes, lighter and more reliable videoendoscopes, and new laryngeal masks that allow visualization of peri-laryngeal tissues and structures.

Nevertheless, and this is an incontrovertible fact, incidents related to airway management continue to occur, both in the operating room setting and, increasingly, in prehospital, emergency, and critical care environments.

L. La Via
Department of General Surgery and Medical Surgical Specialties (CHIRMED), University of Catania, Catania, Italy
e-mail: luigi.lavia@unict.it

D. S. Paternò
UOC Anesthesia and Intensive Care, Giovanni Paolo II Hospital, ASP 7 Ragusa, Ragusa, Italy

M. Sorbello (✉)
UOC Anesthesia and Intensive Care, Giovanni Paolo II Hospital, ASP 7 Ragusa, Ragusa, Italy

Enna Kore University, Enna, Italy
e-mail: massimiliano.sorbello@unikore.it

D. Chiumello, A. De Gasperi (eds.), *Practical Trends in Anesthesia and Intensive Care 2026*, https://doi.org/10.1007/978-3-032-25721-5_16

It is becoming clear that technological advancement is neither the limit nor the means by which to improve safety in airway management and patient outcomes.

Drawing on the lessons learned from aviation, we must recognize the true limitation of technological progress: the human element, now referred to as the human factor.

16.1 Lessons from Aviation

Anesthesia has often been compared to flight; the monitoring phase corresponds to pre-flight checks, induction to takeoff, maintenance, and emergence to cruising and landing. The metaphor is particularly apt, and there are many parallels between the two "flights." A fundamental difference, however, is that anesthesia is a complex, dynamic scenario in which multiple tasks, streams of information, and interpersonal communications intersect; and, not least, patients tend to be less predictable than aircraft in terms of interindividual variability of response [1].

Despite these differences, the metaphor is entirely appropriate, and it also underscores the importance of interaction with monitoring and the influence of communication among the members of the "crew."

The validity of the flight-anesthesia metaphor is further reinforced when considered in light of accident dynamics: on December 29, 1972, Eastern Airlines Flight 401, departing from JFK Airport in New York and bound for Miami, crashed for no apparent reason. Subsequent investigations and access to the black box revealed that the crew became alert and initiated a series of attempts to restore the landing gear, prompted by a cockpit warning light that continued to indicate a malfunction. Examination of the recordings made it clear that the crew *became fixated* on this warning, leading the captain to prolong the flight around the landing strip in an attempt to resolve the issue, *while ignoring* the fuel consumption warning light. We will never know whether the landing gear of EA401 would have ultimately functioned, because the aircraft crashed due to fuel exhaustion. None of the crew members realized this, *fixated* as they were on the landing gear indicator.

This is the first documented example of *fixation error*, which has been and continues to be studied in training courses for civil, military, and space aviation pilots [2], and is often cited as the paradigm of the *human factor* in the dynamics of accidents in complex systems.

Aviation data continue to confirm that crew actions (or omissions) remain the leading single cause of air accidents and that the human factor also plays a fundamental role in other areas, such as inspections, repairs, and air traffic control. This trend is certainly decreasing, and above all, unlike in the past, it is now widely accepted that human error should not be blamed, but rather considered as an inevitable process inherent to human nature and to our physiological cognitive activities (and limitations) [3].

The Augustinian concept of *errare humanum* is therefore more relevant than ever, and its extension, *perseverare autem diabolicum*, is instead the subject of analysis and study of strategies aimed at limiting, counteracting, analyzing, and utilizing the psychological mechanisms underlying error: the *cognitive biases* [4, 5].

Returning to the cockpit, analysis of the dynamics of certain accidents has helped to clarify the underlying mechanisms, also highlighting an important role for *ergonomics*, that is, the interaction between humans and their environment with reference to the devices they use in that environment. Placement, color choices, and shapes can influence ease of use, reduce the incidence of error, and optimize performance, especially under stress [6]. This concept evolves into that of the *cognitive aid*, which, both in the cockpit and in emergency management and decision-making processes in airway management, becomes a decisive element in reducing the incidence of human error. The "remove before flight" tag, large and brightly colored, on the pin that arms the slides on civilian and military aircraft doors, passively *reminds* the crew to perform a certain procedure, simply by its presence or absence. Similarly, and according to the same principle, a *color coding* system is being developed for airway carts, with a precise algorithmic correspondence and intensity for crisis situations (Fig. 16.1).

Another important element has been imported from aviation into the field of airway management, again by analyzing a wealth of evidence that has identified the weak points of a complex system, particularly when it is subjected to high psychophysical stress.

Data provided by Boeing regarding the number of *hull-loss* events, that is, the loss of aircraft, have been analyzed and have provided incontrovertible evidence supporting the routine use of *checklists*, cognitive aid tools used for cross-checking,

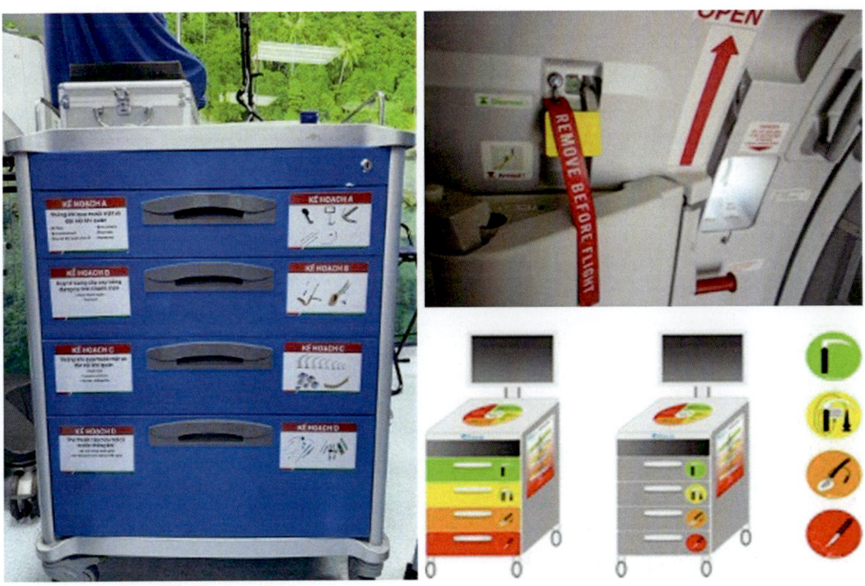

Fig. 16.1 Cognitive aids in airway management

and the cross-verification of crew actions, yet another tool for monitoring and correcting human error.

Recent medical literature suggests that, once the principle of checklists is applied to operating room activities, particularly during pre-induction phases, a reduction in incidents can be achieved, analogous to the aviation sector [7]. Not to mention the similar initiative undertaken by the World Health Organization with the introduction of operating room checklists as part of a *global safety* project. All of this has become an integral part of the "operating room safety manual" adopted by the Italian Ministry of Health as early as 2009 [8] and has since constituted a standard for safety and risk management.

It is now clear that the parallel between aviation and anesthesia, particularly with regard to airway management, is highly appropriate, reflecting the structure of complex systems with a high cognitive load in which human error plays a crucial role in the genesis of incidents. The implementation of corrective factors derived from aviation in airway management has certainly improved the safety and efficiency of procedures, while a fundamental concept remains: the human patient tends to be far less predictable than an aircraft cockpit, and therefore further corrective measures are necessary.

16.2 The Physician as a Human Being

"*The real problem isn't how to stop bad doctors from harming, even killing, their patients. It's how to prevent good doctors from doing so*" [9]. In Gawande's words there is a profound truth: one does not have to be a "bad" doctor to make mistakes.

The human learning mechanism is typically based on the repetition of actions, through a rational process ("analytical behavior") until they form a recognizable *pattern* that becomes ("intuitive behavior") an automatic response. When intuitive, automatic behavior prevails over rational, cognitive behavior, a condition known as *cognitive bias* arises, which in practice becomes what we call "error" [10].

The literature is now unanimous in identifying a long list of cognitive biases (Table 16.1) and equally unanimous in recognizing that they underlie many medical errors [11].

Table 16.1 The main cognitive biases described in the medical literature

Aggregate bias	Gender bias	Psych-out errors
Anchoring	Hindsight bias	Representativeness
Ascertainment bias	Multiple alternatives	Search satisficing
Availability	Omission bias	Sutton's Slip
Base rate neglect	Order effects	Triage-cueing
Commission bias	Outcome bias	Unpacking principle
Confirmation bias	Overconfidence	Vertical line failure
Diagnostic creep	Playing the odds	Visceral bias
Attribution error	Posterior prob.	Ying-Yang out
Gambler's Fallacy	Premature closure	Zebra retreat

A modern approach to safety and risk management in medicine, therefore, must take into account not only the classic mechanisms of error but also the role that the human factor and cognitive biases play in the genesis of incidents.

16.3 Cognitive Biases and Decision-Making Processes

The National Audit Project 4 represented an extremely important study for understanding the nature, dynamics, and corrective elements needed to reduce the incidence of adverse events and incidents in airway management.

The audit, sponsored by the British scientific societies, was conducted over a one-year period, identifying the location and dynamics of incidents.

Among the findings, it was evident that incidents in critical care settings such as the emergency department, accident and emergency, and intensive care unit [12] were certainly numerically fewer than those occurring in the operating room [13]. However, when the data were indexed to the number of procedures, the study clearly showed that incidents in critical care areas were proportionally much more frequent and, above all, associated with higher morbidity and mortality than those observed in the operating room [14].

One of the recurring causes of incidents was the failure to use, or the incorrect interpretation of, capnography, leading clinicians to consider some endotracheal tubes as correctly positioned when they were not, or to (erroneously) interpret abnormal capnographic curves as nonexistent pathological states in the patient. The common denominator in many of these incidents was identified as a series of specific cognitive biases, attributable to well-known behavioral models [15].

Among the main cognitive biases, it is important at this point to mention some of particular relevance in the medical field, especially in airway management.

- Confirmation Bias

- This bias should be understood in the context of "cognitive dissonance" [16], the human tendency to agree with those who agree with us. It is a preferential behavioral pattern that leads to confirmation bias, that is, the act of referring only to perspectives that reinforce our preexisting views. A classic example would be interpreting an abnormal capnographic curve as evidence of bronchospasm while completely dismissing the possibility of esophageal intubation.
- Group Bias
- Similar to the previous one, group bias leads us to overestimate the abilities and value of our own group and to attribute its successes to the group's inherent qualities. It is often summarized by the concept that "a team of experts is not necessarily an expert team."
- Anchoring Bias
- Also known as the "relativity trap," this bias occurs when, in making a decision, we tend to compare only a limited set of elements, "anchoring" ourselves to a value, a preconception, or a diagnosis that is unconsciously used as a reference

point for ongoing assessments, rather than relying on unequivocal or absolute data. The classic case is when, assuming that intubation was performed correctly, one searches for alternative, if not improbable, causes for desaturation or cardiac arrest.

- Gambler's Fallacy
- The gambler's fallacy is the tendency to assign significance to past events and to connect them to current occurrences, so that judgments are deeply influenced by them. This is the typical bias of gamblers (also known as the Monte Carlo bias) and, in medicine, leads to misdirected diagnoses based on previous experiences while ignoring possible, even likely, alternatives.
- Apophenia (Pareidolia)
- This represents a sensory manifestation of confirmation bias, consisting of the brain's tendency to identify familiar shapes in objects; paradigmatic examples include seeing distinct forms in the abstract shapes of clouds, trompe-l'oeil, Rorschach inkblots used in psychiatry, and there are well-known cases that have led to serious incidents in medicine and airway management, particularly in relation to capnography and esophageal intubation ("glottic impersonation") [17].
- Fixation Error
- This occurs as a result of the aforementioned biases and manifests when one clings firmly to a first impression or initial decision, even as conflicting and contradictory evidence accumulates [18]. This leads to the so-called tunnel vision, ignoring possible alternatives, also as a result of selective attention mechanisms [19].
- Projection Bias
- This bias leads us to believe that most people think as we do, often triggering the false consensus bias, whereby we also assume that others not only share our views but also agree with us.
- Negativity Bias
- This bias drives us to pay excessive attention to negative elements, which are mistakenly considered the most important, thus giving greater weight to errors while underestimating successes and acquired competencies.
- Status Quo Bias
- This is a cognitive distortion linked to resistance to change; due to fear of change, there is a tendency to maintain the current state of affairs. It is the classic mechanism whereby, in a difficult airway management situation, one seeks alternative explanations for a clear and decisive clinical-instrumental picture, out of fear of removing the tube and attempting re-intubation.
- Omission Bias
- This bias consists of a systematic tendency to favor omissions over commissions, even when this means exposing oneself to objectively high risks, likely due to an underlying fear of making a wrong choice.
- Loss Aversion Bias
- This is one of the most robust and demonstrable cognitive biases in decision-making, and it consists of the influence on decisions depending on whether the outcome is perceived or experienced as a gain or a loss. A typical, and much

debated, example in this context is the choice of terminology used to refer to cricothyrotomy, which influences its perception as a life-saving maneuver (I will be inclined to perform it) or as the result of a failed or improper airway management (I will not be inclined to perform it) [20, 21].

- Overconfidence Bias
- This bias is related to excessive confidence in our own judgments, often leading us to feel more certain than we actually are. In addition to being "spontaneous," it can also be induced by circumstances, giving rise to the so-called hero complex (the belief that one must "save" the situation through their actions) and "god complex" (the belief that one must become the deus ex machina to resolve the situation; often associated with hierarchical status).
- A corollary manifestation of overconfidence bias, particularly in a team system with a hierarchical structure, is the concept of "authority gradients." This phenomenon occurs when those at lower levels of the hierarchy tend to remain silent or do not fully express their perspective in the decision-making process, inhibited by the higher rank of the person speaking or making the error [22].
- Dunning-Kruger Effect
- This is in some way related to overconfidence bias and is known as the "paradox of ignorance." It leads individuals to overestimate their own skills, knowledge, or abilities precisely when they lack mastery of the subject. Typically, this effect follows a behavioral curve with a negative peak after an incident and a slow curve of recovery and awareness (Fig. 16.2).

A graph illustrating the Dunning-Kruger Effect [23]. The graph has two axes: horizontal axis labeled "Knowledge/Experience" and vertical axis labeled "Confidence." The curve starts low, then rapidly rises to a sharp peak labeled "Mount Stupid," then drops dramatically into a low valley labeled "Valley of Despair," followed by a gradual upward slope labeled "Slope of Enlightenment," finally leveling off at a plateau labeled "Plateau of Sustainability." Use a bold blue line for the curve. Include small icon illustrations: a person with arms crossed confidently at Mount Stupid, a confused person at Valley of Despair, a person studying

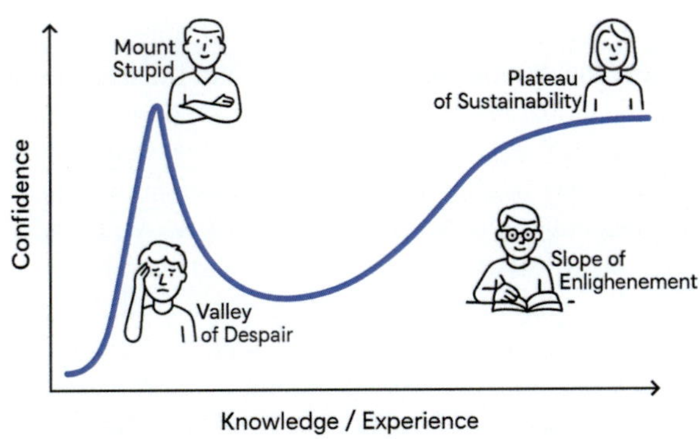

Fig. 16.2 Dunning-Kruger effect (see explanation in the text)

at Slope of Enlightenment, and a calm expert at the plateau. Clean white background, modern sans-serif fonts, professional business presentation style.

We will now examine how these cognitive biases are reflected in airway management and how they can be addressed.

16.4 Cognitive Biases in Airway Management

For many years, airway management has been subject to what, in hindsight, could be defined as a fixation error; the numerous guidelines that have followed the first American Society of Anesthesiologists document in 1993 have, for better or worse, been constructed around a sequence of failures: if intubation failed, a supraglottic device was placed, and if this also failed, the algorithm proceeded further, focusing more on devices than on the actual goal.

Today, it is clear that the goal of airway maneuvers is not intubation itself: we must think in terms of targets, that is, oxygenation, rather than devices (the means to achieve it) [24], in a process that should not be purely sequential but, more appropriately, transitional [25], in light of a well-defined preestablished strategy.

We have long known that no patient dies from failed intubation, but rather from the many (too many) attempts that compromise ventilation or overshadow the patient's only real need: oxygen.

From this perspective, the entire framework of every guideline must be reconsidered in light of the importance of human factors and the prevention of cognitive biases that can result in adverse events.

In this sense, videolaryngoscopy has represented a true cultural evolution, even before a technological one: on the one hand, with appropriate experience, the videolaryngoscope has reduced desaturation, intubation failure, and improved first-pass success [26]; on the other hand, it has enabled a paradigm shift from laryngoscopy as an individual maneuver to a team-based procedure.

This has provided, first and foremost, enormous educational value, as both the instructor and the trainee could share the same view, no longer relying on the often limited feedback from the learner. Secondly, the shared view allowed for targeted assistance during difficulty, for laryngeal manipulation maneuvers, and for sharing the visual field. This last element, in fact, has become a crucial aspect in the recent PUMA guidelines for the prevention of unrecognized esophageal intubation [27]: shifting the responsibility for doubt and the decision to remove the tube from the individual operator to the team has ensured that, after capnography, the videolaryngoscope is the recommended tool to prevent esophageal intubation. With this approach, the likelihood that individual cognitive bias—particularly apophenia and the phenomenon of glottic impersonation—will lead to an incident is minimized, since every decision becomes shared and team-based.

In the same document, the decision to shift the guideline focus from excluding esophageal intubation to actively seeking its confirmation—conceptually, transforming the objective from detecting a failure (missed tracheal intubation) to identifying a success (correctly recognizing esophageal intubation)—becomes an extremely powerful tool to counteract loss aversion bias and confirmation bias [28] through the mechanism of the "nudge" [29].

Unrecognized esophageal intubation is a frequently fatal event, whose incidence has prompted the development of dedicated guidelines by the PUMA working group; the literature shows that such incidents are often linked to nontechnical skills and human factors, to a degree no less significant than technological issues [30], and that biases such as loss aversion bias, confirmation bias, gambler's fallacy, and apophenia have often contributed to the failure to remove a tube erroneously placed in the esophagus or to the misinterpretation of capnographic curves clearly indicative of failed intubation [12, 13], and finally, that there is still considerable limitation, if not resistance, to the adoption of capnography in critical care settings and particularly in intensive care [15], as highlighted by the recent INTUBE study [31].

It is therefore essential, in order to reduce the incidence of this phenomenon, to focus primarily on human factors, and on cognitive and decision-making aspects, even before promoting the adoption of *universal capnography*.

In critical care settings, human factors manifest as communication difficulties, fixation errors, lack of planning, and failure to share and implement strategies and decisions. Time flows differently during a crisis, to the extent that its perception can vary greatly among team members [32].

In this context, the modern approach to complex algorithms should be understood: they must be consulted and studied "in cold blood," away from the crisis, and implemented with cognitive aids that are simple and unambiguous, using icons, symbols, and color codes that do not require effort or cognitive overload during crisis management. A typical example is the so-called Vortex approach developed by the Australian group led by Nicholas Chrimes, which "simplifies" the progression toward non-ventilability and guides the team toward emergency front-of-neck access using a vortex model. This approach is no longer sequential but transitional, meaning that, even from a team-sharing perspective, while one action is being performed (e.g., placement of a supraglottic device due to unexpected laryngoscopic difficulty), another team member prepares the cricothyrotomy set and begins to identify anatomical landmarks for the procedure. In this way, time is anticipated, and the team moves forward in conscious unison, rather than simply following the steps dictated by the vortex [25].

This approach becomes extremely important when analyzing, specifically, the data on cricothyrotomy: the American Society of Anesthesiologists closed claims analysis and data from the UK literature [14] clearly indicate that cricothyrotomy is still underutilized, and that about two-thirds of cricothyrotomies are performed too late to alter the outcome. This highlights a dual problem: on the one hand, the need to improve technical skill (and the literature confirms that just a few manikin exercises are sufficient to master the technique [33]), and on the other, the need to generate situational awareness that prompts the clinician to consider cricothyrotomy. Loss aversion bias, confirmation bias, and overconfidence bias play a significant role in the cognitive process that leads to failure or delay in performing a cricothyrotomy, and it is on these aspects that educational efforts must focus if we are to change the "lived experience" of cricothyrotomy. Emergency oxygenation in the patient with critical hypoxia or asphyxia is a life-saving maneuver; while it is not technically difficult to perform, we must acknowledge that cricothyrotomy is a difficult choice, and it is therefore on cognitive and decision-making tools that we must work to improve the outcome in many cannot intubate–cannot ventilate scenarios.

Similarly, data from NAP4 and the English literature highlight the issue of awake tracheal intubation and the underuse of the flexible bronchoscope [14].

NAP4 [12] clearly indicated that in many cases where flexible bronchoscopy was indicated, and more generally when an awake technique was warranted to manage an anticipated difficult airway, it was not employed, often compromising patient outcomes. Why such reluctance to use an awake technique or the bronchoscope? Certainly, a lack of familiarity and technical proficiency influenced many of the choices reported in NAP4. However, alongside this, as with cricothyrotomy, certain cognitive biases undoubtedly played a crucial role: loss aversion bias, confirmation bias, overconfidence bias, gambler's fallacy, and the hero and god complex.

Even in light of these findings, it is clear that educational efforts must not only promote training in the use of devices and techniques for awake intubation but must also go further. The DAS, aware of the NAP4 results, established a task force that led to the publication of guidelines for awake tracheal intubation [34], and many practical courses have focused on using of the bronchoscope and awake videolaryngoscopy [35].

The current task is to foster awareness of the difficult airway, both anatomical and physiological, and to develop cognitive and decision-making supports that recognize the need for a cautious, "spontaneous breathing-preserving" approach. This includes the creation of algorithms, visual aids, and pain codes to highlight the critical nature of the situation and the need for protective strategies in airway management, as recently recommended by the American Society of Anesthesiologists guidelines for airway management [36].

Therefore, to optimize performance and safety, it is also necessary to address the organization of the environment in which these procedures are performed. For this reason, the concept of *ergonomics* is increasingly discussed, as the human factor can be defined as "the study of the interrelationship between human beings, the tools they use, and the environment that surrounds them" [37].

For these reasons, a modern architectural setting in critical care must take into account the positioning of tables and monitors; it should facilitate direct eye contact among team members to optimize two-way communication, streamline workflows, and make access to equipment more intuitive. Timekeeping clocks on one side, and carts organized according to color codes or other cognitive aids on the other, should enhance human-environment interaction. In this regard, the recent guidelines for airway management in critical care settings produced by the UK Difficult Airway Society (DAS) go beyond listing procedures or devices: they specify the positions of team members around the patient (identifying the "airway manager," "hemodynamic manager," "team leader," and "runner") and provide dedicated checklists as cognitive aids [38].

The need to implement these resources is driven by extensive evidence in the literature, especially in critical care. Intensive care units are environments of high instrumental, interpersonal, and emotional complexity, where the conditions that can lead to cognitive bias are statistically much more frequent.

In the words of Walsh, intensive care is an environment of high cognitive complexity, where the amount of information required by the clinician to make the correct decision often exceeds the amount of information an individual can process simultaneously [39].

Intensive care is also a setting that, while allowing a certain familiarity with the environment and team members—due to the larger team size compared to the emergency department or operating room—can foster mechanisms of non-designated task assignment or a sense of relative reassurance linked to the "dilution" of responsibility within a larger team and in an environment inherently characterized by the presence and regular occurrence of severe complications.

Recent literature has definitively brought this reality to light, providing figures that were previously only perceived but now have a precise dimension.

NAP4 [12, 13] and the INTUBE study [31] have, for the first time, clearly demonstrated the impact of the human factor and nontechnical skills in the genesis of incidents; INTUBE measured the incidence of cardiac arrest associated with airway management, placing it at a concerning approximately 3%, with a prevalence of nearly one in two patients experiencing hemodynamic events of varying severity associated with airway management. Furthermore, the INTUBE study revealed the underuse of capnography (only 17%), the role of videolaryngoscopy depending on the center's expertise [40] and the role of propofol in the pathogenesis of cardiocirculatory events [41], highlighting the need to intervene not only on individual aspects (drugs, monitoring, procedures) but also on the underlying human factors that drive and determine these situations and the choices or omissions made.

Why, if so many physicians are aware of the cardiodepressive effects of propofol, do they continue to use it? Why do many anesthesiologists, despite being fully aware of the importance of capnography in confirming successful intubation, use it so infrequently in critical care settings?

In light of these considerations, it becomes clearly necessary to review and expand the tools of specialist training. Alongside the essential need to provide technical competencies and practical skills specific to the various devices, it is now equally indispensable to train future specialists in the crucial aspects of human factors and nontechnical skills. Thus, simulation becomes the essential tool for comprehensive training [42].

A context in which organizational and communication skills can be tested, where crises can be simulated, team interactions during crises can be observed, and the potential and benefits of using decision-making and cognitive aids for crisis management and resolution can be evaluated [43].

16.5 Conclusions

The role of human factors in anesthesia, and particularly in airway management, is now a well-established [44, 45], and widely recognized element, with increasing acknowledgment in international guidelines [46]. The Difficult Airway Society has developed a dedicated guideline for the implementation of human factors in anesthesia [47], for physician training, and for the prevention of errors associated with cognitive biases, recognizing the unavoidable need to address these issues to improve the safety of both patients and healthcare providers [48–51].

The evolution of airway management guidelines, including within the PUMA (Project for Universal Airway Management) initiative, recognizes the decisive importance of human factors, identifying the need to address language, the complexity of algorithms, the importance of teamwork, and the operational environment itself [52–54].

In a world of rapidly evolving technology, where artificial intelligence is also making its way into Medicine, it is crucial to remember that the true limit to technological advancement is the human being who uses it. It is on this front that organizational and educational efforts must be focused to maximize outcomes and patient safety.

If we want airway management to reach the safety standards of modern aeronautics, we must embrace the lessons of aviation pioneers, remembering that both in the sky and in the operating room, what makes the difference are human factors and our humanity.

References

1. Heard G. Errors in medicine: a human factors perspective. Australasian Anaesthesia, no. 2005, Australian and New Zealand College of Anaesthetists; 2005, pp. 1–11. https://search.informit.org/doi/10.3316/informit.490623210425261.
2. Lauber JK. In: HW Orlady, HC Foushee, eds. NASA Conference Publication 2455; 1987.
3. Toff NJ. Human factors in anaesthesia: lessons from aviation. Br J Anaesth. 2010;105(1):21–5. https://doi.org/10.1093/bja/aeq127.
4. Jala S, Fry M, Elliott R. Cognitive bias during clinical decision-making and its influence on patient outcomes in the emergency department: a scoping review. J Clin Nurs. 2023;32(19–20):7076–85. https://doi.org/10.1111/jocn.16845.
5. Beldhuis IE, Marapin RS, Jiang YY, Simões de Souza NF, Georgiou A, Kaufmann T, Castela Forte J, van der Horst ICC. Cognitive biases, environmental, patient and personal factors associated with critical care decision making: a scoping review. J Crit Care. 2021;64:144–53. https://doi.org/10.1016/j.jcrc.2021.04.012.
6. Wu X, Wanyan X, Zhuang D. Pilot's visual attention allocation modeling under fatigue. Technol Health Care. 2015;23 Suppl 2:S373–81. https://doi.org/10.3233/THC-150974.
7. Jelacic S, Bowdle A, Nair BG, Togashi K, Wu C, Boorman DJ, Cain KC, Lang JD, Dellinger EP. The effects of an aviation-style computerised pre-induction anaesthesia checklist on pre-anaesthetic set-up and non-routine events. Anaesthesia. 2019;74(9):1138–46. https://doi.org/10.1111/anae.14707.
8. https://www.salute.gov.it/imgs/C_17_pubblicazioni_1119_allegato.pdf
9. Gawande A. When doctors make mistakes. The New Yorker, 1 February 1999. p. 40–55.

10. Stiegler MP, Tung A. Cognitive processes in anesthesiology decision making. Anesthesiology. 2014;120(1):204–17. https://doi.org/10.1097/ALN.0000000000000073.
11. Saposnik G, Redelmeier D, Ruff CC, Tobler PN. Cognitive biases associated with medical decisions: a systematic review. BMC Med Inform Decis Mak. 2016;16(1):138. https://doi.org/10.1186/s12911-016-0377-1.
12. Cook TM, Woodall N, Harper J, Benger J; Fourth National Audit Project. Major complications of airway management in the UK: results of the Fourth National Audit Project of the Royal College of Anaesthetists and the Difficult Airway Society. Part 2: intensive care and emergency departments. Br J Anaesth. 2011;106(5):632–42. https://doi.org/10.1093/bja/aer059.
13. Cook TM, Woodall N, Frerk C; Fourth National Audit Project. Major complications of airway management in the UK: results of the Fourth National Audit Project of the Royal College of Anaesthetists and the Difficult Airway Society. Part 1: anaesthesia. Br J Anaesth. 2011;106(5):617–31. https://doi.org/10.1093/bja/aer058.
14. Cook TM, MacDougall-Davis SR. Complications and failure of airway management. Br J Anaesth. 2012;109 Suppl 1:i68–85. https://doi.org/10.1093/bja/aes393.
15. Russotto V, Cook TM. Capnography use in the critical care setting: why do clinicians fail to implement this safety measure? Br J Anaesth. 2021;127(5):661–4. https://doi.org/10.1016/j.bja.2021.08.010.
16. Skinner BF. Some contributions of an experimental analysis of behavior to psychology as a whole. Am Psychol. 1953;8(2):69–78.
17. Kovacs G, Duggan LV, Brindley PG. Glottic impersonation. Can J Anaesth. 2017;64(3):320. https://doi.org/10.1007/s12630-016-0804-x.
18. Schwid HA, O'Donnell D. Anesthesiologists' management of simulated critical incidents. Anesthesiology. 1992;76(4):495–501. https://doi.org/10.1097/00000542-199204000-00002.
19. Fioratou E, Flin R, Glavin R. No simple fix for fixation errors: cognitive processes and their clinical applications. Anaesthesia. 2010;65(1):61–9. https://doi.org/10.1111/j.1365-2044.2009.05994.x.
20. Cooper S. "We need to cut the neck!": confronting psychological and moral distress during emergency cricothyrotomy. Narrat Inq Bioeth. 2013;3(2):E5–9. https://doi.org/10.1353/nib.2013.0051.
21. Booth AWG, Vidhani K. Human factors can't intubate can't oxygenate (CICO) bundle is more important than needle versus scalpel debate. Br J Anaesth. 2017;118(3):466–8. https://doi.org/10.1093/bja/aex021.
22. Friedman Z, Hayter MA, Everett TC, Matava CT, Noble LM, Bould MD. Power and conflict: the effect of a superior's interpersonal behaviour on trainees' ability to challenge authority during a simulated airway emergency. Anaesthesia. 2015;70(10):1119–29. https://doi.org/10.1111/anae.13191.
23. https://onlinepethealth.com/the-dunning-kruger-effect/
24. Sorbello M, Afshari A, De Hert S. Device or target? A paradigm shift in airway management: implications for guidelines, clinical practice and teaching. Eur J Anaesthesiol. 2018;35(11):811–4. https://doi.org/10.1097/EJA.0000000000000893.
25. Chrimes N, Higgs A, Rehak A. Lost in transition: the challenges of getting airway clinicians to move from the upper airway to the neck during an airway crisis. Br J Anaesth. 2020;125(1):e38–46. https://doi.org/10.1016/j.bja.2020.04.052.
26. Hansel J, Rogers AM, Lewis SR, Cook TM, Smith AF. Videolaryngoscopy versus direct laryngoscopy for adults undergoing tracheal intubation: a Cochrane systematic review and meta-analysis update. Br J Anaesth. 2022;129(4):612–23. https://doi.org/10.1016/j.bja.2022.05.027.
27. Chrimes N, Higgs A, Hagberg CA, Baker PA, Cooper RM, Greif R, Kovacs G, Law JA, Marshall SD, Myatra SN, O'Sullivan EP, Rosenblatt WH, Ross CH, Sakles JC, Sorbello M, Cook TM. Preventing unrecognised oesophageal intubation: a consensus guideline from the Project for Universal Management of Airways and international airway societies. Anaesthesia. 2022;77(12):1395–415. https://doi.org/10.1111/anae.15817.

28. Sorbello M, De Jong A, De Robertis E, Greif R. Dubito ergo sum. From philosophy towards prevention of unrecognised oesophageal intubation. Eur J Anaesthesiol. 2023;40(5):310–2. https://doi.org/10.1097/EJA.0000000000001822.
29. Bourdeaux CP, Thomas MJ, Gould TH, Malhotra G, Jarvstad A, Jones T, Gilchrist ID. Increasing compliance with low tidal volume ventilation in the ICU with two nudge-based interventions: evaluation through intervention time-series analyses. BMJ Open. 2016;6(5):e010129. https://doi.org/10.1136/bmjopen-2015-010129.
30. Honardar MR, Posner KL, Domino KB. Delayed detection of esophageal intubation in anesthesia malpractice claims: brief report of a case series. Anesth Analg. 2017;125(6):1948–51. https://doi.org/10.1213/ANE.0000000000001795.
31. Russotto V, Myatra SN, Laffey JG, Tassistro E, Antolini L, Bauer P, Lascarrou JB, Szuldrzynski K, Camporota L, Pelosi P, Sorbello M, Higgs A, Greif R, Putensen C, Agvald-Öhman C, Chalkias A, Bokums K, Brewster D, Rossi E, Fumagalli R, Pesenti A, Foti G, Bellani G; INTUBE Study Investigators. Intubation practices and adverse peri-intubation events in critically ill patients from 29 countries. JAMA. 2021;325(12):1164–72. https://doi.org/10.1001/jama.2021.1727.
32. Cemalovic N, Scoccimarro A, Arslan A, Fraser R, Kanter M, Caputo N. Human factors in the emergency department: is physician perception of time to intubation and desaturation rate accurate? Emerg Med Australas. 2016;28(3):295–9. https://doi.org/10.1111/1742-6723.12575.
33. Onrubia X, Frova G, Sorbello M. Front of neck access to the airway: a narrative review. Trends Anaesth Crit Care. 2018;22:45 55. https://doi.org/10.1016/j.tacc.2018.06.001.
34. Ahmad I, El-Boghdadly K, Bhagrath R, Hodzovic I, McNarry AF, Mir F, O'Sullivan EP, Patel A, Stacey M, Vaughan D. Difficult Airway Society guidelines for awake tracheal intubation (ATI) in adults. Anaesthesia. 2020;75(4):509–28. https://doi.org/10.1111/anae.14904.
35. Sorbello M, Saracoglu KT, Cortese G, Onrubia X, Pereira AI, Canbay O, Saracoglu A, Michalek P, Charco Mora P, Timmermann A, Greif R. Back home full in oxygen after Antalya: a report of the European Airway Conference 2023. Trends Anaesth Crit Care. 2022;47:20–6.
36. Apfelbaum JL, Hagberg CA, Connis RT, Abdelmalak BB, Agarkar M, Dutton RP, Fiadjoe JE, Greif R, Klock PA, Mercier D, Myatra SN, O'Sullivan EP, Rosenblatt WH, Sorbello M, Tung A. 2022 American Society of Anesthesiologists practice guidelines for management of the difficult airway. Anesthesiology. 2022;136(1):31–81. https://doi.org/10.1097/ALN.0000000000004002.
37. Weinger MB, Pantiskas C, Wiklund M, Carstensen P. Incorporating human factors into the design of medical devices. JAMA. 1998;280:1484.
38. Higgs A, McGrath BA, Goddard C, Rangasami J, Suntharalingam G, Gale R, Cook TM; Difficult Airway Society; Intensive Care Society; Faculty of Intensive Care Medicine; Royal College of Anaesthetists. Guidelines for the management of tracheal intubation in critically ill adults. Br J Anaesth. 2018;120(2):323–52. https://doi.org/10.1016/j.bja.2017.10.021.
39. Walsh T, Beatty PC. Human factors error and patient monitoring. Physiol Meas. 2002;23(3):R111–32. https://doi.org/10.1088/0967-3334/23/3/201.
40. Russotto V, Lascarrou JB, Tassistro E, Parotto M, Antolini L, Bauer P, Szułdrzyński K, Camporota L, Putensen C, Pelosi P, Sorbello M, Higgs A, Greif R, Grasselli G, Valsecchi MG, Fumagalli R, Foti G, Caironi P, Bellani G, Laffey JG, Myatra SN, INTUBE Study Investigators. Efficacy and adverse events profile of videolaryngoscopy in critically ill patients: subanalysis of the INTUBE study. Br J Anaesth. 2023;131(3):607–16. https://doi.org/10.1016/j.bja.2023.04.022.
41. Russotto V, Tassistro E, Myatra SN, Parotto M, Antolini L, Bauer P, Lascarrou JB, Szułdrzyński K, Camporota L, Putensen C, Pelosi P, Sorbello M, Higgs A, Greif R, Pesenti A, Valsecchi MG, Fumagalli R, Foti G, Bellani G, Laffey JG. Peri-intubation cardiovascular collapse in critically ill patients: insights from the INTUBE Study. Am J Respir Crit Care Med. 2022;206(4):449–58. https://doi.org/10.1164/rccm.202111-2575OC.
42. Salas E, Wilson KA, Burke CS, Priest HA. Using simulation-based training to improve patient safety: what does it take? Jt Comm J Qual Patient Saf. 2005;31(7):363–71. https://doi.org/10.1016/s1553-7250(05)31049-x.

43. Dow AW, Salas E, Mazmanian PE. Improving quality in systems of care: solving complicated challenges with simulation-based continuing professional development. J Contin Educ Heal Prof. 2012;32(4):230–5. https://doi.org/10.1002/chp.21150.
44. Jones CPL, Fawker-Corbett J, Groom P, Morton B, Lister C, Mercer SJ. Human factors in preventing complications in anaesthesia: a systematic review. Anaesthesia. 2018;73(Suppl 1):12–24. https://doi.org/10.1111/anae.14136.
45. Kelly FE, Frerk C, Bailey CR, Cook TM, Ferguson K, Flin R, Fong K, Groom P, John C, Lang AR, Meek T, Miller KL, Richmond L, Sevdalis N, Stacey MR. Human factors in anaesthesia: a narrative review. Anaesthesia. 2023;78(4):479–90. https://doi.org/10.1111/anae.15920.
46. Edelman DA, Duggan LV, Lockhart SL, Marshall SD, Turner MC, Brewster DJ. Prevalence and commonality of non-technical skills and human factors in airway management guidelines: a narrative review of the last 5 years. Anaesthesia. 2022;77(10):1129–36. https://doi.org/10.1111/anae.15813.
47. Kelly FE, Frerk C, Bailey CR, Cook TM, Ferguson K, Flin R, Fong K, Groom P, John C, Lang AR, Meek T, Miller KL, Richmond L, Sevdalis N, Stacey MR. Implementing human factors in anaesthesia: guidance for clinicians, departments and hospitals: Guidelines from the Difficult Airway Society and the Association of Anaesthetists: Guidelines from the Difficult Airway Society and the Association of Anaesthetists. Anaesthesia. 2023;78(4):458–78. https://doi.org/10.1111/anae.15941.
48. Croskerry P. The importance of cognitive errors in diagnosis and strategies to minimize them. Acad Med. 2003;78(8):775–80. https://doi.org/10.1097/00001888-200308000-00003.
49. Fuchs A, Nekhendzy V, Greif R. The evolving landscape of airway education in anesthesia for head and neck surgery. Curr Opin Anaesthesiol. 2025;38(6):817–24. https://doi.org/10.1097/ACO.0000000000001572.
50. Marchesini V, Asai T, Disma N. Cognitive errors in paediatric difficult airway management: a step into the unknown. Br J Anaesth. 2025;135(5):1394–6. https://doi.org/10.1016/j.bja.2025.06.002.
51. Mohanty PK. Human factors in difficult airway management: an anaesthetist's perspective. Natl J Maxillofac Surg. 2025;16(1):1–2. https://doi.org/10.4103/njms.njms_13_25. Epub 2025 Apr 28.
52. Chrimes N, Higgs A, Law JA, Baker PA, Cooper RM, Greif R, Kovacs G, Myatra SN, O'Sullivan EP, Rosenblatt WH, Ross CH, Sakles JC, Sorbello M, Hagberg CA. Project for Universal Management of Airways - part 1: concept and methods. Anaesthesia. 2020;75(12):1671–82. https://doi.org/10.1111/anae.15269.
53. Weingart SD, Barnicle RN, Malik S, Tanzi M, Wright B, McKenna P, Frost M, Lu C, King C, Singer A, Bracey A. The airway lead and the creation of a comprehensive emergency airway quality program. J Emerg Med. 2025;72:104–11. https://doi.org/10.1016/j.jemermed.2024.11.010.
54. Grigg E. Improving anesthesia safety: a human factors approach to feedback and system constraints. Curr Opin Anaesthesiol. 2025;38(6):769–75. https://doi.org/10.1097/ACO.0000000000001561.

17 Role of Echocardiography in Hemodynamic Instability

Marco Cinicola, Francesca Pompei, Veronica Basso, Emilia Moro, Silvia Rogante, and Luigi Tritapepe

17.1 Introduction

Critically ill patients admitted to the Intensive Care Unit experience hemodynamic instability due to cardiovascular alterations associated with the most common ICU pathologies (septic, cardiogenic, and obstructive shock; respiratory failure; trauma, renal, hepatic, or multiorgan failure; etc.). One of the main warning signs is hypotension, often accompanied by tissue hypoperfusion, which requires correction. Clearly, hemodynamic monitoring in these conditions is a top priority and is essential for diagnosing the underlying cause of instability, whether it is related to preload, afterload, or contractility. Especially in shock states, continuous hemodynamic monitoring, whether invasive or not, allows categorization of vasoplegia, hypovolemia, and low cardiac output states. The introduction of echocardiography and ultrasound in general has enabled us to increase diagnostic attention to anatomical (valvular disease, pericardial, and vascular disorders) or functional (left or right ventricular dysfunction, diastolic dysfunction) pathologies that can generate the aforementioned clinical categories, but which require different therapeutic approaches.

M. Cinicola · F. Pompei · V. Basso · E. Moro · S. Rogante · L. Tritapepe (✉)
Department of Anesthesia and Intensive Care, Emergency and Acceptance Department, San Camillo-Forlanini Hospital, Rome, Italy
e-mail: mcinicola@scamilloforlanini.rm.it; fpompei@scamilloforlanini.rm.it; vbasso@scamilloforlanini.rm.it; emoro@scamilloforlanini.rm.it; srogante@scamilloforlanini.rm.it; luigi.tritapepe@uniroma1.it

D. Chiumello, A. De Gasperi (eds.), *Practical Trends in Anesthesia and Intensive Care 2026*, https://doi.org/10.1007/978-3-032-25721-5_17

17.2 Role of Echocardiography

The use of echocardiography in the Intensive Care Unit is relatively recent, linked to the miniaturization of ultrasound machines and the resulting reduction in costs, but above all to a cultural shift regarding the utility of echocardiography in the hands of those already managing critically ill patients. Real-time visualization of cardiac function allows, after a rapid assessment of the heart's involvement in hemodynamic instability, accurate and noninvasive measurement of hemodynamic variables. In addition to its use in diagnosing hemodynamic decompensation syndromes, echocardiography can be employed as a semicontinuous monitoring system, enabling assessment of cardiac output adequacy, positive fluid responsiveness, and improvement in cardiac performance, the measurement of intracavitary pressures, and, above all, the effects of ventilation on hemodynamic status. Since the use of echocardiography does not conflict with hemodynamic monitoring, but rather certifies its use and validity, the new concept of "echodynamics" is gaining ground among intensivists. We will therefore attempt to describe some of the most important hemodynamic parameters that can be obtained in the Intensive Care Unit in patients with hemodynamic instability. There are guidelines, clearly described and supported by extensive literature, that define the paradigmatic cases in which echocardiography should be used [1]. These paradigmatic cases are classified as appropriateness class A, such as unexplained hypotension, respiratory failure with hemodynamic instability, pulmonary embolism or suspected pulmonary embolism, and myocardial ischemia/infarction. The superiority of echocardiography in these situations, both due to its noninvasiveness in the case of transthoracic echocardiography (TTE) [2, 3] and its semi-invasive nature in the case of transesophageal echocardiography (TEE) [4], is demonstrated by the ability to assess in real time the cause of hemodynamic instability, as well as to visualize the morphology and function of the cardiac chambers. Current technological advances applied to echocardiography allow most patients to be studied via the transthoracic approach, using standard windows and planes from which clinically applicable conclusions can be drawn (Fig. 17.1).

Two-dimensional (2D) echocardiography allows visualization of most cardiac structures, enabling assessment of the morphology and size of the right and left chambers, the cardiac walls, and the presence of masses within the cardiac chambers. This information is fundamentally qualitative, and Doppler ultrasound in its various modes (pulsed, continuous, and color) is necessary to obtain information on the direction and velocity of blood flow in the different chambers and major vessels. By knowing the flow velocity and simplifying the Bernoulli equation, we can calculate the pressure gradient between chambers, determine valve areas, and assess the intracavitary pressures of the different cardiac chambers (Fig. 17.2).

TEE [4] is reserved for situations in which the available window is inadequate or suboptimal for TTE (obese patients, COPD, mechanically ventilated, post-thoracic surgery, etc.); when we need to evaluate structures that are difficult to examine with TTE (e.g., the atrial appendages, thoracic aorta, or prosthetic valves); or when a diagnosis requires high-quality imaging, as in acute aortic syndrome, endocarditis

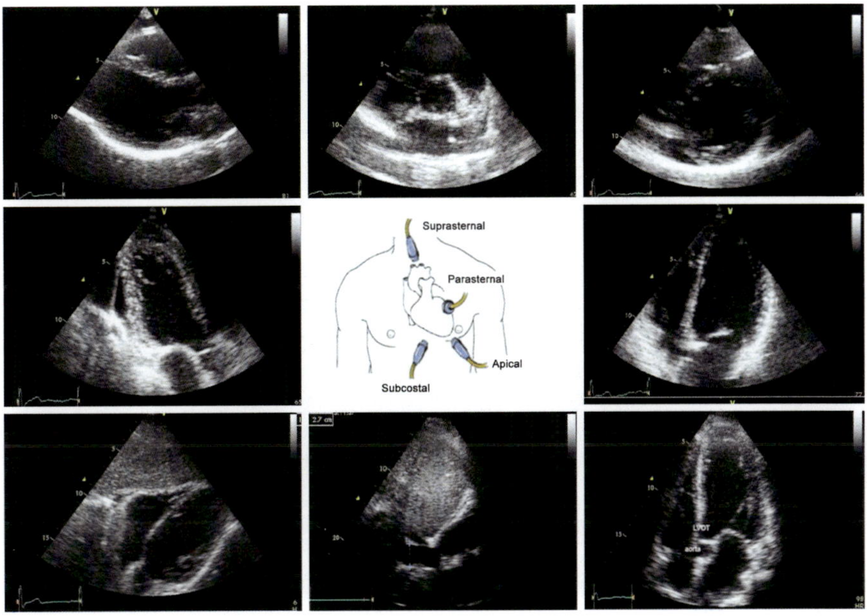

Fig. 17.1 Various transthoracic echocardiographic views

Fig. 17.2 Illustration of the Bernoulli equation

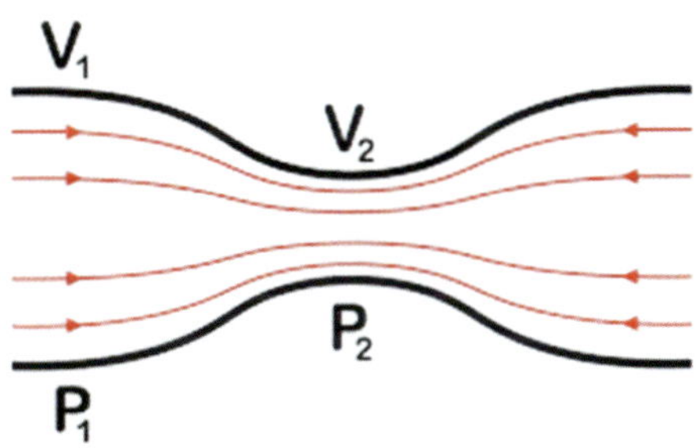

and its complications, and the detection of thrombi, masses, or prosthetic dysfunction. A common refrain among non-echocardiographer clinicians is that echocardiography has a major limitation in being operator-dependent. Our scientific society, SIAARTI, has long been committed to echocardiographic training for anesthesiologists and intensivists, precisely to enable everyone to perform at least a basic echocardiographic examination that, in situations of severe hemodynamic instability, allows rapid recognition of conditions that may quickly deteriorate if not diagnosed or if treated incorrectly. In this context, a basic two-dimensional echocardiographic study allows us to confirm or rule out clinical situations based on binary (yes/no) answers to ensure the need for urgent treatment. A series of basic questions must be considered when performing echocardiography in the critically ill patient in shock: Is the heart involved? Is the dysfunction in the right or left heart? Is the patient adequately filled? Another very interesting aspect is the ability to rapidly assess, with echocardiography, the positive effects of targeted therapy. The intensive care literature demonstrates the utility of echocardiography in obtaining hemodynamic measurements that can be used both for diagnostic purposes and to analyze variability and changes induced by applied treatments.

17.3 Left Ventricle

One of the classic questions when facing a patient with hemodynamic instability is: Is this a cardiac problem? And if so, is left ventricular function (LVF) impaired? Assessment of left ventricular function is one of the fundamental elements for intelligently managing hemodynamic instability and thus making an informed choice between volume replacement and inotropic/vasopressor drugs [5]. Many clinical conditions, initially or apparently noncardiac, ultimately affect the left ventricle, such as pancreatitis, sepsis, neurogenic disorders, intoxications, anaphylaxis, and brain death. In septic shock in particular, there is a high incidence of left ventricular systolic and diastolic dysfunction in over 40% of patients [6]. This is also due to the inappropriate use of drugs and fluids, which can affect left ventricular function. The quantitative methods used to estimate left ventricular systolic function with echocardiography include linear measurements in M-mode, two-dimensional measurements in 2D mode, and calculations derived from intracardiac flows using Doppler echocardiography (Fig. 17.3).

The assessment of LVF should first and foremost be performed visually (eyeball method) to immediately recognize a normal geometry or a dilated heart with regular motion, that is, walls that synchronously move closer together and thicken during contraction. In this way, it is possible to initially differentiate between normal, depressed, or severely depressed contraction by referring to the geometric difference between systole and diastole. This first step already allows for differentiation of therapy, especially fluid management. The subjective visual estimation of ejection fraction (EF) is widely used in daily clinical practice, although experience is required on the part of the intensivist to determine the different degrees of dysfunction (<30% severely depressed, >30% to <40% moderately depressed, >40% to <55% mildly depressed, and > 55% normal), with an acceptable correlation with quantitative determinations [2, 3]. Extreme values are easily identifiable. In this context, a group of intensivists with 2 hours of theoretical training and only 4 hours of practice, using a portable echocardiograph, were able to correctly identify normal LVF in 92% of cases and depressed LVF in 80% of cases. The most common error

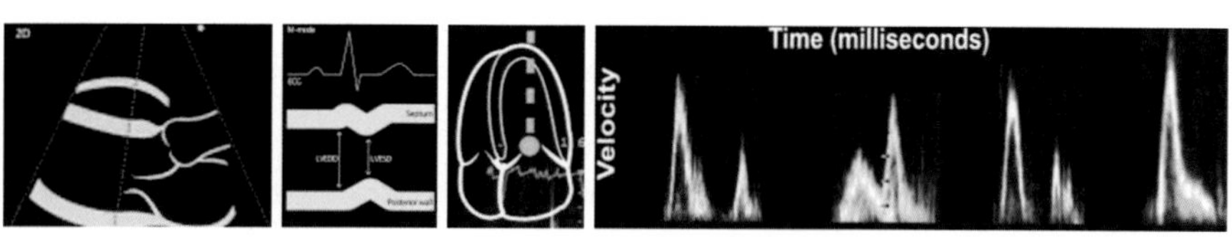

Fig. 17.3 Methods for assessing left ventricular function

is overestimation of left ventricular function. Going into further detail, the assessment of left ventricular function (LVF) may involve linear measurements, area measurements, and finally volume measurements. For these measurements, both one-dimensional (M-mode) and two-dimensional (2D) techniques are used. The combination of these two methods allows, in the parasternal long-axis view, for a perpendicular section of the left ventricle to be obtained, enabling measurement not only of wall thicknesses but, most importantly, of diastolic and systolic diameters. To accurately determine where to place the diastolic and systolic cuts of the left ventricle, the electrocardiogram is used (the diastolic diameter coincides with the peak of the R wave on the ECG trace, while the systolic diameter corresponds to the point of maximum excursion of the endocardial margin). Clearly, the more perpendicular the M-mode cut is to the ventricle, the more accurate the measurement. From these measurements, the shortening fraction (SF) can be obtained: SF = (Dd − Ds)/Dd × 100 (Fig. 17.4), which expresses the percentage relationship between the standardized diastolic and systolic diameters relative to the diastolic diameter (normal value >30%). This technique has significant limitations in cases of non-global structural and functional abnormalities (ischemic heart disease) or when the imaging plane does not meet the required perpendicularity between the cardiac walls. It is therefore highly operator-dependent. The methodology is also influenced by preload and contractility and assesses only the function of the segments intersected by the ultrasound beam. Consequently, left ventricular function is estimated assuming symmetric contraction. However, the parameters are easy to obtain, reproducible, and reliable for functional assessment, as no mathematical model needs to

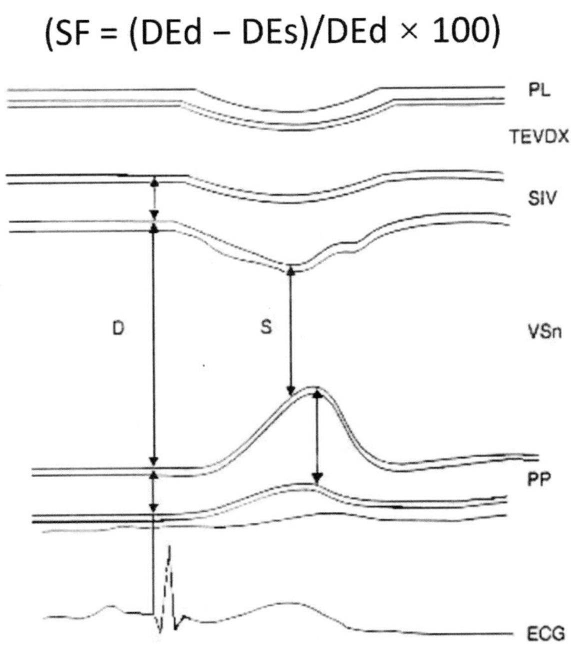

Fig. 17.4 M-mode assessment of cardiac diameters

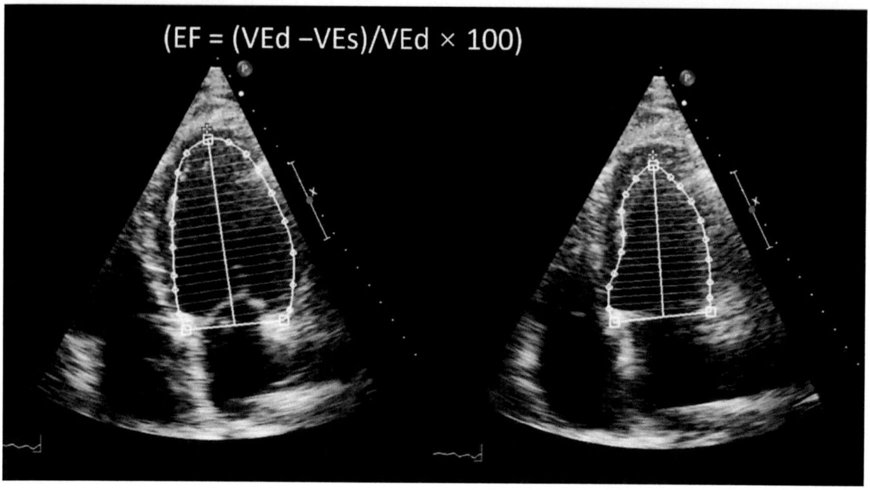

Fig. 17.5 Measurement of EF using the Simpson method

be assumed. An assessment of diastolic and systolic areas in the parasternal short-axis view allows evaluation of the fractional area change (FAC) of the left ventricle: FAC = (Area D − Area S)/Area D × 100 (normal values >40%) [2, 3]. It is intuitive that if the two areas differ greatly, despite being affected by volume load, this indicates good LVF. As experience increases, it becomes possible to measure the ejection fraction, which relates the end-diastolic ventricular volume (EDV) to the end-systolic ventricular volume (ESV), standardized to the end-diastolic volume (EF = (EDV − ESV)/EDV × 100) (Fig. 17.5).

This type of measurement considers the left ventricular ellipse as composed of a series of disks stacked from the base to the apex of the heart (Simpson's method), which, when measured together by tracing the endocardial border and excluding the papillary muscles, represent the volume of the left ventricle. This measurement must be performed in 2D, considering both the four-chamber and two-chamber views and averaging the two measurements. A complex formula, implemented in the ultrasound software and thus immediately available as a value, allows calculation of the end-systolic volume (ESV) and end-diastolic volume (EDV), and thus the ejection fraction derived from the formula: EF = (EDV − ESV)/EDV. The main limitations of the method are the difficulty, in many cases, of delineating the endocardial border and creating a true apical sagittal plane (which is thinner than the surrounding level), where it is very common to obtain a tangential rather than orthogonal two-chamber apical acquisition relative to the four-chamber apical view. These methods analyze LVF globally, but can also be used to assess segmental systolic function. In fact, dividing the myocardium into basal, mid, and apical segments in both apical long-axis views (4C, 2C, and 3C) and short-axis (parasternal) views allows for the evaluation of thickening and contraction in these 17 segments, thereby enabling the identification of areas of hypokinesia, dyskinesia, or akinesia and correlating these kinetic abnormalities with the different coronary perfusion territories of the explored regions.

17.4 Right Ventricle

The right ventricle can be considered almost the most affected ventricle in critical care pathologies due to its functional dependence on ventilatory issues [7]. The questions an intensivist faces in cases of hemodynamic instability are: Is the patient's right ventricle normal? Is it functioning? Is there acute cor pulmonale? The function of the right ventricle, which is difficult to assess hemodynamically, has long been neglected due to limited understanding and its assessment being almost exclusively based on pressure and flow measurements (Swan-Ganz catheter). As a result of these shortcomings in measurement and reproducibility, echocardiography has become an indispensable tool for functional assessment of the right ventricle. Under normal conditions, the right ventricle (RV) functions as a low-pressure chamber, highly adaptable to volume overload but with limited response to increases in pressure within the pulmonary arterial system. This is particularly important in diagnosing right ventricular failure associated with pulmonary embolism, acute respiratory distress syndrome (ARDS), cardiac tamponade, and all situations in which heart-lung interactions, influenced by intrathoracic pressure changes from mechanical ventilation, lead to right-sided heart failure [7]. By using different imaging planes and despite anatomical and technical challenges (the RV's complex geometry, irregular crescent shape, thin walls, irregular endocardial surface with a moderator band and trabeculae that make endocardial border identification difficult), echocardiography allows for the study of the global right heart chambers, particularly with two-dimensional imaging, which guides M-mode measurements and the orientation of the ultrasound beam in Doppler techniques (Fig. 17.6).

Various views allow for measurement of right ventricular diameters (M-mode) and areas (2D). Additionally, both in apical and subcostal 4C views and in parasternal short-axis, we can assess the interdependence of the two ventricles and their geometric relationship with the left ventricle [8]. In the parasternal long-axis view, the visible portion of the right ventricle allows measurement of the maximum diameter, which should not exceed 30 mm (normal range 9–26 mm); this measurement enables the identification of right ventricular dilation. This diameter can change rapidly with fluid challenge and thus serves as an indicator of the effectiveness of volume resuscitation in correcting hemodynamic instability. Furthermore, in the 4C view, we can assess the size of the right atrium and the orientation of the interatrial and interventricular septa, which reflect pressure increases in the examined chambers. In general, several studies have demonstrated the feasibility of measuring diameters, determining areas by planimetry, and calculating ejection fraction, although this is challenging due to the RV's geometry. In this context, various methods have been developed involving the measurement of different diameters, which are poorly reproducible in routine emergency practice. For these reasons, the relative dimensional relationship between RV and LV at end-diastole is analyzed

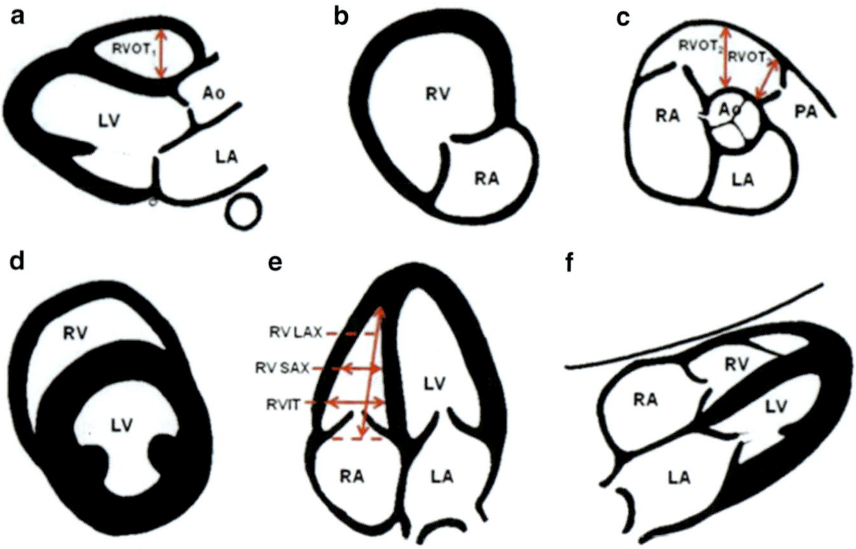

Fig. 17.6 Various views for the assessment of the right ventricle

(normal ratio < 0.6 with RV < LV; moderate RV dilation = LV; severe RV dilation RV > LV, with ratio > 1). Special attention should be paid to the assessment of the interventricular septum (IVS), the muscular wall separating the right ventricle (RV) from the left ventricle (LV) [8]. Although anatomically and functionally part of the LV, in certain pathological conditions, it bows toward the left, resulting in left ventricular hypodiastolia, which is difficult to correct with fluid therapy. The IVS diameter in diastole is 7–11 mm, which is three times greater than the diameter of the RV free wall, with a systolic thickening of 35%. Echocardiography is the only technique that allows us to study interventricular dynamics and interdependence. IVS motion can be analyzed using two-dimensional echocardiography, particularly in the parasternal short-axis view at the level of the mitral valve. The LV appears as a circular structure and the septum as an arc comprising 2/5 of the circumference. Under normal conditions, the IVS is convex toward the RV and concave toward the LV, maintaining this morphology throughout the cardiac cycle. Abnormalities in motion, such as paradoxical systolic movement or the configuration of the RV in both systole and diastole, can be used to identify the presence of diastolic or systolic overload. In cases of RV diastolic overload, the IVS flattens during diastole, as RV diastolic pressure equals or exceeds that of the LV. Systolic overload, in the presence of higher pressure in the RV compared to LV, is identified by the presence of a flattened septum (D shape, Fig. 17.7).

both in systole and diastole, with reduced dynamics. The analysis of segmental contractility abnormalities becomes particularly important in right ventricular infarction, which is typically characterized by akinesia or dyskinesia of some of the surfaces explored in different views. When the right ventricle is larger than the left,

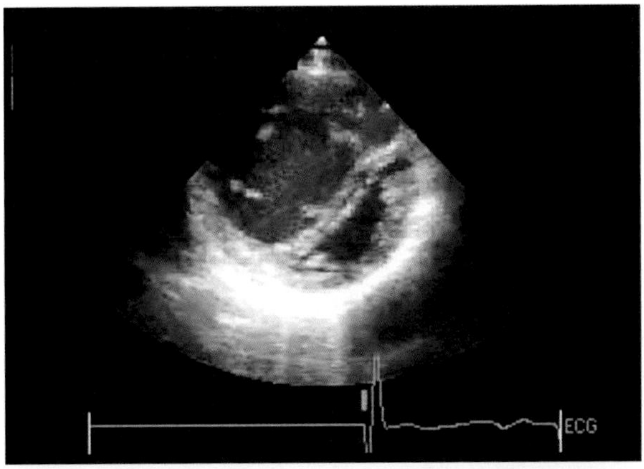

Fig. 17.7 D shape of the left ventricle

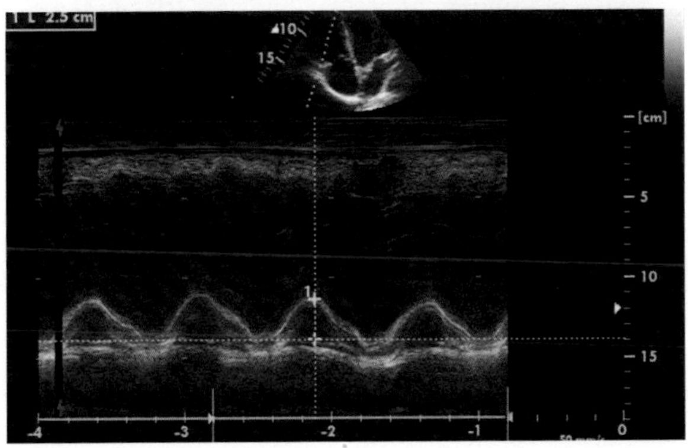

Fig. 17.8 TAPSE

with a hypokinetic mid-free wall and a hyperkinetic apical wall of the right ventricle (McConnell's sign), a systolic pulmonary artery pressure of 50 mmHg, and significant tricuspid regurgitation, pulmonary embolism can be hypothesized as the causal event of hemodynamic instability. These signs are clearly related to the increased pressure generated in the right heart chambers. Considering the contractile movement of the right ventricle, which differs from that of the left ventricle—after diastolic filling, the blood flow is propelled toward the pulmonary artery by a piston-like movement—it is possible to simplify the assessment of right ventricular function using M-mode on the lateral portion of the tricuspid annulus. The tricuspid annular plane systolic excursion (TAPSE, Fig. 17.8) is measured in M-mode and represents the excursion or distance of the tricuspid annulus displacement from end-diastole to end-systole [9].

This simple measurement, validated in the literature, is not affected by heart rate (HR) but is influenced by preload and afterload. It remains a straightforward method for assessing right ventricular contractility. Values below 15 mm are considered pathological and carry a negative prognostic significance. More accurate is the measurement of the peak systolic velocity of the S wave using tissue Doppler imaging

(TDI), performed at the lateral wall of the right ventricle in the apical four-chamber view. A positive wave is recorded after the QRS and is preceded by another, shorter wave corresponding to isovolumetric contraction. Normal values are considered to be 15 ± 2 cm/s, while right ventricular dysfunction is defined as <10 cm/s. Using echocardiography in its M-mode and 2D modalities, we can obtain both direct and indirect data related to pulmonary hypertension, suspect its presence even though the assessment is not quantitative, and study its effects on the cardiac valves and right heart chambers. Doppler echocardiography is the technique that provides information and quantification of pulmonary hypertension. Analysis of the morphology of the pulmonary flow can be performed in the parasternal short-axis view at the base of the heart, placing the pulsed Doppler sample volume at the level of the pulmonary valve. Under normal conditions, a triangular wave is observed, which gradually accelerates with a peak in mid-systole, followed by a slow decline ending just before valve closure (type I). The presence of a midsystolic notch is indicative of severe pulmonary hypertension (type III), with a sensitivity of 56% and a specificity of 100% for PAP > 50 mmHg. This measurement, which is not easy to obtain, is nonetheless a highly reliable method for quantifying pulmonary hypertension. More simply, we can take advantage of the presence of tricuspid regurgitation, which generates a regurgitant flow into the right atrium, clearly visible with color Doppler. In the four-chamber view, this regurgitation can be quantified with continuous-wave Doppler because the projection allows perfect alignment of the Doppler with the direction of the regurgitant jet. In this way, by measuring the maximum velocity of the regurgitant jet in m/s, the transvalvular pressure gradient between the right atrium (RA) and right ventricle (RV) can be calculated using the modified Bernoulli equation: $PRV - PRA = 4 \times Vmax^2$. The right ventricular systolic pressure is equal to the sum of the systolic gradient between RA and RV plus the right atrial pressure (RAP) and, in the absence of right atrial outflow tract obstruction, is equal to the systolic pressure of the pulmonary artery, so: $PAP = 4 \times Vmax^2 + RAP$ [10]. Several alternatives are available to determine the mean right atrial pressure to be added to the gradient, such as:

- Use of a central venous catheter
- Use of the diameter of the inferior vena cava (IVC) (normal diameter 16 ± 2 mm) and its inspiratory collapse index (IC), due to the good correlation between these parameters and right atrial pressure

An IVC ≤ 21 mm with IC > 50% estimates an RA pressure between 0 and 5 mmHg, while an IVC > 21 mm and a non-collapsible vein indicate a pressure ≥ 15 mmHg. The reliability of this estimate is well established in the literature; however, there are technical limitations in patients admitted to intensive care. In particular, mechanical ventilation complicates the technique due to the absence of an adequate echocardiographic window. In non-ventilated patients, the presence of dyspnea and the inability to tolerate the left lateral decubitus position are the main obstacles. In the presence of arrhythmias, particularly atrial fibrillation, it is necessary to average measurements over 5–10 beats. Despite these limitations, the measurement of pulmonary artery systolic pressure by Doppler echocardiography is reliable, with good correlation to invasive methods [11].

17.5 Cardiac Output (CO)

Patients in the Intensive Care Unit need to adjust their cardiac output, or more precisely their stroke volume, to meet the metabolic demands imposed by their underlying conditions. Naturally, one of the intensivist's key questions is to determine the cardiac output and assess whether it is adequate. Classic invasive hemodynamic monitoring (including both pulmonary or transpulmonary dilution techniques and pulse contour analysis) as well as noninvasive methods (digital pressure clamp, bioreactance, etc.) allow for continuous monitoring of this parameter, proving fundamental and almost irreplaceable. The limitation of classic monitoring is that it categorizes low or high output states without providing diagnostic insight into the underlying cause, which may be related to alterations in preload, afterload, or, much less directly, contractility. Echocardiography, with certain limitations, can provide an estimate of cardiac output with the distinct advantage of also offering insight into the cause of its alteration. However, cardiac output measurement by echocardiography is a spot measurement, not continuous, and cannot replace CO monitoring in the critically ill patient. Cardiac output is an estimate of the global function of the cardiovascular system and is calculated as the product of heart rate (HR) and stroke volume (SV). According to the principles of classical hydrodynamics, the volume passing through a given section can be calculated by multiplying the area of the section (Area, cm^2) by the time-velocity integral (VTI, cm) of the flow through it; this represents the systolic distance traveled by the blood during the measured time period: SV = A × VTI (Fig. 17.9) [12, 13].

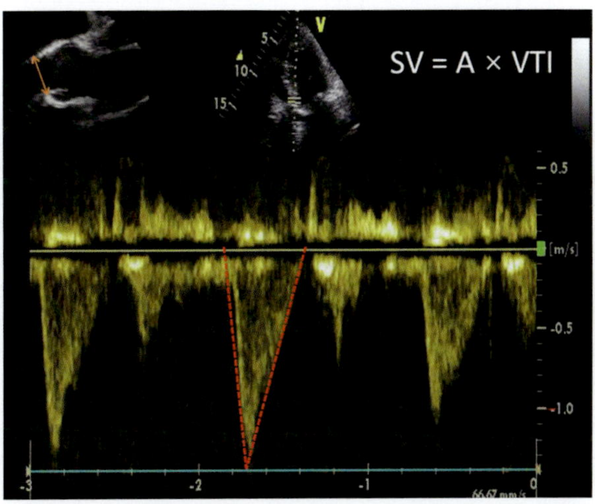

Fig. 17.9 Method for measuring cardiac output with transthoracic echocardiography

The area most commonly used for this purpose in clinical practice is the area of the aortic valve annulus. The annular diameter (D) is measured at the insertion of the valve cusps or leaflets, which in most cases is best visualized in the parasternal long-axis view of the left ventricle in TTE and/or the mid-esophageal two-chamber view in TEE, assuming a circular geometry. To this end, the area is zoomed in at the onset of systole, measuring from the insertion or junction of the anterior cusp on the endocardium to the same point on the posterior cusp: area = $\pi \times (D/2)^2 = 0.785 \times D^2$. The stroke volume is thus determined by calculating the volume of blood passing through the aortic valve with each beat. Pulsed Doppler provides the flow velocity spectrum at this level, using the apical five-chamber or three-chamber view, which allows for a more parallel alignment between the flow direction and the Doppler beam. In aortic valve disease, due to the difficulty in accurately identifying the effective diameter, it is preferable to use the diameter of the left ventricular outflow tract (LVOT), also considering its structural integrity despite volumetric changes in the left ventricle. The flow measurement (VTI) of the LVOT is performed by placing the sample volume near the valve area, on the ventricular side. Normal values range from 18 to 23 cm; a value of <12 cm indicates low output [12, 13]. Currently, all echocardiography systems provide the VTI (in cm) when the Doppler signal curve is traced using the built-in measurement software. Thus, CO (cm^3 /min) = $0.785 \times D^2$ (cm^2) × VTI (cm/beat) × HR (beats/min). Despite the assumptions underlying this method and the need for careful, high-quality imaging, it has shown acceptable overall correlation with invasive techniques, although with considerable individual variability and the requirement for a normal LVOT and absence of significant aortic regurgitation. The main limitation is error in measuring the subaortic annular diameter (LVOT), particularly since this error is amplified by squaring the measurement (i.e., raising it to the second power) (Fig. 17.9). The mean flow velocity in the LVOT is an extremely useful parameter for estimating cardiac index, and especially for monitoring changes that occur in response to new hemodynamic situations or following treatment. Furthermore, the aortic VTI, in cases of mechanical ventilation and hypovolemia, fluctuates between maximum and minimum values during the ventilatory cycle, providing an indication of fluid responsiveness.

17.6 Pressures and Diastolic Function

Without entering into the longstanding debate over pressures and volumes in hemodynamic monitoring, it is important to recall the role of pressure monitoring, which can ensure or reduce flow to and from a cardiac chamber and the peripheral circulation. So, can we estimate filling pressures with echocardiography? Although the literature has shown that isolated pressure measurements, such as CVP or wedge pressure, are not highly reliable, we believe that when these are combined with measurements of stroke volume and vascular resistance, they can still play a significant role in assessing the need for volume replacement. However, it is essential to emphasize that knowledge of both function and morphology—that is, the morpho-functional characteristics—of the left and right ventricles, which only echocardiography can provide, is indispensable. Thus, in a patient with hemodynamic instability, knowledge of the pulmonary capillary wedge pressure is fundamental when integrated with important data such as the anatomical characteristics of the left ventricle (hypertrophic/dilated) and its overall function. The wedge pressure is an indicator of preload and left ventricular function and has diagnostic applications, allowing us to distinguish between different etiologies of pulmonary edema. Educationally, preload is correlated with the left ventricular end-diastolic volume, and the pressure generated by this volume is assimilated to the left atrial pressure, which in turn correlates with the wedge pressure. Since this pressure equilibrium is established during the various phases of diastole, the use of Doppler can allow us to estimate these pressures non-invasively (Table 17.1) [14].

The filling flow across the mitral valve during diastole allows assessment of left ventricular filling, which is evaluated by pulsed-wave Doppler (Pw) by placing the sample volume at the free edge of the mitral valve leaflets in the apical four-chamber view. At each time point during diastolic filling, the velocity represented by the wave reflects the instantaneous pressure gradient between the left atrium and the left ventricle, in accordance with the Bernoulli equation. The Doppler velocity spectrum consists of two waves if the patient is in sinus rhythm: the E wave (Early), corresponding to rapid protodiastolic filling, and the A wave (Atrial), dependent on atrial contraction [14]. Similarly, by placing the pulsed Doppler sample volume between the mitral valve and the left ventricular outflow tract in the apical five-chamber view, using color Doppler as a guide to flow direction, the systolic flow curve at that level can be obtained, allowing measurement of the isovolumic relaxation time (IVRT). Its duration is measured from the closure artifact of the aortic flow to the onset of mitral flow (E wave). Typically, the normal mitral inflow curve in a middle-aged individual shows an E wave (velocity 80 ± 16 cm/s) slightly greater than the A wave (56 ± 13 cm/s), with an E/A ratio > 1, an E wave deceleration time (DT) of about 180 ms (199 ± 32), and an IVRT around 90 ms (69 ± 12 ms). By simultaneously recording the diastolic filling waves of the left ventricle and the systolic flow curve, a comprehensive representation of the cardiac cycle is obtained. The interaction between diastolic filling flow (generating the E and A waves on pulsed Doppler) and the elastic properties of the left ventricle (compliance) determines the diastolic characteristics of the left ventricle that can describe specific patterns. The onset of diastolic dysfunction involves conditions of impaired ventricular relaxation and altered ventricular filling, which are clearly dependent on and

Table 17.1 Estimation of LAP using Doppler parameters

Doppler parameters	Threshold value	Predicted LAP	Specificity	Positive predictive value
E/A	>2	>18 mmHg	–	100%
DT	<175 ms	=18 mmHg	94%	–
E/e′	>15 >7 >7.5	>18–20 mmHg =13 mmHg =15 mmHg	88% 92% 81%	– – –
E/Vp	>2 >2.6	=13 mmHg >18 mmHg		

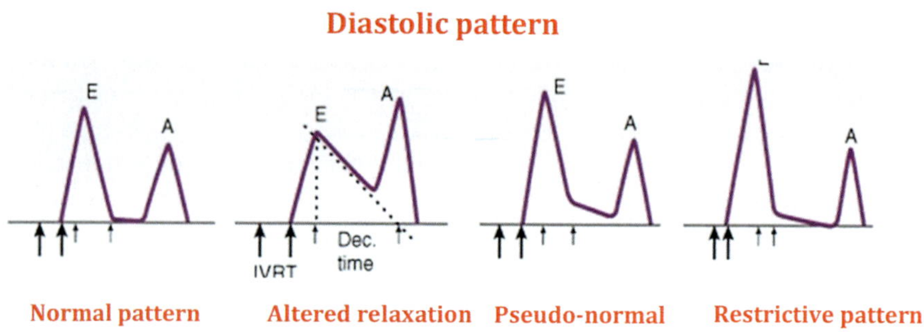

Fig. 17.10 Diastolic patterns on pulsed-wave transmitral Doppler

result in increased left atrial pressure (LAP). Consequently, the morphology of the curve is modified by various factors, such as existing hemodynamic conditions, heart rate, and age. Its features and the evolution of filling patterns in relation to the degree of diastolic dysfunction are summarized in Fig. 17.10.

The mitral inflow velocity curve is technically very simple to obtain, reproducible, and easy to perform at the patient's bedside. An E/A ratio ≥ 2 has low sensitivity (52%) but high specificity (100%) for detecting LAP ≥20 mmHg. If associated with a DT < 180 ms, LAP is ≥20 mmHg, with both sensitivity and specificity of 100%. These conditions are valid in patients with reduced EF, while in patients with preserved function—thus with normal ventricular relaxation—these findings lose some of their significance. The assessment of diastolic function cannot be limited to the simple, though effective in some contexts, transmitral Doppler, but requires multiple evaluations that demand greater echocardiographic expertise. The early diastolic inflow velocity can be assessed using color M-mode, which highlights, in the apical 4C view, the slope of the left ventricular inflow velocity (Propagation Velocity, Vp). After freezing the image, Vp is measured as the gradient of the line separating the first aliasing of early diastolic flow (blue/red transition) from the mitral annulus to the apex of the ventricle (normal >60 cm/s) (Fig. 17.11).

By combining various parameters obtained from different measurement techniques, reliable estimates of LAP can be achieved. The ratio between the peak velocity of the E wave on transmitral Doppler and the propagation velocity (E/Vp) > 2.5 predicts an LAP >15 mmHg. This measurement is less affected by loading conditions but loses predictive value in the presence of atrial fibrillation. Its predictive capacity is also lost in ventricular dysfunction (cardiomyopathies, stenosis, or the presence of a mitral valve prosthesis).

17.6.1 Tissue Doppler Imaging (TDI)

One application of Doppler is the measurement of myocardial contraction and relaxation velocities, rather than the velocity of red blood cell flow. Pulsed Doppler sampling of the myocardium at the level of the mitral annulus in septal or lateral position in the 4C view reflects the movement of the longitudinal cardiac fibers.

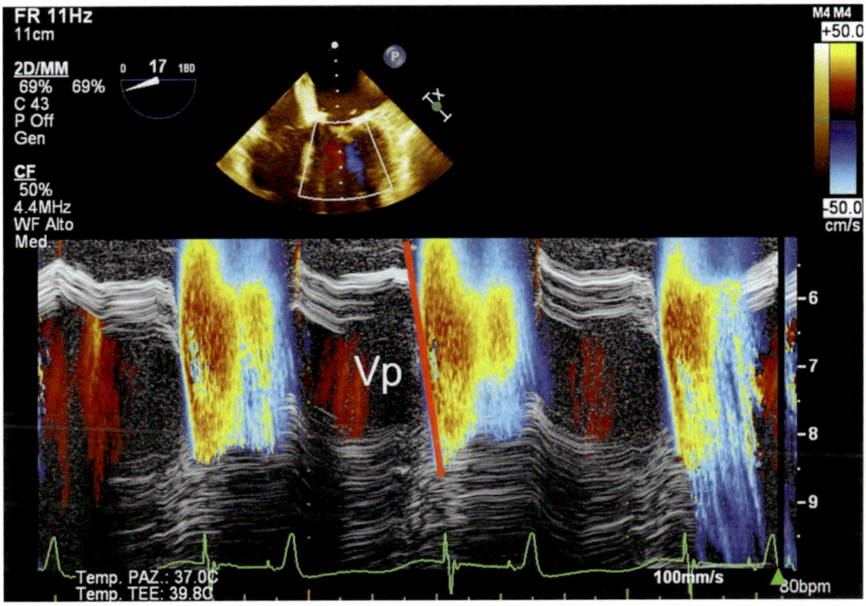

Fig. 17.11 Representation of Vp on color M-mode

This Doppler modality is Tissue Doppler Imaging (TDI), which is better able to assess diastolic function, as it is less affected by loading conditions [15]. Tissue Doppler can also be applied to the tricuspid annulus, providing valuable information on right ventricular function. The waves generated by TDI measure systolic and diastolic velocities (approximately 1/10 of blood flow velocity) and specifically include:

- S′, systolic wave, which shows two components in some patients and represents isovolumetric contraction and the ejection phase of systole. A peak systolic velocity S′ > 9 cm/s predicts an EF >50% with a sensitivity of 88% and a specificity of 97%.
- e′, early diastolic wave, representing the rapid filling phase.
- a′, late diastolic wave, representing the late filling phase and atrial contraction (Fig. 17.12) [16–18].

TDI requires greater expertise, but given its lower dependence on loading conditions, it is very useful in revealing pseudonormalized patterns on transmitral Doppler or in cases of atrial fibrillation. Special attention should be paid to patients with prosthetic valves or mitral annular calcification. The ratio between the peak velocity of the E wave and that of the e′ wave (E/e′) can provide information on left atrial pressure (LAP). An E/e′ ratio > 15 indicates a LAP >18–20 mmHg [16–19]. Other data, including pulmonary vein flow (PVF) or combined parameters, can be used in cases where the mitral filling pattern presents some of the aforementioned

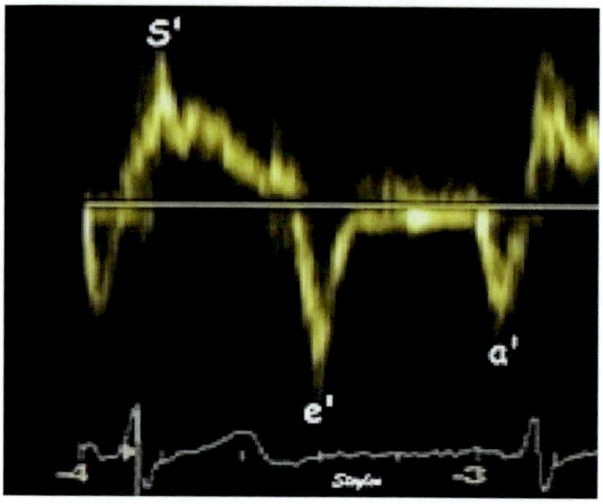

Fig. 17.12 TDI image of the mitral annulus

limitations. It is important to remember that all these measurements can be rapidly obtained at the bedside using transthoracic echocardiography and can be repeated as often as necessary. Finally, attention should be paid to left atrial size, as increased dimensions are always associated with diastolic dysfunction.

17.7 Preload

The greatest debate in intensive care medicine concerns preload. Which indicators should be considered: pressures, volumes, or an integration of both measurements? In practice, the question every intensivist faces in the presence of hemodynamic instability is: Is the patient full or empty? And is the heart preload-dependent? We have learned that dynamic indices related to heart-lung interaction, while never indicating the patient's actual volemic status, can identify which patients, classified as fluid responders, may benefit from volume replacement to improve stroke volume [20]. Echocardiography plays an effective role in this assessment. In fact, certain measurements (left ventricular end-diastolic area and volume) have been proposed as reliable indices of preload. Specifically, when the indexed left ventricular end-diastolic area measures <5.5 cm^2/m^2, we can state with certainty that the patient is hypovolemic. Many diametric (right-sided), Doppler, and dimensional measurements of the cardiac chambers can indicate which patients may be considered susceptible to volume expansion (low preload), but above all, dynamic changes in flow can indicate a positive response to fluid loading in fluid responders. Echocardiographic assessment offers many advantages over traditional hemodynamic measurements (PPV, SVV, SPV) [21] because it combines these indices with cardiac morphology and function. In fact, we can construct a Frank-Starling curve using the various parasternal short-axis views of the left ventricles of our patients.

17.7.1 Analysis of the Inferior Vena Cava (IVC) Diameter

The subcostal view often allows assessment of the inferior vena cava and suprahepatic veins, providing an indirect estimate of right atrial pressure. Variations in intra-abdominal pressure and respiration rapidly alter its volume. During inspiration, venous return increases and the IVC diameter decreases. The size and reduction in diameter during inspiration (collapse index: maximum diameter in expiration minus minimum diameter in inspiration divided by maximum diameter in expiration) correlate with mean right atrial pressure. The IVC respiratory variability index has been defined as $Dmax - Dmin/(Dmax + Dmin)/2 \times 100$, where Dmax and Dmin are the maximum and minimum IVC values, respectively, during a mechanical respiratory cycle (Fig. 17.13) [22].

Observing a variation in IVC diameter $\geq 12\%$ allows us to distinguish between responders and nonresponders to volume expansion, with high sensitivity and specificity. Assessment of the IVC during spontaneous breathing appears adequate for estimating fluid responsiveness if it detects a small IVC with a high collapsibility index; this low reliability compared to what is observed in intubated patients appears to be related to the variability in respiratory rate and amplitude, to which must be added the variability in diastolic filling during arrhythmia (atrial fibrillation). For a long time, we reasoned according to the full/empty logic: a small and collapsible IVC was considered synonymous with a "depleted" patient, while a dilated and hyporeactive IVC characterized a "full" patient. While the first statement is currently accepted, the second is only partially true. In fact, there are several pathological conditions that can influence the degree of IVC collapsibility: in particular, in the presence of conditions that increase CVP (tension pneumothorax, cardiac tamponade, application of PEEP, chronic cor pulmonale, right ventricular infarction, pulmonary embolism, severe tricuspid regurgitation, cardiac contusion, ARDS, abdominal compartment syndrome), the IVC becomes dilated and hyporeactive, but this does not exclude the possibility that the patient is still fluid responsive [21].

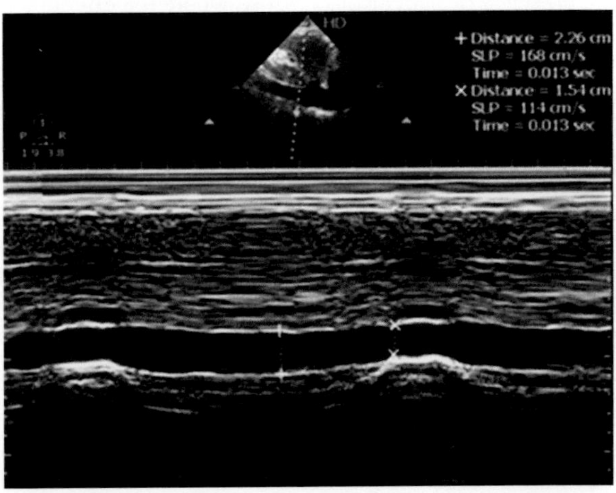

Fig. 17.13 IVC in M-mode

17.7.2 Analysis of Superior Vena Cava (SVC) Diameter Variability

In mechanically ventilated patients, transesophageal echocardiography can be used to assess the inspiratory increase in pleural pressure during lung insufflation, which produces a total or partial collapse of the SVC. Observation of this collapse suggests that, at this point, the external pressure exerted by the thoracic cavity on the superior vena cava exceeds the venous pressure. In this context, it has been shown that a variability in SVC diameter greater than 36% predicts a positive response to volume expansion, with a sensitivity of 90% and a specificity of 100% [23].

17.7.3 Analysis of Aortic Peak Flow Velocity (PFV) Variation

This parameter is obtained by recording the aortic flow in the left ventricular outflow tract (see cardiac output). A PFV variation value (PVmax − PVmin/PVmax + PVmin/2 × 100) of 12% can also be used in the assessment of volume expansion [24].

17.7.4 Passive Leg Raising (PLR)

An alternative to the fluid challenge for inducing a change in preload is Passive Leg Raising: this maneuver is comparable to an "autotransfusion" and can be performed simply by raising the patient's lower limbs while in a semi-recumbent position by tilting the bed for a few minutes. This results in the recruitment of approximately 300–500 cc of "unstressed" blood without infusing fluids. The assessment of fluid responsiveness can be performed using a continuous and invasive SV monitoring method (preferable) or a noninvasive (echocardiographic) method, carried out before, during, and after the maneuver, bearing in mind that the maximum hemodynamic effect of PLR occurs within one minute [25]. PLR has its limitations: it cannot be performed in patients with trauma, abdominal compartment syndrome, or in the presence of pain or discomfort, where the effect of volume expansion is reduced due to catecholaminergic activation [26]. The advantages are the possibility of performing the maneuver even in the presence of arrhythmia, during spontaneous breathing, and above all, inducing a change in preload without administering fluids that could be potentially harmful if the patient is not a fluid responder (the hemodynamic effect of the maneuver is self-limiting). Echocardiography, in addition to providing targeted information for the diagnostic assessment of shock and a visual estimation of the systolic function of both ventricles, can, in expert hands, be used to assess SV and CO and, above all, any changes induced by dynamic tests (fluid challenge, PLR, variations related to the respiratory cycle during spontaneous breathing or mechanical ventilation, the End Expiratory Occlusion Test). Cardiac output, by virtue of the continuity equation (already described in the Cardiac Output section), is equal to the product of the cross-sectional area of the left ventricular outflow tract and the aortic VTI measured with pulsed Doppler at the outflow tract in the apical five-chamber view [24]. The change in VTI (or more generally in SV) following PLR provides valuable information on the positive predictive value of the maneuver for the patient's volume status.

17.8 Practical Aspects

Fluid management has progressively shifted towards a more dynamic and functional approach based on the prediction of fluid responsiveness (FR), in order to improve efficacy and benefits and limit the harmful effects of fluids. The application of an optimal threshold for validated parameters above which the patient may be fluid responsive generates a "gray zone." Therefore, the goal of intensivists should be to adapt the threshold to the respective sensitivity and specificity required to predict FR, according to the patient's condition. Intensivists should consider being highly specific in severely hypoxemic patients, in whom fluids may be significantly harmful, and primarily sensitive in patients without blood gas abnormalities, since maintaining a non-optimal volume could be harmful in this case. Applying an approach continuous prediction of FR, that is, how much the cardiac output is expected to increase after a fluid bolus, rather than the classic binary approach of whether the patient will be a "responder" or not, may be more effective. Echocardiography is fundamental for the management of patients with respiratory or circulatory failure. Many echocardiographic parameters have been proposed to predict FR. Measurement of the aortic velocity time integral (VTI) correlates with stroke volume and is sufficiently accurate to detect small changes in ejection volume, with a precision of 6–4% when measured in a single heartbeat or averaged over three heartbeats, respectively, in patients in sinus rhythm without the influence of ventilation type. This measurement requires good alignment with the ejection flow. Here, we propose how to use echocardiography to predict FR and differentiate among three situations: a patient with adequate volume, a hypovolemic patient, and a patient who can still respond to fluids despite adequate volemia. In the first scenario, fluid administration should not be considered and may even be contraindicated; echocardiographic parameters indicate that the patient is already overfilled and congested (no variation in SVV; IVC > 2.5 cm and non-collapsible). In the second, fluid administration should be strongly considered: echocardiographic parameters suggest that the patient is likely hypovolemic and therefore fluid responsive (IVC < 2 cm with more than 50% collapse; marked SVV, left ventricular end-diastolic area with papillary muscle kissing). In the last scenario, fluid administration may be optional; hypovolemia has already been corrected, but echocardiographic parameters indicate that cardiac output could still increase to some extent after a fluid bolus (change in aortic VTI with PLR). However, several key points should be discussed first: (i) echocardiography must be interpreted as a whole, while most parameters are unfortunately validated in isolation; (ii) intensivists do not treat an ultrasound image but a patient, and echocardiography is merely an aid; (iii) in many cases, intensivists simply need to administer fluids, as during hemorrhage or in the very early phase of septic shock; and (iv) echocardiography is limited and does not provide direct information on organ perfusion.

17.9 Operational Aspects

The patient should not be given fluids when:

1. The right ventricle (RV) is severely dilated (the right ventricle is larger than the left ventricle (LV)), with or without paradoxical septal motion. Administering more fluids may be harmful even in cases of less severe right ventricular dilation, while the optimal threshold for the RV/LV end-diastolic area ratio is unknown.
2. The end-expiratory diameter of the inferior vena cava (IVC) is greater than 25–27 mm. This reflects significant congestion, with effects on the liver and kidneys. It is associated with 80–90% of fluid nonresponders.
3. An echocardiographic pattern of cardiogenic shock is observed, with low LVEF and elevated left ventricular filling pressure (restrictive mitral pattern with $E/A > 1.8$ and/or $E/e' > 15$). In septic shock, however, despite reduced LVEF, patients may still be fluid responders, but in this case, left ventricular filling pressure will not be increased (no restrictive mitral pattern and even $E/A < 1$).
4. Significant mitral or aortic regurgitation is observed. For grading of valvular disease, in addition to assessing ventricular dilation, a more detailed echocardiographic evaluation is required, but in general, great caution is needed when administering fluids.

The patient should be given fluids when:

1. A left ventricle with "papillary muscle kissing" is observed. This is associated with left ventricular hyperkinesia and a low end-diastolic area (<5.5 cm^2/m^2); in profound vasoplegia, the left ventricle remains hyperkinetic, but its end-diastolic area is normal, while the end-systolic area is greatly reduced; this does not require further fluids. Dynamic obstruction of the left ventricular outflow tract (LVOT) may also be observed and should be corrected with fluids, with or without beta-blockers. In the case of right ventricular failure, leftward shift of the IVS leads to left ventricular hypodiastolia, but fluid administration is not recommended.
2. The diameter of the inferior vena cava is <10 mm. This is usually associated with low central venous pressure, and 90% of patients respond to fluids.
3. The decrease in the diameter of the superior vena cava (SVC) is greater than 31% during ventilation, or is more evident when partial or complete collapse of the SVC is observed. Its specificity in predicting a fluid response is 90%. This has been validated only in mechanically ventilated patients without any spontaneous effort and requires transesophageal echocardiography.

Fluid administration is uncertain when:

1. The measured echocardiographic parameters fall within a gray zone. Although fluid responsiveness is confirmed by the VTI value after PLR, this information

should be complemented with the patient's clinical presentation, for example, if they are hypoxemic.

2. Mild respiratory variations of the SVC are observed. Here, the sensitivity in predicting a significant increase in aortic VTI is close to 90%, but specificity is very low (25%). The greater the respiratory variation, the greater the expected increase in aortic VTI.
3. An increase in peak aortic velocity is observed during ventilation. This has only been validated in mechanically ventilated patients without spontaneous effort. This is the most sensitive parameter; it reflects the preload dependence of the left ventricle, similar to pulse pressure variations, and can occur in nonresponsive patients with severe right ventricular dilation. Therefore, it cannot be interpreted without information on RV size. The greater the respiratory variation, the greater the expected increase in aortic VTI in patients without RV impairment.
4. In case of doubt, or in combination, a passive leg raise (PLR) can be performed. The patient is very likely to be fluid responsive when PLR induces an increase in aortic VTI greater than 10% within 1 minute from the start of the maneuver (Fig. 17.14).

PLR is considered an excellent method for assessing fluid responsiveness, especially when other parameters are not available, but it has its own limitations (high intra-abdominal pressure). It mimics a fluid challenge (300 mL is mobilized from the legs and abdomen to the thorax) and allows intensivists to include severely hypoxemic patients in clinical research on fluid management. A mini fluid challenge

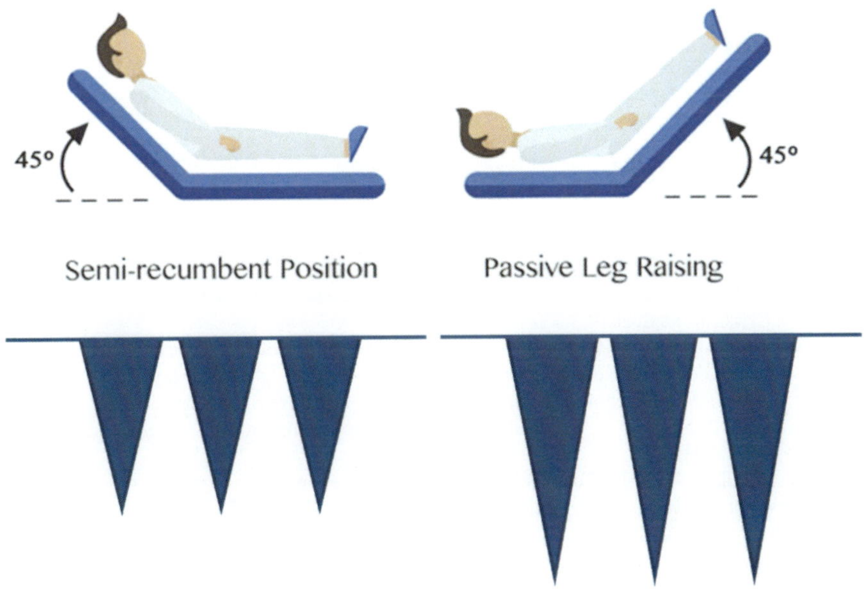

Fig. 17.14 Change in aortic VTI after PLR

with 100 mL of saline and assessment of aortic VTI has also been proposed. Finally, although respiratory variations of the IVC are widely used, they cannot accurately predict fluid responsiveness. In spontaneously breathing patients, the collapsibility index of the inferior vena cava depends on the level of inspiratory effort, and in mechanically ventilated patients, the distensibility index of the inferior vena cava is obtainable in only 78% of patients and has poor predictive performance.

17.10 Conclusions

Echocardiography is ideal for guiding fluid resuscitation in critically ill patients. It can be used to assess fluid responsiveness by evaluating the left ventricle, aortic outflow, inferior vena cava, and right ventricle. Static measurements and dynamic variables based on heart-lung interactions combine to predict and measure fluid responsiveness and to assess the response to intravenous fluid resuscitation. In-depth knowledge of these variables, the underlying physiology, and the pitfalls of their use allows echocardiography to safely assess these patients and, in combination with clinical judgment, to manage them appropriately. The question of whether the patient will improve with fluids, additional vasopressors, or inotropes can be difficult to answer. Echocardiography provides many answers for a data-driven approach to address this issue. Clearly, learning echocardiographic measurement techniques is challenging, but the scientific society SIAARTI and the residency programs in Anesthesia and Intensive Care, having recognized these needs, have been working for many years to promote a culture of echocardiographic training.

References

1. Chew MS. Haemodynamic monitoring using echocardiography in the critically ill: a review. Cardiol Res Pract. 2012;2012:139537.
2. Beaulieu Y, Marik PE. Bedside ultrasonography in the ICU: part 1. Chest. 2005;128:881–95.
3. Beaulieu Y, Marik PE. Bedside ultrasonography in the ICU: part 2. Chest. 2005;128:1766–81.
4. Slama MA, Novara A, Van de Putte P, et al. Diagnostic and therapeutic implications of transesophageal echocardiography in medical ICU patients with unexplained shock, hypoxemia, or suspected endocarditis. Intensive Care Med. 1996;22:916–22.
5. Zerbib Y, Maizel J, Slama M. Echocardiographic assessment of left ventricular function. J Emerg Crit Care Med. 2019;3:33.
6. Boissier F, Razazi K, Seemann A, et al. Left ventricular systolic dysfunction during septic shock: the role of loading conditions. Intensive Care Med. 2017;43:633–42.
7. Orde S, Slama M, Yastrebov K, Mclean A, Huang S. Subjective right ventricle assessment by echo qualified intensive care specialists: assessing agreement with objective measures. Crit Care. 2019;23(1):70.
8. Salinas P, Dieiev V. Critical care echocardiography: assessing left and right ventricular function in the intensive care unit. Semin Ultrasound CT MRI. 2023;45:58–73.
9. Lahham S, Lee C, Ali Q, et al. Tricuspid Annular Plane of Systolic Excursion (TAPSE) for the evaluation of patients with severe sepsis and septic shock. West J Emerg Med. 2020;21(2):348–52.

10. Slama M, Maizel J. Echocardiographic measurement of ventricular function. Curr Opin Crit Care. 2006;12:241–8.
11. Axler O, Megarbane B, Lentschener C, et al. Comparison of cardiac output measured with echocardiographic volumes and aortic Doppler methods during mechanical ventilation. Intensive Care Med. 2003;29:208–17.
12. Zhang Y, Wang Y, Shi J, Hua Z, Xu J. Cardiac output measurements via echocardiography versus thermodilution: a systematic review and meta-analysis. PLoS One. 2019;14(10):e0222105.
13. Gonzalez FA, Santonocito C, Maybauer MO, et al. Diastology in the intensive care unit: challenges for the assessment and future directions. Echocardiography. 41(2):e15773.
14. Nagueh SF, Smiseth OA, Appleton CP, et al. Recommendations for the evaluation of left ventricular diastolic function by echocardiography: an update from the American Society of Echocardiography and the European Association of Cardiovascular Imaging. Eur Heart J Cardiovasc Imaging. 2016;17:1321–60.
15. Nagueh SF, Middleton KJ, Kopelen HA, et al. Doppler tissue imaging: a noninvasive technique for evaluation of left ventricular relaxation and estimation of filling pressures. J Am Coll Cardiol. 1997;30:1527–33.
16. Mishiro Y, Oki T, Yamada H, et al. Evaluation of left ventricular contraction abnormalities in patients with dilated cardiomyopathy with the use of pulsed tissue Doppler imaging. J Am Soc Echocardiogr. 1999;12:913–20.
17. Slama M, Susic D, Varagic J, et al. Diastolic dysfunction in hypertension. Curr Opin Cardiol. 2002;17:368–73.
18. Combes A, Arnoult F, Trouillet JL. Tissue Doppler imaging estimation of pulmonary artery occlusion pressure in ICU patients. Intensive Care Med. 2004;30:75–81.
19. Vignon P, Mentec H, Terre S, et al. Diagnostic accuracy and therapeutic impact of transthoracic and transesophageal echocardiography in mechanically ventilated patients in the ICU. Chest. 1994;106:1829–34.
20. Michard F. Predicting fluid responsiveness in ICU patients: a critical analysis of the evidence. Chest. 2002;121:2000–8.
21. Jardin F, Vieillard-Baron A. Ultrasonographic examination of the venae cavae. Intensive Care Med. 2006;32:203–6. https://doi.org/10.1007/s00134-005-0013-5.
22. Airapetian N, Maizel J, Alyamani O, Mahjoub Y, Lorne E, Levrard M, Ammenouche N, Seydi A, Tinturier F, Lobjoie E, et al. Does inferior vena cava respiratory variability predict fluid responsiveness in spontaneously breathing patients? Crit Care. 2015;19:400. https://doi.org/10.1186/s13054-015-1100-9.
23. Vieillard-Baron A, Chergui K, Rabiller A, Peyrouset O, Page B, Beauchet A, Jardin F. Superior vena caval collapsibility as a gauge of volume status in ventilated septic patients. Intensive Care Med. 2004;30:1734–9.
24. Miller A, Mandeville J. Predicting and measuring fluid responsiveness with echocardiography. Echo Res Pract. 2016;3(2):G1–G12.
25. Cavallaro F, Sandroni C, Marano C, La Torre G, Mannocci A, De Waure C, Bello G, Maviglia R, Antonelli M. Diagnostic accuracy of passive leg raising for prediction of fluid responsiveness in adults: systematic review and meta-analysis of clinical studies. Intensive Care Med. 2010;36:1475–83.
26. Muller L, Toumi M, Bousquet P-J, Riu-Poulenc B, Louart G, Candela D, Zoric L, Suehs C, de La Coussaye JE, Molinari N, et al. An increase in aortic blood flow after an infusion of 100 ml colloid over 1 minute can predict fluid responsiveness: the mini-fluid challenge study. Anesthesiology. 2011;115:541–7.

Assessment and Admission Criteria in the Intensive Care Unit

18

Luciana Mascia, Rosanna D'Albo, and Irene Cavalli

18.1 Introduction

The field of Intensive Care Medicine has achieved significant milestones in the treatment of patients with complex disorders. Alongside these advances, however, there has been growing awareness of the morbidity that persists after critical illness. Indeed, admission to the Intensive Care Unit (ICU) alters the patient's "life trajectory" and often represents a traumatic experience for the entire family. Transparent and public sharing of the issues that persist after ICU discharge is essential to obtain informed consent for initiating and continuing intensive care, to align medical treatment with the values of the patient and family, and to ensure widespread awareness of the substantial human and economic costs associated with these outcomes.

On the other hand, the possibility of admission to the ICU—a unit associated with high human, emotional, and economic costs—also depends on the availability of resources allocated for patient care. Taken together, these considerations form some of the foundations for a proper assessment of ICU admission criteria.

The initial planning of intensive care treatment is designed to address a life-threatening illness, stabilize vital functions, develop a treatment strategy, and alleviate severe clinical symptoms. After the first days of ICU admission, in addition to evaluating the response to treatment, it is necessary to assess the alignment between the interventions provided and the patient's preferences and values. These preferences and values must therefore be known to the ICU clinical team. For patients

L. Mascia (✉)
Department of Experimental Medicine, University of Salento, Lecce, Italy
e-mail: luciana.mascia@unisalento.it

R. D'Albo · I. Cavalli
Department of Medical and Surgical Sciences, Alma Mater Studiorum, University of Bologna, Bologna, Italy
e-mail: rosanna.dalbo@studio.unibo.it; irene.cavalli@aosp.bo.it

D. Chiumello, A. De Gasperi (eds.), *Practical Trends in Anesthesia and Intensive Care 2026*, https://doi.org/10.1007/978-3-032-25721-5_18

without legally binding advance directives and/or legally appointed surrogates, relatives or close contacts serve as sources of information and may act as legal surrogates. However, during family meetings, discussions about preferences, patient values, and realistic care goals may not be conclusive. The optimal timing for initiating such discussions may not be clear, as family members face emotional conflicts, distress, and, in some cases, guilt when they are involved in decisions to limit life-supporting treatments (LST) [1]. An appropriate level of communication and support, with transparent discussions about what is achievable in the context of the patient's preferences and values, is essential: each patient should be offered only those treatments whose expected effects are consistent with their preferences. This underscores the need to establish criteria to guide clinicians in deciding whether to admit a patient and in allocating available resources.

18.1.1 Current Admission Criteria

Currently, the principles guiding the decision to proceed with intensive care in a patient are essentially twofold: triage and futility [2].

- *Triage*: After the initial assessment, admission is determined based on clinical severity and thus the likelihood that the patient will benefit from intensive care. In this way, only those patients who, in the clinical judgment of the physician performing the triage, are likely to benefit from ICU care should be admitted, while admission should be avoided for patients deemed too ill to benefit from intensive care or sufficiently stable in terms of vital organ function.
- *Futility*: In this case, intensive care is considered useless and inappropriate for the patient, whose clinical condition is too severe to benefit from ICU care. Ethical and professional considerations also play a role here (primum non nocere).

As a result, the decision-making process aims to ensure that the patient derives benefit from intensive care. However, this approach requires a clear definition of "benefit"; it, therefore, remains to be determined what constitutes benefit from intensive care and who is responsible for defining this objective.

During the SARS-CoV-2 pandemic, ICU admission criteria were constrained by the discrepancy between the demand for intensive care, the resources available, and thus the ability to provide adequate care [3]. This discrepancy heightened the tendency to discriminate based on age or disability, despite efforts to establish the most ethical guidelines possible [4]. The urgency of ensuring social equity in triage and resource allocation became increasingly apparent. The challenge of objectively defining the "benefit" of intensive care is particularly evident in complex patients with multiple comorbidities, advanced age, and/or disabilities.

18.1.2 Severity Scores and Prognosis

The presence of multiple comorbidities often makes intensive management challenging, due to adverse effects and risks associated with therapies, invasive procedures, and the ICU environment itself. Furthermore, in these situations, the goal of intensive care becomes uncertain, as does the likelihood that these patients will benefit from it. The use of severity scores is, therefore, a crucial aspect of this assessment.

Among the indices proposed in the literature, the Charlson Comorbidity Index is a score that predicts patient mortality based on existing comorbidities [5]. It was validated to assess short-term mortality risk in patients enrolled in longitudinal studies. Seventeen categories of comorbidities are considered, each assigned a score of 1, 2, 3, or 6 according to the risk of death associated with that condition. The score also increases with the patient's age.

This score can be integrated with severity scores specifically used in intensive care settings, such as APACHE or SAPS [6]. These are among the most widely used and incorporate vital signs and clinical data to outline the clinical condition at admission and estimate the probability of death in intensive care. The use of these scores dates back to the 1980s [7, 8], and over time, they have undergone several revisions in parallel with advances in the field and the evolution of statistical techniques. In fact, APACHE and SAPS have reached their fourth [9] and third [10] versions, respectively. Both consider the worst recorded values of relevant physiological variables to generate a score correlated with the probability of death in the ICU. Notably, SAPS also takes into account the patient's geographic region of origin, dividing the world into five areas. The constant updating of these scores is driven by the need to adapt predictive models to patient populations whose characteristics change over time, from average age to prevalent comorbidities and, finally, to the most frequent diagnoses leading to ICU admission. In this regard, a significant innovation of SAPS 3 is the assignment of a score based on 20 physiological variables that consider the patient's clinical condition prior to ICU admission, the reason for admission, and the patient's deterioration within 1 hour before or after admission. For this reason, the latest version of SAPS differs from its predecessors and from other scores by giving greater weight to the patient's baseline condition, compared, for example, to APACHE, which instead considers the first 24 hours of admission to assign the score. The application of these scores is a valuable tool for clinicians in addressing the most complex issues regarding the appropriateness of admitting patients for whom the real benefit of intensive care is not always evident. However, it is important to emphasize that these should not be the sole guide in initiating or continuing intensive treatment. Over the years, their most significant limitations have often been highlighted. First, these scores demonstrate their strongest predictive power only when applied to populations that closely resemble those on which they were originally validated; otherwise, their accuracy in predicting mortality becomes very low. Second, their accuracy largely depends on the quality of the data collected, how these are integrated into the models, and how missing data are interpreted. Third, some studies have pointed out that these prognostic scores have intrinsic biases: two examples are the use of automated data recording systems, which systematically assign higher scores [11], and variability in the frequency of data collection during the 24-hour window considered [12].

For all these reasons, these scores are not sufficient on their own but should rather support the clinician's ability to integrate information from each patient's baseline condition and preferences to ensure the best possible outcome.

18.1.3 Chronological and Biological Age: Ageism

"Ageism" refers to stereotypes (how we think), prejudices (how we feel), and discrimination (how we act) directed toward others and ourselves based on chronological age.

With a global population characterized by an increasingly higher average age, especially in the Western world, the need for ICU admission among older patients is steadily rising. This need often clashes with limited resource availability. All this inevitably leads to a tendency to "discriminate" against older age groups, due to the perception of resource waste for patients whose benefit from ICU admission is seen as limited or negligible [13]. However, this tendency requires careful analysis. First, a distinction must be made between chronological and biological age, as these often do not coincide. Chronological age alone is frequently used as a decision-making parameter in assigning certain treatments to patients, even though there is often no evidence supporting a linear increase in risk with advancing age, nor clear age thresholds beyond which a treatment should be considered inappropriate. A recent meta-analysis has shown that even in determining eligibility for invasive treatments such as extracorporeal support for severe respiratory failure (VV-ECMO), there is no clear age cut-off, but rather a linear relationship with increased risk. Moreover, since, unlike in the hospital setting, mortality in the ICU among patients undergoing VV-ECMO increases linearly with age, it is necessary to investigate these outcomes over a longer term [14].

In the surgical field, the possibility of operating on very elderly patients (e.g., femoral fracture) presupposes that intensive care units are prepared to admit this type of patient in the postoperative period [15]. A further distinction must be made between elective and emergency surgery, as in the former case it is possible to assess the risks associated with the surgical procedure, decide on the type of surgery, and even consider not proceeding and opting for more conservative measures; in the latter case, there is often no opportunity to make these assessments calmly and with the involvement of the patient and family.

To date, some studies have shown that, on average, the rate of non-admission to the ICU increases with age, as does the mortality rate. Nevertheless, there is considerable variability in ICU admission rates for older patients among different countries [16] and even among centers within the same country [17]. The reasons for this variability are unclear, likely reflecting only differing clinical opinions. However, these differences have not been associated with either mortality or persistent functional decline in patients after admission. Despite reluctance to admit older patients to the ICU, a study conducted in 11 European intensive care units [16] demonstrated that these patients actually derive the greatest benefit in terms of 28-day mortality from intensive care. Unfortunately, this does not always translate into an improvement in quality of life and again raises uncertainty about the overall goal of intensive treatment.

18.1.4 Patients with Disabilities: Ableism

"Ableism" refers to any discrimination, prejudice, or marginalization against people with disabilities. A class of patients that is in fact "silently" discriminated against in access to care, and particularly to intensive care, is that of people with disabilities (neurological, psychiatric, physical, and autism) [18, 19]. The reluctance to admit these patients to the ICU stems from a series of deeply rooted societal and medical biases, foremost among them the idea that a person with a disability has a lower quality of life than a person without a disability (which also affects the perceived appropriateness of allocating resources to these patients). This belief has often been described as unconscious ableism: the notion that the life of a person with a disability is less valuable than that of a person without a disability.

All of this occurs "silently" in our daily lives, even though, for example, in the United States, the Department of Health and Human Services has publicly stated that such decisions violate the law protecting citizens with disabilities. The situation is further complicated by the very frequent communication difficulties these patients experience and the presumption by medical teams or even family members that they always know what is best for the patient and that the patient is incapable of participating in decisions about their own care. This often results in the complete inability of patients with disabilities to fully express their will for self-determination—a right that, on the contrary, should always be guaranteed. This also undermines the establishment of the doctor-patient relationship of trust that should be the foundation of every medical act. The distance from patients with disabilities is further increased by the limited knowledge of these conditions, even among intensive care physicians themselves. To ensure equitable access to care for these patients, it is essential first to recognize that the ultimate goal of intensive care is to return them to their clinical condition prior to the acute event that necessitated admission. Achieving this requires increasing clinicians' training and their level of "comfort" with these conditions, not only from a technical and medical perspective. Clinicians must also understand the needs of these patients in a holistic way, including emotional and social aspects, and learn to communicate with them in order to obtain consent that is as free and informed as possible. Only in this way can true inclusion be achieved and clinical practice be centered on the individual and their needs [20].

18.1.5 Frailty

Frailty is defined as "a dynamic state affecting an individual who experiences losses in one or more functional domains (physical, psychological, social), due to the influence of multiple variables that increase the risk of adverse health outcomes" [21]. According to this emerging concept, frail patients are those who exhibit a series of characteristics resulting from the loss of homeostatic mechanisms, making them more vulnerable to adverse events and less able to recover afterwards [22]. Frailty is therefore not a disease diagnosis per se but requires a comprehensive assessment of the patient. The assessment of frailty is not yet fully standardized: in some cases it is based on existing comorbidities, in others on the presence of certain features such as a tendency to fatigue, weight loss, or dependence on others for daily activities; however, the best score proposed in the literature is the "Clinical Frailty Scale," which has also been correlated with the degree of dementia [23]. Since frailty has also been associated with mortality, considering this global parameter in the assessment of the patient and their need for intensive care could be a reasonable approach also from the perspective of resource rationalization. However, it should be noted that even in this way, the issues of discrimination, ableism, and ageism would not be fully addressed. In fact, people are often considered "frail" based on age, and furthermore, classifying people with disabilities using the same scores applied to patients without disabilities would represent a clear selection error.

18.1.6 Shared Decision-Making Model

In light of the considerations outlined above, for patients in a critical clinical condition for whom an intensive care stay of more than 48 hours is anticipated, clarifying the patient's preferences regarding the level of care is essential for the patient, the surrogate decision-maker, and healthcare professionals. Scheduled meetings with the family have been associated with greater satisfaction with the decision-making process, though not with overall satisfaction with the care provided [24]. In a randomized study, a family support intervention did not reduce symptoms of anxiety and depression among families, but did improve families' assessment of communication [25]. Meaningful discussions about care goals require that families have a good understanding of life-sustaining treatments (LST), the level and intensity of support provided, and the patient's critical status [3, 26]. In addition, intensive care staff must identify the strategies by which each patient and family chooses to cope with the situation. When there is consensus that LSTs do not provide benefit, they should be withheld or withdrawn. In these situations in particular, structured support and communication are important to reduce the risk of complicated grief, anxiety, and symptoms of post-traumatic stress disorder among relatives.

The decision to "de-escalate" therapy, limit care, or withdraw ongoing treatments is a daily choice for the clinician. This entails a significant emotional and moral burden and therefore requires special attention. Usually, the decision is never made autonomously by the clinician but is always the result of a shared choice between the treating physician, who proposes a therapeutic plan or deems a certain treatment no longer appropriate, and the wishes of the patient or their representative: at this point, the clinician shares the best decision to safeguard the patient's dignity. This model is defined as "shared decision-making" (SDM), a decision-making model based on ongoing dialogue between clinician and patient, grounded in respect for the principles of autonomy and dignity of the patient [27, 28].

SDM is a collaborative process that enables the clinician and the patient or their delegate to jointly decide on the overall goals of care, based primarily on the best available scientific evidence and the patient's goals and expectations for quality of life [28]. The SDM model is based on three fundamental principles: information exchange, deliberation, and the decision on a specific therapeutic plan [28, 29]. The clinician then has the fiduciary duty to use their clinical experience and judgment in the daily management of the patient, in accordance with the general goals and preferences of the patient.

A systematic review [30] reported a positive correlation between the SDM model and various affective-cognitive, behavioral, or health-related aspects of the patient, albeit with limitations mainly due to the observational nature of the studies analyzed [30].

The shared decision-making model should be implemented not only between the clinician and the patient or their delegate, but also primarily among clinicians, especially those from different specialties. Several studies have shown that implementing this model among clinicians from different specialties can improve patient clinical outcomes, increase professional satisfaction while reducing the risk of burnout, and decrease both patient length of stay and the error rate for individual patients [31, 32].

When discussing the shared decision-making model, a fundamental aspect that clinicians must consider is communication with patients or their relatives/delegates. Effective communication enables patients/relatives to better understand their problems and the possible therapeutic options; this results in better adherence to the proposed therapeutic plan, reduced stress and anxiety for patients, and improved well-being for the clinician as well [33, 34].

A review article [35] investigated the effects of communication based on a structured model compared to communication left to the discretion of each clinician regarding the decision to withdraw care in patients admitted to intensive care. This review, although with low levels of evidence due to the limited number of randomized studies included, showed that communication based on a structured model increases the clarity of discussions about care goals with patients/relatives, reduces patient length of stay in intensive care, and lowers healthcare costs by reducing inappropriate resource use. The recent guidelines of the European Society of Intensive Care Medicine [1] on end-of-life and palliative care devote an entire section to the importance of communication with relatives, emphasizing in particular that programs aimed at clinicians to acquire the necessary skills for effective communication can reduce anxiety, depression, and symptoms of post-traumatic stress disorder in relatives of patients undergoing end-of-life care. Furthermore, the same guidelines highlight the importance of using written communication tools to support verbal communication [1, 33].

Several models have been proposed for communication structures. One of the simplest models is based on the ABCDE rule [27] (Accuracy, Brevity, Clarity, Delivery, Empathy), that is, accuracy, brevity of information, clarity of information, communication using appropriate nonverbal language, and empathy with interlocutors. Another proposed approach is the *who, what, when, where, how* [34] method. This method suggests following five steps when planning communication with family members, starting with who (*who*) the patient would like to have present during the meeting; what (*what*) the topic of the meeting is, meaning the clinician must be clear about the objective of the conversation to ensure it is clear and effective; when (*when*) it is appropriate to hold the meeting, referring to dedicating the necessary time to listen, reflect, and ensure understanding of what is being communicated; where (*where*) a suitable, comfortable, and private place to conduct the meeting; how (*how*) to structure and conduct the meeting, preferably starting with a semi-structured discussion to achieve the proposed communication objectives, but also being flexible according to the dynamics and needs of the patient, adapting communication accordingly.

Therefore, when intensive care is required for one or more organ instabilities in a patient, the priority is to determine whether intensive care is proportionate for that patient at that specific point in their clinical history; the initiation of a care plan aimed at restoring organ failure or a care plan focused on palliation must be shared in all its aspects between the clinician and the patient or their proxy, respecting the patient's autonomy and self-determination; finally, at every stage of the patient's clinical course and throughout the care and/or palliative process, effective and structured communication by the clinician improves adherence to the therapeutic plan, reduces stress for the patient and their proxy, and decreases average length of stay as well as inappropriate use of resources.

This approach can therefore be summarized in the following points: (1) "patient-centered care," (2) satisfaction with the decision-making process, and (3) attention to mental health symptoms (depression, grief, and post-traumatic stress disorder [PTSD]).

18.1.7 Advance Directives (AD) and Informed Consent

Law No. 219 of December 22, 2017 [36], establishes, through eight articles, the regulations regarding informed consent, advance directives (AD), and shared care planning for adult, minor, and incapacitated patients. Specifically, the law states in its initial articles the importance of informed consent, reiterating the clinician's obligation to provide clear, explicit, and comprehensive information on every aspect of the diagnostic and therapeutic process. In particular, the law reaffirms the dignity and self-determination of the patient, stating that no medical treatment may be initiated or continued unless explicitly accepted by the individual concerned. Article 1 of Law 2017/219 also emphasizes the competence, professional autonomy, and responsibility of the physician in proposing or refusing a specific treatment deemed not beneficial for the patient. In this regard, the law explicitly states that, in cases of patients with a poor prognosis or who are dying, the physician must refrain from administering unreasonable care or disproportionate treatments. In emergency situations where the individual is unable to provide consent for a specific treatment, necessary care will be provided to stabilize the patient, always respecting their wishes where these are readily available. In this context, the law explicitly allows for the drafting of "advance directives (AD)," that is, an expression of will regarding healthcare, after receiving adequate medical information about the consequences of one's choices, and thus the need to express consent or refusal for specific diagnostic, therapeutic, or individual medical treatments. Advance directives may be revoked by the individual at any time or may be disregarded in whole or in part by the physician, in agreement with the proxy if one is designated in the AD, in cases of clear inconsistency or if they do not correspond to the current clinical condition when, at the time of signing, possible treatments capable of offering real chances of survival and improved quality of life were not foreseeable. In the final part of the law, Article 5 addresses the issue of shared care planning. This aspect is fundamental as it provides for the planning and sharing between the individual and the physician of a care plan that can be updated and/or modified jointly as the underlying disease evolves.

18.1.8 Proportionality of Care

To address all the critical issues discussed so far, it is necessary to start from the beginning and attempt to establish the endpoint of an ICU admission. In seeking to answer the initial question, it is reasonable to state that the goal of ICU admission is to enable the patient with one or more organ failures to overcome the acute phase of illness and facilitate a return to a dignified and acceptable quality of life for the patient. In this context, not all patients with organ instability are eligible for intensive treatments, nor do all accept intensive treatments if these are deemed unlikely to ensure a return to an acceptable level of autonomy and quality of life. To achieve this goal, intensive care must be proportional, that is, able to ensure the patient overcomes the acute phase of illness and returns to a decent quality of life.

The concept of "proportionality of care" encompasses three fundamental aspects:

- The assumption that a given treatment can actually be of benefit to the patient
- The involvement of the patient in the decision-making process regarding the therapeutic plan and the acceptance of a specific treatment that the patient perceives as capable of improving their quality of life
- The ability to refrain from initiating any therapeutic pathway or to modify ongoing treatments toward palliative care when these become disproportionate and no longer provide any reasonable benefit to the patient [24]

Therefore, "proportionality of care" refers to a care plan for a specific patient at a specific point in their clinical history, which is able to improve not only the current clinical condition but also restore a dignified quality of life. This latter aspect is fundamental because, even when appropriate, a given treatment that is not accepted or perceived by the patient as capable of improving their quality of life is not proportional for that specific patient.

The ultimate goal of a care plan is always to ensure the patient's dignity. Therefore, when a care plan is unable to restore organ function—for example, in patients who no longer respond to maximal treatments or in patients who, although still having some autonomous vital functions, are considered "dying" due to the precariousness of those functions—the care plan should shift toward a "palliative care" approach, a clinical management that allows the dying person to experience the end of life with dignity and without suffering [24, 25].

A "proportional care" plan is fundamentally based on a shared decision-making model with the patient, respecting their autonomy and dignity at all times.

18.2 Conclusion

In conclusion, the criteria for determining the need for ICU admission should primarily take into account the patient's wishes and then their overall clinical history, in order to obtain the most comprehensive picture possible of post-admission prospects. In more complex cases, which often involve elderly, frail individuals with multiple comorbidities who are frequently unable to express their consent or wishes due to their condition, such decisions should not be left to a single physician, especially if that physician is encountering the patient for the first time. On the contrary, it would be more appropriate for the decision to admit a patient to the ICU to result from a collegial decision-making process, in which the medical opinions of those who have followed the patient throughout their course, up to the acute event necessitating intensive care, are considered. For this reason, the general practitioner, specialists, any referring oncologist, and the intensivist who will be responsible for the patient in the event of admission should all be involved in the decision.

In some more severe and acute cases, it may be appropriate to consider postponing the decision regarding the proportionality of intensive treatment until after the patient has been stabilized. In this way, the aim would be to resolve at least the acute condition, and then, with greater calm and as much information as possible, decide whether intensive treatment is appropriate.

In any case, it is essential to take into account the wishes of the patient or their designated representatives. Communication among clinicians and with the patient's family completes this process of shared decision-making, ensuring that the burden of the choice does not fall on a single individual but is the result of a collective process. What must absolutely be avoided, in order to respect the rights of both patients and physicians and their professionalism, is the uncritical activation of a sort of "conveyor belt" [26] on which patients are automatically transferred by virtue of protocols, numerical values, and thresholds that overwhelm physicians and prevent them from making ethical therapeutic choices.

References

1. Kesecioglu J, et al. European Society of Intensive Care Medicine guidelines on end of life and palliative care in the intensive care unit. Intensive Care Med. 2024; https://doi.org/10.1007/s00134-024-07579-1.
2. Joynt GM, Gomersall CD, Tan P, Lee A, Cheng CA, Wong EL. Prospective evaluation of patients refused admission to an intensive care unit: triage, futility and outcome. Intensive Care Med. 2001;27(9):1459–65. https://doi.org/10.1007/s001340101041.
3. Joebges S, Biller-Andorno N. Ethics guidelines on COVID-19 triage—an emerging international consensus. Crit Care. 2020;24(1):201. https://doi.org/10.1186/s13054-020-02927-1.
4. Craxì L, Vergano M, Savulescu J, Wilkinson D. Rationing in a pandemic: lessons from Italy. Asian Bioeth Rev. 2020;12(3):325–30. https://doi.org/10.1007/s41649-020-00127-1.
5. Charlson ME, Pompei P, Ales KL, MacKenzie CR. A new method of classifying prognostic comorbidity in longitudinal studies: development and validation. J Chronic Dis. 1987;40(5):373–83. https://doi.org/10.1016/0021-9681(87)90171-8.
6. Vincent J-L, Moreno R. Clinical review: scoring systems in the critically ill. Crit Care. 2010;14(2):207. https://doi.org/10.1186/cc8204.
7. Le Gall J-R, et al. A simplified acute physiology score for ICU patients. Crit Care Med. 1984;12(11):975–7. https://doi.org/10.1097/00003246-198411000-00012.
8. Knaus WA, Zimmerman JE, Wagner DP, Draper EA, Lawrence DE. APACHE-acute physiology and chronic health evaluation: a physiologically based classification system. Crit Care Med. 1981;9(8):591–7. https://doi.org/10.1097/00003246-198108000-00008.
9. Zimmerman JE, Kramer AA, McNair DS, Malila FM. Acute Physiology and Chronic Health Evaluation (APACHE) IV: hospital mortality assessment for today's critically ill patients. Crit Care Med. 2006;34(5):1297–310. https://doi.org/10.1097/01.CCM.0000215112.84523.F0.
10. Moreno RP, et al. SAPS 3--From evaluation of the patient to evaluation of the intensive care unit. Part 2: development of a prognostic model for hospital mortality at ICU admission. Intensive Care Med. 2005;31(10):1345–55. https://doi.org/10.1007/s00134-005-2763-5.
11. Bosman RJ, Oudemane van Straaten HM, Zandstra DF. The use of intensive care information systems alters outcome prediction. Intensive Care Med. 1998;24(9):953–8. https://doi.org/10.1007/s001340050695.
12. Suistomaa M, Kari A, Ruokonen E, Takala J. Sampling rate causes bias in APACHE II and SAPS II scores. Intensive Care Med. 2000;26(12):1773–8. https://doi.org/10.1007/s001340000677.
13. Christensen K, Hansen TG, Rasmussen LS. Intensive care units and the oldest-old: are we doing good, too little, or too much? Acta Anaesthesiol Scand. 2013;57(6):681–3. https://doi.org/10.1111/aas.12110.
14. Tonetti T, et al. Role of age as eligibility criterion for ECMO in patients with ARDS: meta-regression analysis. Crit Care. 2024;28(1):278. https://doi.org/10.1186/s13054-024-05074-z.
15. Melegari G, et al. Postoperative cognitive worsening in seniors with an age above life expectancy: a prospective longitudinal study. Minerva Anestesiol. 2024;90(3) https://doi.org/10.23736/S0375-9393.23.17572-9.
16. Sprung CL, et al. The Eldicus prospective, observational study of triage decision making in European intensive care units. Part II: intensive care benefit for the elderly. Crit Care Med. 2012;40(1):132–8. https://doi.org/10.1097/CCM.0b013e318232d6b0.
17. Boumendil A, et al. Variability of intensive care admission decisions for the very elderly. PLoS One. 2012;7(4):e34387. https://doi.org/10.1371/journal.pone.0034387.
18. Taccone FS. Ableism in the intensive care unit. Intensive Care Med. 2023;49(7):898–9. https://doi.org/10.1007/s00134-023-07084-x.
19. Morris MA. Death by ableism. N Engl J Med. 2023;388(1):5–7. https://doi.org/10.1056/NEJMp2212109.
20. Mello MM, Persad G, White DB. Respecting disability rights - toward improved crisis standards of care. N Engl J Med. 2020;383(5):e26. https://doi.org/10.1056/NEJMp2011997.

21. Wilkinson DJC. Frailty triage: is rationing intensive medical treatment on the grounds of frailty ethical? Am J Bioeth. 2021;21(11):48–63. https://doi.org/10.1080/15265161.2020.1851809.
22. Ranzani OT, Besen BAMP, Herridge MS. Focus on the frail and elderly: who should have a trial of ICU treatment? Intensive Care Med. 2020;46(5):1030–2. https://doi.org/10.1007/s00134-020-05963-1.
23. Rockwood K. A global clinical measure of fitness and frailty in elderly people. Can Med Assoc J. 2005;173(5):489–95. https://doi.org/10.1503/cmaj.050051.
24. Bibas L, Peretz-Larochelle M, Adhikari NK, Goldfarb MJ, Luk A, Englesakis M, Detsky ME, Lawler PR. Association of Surrogate Decision-making Interventions for Critically Ill Adults With Patient, Family, and Resource Use Outcomes: A Systematic Review and Meta-analysis. JAMA Netw Open. 2019;2(7):e197229. https://doi.org/10.1001/jamanetworkopen.2019.7229.
25. Cook D, Rocker G. Dying with dignity in the intensive care unit. N Engl J Med. 2014;370(26):2506–14. https://doi.org/10.1056/NEJMra1208795.
26. Elia F, Aprà F. Walking away from conveyor-belt medicine. N Engl J Med. 2019;380(1):8–9. https://doi.org/10.1056/NEJMp1810681.
27. Supporting Clinical Decision Making. [Online]. Available: https://www.moralbalance.org.
28. Kon AA, Davidson JE, Morrison W, Danis M, White DB. Shared-decision-making-in-intensive-care-units-executive-summary-of-the-american-college-of-critical. care mwedicine and American Thoracic Society Policy statements. Crit Care Med. 2016;44:188–201.
29. Elwyn G, et al. Shared decision making: a model for clinical practice. J Gen Intern Med. 2012;27(10):1361–7. https://doi.org/10.1007/s11606-012-2077-6.
30. Shay LA, Lafata JE. Where is the evidence? A systematic review of shared decision making and patient outcomes. Med Decis Making. 2015;35(1):114–31. https://doi.org/10.1177/0272989X14551638.
31. Braam A, Buljac-Samardzic M, Hilders CGJM, van Wijngaarden JDH. Collaboration between physicians from different medical specialties in hospital settings: a systematic review. J Multidiscip Healthc. 2022;15:2277–300. https://doi.org/10.2147/JMDH.S376927.
32. Dobler CC, West CP, Montori VM. Can shared decision making improve physician well-being and reduce burnout? Cureus. 2017; https://doi.org/10.7759/cureus.1615.
33. Maguire P, Pitceathly C. Key communication skills and how to acquire them. BMJ. 2002;325(7366):697–700. https://doi.org/10.1136/bmj.325.7366.697.
34. Pfeifer M, Head BA. AMA Journal of Ethics ® Number 8: E724-731 MEDICAL EDUCATION which critical communication skills are essential for interdisciplinary end-of-life discussions? 2018. [Online]. Available: https://www.amajournalofethics.org.
35. Oczkowski SJW, Chung H-O, Hanvey L, Mbuagbaw L, You JJ. Communication tools for end-of-life decision-making in the intensive care unit: a systematic review and meta-analysis. Crit Care. 2016;20:97. https://doi.org/10.1186/s13054-016-1264-y.
36. Law n. 219/2017 "Norme in materia di consenso informato e di disposizioni anticipate di trattamento" [Provisions for informed consent and advance directives]. Gazzetta Ufficiale della Repubblica Italiana S.G. n. 12, 16 January 2018. https://www.gazzettaufficiale.it/eli/id/2018/1/16/18G00006/sg.

19 Rationalization of Opioid Use in Intensive Care

Giovanni Misseri, Matteo Piattoli, Alice Mirasola, and Cesare Gregoretti

19.1 Introduction

Since the early days of critical care medicine, numerous clinical studies, systematic literature reviews, and guidelines have enhanced our understanding of the importance of optimal pain control and sedation management in patients admitted to intensive care [1]. Whereas in the past it was believed that critically ill patients benefited from deep analgosedation—effectively putting the body in "stand-by" mode to allow the disease to run its course and resolve with appropriate organ support and targeted therapies—it is now well established that uncontrolled application of analgosedation protocols can prolong ICU stays and thus delay clinical improvement [2].

The goal of appropriate analgosedation in critically ill patients is to ensure comfort, enable the performance of more or less invasive and painful procedures, all while maintaining safety. Acute pain and agitation contribute to the development of distress, chronic pain, and post-traumatic stress syndrome, which may persist even after discharge from intensive care [3, 4]. In addition, the physiological responses to

G. Misseri
Anesthesia and Intensive Care Unit - "G. Giglio" Foundation Institute, Palermo, Italy

M. Piattoli
Department of Internal Clinical, Anesthesiological and Cardiovascular Sciences, Umberto I Hospital, Sapienza University of Rome, Rome, Italy

A. Mirasola
Anesthesia and Intensive Care Unit, San Giovanni di Dio Hospital, Agrigento, Italy

C. Gregoretti (✉)
Anesthesia and Intensive Care Unit - "G. Giglio" Foundation Institute, Palermo, Italy

School of Medicine and Surgery, Saint Camillus International Medical University in Rome – UniCamillus, Rome, Italy
e-mail: c.gregoretti@gmail.com

D. Chiumello, A. De Gasperi (eds.), *Practical Trends in Anesthesia and Intensive Care 2026*, https://doi.org/10.1007/978-3-032-25721-5_19

chronic pain lead to increased oxygen consumption, elevated endogenous catecholamine release, and hypermetabolism [4, 5]. Analgesics and sedatives are commonly administered to mitigate these responses, but require an individualized approach, balancing the potential harmful effects of prolonged analgosedation, which include delirium, weakness, difficult weaning from mechanical ventilation, and consequently, increased mortality [2].

Opioids represent a class of drugs useful in the management of pain and sedation, especially in clinical settings such as intensive care, where patients increasingly require a personalized approach to treatment. However, their use presents a series of challenges related to side effects, the risk of dependence and tolerance, and the management of withdrawal syndrome. The aim of rationalizing opioid use in intensive care is to ensure optimal pain control and adequate analgosedation, while minimizing adverse effects and optimizing available resources. Taking into account key clinical studies and introducing the concept of *opioid stewardship*, we will consider which strategies for pain and sedation management should be implemented in intensive care, the pros and cons of opioid use, and how these may affect outcomes in critically ill patients, even after discharge.

19.2 Assessment and Monitoring of Pain and Sedation Depth in Intensive Care

Most patients report pain during their stay in intensive care. Pain is multifactorial and may be caused by the underlying illness for which the patient is admitted to intensive care, by invasive treatments, and by standard care procedures [6]. The definition of pain, understood as a sensory and unpleasant emotional state induced by external and/or internal noxious stimuli, thus allows us to understand pain as an experience influenced by physiological and psychological pathways that interact to produce it. The experience of pain is not limited to "awake" patients, as pain has been reported as a significant memory among patients discharged from intensive care units [7]. For both psychological and physiological reasons, especially when patients are unable to fully express and describe their experiences, it is important to assess and treat pain in the intensive care setting using validated *scoring systems*. Therefore, it is essential that nurses and physicians are able to monitor and detect pain using these tools, titrate analgesic doses, minimize excessive use and serious side effects, and detect medical complications during the ICU stay. Although pain management is a high priority and the first component in major *bundles* in intensive care [8], there is a lack of evidence to assist clinicians in the objective identification of pain and its optimal management. Pain monitoring is associated with improved outcomes (reduced use of sedatives, shorter duration of mechanical ventilation, and reduced length of stay) [2, 6] and should be tailored to the patient's condition, adopting personalized pharmacological and non-pharmacological *patient-tailored* strategies. Moreover, the same tool should be used in a given patient with a given condition to monitor changes over time.

Pain is a personal experience and, whenever possible, patient self-assessment should be obtained (gold standard). Common scales for self-assessment of pain include the verbal description scale (VDS), the visual analog scale (VAS), and the 0–10 numeric rating scale (NRS). The NRS has demonstrated greater sensitivity in detecting pain compared to the simple YES/NO question, the VDS, and the VAS [9]. All these scales are well validated and recommended by current guidelines, but their use is limited to patients who are able to communicate (including non-verbal communication) with healthcare staff. However, self-reporting of pain becomes impossible in deeply sedated patients or may yield unreliable information in patients with delirium. In these situations, alternative pain assessment relies on observation of patient behaviors. Among the validated tools for patients unable to communicate verbally or non-verbally, which objectively quantify and qualify pain in these patients [2], two have demonstrated robust psychometric performance and are available in several translations, with the highest validity and reliability for pain monitoring in critically ill patients, allowing for optimization of analgesic administration and titration: the Critical Care Observation Pain Tool (CPOT) and the Behavioral Pain Scale (BPS) [2]. These scales help standardize the observation of pain-indicative behaviors (facial expressions, movements/muscle tone, vocalization, or compliance with mechanical ventilation). CPOT and BPS have been validated in ICU patients with various conditions, both intubated and non-intubated, sedated or delirious, and in patients with brain injuries [6]. Neuromuscular blocking agents (NMBAs) are used in conjunction with deep analgesia-sedation in severe neurological or respiratory conditions. In such cases, behavioral scales cannot be used, and it is therefore recommended to discontinue these drugs to assess pain and sedation [10]. In these situations, alternative pain assessment methods must be explored. During neuromuscular blockade in critically ill patients, changes in continuous monitoring of vital signs (e.g., heart rate, blood pressure) are used to guide decisions regarding analgesic-sedative titration. However, vital signs alone are not valid indicators of pain intensity [6]. New electrophysiological devices have been developed for monitoring nociception and pain, which could be used in situations where validated assessment scales cannot be applied [11]. These devices are based on the measurement of physiological markers related to sympathetic-parasympathetic responses (e.g., pupillary dilation, heart rate variability, sweating). A new multiparametric assessment tool, the Nociception Level Index (NOL) [12], has been developed based on the assumption that combining multiple physiological parameters is superior to their individual use. The NOL simultaneously integrates HRV, photoplethysmographic waveform amplitude, skin conductance, and temperature. Pilot studies have shown that the NOL may discriminate between painful and non-painful care procedures and has been associated with NRS and CPOT scores. Although promising, due to the lack of research studies, these devices cannot be recommended for analgesia titration in intensive care, because of the risk of opioid overuse due to the high sensitivity of these devices to nociceptive stimuli. Overall, the clinical benefits on patient outcomes of all available monitoring devices (developed mainly for anesthetized patients) still need to be further investigated in the intensive care setting. Their use in critically ill patients may be considered on a case-by-case basis with regular evaluation, particularly for analgesia titration.

Opioids often play a crucial role in sedation in intensive care, whether used alone or in combination with other sedative drugs. Some of the earliest published studies in intensive care highlight the role of analgosedation in alleviating anxiety in critically ill patients, reducing oxygen consumption, and facilitating nursing care, resulting in widespread use among patients requiring mechanical ventilation [13]. Patient agitation is often the underlying reason for the need for sedation. Therefore, before initiating the administration of analgosedative drugs, interventions aimed at reducing patient anxiety should be considered, such as mobilization, adequate control of pain from invasive and care-related procedures, reduction of dyspnea and air hunger, and also taking into account the possibility that the patient has developed withdrawal and/or tolerance to ongoing pharmacological treatments [4].

Sedation and agitation, however, can be difficult to distinguish, and scales that quantify sedation always include an assessment of agitation. When deciding to initiate or continue therapy with analgosedative drugs, alongside pain management, the patient's level of sedation and agitation should be assessed using validated tools that improve communication and understanding among team members and help achieve the desired therapeutic goals. These goals should be reassessed at least daily, so that pharmacological and non-pharmacological strategies can be adjusted according to the patient's response. Moreover, as with pain, there is interindividual variability in response to administered sedatives, driven by pharmacokinetic and pharmacodynamic mechanisms in the critically ill patient. In contrast to pain assessment, tools for evaluating sedation and agitation and guidelines for sedation strategies are well validated and based on large randomized controlled trials. However, it is important to emphasize that the two assessments (pain intensity and sedation) cannot be separated and are therefore interdependent in the management of critically ill patients.

Validated and commonly used sedation and agitation assessment scales in intensive care include the Richmond Agitation-Sedation Scale (RASS) [14] and the Riker Sedation-Agitation Scale (SAS) [15]. These scales remain the gold standard for sedation monitoring. Processed electroencephalogram monitoring systems, frequently used to monitor the depth of anesthesia in the operating room, have been introduced into clinical practice in intensive care to monitor the depth of sedation. Their use is currently most appropriate for patients who cannot be assessed using the standard scales, such as paralyzed patients. However, limitations such as interindividual variability, reduced reliability in elderly patient populations, costs, and movement artifacts currently limit their widespread use, and their application is often complementary to subjective assessments [16].

The success of pain and sedation assessments with drug titration has led to a reduction in the dose and duration of opioid and sedative administration, less time spent in deep sedation, reduced pain, and an overall improvement in outcomes, including the duration of invasive mechanical ventilation, length of stay, mortality, and overall costs [4, 17, 18]. This has led to the coining of the term analgosedation, referring to the clinical practice of prioritizing analgesia and reducing overall sedation by using the lowest dose necessary to achieve intensive care treatment goals [19].

19.3 Opioids in the Critically Ill Patient: From Pain Control to Sedation in Intensive Care

Opioids are among the most commonly administered drugs to critically ill patients in intensive care. It is estimated that opioids are administered to nearly 80% of patients undergoing mechanical ventilation [20, 21]. The primary indication is the treatment of acute pain or discomfort. The causes of acute pain are complex, often synergistic with other factors, and include the underlying condition for which the patient is admitted to intensive care (such as sepsis, trauma, burns, surgery), the use of medical devices, and the performance of procedures to facilitate supportive therapies (e.g., the presence of an endotracheal tube, urinary catheter, prolonged immobility), mobilization, hygiene, care of pressure ulcers, airway suctioning, and management of vascular access. Other causes of acute pain with multifactorial psychosocial components in the critically ill patient include delirium, sleep deprivation, anxiety and fear, social isolation, depression, and post-traumatic stress disorder. Acute pain is common in severely ill patients, with 80% reporting moderate to severe pain during their stay in intensive care [4, 22, 23]. Furthermore, about half of intensive care patients, both medical and surgical, report moderate to severe pain at rest [23]. Opioids are recommended as first-line analgesics for non-neuropathic pain in critically ill patients [2].

The most commonly used opioid formulations in intensive care include morphine derivatives and synthetic formulations such as fentanyl and remifentanil. Over the past two decades, there has been a shift in the preferred drugs used for analgosedation in ventilated intensive care patients. While morphine was once preferred over synthetic opioids such as fentanyl, sufentanil, alfentanil, and remifentanil [23], over time fentanyl has become more popular than the other opioids [24]. The reasons for this change have not been extensively studied, but may be related to the perception of a more favorable pharmacokinetic profile, the lack of accumulation of active metabolites in patients with severe and irreversible organ dysfunction, and the reduced incidence of adverse events (such as nausea and vomiting, urinary retention, and constipation). It is likely that all these factors play a role in the prescribing decision-making process. Geographic variation in the type of opioid prescribed in intensive care has also been observed: the drugs most commonly used for analgosedation of critically ill patients in Australia and New Zealand [25] are morphine and fentanyl (with ventilated patients receiving fentanyl (80%), morphine (30%), and alfentanil (7.6%)); in France [26], approximately 40% of patients are treated with sufentanil, 25% with fentanyl, and 20% with morphine. In a European survey on opioid use in intensive care [27], morphine was preferred over fentanyl and sufentanil in Norway, the United Kingdom, Ireland, Sweden, Switzerland, the Netherlands, Spain, and Portugal; conversely, fentanyl was preferentially used in France, Germany, and Italy. Although this survey was conducted more than 20 years ago and preferences may have changed over time, the study highlights a certain degree of geographic variability in clinical practice. To date, there is a lack of large comparative effectiveness studies and clinical trials aimed at comparing the different classes of opioids used for analgosedation in intensive care units.

19.3.1 Pain Management in Critically Ill Patients

Patients admitted to intensive care undergo numerous diagnostic and therapeutic procedures every day [28]. In a large, prospective, cross-sectional, multicenter study on the intensity of pain associated with 12 different procedures in 192 intensive care units across 28 participating countries, the authors found that the most painful procedures included removal of surgical and chest drains, and arterial catheterization. Often, even basic hygiene care and patient mobilization can cause painful stimuli and discomfort [29]. Therefore, adequate pain control is essential, preferably through a multimodal analgesic approach that leverages the action of opioids in combination with NSAIDs or the use of regional anesthesia techniques. Multimodal pain management is even more important in patients undergoing surgery and admitted to intensive care.

Considering pain caused by diagnostic and therapeutic procedures, one study compared the efficacy of remifentanil 0.5 mcg/kg versus placebo for the treatment of pain associated with chest drain removal. This study demonstrated that pain was significantly better controlled in patients who received remifentanil compared to those treated with placebo [30].

In surgical patients, morphine is widely used to control moderate to severe postoperative pain, and the use of repeated and intravenous bolus administrations of morphine generally allows for rapid titration of the dose required for adequate pain relief [31]. The essential principle of a titration regimen is to adjust the dose of morphine to the level of pain observed, taking into account comorbidities, patient age, and the presence of obesity. The optimal regimen in the postoperative setting may involve the administration of both a lipophilic opioid such as fentanyl for rapid pain control and morphine for a longer-lasting effect. However, studies on this combination exist, and its risk/benefit ratio remains a subject of debate [32]. The patient's sensitivity to pain remains the most important cause of variability in the required morphine dose. This is the main justification for using morphine titration to achieve adequate analgesia in each patient. A study on morphine titration in the postoperative period attempted to identify covariates that significantly influence the dose required to achieve analgesia and sedation. The ED50 of morphine for analgesia was approximately 10.2 mg [33]. Factors that reduced the ED50 included: a low VAS score, a short interval between awakening and the first titration dose, and the administration of nonsteroidal anti-inflammatory drugs (NSAIDs) at the end of surgery. Any titration protocol should define the pain score threshold required to administer morphine, the total dose of morphine boluses administered, the interval between doses, the point at which titration should be stopped, and the maximum dose of morphine to be reached. A study conducted on over 3000 postoperative patients in the PACU (post-anesthesia care unit) revealed that patients with higher initial VAS scores required incremental doses of morphine to achieve an acceptable level of pain control. The mean dose for pain relief was 0.17 mg/kg with a median of four boluses (range: 1–20) [34].

As previously emphasized, the use of opioids is recommended as part of a broader multimodal approach that includes additional drugs such as NSAIDs, gabapentinoids, paracetamol, regional analgesia/anesthesia techniques, and non-pharmacological adjuvants (e.g., relaxation techniques, meditation, and psychological support) [4]. Alternative interventions to avoid the use of opioids may include optimizing patient-ventilator synchrony, repositioning and mobilizing the patient to relieve discomfort, and maintaining the sleep-wake cycle. Recently, ketamine [35] has gained popularity, mainly due to its potential opioid-sparing effects and overall safety profile; however, concerns remain regarding side effects such as delirium, nightmares, and laryngospasm, which may be reduced when used at lower or subanesthetic doses.

19.3.2 The Use of Opioids for Analgosedation in Critically Ill Patients

The pillars of analgosedation in intensive care include the use of multimodal pharmacotherapeutic regimens for pain control, frequent assessment of pain intensity and depth of sedation, daily interruption of sedative drug administration, and a personalized therapeutic approach utilizing *short-acting* pharmacological agents. The target, whenever possible, should be *light sedation* [2, 4, 36]. Moreover, an increasing number of studies demonstrate that the presence of family members provides a significant contribution in limiting the incidence of delirium, and has a genuine anxiolytic and reorienting effect for the critically ill patient [19]. These *bundles* have evolved to offer the best possible care to severely ill patients. However, their adoption has been negatively affected by slow dissemination and the COVID-19 pandemic [24, 37]. Drug shortages, resource constraints, staff safety, workforce shortages, limited knowledge of the disease, and the mistaken belief that patients with severe respiratory failure due to COVID-19 required deep analgosedation have contributed to changes in clinical practice, including increased use of benzodiazepines and reduced adherence to daily sedation interruptions.

The goal of light sedation is to maintain the patient in a state of calm, cooperation, and comfort (the 3C rule) [19]. Ideally, the patient should remain alert, able to maintain eye contact, interact with caregivers and family members, and participate in physical rehabilitation therapy, while also being able to rest without interruption. This state, equivalent to a Richmond Agitation Sedation Scale (RASS) score of −1/0 [14], has been shown to have several favorable clinical effects [2, 38]. Agitation in the intensive care patient may result from many factors, including pain, delirium, anxiety, drug withdrawal syndromes, poor synchrony with mechanical ventilation, and pressure ulcers. Emphasis should always be placed on diagnosing and promptly identifying the causes of agitation, rather than simply treating the symptoms, which could lead to the use of inadequate analgosedation protocols. Suboptimal pain management should also be considered an important factor in agitation and should therefore be addressed accordingly, without masking the signs of agitation. Attention should also be paid to ruling out organic and pathophysiological factors as causes of agitation, such as decreased cerebral perfusion, severe hypoxemia, sepsis, fever, electrolyte imbalances, sleep disturbances, and drug administration, all of which can cause brain dysfunction and altered mental status. In these cases, short-term sedation may be necessary until the acute conditions described above are resolved. The presence or absence of delirium should be objectively assessed using a validated clinical tool, such as the Confusion Assessment Method for the ICU (CAM-ICU) [39].

Analgosedation in critically ill patients may involve two distinct strategies that, in practice, represent significantly different approaches: (1) analgesia-first sedation, in which opioid analgesia is used before the administration of a sedative, or (2) analgesia-based sedation, in which the analgesic is used in place of sedatives [40]. Analgesia-based sedation goes beyond the concept of addressing pain first and uses opioids to manage agitation or facilitate mechanical ventilation. Estimates from the study by Duprey et al. [41] reflect a shift in practice toward analgesia-based sedation, where the average opioid dose increased approximately tenfold from 2017 to 2019 compared to 2015–2016 (478 mg versus 56 mg), and patients were more likely to receive an opioid at a higher median dose on days when pain scores were not documented. This trend was also observed in non-arousable patients, who were more likely to receive an opioid (at the highest median dose).

Fentanyl and sufentanil are lipophilic drugs and therefore have a rapid onset. However, greater lipophilicity also results in an increased volume of distribution, thereby raising the risk of accumulation and delayed recovery after prolonged administration. In contrast, remifentanil (a fentanyl derivative) is a short-acting opioid with unique properties. Unlike other opioids that require hepatic biotransformation and renal elimination, remifentanil is metabolized by nonspecific plasma esterases. The context-sensitive half-life (i.e., the time required for the plasma concentration of the drug to decrease by 50% after cessation of an infusion) of remifentanil is short (3.2 minutes), even after a prolonged infusion (> 8 hours) [42]. Therefore, analgesia-based sedation with remifentanil has been introduced as an option for critically ill patients in intensive care. Moreover, its half-life is not only independent of the duration of infusion but also of organ function. For these reasons, it has been studied as a sedative agent in intensive care, predominantly among surgical patients, in comparison with midazolam alone, midazolam with fentanyl, fentanyl alone, and morphine [43–46]. Although remifentanil has been associated, in these small studies, with a reduction in days of mechanical ventilation and length of stay in intensive care, it has not yet been evaluated in a large and heterogeneous population of critically ill patients, and it is currently not a common choice in most intensive care units. In studies comparing remifentanil and morphine, the former was associated with faster achievement of sedation targets, reduced use of supplemental medications, and shorter duration of mechanical ventilation [45]. Prolonged use of remifentanil may contribute to hyperalgesia (pain disproportionate to the stimulus) upon discontinuation and to glycine toxicity when used in patients with impaired renal metabolism, depending on the formulation used [4]. When fentanyl was compared with remifentanil, patients showed equal time to achieve sedation targets, no difference in extubation times, and reported improved pain after extubation [47]; however, patients receiving fentanyl required more frequent administration of additional sedatives compared to those receiving remifentanil [48]. Overall, fentanyl and its derivatives have superior properties (e.g., safety, tolerability, short duration of action, easy titratability, efficacy at equipotent doses) for use in intensive care, but no data clearly support one of these drugs over another. However, meperidine, codeine, and morphine have clear contraindications in specific patient populations. Meperidine carries an increased risk of adverse drug reactions and neurotoxic effects, particularly in patients with renal failure. Morphine also undergoes renal metabolism to an active metabolite (morphine-3-glucuronide) that can prolong sedation and contribute to respiratory depression and neuroexcitatory side effects such as myoclonus. Codeine is used less frequently due to its low analgesic potency and hepatic metabolism to morphine, and therefore has a risk profile similar to morphine in this population.

The use of opioid-based analgosedation is also indicated in critically ill patients receiving noninvasive respiratory support. Opioids do not depress respiratory drive, but they do affect respiratory timing. While they may improve dyspnea, they could also lead to the development of apnea, and therefore their use must always be guided by careful monitoring [49].

Despite the clear benefit of opioids in facilitating invasive therapies, prolonged opioid infusions, as is common in patients undergoing mechanical ventilation, can be harmful. Prolonged duration of opioid-based analgosedation can lead to short-term adverse effects such as delirium, acute opioid tolerance, opioid-induced hyperalgesia, immunosuppression with increased risk of infections, iatrogenic withdrawal syndrome upon abrupt discontinuation, and long-term effects such as persistent opioid use and its potential role in the development of chronic pain in patients discharged from intensive care (Table 19.1).

Table 19.1 Pharmacokinetics and pharmacodynamics properties of the most commonly used opioids in intensive care. Indicated dosages derive from analysed literature (dose may change according to reference source)

Opioids	Loading dose	Maintenance dose	Onset	Characteristics
Fentanyl	1–2 mcg/kg (25–100 mcg)	0.35–0.5 mcg/kg every 0.5–1 hour (25–50 mcg) and/or 0.7–10 mcg/kg/h by continuous infusion. In most patients: 1–3 mcg/kg/h by continuous infusion (with IV boluses as needed)	< 1–2 min	*Advantages*: potent analgesic effect, with immediate onset and less hemodynamic impact (compared to other opioids). Hepatic metabolism (CYP3A4) to inactive metabolites *Disadvantages*: lipophilic drug, with risk of accumulation in adipose tissue, especially with continuous infusion or high doses. At high doses, chest wall rigidity may occur
Morphine	2–10 mg	2–4 mg every 1–2 hours, or 2–30 mg/h by infusion	5–10 min	*Advantages*: non-CYP-related metabolism (glucuronidation); allows for drug titration until effective doses are reached (especially in acute post-surgical and post-procedural pain and in breakthrough pain) *Disadvantages*: in hepatic and/or renal dysfunction, risk of accumulation. Metabolites are active, with potential adverse effects and excessive sedation. Histamine release, vasodilation, hypotension, and bradycardia can be significant adverse effects
Remifentanil	Generally not used in intensive care patients; risk of excessive bradycardia and hypotension	0.05–0.25 mcg/kg/min	1–3 min	*Advantages*: ultra-short acting; context-sensitive half-life of about 3 min; metabolized by nonspecific plasma esterases to inactive metabolites; TCI (target-controlled infusion) administration possible *Disadvantages*: upon discontinuation, risk of hyperalgesia; risk of glycine accumulation toxicity (in renal failure)

19.4 Opioid Stewardship in Intensive Care

The term *stewardship* is found in many aspects of healthcare and, more specifically in pharmacology, in relation to the rational use of antimicrobials and opioids. Opioid stewardship is modeled after the approach developed for antibiotics, with which it shares many similarities. In 2017, the United States Department of Health and Human Services declared the opioid crisis a national emergency. As a direct consequence, hospitals and healthcare systems are seeking and developing methods to address this crisis through the implementation of tools to help healthcare professionals provide appropriate opioid therapies. According to the Institute of Safe Medication Practices (ISMP) of Canada, *opioid stewardship* can be defined as the set of "coordinated and designed interventions to improve, monitor, and evaluate opioid use in order to support and protect human health" [50]. Appropriate opioid stewardship is based on the acquisition of specific skills in the management of complex pain. This includes understanding the pharmacology of analgesics and their therapeutic application, using appropriate tools to rationalize opioid prescribing, adequate monitoring, and surveillance of the beneficial and/or adverse effects of these drugs.

During hospitalization, opioids remain a cornerstone of therapy for patients undergoing surgical procedures or in intensive care, in the treatment of acute pain conditions or refractory to alternative therapies. Postoperative pain control has been the subject of numerous studies and guidelines, receiving renewed attention in light of the current opioid crisis. Conversely, although several guidelines and recommendations are available for the treatment and assessment of pain in intensive care, the supporting clinical evidence is limited and often based on extrapolations from studies on postoperative pain management. Moreover, such evidence is particularly scarce when considering pain management strategies during the transition phase from intensive care to the hospital ward and ultimately to discharge home.

Opioid prescription at discharge following surgery has been widely investigated and addressed in recommendations, as inappropriate prescribing is very common, although it often depends on the type of procedure the patient has undergone [51, 52]. Furthermore, post-discharge opioid use is frequently anticipated and planned, starting from opioid-based therapeutic plans implemented during hospitalization and prior to discharge [53]. However, data regarding opioid prescriptions at discharge after an intensive care unit (ICU) stay are limited: in a study involving 120 patients aged 65 years or older, previously admitted to the ICU for respiratory failure or shock, it was found that 59% of the opioids present in therapy at discharge—and later deemed inappropriate—were prescribed for the first time during the ICU stay [54]. Opioids accounted for only 12% of these therapies, but in 73% of cases, their administration was initiated in the ICU. Although there is less information on opioid prescribing at discharge after intensive care compared to surgical admissions, CDC recommendations regarding discharge prescription limitations should also apply to opioid-naïve patients discharged after an ICU stay [22].

A possible solution to the excessive prescription of opioids for acute pain control in intensive care is the adoption of multimodal pain management strategies. In this context, appropriate pain assessment and management can be facilitated by a multidisciplinary approach involving physicians, nursing staff, and clinically trained pharmacists specializing in pain management. Opioid use should be subject to ongoing reassessment, especially during transitions of care. This is because non-opioid agents may become more suitable alternatives as pain severity decreases and the organ dysfunction that led to ICU admission resolves. Additionally, follow-up should be considered for patients after discharge, particularly when opioid administration is continued. The involvement of clinical pharmacists in post-ICU follow-up (e.g., recovery centers) can help identify pain control issues and adverse effects associated with opioid use [55].

We can therefore state that the priorities of an *opioid stewardship* program are twofold: to appropriately treat acute pain and/or exacerbations of chronic pain during ICU/hospital admissions, and to limit misuse and improve opioid utilization. It is not surprising that efforts to control the opioid epidemic have focused on limiting inappropriate opioid prescriptions at discharge. Indeed, it has been shown that opioid prescribing at discharge contributes to the chronic use of these drugs and to the development of dependence and tolerance [47].

In conclusion, effective *opioid stewardship* programs in intensive care must be based on multidisciplinary approaches involving physicians, pharmacists, nurses, and pain specialists (Fig. 19.1). The collaboration of these professionals is aimed at implementing evidence-based protocols that enable careful selection of the opioid to be used, appropriate dosing, monitoring of pain intensity, and reduction of inappropriate analgesic prescriptions [56]. These programs emphasize multimodal strategies that utilize non-opioid medications such as acetaminophen, NSAIDs, alpha-2 antagonists, ketamine, and regional anesthesia techniques to minimize opioid requirements [57]. Alongside careful patient monitoring using validated tools and scales, pharmacokinetic considerations are central to opioid management in intensive care, as critical illness frequently alters drug metabolism and clearance,

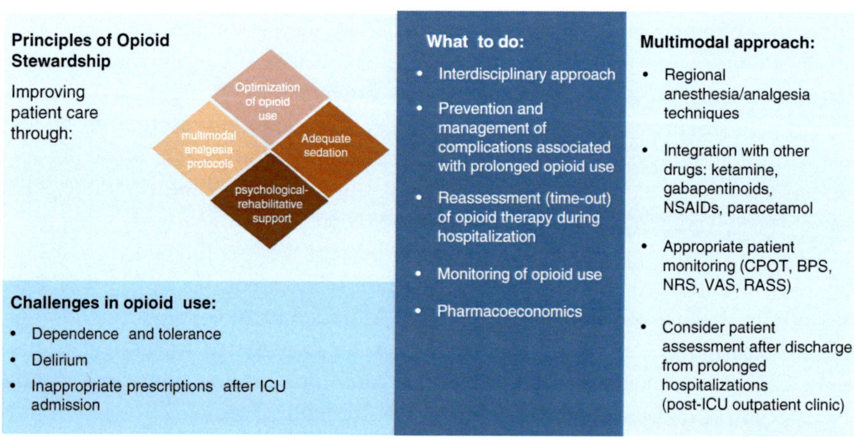

Fig. 19.1 Opioid Stewardship in ICU

potentially leading to metabolite accumulation or ineffective dosing [58]. Special attention must be paid to patients with hepatic or renal impairment. In these cases, opioid metabolites may accumulate and cause adverse effects ranging from prolonged sedation to neurotoxicity. From a management perspective, continuous quality improvement initiatives—monitoring opioid utilization patterns, protocol adherence, adverse events, and early identification of opportunities to improve prescribing and management practices—can enhance the use of these drugs and the indications for which they are prescribed. As the healthcare system continues to confront the growing opioid epidemic, *opioid stewardship* programs in intensive care could play a protective role for vulnerable patients, both by ensuring adequate pain control and by limiting unwarranted opioid exposure, thereby improving outcomes for critically ill patients, such as reducing days on mechanical ventilation, reduction in intensive care unit length of stay, prevention of the development of chronic pain syndromes after intensive care, and limitation of persistent opioid use following critical illness [59, 60].

19.5 Conclusions

Increasing scientific evidence supports a rationalization of opioid use in the management of critically ill patients in the intensive care unit. The best clinical outcomes are achieved when a multimodal approach, incorporating both pharmacological and non-pharmacological strategies, is employed for pain control and for achieving and optimizing sedation targets. Adequate monitoring and rational use of opioids allow for a reduction in adverse effects while enhancing their benefits. The management of pain and agitation with short-acting drugs, continuously titrated based on the patient's clinical assessments, is associated with improved short- and long-term outcomes after discharge. The development of protocols based on data from various studies over recent decades has changed the way we manage patients and improved outcomes in intensive care units worldwide. The identification of appropriate drugs for specific patient populations based on existing comorbidities (e.g., patients with heart failure, transplant recipients, or those with substance use disorders) and the critical illnesses being treated (e.g., patients admitted to intensive care after major surgery, trauma, or neurological conditions) will continue to evolve as our understanding of critical illness, opioid use in intensive care, and associated clinical outcomes increases. The implementation of *opioid stewardship* programs in intensive care, therefore, is increasingly indicated and forms the basis for the rationalization and optimization of their use.

References

1. Shapiro BA, Warren J, Egol AB, Greenbaum DM, Jacobi J, Nasraway SA, et al. Practice parameters for intravenous analgesia and sedation for adult patients in the intensive care unit: an executive summary. Society of Critical Care Medicine. Crit Care Med. 1995;23(9):1596–600.

2. Devlin JW, Skrobik Y, Gélinas C, Needham DM, Slooter AJC, Pandharipande PP, et al. Clinical practice guidelines for the prevention and management of pain, agitation/sedation, delirium, immobility, and sleep disruption in adult patients in the ICU. Crit Care Med. 2018;46(9):e825.
3. Devine H, Quasim T, McPeake J, Shaw M, Mccallum L, Mactavish P. Chronic pain in intensive care unit survivors: incidence, characteristics and side-effects up to one-year post-discharge. J Rehabil Med. 2019;51:451.
4. Boncyk C, Rolfsen ML, Richards D, Stollings JL, Mart MF, Hughes CG, et al. Management of pain and sedation in the intensive care unit. BMJ. 2024;387:e079789.
5. Burton AR, Fazalbhoy A, Macefield VG. Sympathetic responses to noxious stimulation of muscle and skin. Front Neurol. 2016;7:109.
6. Chanques G, Gélinas C. Monitoring pain in the intensive care unit (ICU). Intensive Care Med. 2022;48(10):1508–11.
7. van de Leur JP, van der Schans CP, Loef BG, Deelman BG, Geertzen JH, Zwaveling JH. Discomfort and factual recollection in intensive care unit patients. Crit Care. 2004;8(6):R467–73.
8. Pun BT, Balas MC, Barnes-Daly MA, Thompson JL, Aldrich JM, Barr J, et al. Caring for critically ill patients with the ABCDEF bundle: results of the ICU liberation collaborative in over 15,000 adults. Crit Care Med. 2019;47(1):3.
9. Chanques G, Viel E, Constantin JM, Jung B, de Lattre S, Carr J, et al. The measurement of pain in intensive care unit: comparison of 5 self-report intensity scales. Pain. 2010;151(3):711–21.
10. Murray MJ, DeBlock H, Erstad B, Gray A, Jacobi J, Jordan C, et al. Clinical practice guidelines for sustained neuromuscular blockade in the adult critically ill patient. Crit Care Med. 2016;44(11):2079.
11. Ledowski T. Objective monitoring of nociception: a review of current commercial solutions. BJA Br J Anaesth. 2019;123(2):e312–21.
12. Gélinas C, Shahiri TS, Richard-Lalonde M, Laporta D, Morin JF, Boitor M, et al. Exploration of a multi-parameter technology for pain assessment in postoperative patients after cardiac surgery in the intensive care unit: the Nociception Level Index (NOL)TM. J Pain Res. 2021;14:3723.
13. Merriman HM. The techniques used to sedate ventilated patients. A survey of methods used in 34 ICUs in Great Britain. Intensive Care Med. 1981;7(5):217–24.
14. Ely EW, Truman B, Shintani A, Thomason JWW, Wheeler AP, Gordon S, et al. Monitoring sedation status over time in ICU patients: reliability and validity of the Richmond Agitation-Sedation Scale (RASS). JAMA. 2003;289(22):2983.
15. Riker RR, Picard JT, Fraser GL. Prospective evaluation of the sedation-agitation scale for adult critically ill patients. Crit Care Med. 1999;27(7):1325.
16. Rasulo FA, Hopkins P, Lobo FA, Pandin P, Matta B, Carozzi C, et al. Processed electroencephalogram-based monitoring to guide sedation in critically ill adult patients: recommendations from an international expert panel-based consensus. Neurocrit Care. 2023;38(2):296–311.
17. Wongtangman K, Santer P, Wachtendorf LJ, Azimaraghi O, Baedorf Kassis E, Teja B, et al. Association of sedation, coma, and in-hospital mortality in mechanically ventilated patients with coronavirus disease 2019-related acute respiratory distress syndrome: a retrospective cohort study. Crit Care Med. 2021;49(9):1524–34.
18. Rozendaal FW, Spronk PE, Snellen FF, Schoen A, van Zanten ARH, Foudraine NA, et al. Remifentanil-propofol analgo-sedation shortens duration of ventilation and length of ICU stay compared to a conventional regimen: a centre randomised, cross-over, open-label study in The Netherlands. Intensive Care Med. 2009;35(2):291–8.
19. Vincent JL, Shehabi Y, Walsh TS, Pandharipande PP, Ball JA, Spronk P, et al. Comfort and patient-centred care without excessive sedation: the eCASH concept. Intensive Care Med. 2016;42:962.

20. Girard TD, Thompson JL, Pandharipande PP, Brummel NE, Jackson JC, Patel MB, et al. Clinical phenotypes of delirium during critical illness and severity of subsequent long-term cognitive impairment: a prospective cohort study. Lancet Respir Med. 2018;6(3):213–22.
21. Wunsch H, Hill AD, Fu L, Fowler RA, Wang HT, Gomes T, et al. New opioid use after invasive mechanical ventilation and hospital discharge. Am J Respir Crit Care Med [Internet]. 2020 Aug 15 [cited 2025 Mar 7];202(4). Available from: https://pubmed.ncbi.nlm.nih.gov/32348694/.
22. Erstad BL, Puntillo K, Gilbert HC, Grap MJ, Li D, Medina J, et al. Pain management principles in the critically ill. Chest. 2009;135(4):1075–86.
23. Moran BL, Myburgh JA, Scott DA. The complications of opioid use during and post–intensive care admission: a narrative review. Anaesth Intensive Care. 2022;50(1–2):108–26.
24. Payen JF, Chanques G, Futier E, Velly L, Jaber S, Constantin JM. Sedation for critically ill patients with COVID-19: which specificities? One size does not fit all. Anaesth Crit Care Pain Med. 2020;39(3):341.
25. O'Connor M, Bucknall T, Manias E. Sedation management in Australian and New Zealand intensive care units: doctors' and nurses' practices and opinions. Am J Crit Care. 2010;19(3):285–95.
26. Payen JF, Chanques G, Mantz J, Hercule C, Auriant I, Leguillou JL, et al. Current practices in sedation and analgesia for mechanically ventilated critically ill patients: a prospective multicenter patient-based study. Anesthesiology. 2007;106(4):687.
27. Soliman HM, Mélot C, Vincent JL. Sedative and analgesic practice in the intensive care unit: the results of a European survey. Br J Anaesth. 2001;87(2):186–92.
28. Pota V, Coppolino F, Barbarisi A, Passavanti MB, Aurilio C, Sansone P, et al. Pain in intensive care: a narrative review. Pain Ther. 2022;11(2):359–67.
29. Puntillo KA, Morris AB, Thompson CL, Stanik-Hutt J, White CA, Wild LR. Pain behaviors observed during six common procedures: results from thunder project II. Crit Care Med. 2004;32(2).421–7. https://doi.org/10.1097/01.CCM.0000108875.35298.D2.
30. Casey E, Lane A, Kuriakose D, McGeary S, Hayes N, Phelan D, Buggy D. Bolus remifentanil for chest drain removal in ICU: a randomized double-blind comparison of three modes of analgesia in post-cardiac surgical patients. Intensive Care Med. 2010;36(8):1380–5. https://doi.org/10.1007/s00134-010-1836-2.
31. Aubrun F, Mazoit JX, Riou B. Postoperative intravenous morphine titration. Br J Anaesth. 2012;108(2):193–201.
32. Dahmani S, Dupont H, Mantz J, Desmonts JM, Keita H. Predictive factors of early morphine requirements in the post-anaesthesia care unit (PACU). Br J Anaesth. 2001;87(3):385–9.
33. Kalvass JC, Olson ER, Cassidy MP, Selley DE, Pollack GM. Pharmacokinetics and pharmacodynamics of seven opioids in P-glycoprotein-competent mice: assessment of unbound brain EC50,u and correlation of in vitro, preclinical, and clinical data. J Pharmacol Exp Ther. 2007;323(1):346–55. https://doi.org/10.1124/jpet.107.119560.
34. Aubrun F, Langeron O, Quesnel C, Coriat P, Riou B. Relationships between measurement of pain using visual analog score and morphine requirements during postoperative intravenous morphine titration. Anesthesiology. 2003;98(6):1415–21. https://doi.org/10.1097/00000542-200306000-00017.
35. Assouline B, Tramèr MR, Kreienbühl L, Elia N. Benefit and harm of adding ketamine to an opioid in a patient-controlled analgesia device for the control of postoperative pain: systematic review and meta-analyses of randomized controlled trials with trial sequential analyses. Pain. 2016;157(12):2854–64.
36. DAS-Taskforce 2015, Baron R, Binder A, Biniek R, Braune S, Buerkle H, et al. Evidence and consensus based guideline for the management of delirium, analgesia, and sedation in intensive care medicine. Revision 2015 (DAS-Guideline 2015) - short version. Ger Med Sci GMS E-J. 2015;13:Doc19.

37. Kapp CM, Zaeh S, Niedermeyer S, Punjabi NM, Siddharthan T, Damarla M. The use of analgesia and sedation in mechanically ventilated patients with COVID-19 acute respiratory distress syndrome. Anesth Analg. 2020;131(4):e198–200.
38. Barr J, Fraser GL, Puntillo K, Ely EW, Gélinas C, Dasta JF, et al. Clinical practice guidelines for the management of pain, agitation, and delirium in adult patients in the intensive care unit. Crit Care Med. 2013;41(1):263–306.
39. Ely EW, Margolin R, Francis J, May L, Truman B, Dittus R, et al. Evaluation of delirium in critically ill patients: validation of the confusion assessment method for the Intensive Care Unit (CAM-ICU). Crit Care Med. 2001;29(7):1370–9.
40. Murray BP, Newsome AS. Opioids for sedation: has the pendulum swung too far? Am J Respir Crit Care Med. 2021;204(5):611.
41. Duprey MS, Dijkstra-Kersten SMA, Zaal IJ, Briesacher BA, Saczynski JS, Griffith JL, et al. Opioid use increases the risk of delirium in critically ill adults independently of pain. Am J Respir Crit Care Med. 2021;204(5):566–72.
42. Beers R, Camporesi E. Remifentanil update: clinical science and utility. CNS Drugs. 2004;18(15):1085–104.
43. Muellejans B, Matthey T, Scholpp J, Schill M. Sedation in the intensive care unit with remifentanil/propofol versus midazolam/fentanyl: a randomised, open-label, pharmacoeconomic trial. Crit Care Lond Engl. 2006;10(3):R91.
44. Breen D, Karabinis A, Malbrain M, Morais R, Albrecht S, Jarnvig IL, et al. Decreased duration of mechanical ventilation when comparing analgesia-based sedation using remifentanil with standard hypnotic-based sedation for up to 10 days in intensive care unit patients: a randomised trial [ISRCTN47583497]. Crit Care Lond Engl. 2005;9(3):R200–10.
45. Dahaba AA, Grabner T, Rehak PH, List WF, Metzler H. Remifentanil versus morphine analgesia and sedation for mechanically ventilated critically ill patients: a randomized double blind study. Anesthesiology. 2004;101(3):640–6.
46. Spies C, Macguill M, Heymann A, Ganea C, Krahne D, Assman A, et al. A prospective, randomized, double-blind, multicenter study comparing remifentanil with fentanyl in mechanically ventilated patients. Intensive Care Med. 2011;37(3):469–76.
47. Oyler D, Bernard AC, VanHoose JD, Parli SE, Ellis CS, Li D, et al. Minimizing opioid use after acute major trauma. Am J Health-Syst Pharm. 2018;75(3):105–10.
48. Muellejans B, López A, Cross MH, Bonome C, Morrison L, Kirkham AJ. Remifentanil versus fentanyl for analgesia based sedation to provide patient comfort in the intensive care unit: a randomized, double-blind controlled trial [ISRCTN43755713]. Crit Care. 2003;8(1):R1.
49. Grieco DL, Maggiore SM, Roca O, Spinelli E, Patel BK, Thille AW, et al. Non-invasive ventilatory support and high-flow nasal oxygen as first-line treatment of acute hypoxemic respiratory failure and ARDS. Intensive Care Med. 2021;47(8):851–66.
50. Uritsky TJ, Busch ME, Chae SG, Genord C. Opioid stewardship: building on antibiotic stewardship principles. J Pain Palliat Care Pharmacother. 2021;34(4):181–3.
51. Chen EY, Marcantonio A, Tornetta P. Correlation between 24-hour predischarge opioid use and amount of opioids prescribed at hospital discharge. JAMA Surg. 2018;153(2):e174859.
52. Feinberg AE, Chesney TR, Srikandarajah S, Acuna SA, McLeod RS. Best practice in surgery group. opioid use after discharge in postoperative patients: a systematic review. Ann Surg. 2018;267(6):1056–62.
53. Hill MV, Stucke RS, Billmeier SE, Kelly JL, Barth RJ. Guideline for discharge opioid prescriptions after inpatient general surgical procedures. J Am Coll Surg. 2018;226(6):996–1003.
54. Morandi A, Vasilevskis E, Pandharipande PP, Girard TD, Solberg LM, Neal EB, et al. Inappropriate medication prescriptions in elderly adults surviving an intensive care unit hospitalization. J Am Geriatr Soc. 2013;61(7):1128–34.

55. Stollings JL, Bloom SL, Wang L, Ely EW, Jackson JC, Sevin CM. Critical care pharmacists and medication management in an ICU recovery center. Ann Pharmacother. 2018;52(8):713–23.
56. Waldfogel JM, Rosen M, Sharma R, Zhang A, Bass EB, Dy SM. Opioid stewardship: rapid review. In: Making healthcare safer IV: a continuous updating of patient safety harms and practices [internet]. Rockville: Agency for Healthcare Research and Quality (US); 2023 [cited 2025 Mar 10]. Available from: http://www.ncbi.nlm.nih.gov/books/NBK598858/.
57. McEvoy MD, Raymond BL, Krige A. Opioid-sparing perioperative analgesia within enhanced recovery programs. Anesthesiol Clin. 2022;40(1):35–58.
58. Smith BS, Yogaratnam D, Levasseur-Franklin KE, Forni A, Fong J. Introduction to drug pharmacokinetics in the critically ill patient. Chest. 2012;141(5):1327–36.
59. Huang A, Azam A, Segal S, Pivovarov K, Katznelson G, Ladak SS, et al. Chronic postsurgical pain and persistent opioid use following surgery: the need for a transitional pain service. Pain Manag. 2016;6(5):435–43.
60. Kurteva S, Abrahamowicz M, Gomes T, Tamblyn R. Association of opioid consumption profiles after hospitalization with risk of adverse health care events. JAMA Netw Open. 2021;4(5):e218782.

Post-anoxic Coma

20

Claudio Sandroni

Abbreviations

AED	Automated external defibrillator
ALS	Advanced Life Support
BLS	Basic Life Support
CPR	Cardiopulmonary resuscitation
ECG	Electrocardiogram
ECPR	Extracorporeal cardiopulmonary resuscitation
ERC	European Resuscitation Council
$ETCO_2$	End-tidal carbon dioxide
IHCA	In-hospital cardiac arrest
ILCOR	International Liaison Committee on Resuscitation
OHCA	Out-of-hospital cardiac arrest
PEA	Pulseless electrical activity
PEEP	Positive end-expiratory pressure
pVT	Pulseless ventricular tachycardia
ROSC	Return of spontaneous circulation
VF	Ventricular fibrillation

C. Sandroni (✉)
Department of Intensive Care, Emergency Medicine, and Anesthesiology, Fondazione Policlinico Universitario A. Gemelli-IRCCS – Università Cattolica del Sacro Cuore, Rome, Italy
e-mail: claudio.sandroni@unicatt.it

D. Chiumello, A. De Gasperi (eds.), *Practical Trends in Anesthesia and Intensive Care 2026*, https://doi.org/10.1007/978-3-032-25721-5_20

20.1 Introduction

Anoxia is the second most common cause of non-traumatic coma in patients admitted to intensive care [1]. In almost all cases, anoxia is caused by cardiac arrest. Causes of isolated cerebral anoxia without cardiac arrest are much rarer and include drowning, strangulation, or carbon monoxide poisoning [2]. In patients resuscitated from cardiac arrest, hypoxic-ischemic brain injury (HIBI) is the leading cause of acute-phase death and long-term disability among patients discharged alive from the hospital [3]. This chapter—unless otherwise specified—addresses post-anoxic coma following cardiac arrest, including its pathophysiology, clinical presentation, intensive care management, and short- and long-term prognosis.

20.2 Pathophysiology

HIBI typically develops in two phases [4]: primary (ischemic) injury and secondary (reperfusion) injury, which occur during cardiac arrest and after restoration of cerebral perfusion, respectively.

20.2.1 Primary Injury: Ischemia

Cardiac arrest causes the immediate cessation of blood flow to all organs. This no-flow phase lasts until cardiopulmonary resuscitation (CPR) restores partial reperfusion. When a patient in cardiac arrest is resuscitated, systemic circulation is partially restored, but cardiac output reaches only 20–25% of normal values. This low-flow phase extends from the start of cardiopulmonary resuscitation to the return of spontaneous circulation (*ROSC*) or the initiation of extracorporeal circulation (*ECPR*).

From the onset of the no-flow phase, the lack of oxygen immediately interrupts the aerobic metabolism. Since neurons lack intrinsic energy reserves to withstand ischemia, cardiac arrest is followed by rapid depletion of adenosine triphosphate (ATP) [4] and consequent failure of the Na^+/K^+ ATP-dependent ion exchange pump located on the cell membrane. This pump, essential for maintaining the physiological polarity of the membrane, expels sodium ions from the cell while simultaneously importing potassium ions into the intracellular compartment. This exchange requires energy supplied by ATP, as it occurs against the transmembrane concentration gradient. The sudden cessation of Na^+/K^+ pump activity leads to a massive passive influx of sodium and water into the intracellular compartment, resulting in cellular swelling (cytotoxic edema). Animal studies have shown that cytotoxic edema develops very early, being detectable by magnetic resonance imaging already during cardiac arrest and resuscitation [5]. Simultaneously with the influx of sodium, there is also a passive efflux of potassium. The cell membrane depolarizes, which triggers the opening of voltage-dependent Ca^{++} channels, resulting in a passive influx of calcium ions. The increase in intracellular calcium is important for subsequent reperfusion injury, as explained later.

Cerebral blood flow (*CBF*) during the low-flow phase has not been directly measured in humans, but it is believed to remain largely below the level required to maintain cellular integrity. Therefore, it is likely that further progression of ischemic brain injury may occur during the low flow phase [6].

20.2.2 Secondary Injury: Reperfusion

Reperfusion of the ischemic cerebrovascular bed following ROSC triggers a series of mechanisms leading to secondary brain injury. These mechanisms are complex, but among them, the increase in intracellular Ca^{++} induced by the release of excitatory neurotransmitters plays a particularly important role. This phenomenon adds to the passive influx of Ca^{++} that occurred during the ischemic phase, and leads on one hand to the activation of Ca^{++} -dependent lytic enzymes (proteases, phospholipases) causing neuronal damage and apoptosis, and on the other hand to mitochondrial dysfunction with consequent cellular energy deficit and release of reactive oxygen species, which further increase neuronal damage and establish a vicious cycle ultimately resulting in cell death.

In the hours or days following cardiac arrest, patients in post-anoxic coma develop further reperfusion-related brain injury due to the activation of inflammatory processes [7]. The cells responsible for this are both microglia [8] and circulating leukocytes, which adhere to endothelial cells of the cerebral microcirculation and migrate into brain tissue, releasing cytokines. The resulting effect is an increase in blood-brain barrier permeability, resulting in vasogenic edema that adds to the previously described cytotoxic edema. These mechanisms explain the alterations in brain tissue—especially affecting the gray matter—visible on neuroimaging in patients with post-anoxic coma, and their progressive evolution in the first days after cardiac arrest.

20.2.3 Cerebral Blood Flow in the Acute Phase of Post-anoxic Coma

Predominantly, experimental evidence has shown that, after a transient hyperemia, CBF following ROSC decreases to less than 50% of pre-arrest values [6]. However, it is still uncertain whether this hypoperfusion contributes to worsening brain injury in patients with post-anoxic coma. Some clinical studies have shown that both cerebral oxygen consumption [9] and the cerebral oxygen extraction fraction were reduced 24–72 h after cardiac arrest [10], suggesting that the coupling between CBF and oxygen demand was nonetheless maintained. However, more recent clinical studies [11], conducted with intraparenchymal microcatheters, have revealed that about half of patients in post-anoxic coma exhibited tissue hypoxia (measured as brain tissue oxygen pressure ($PbtO_2$) below 20 mmHg) at 13–40 h after arrest, and that this hypoxia was associated with the release of neuronal injury biomarkers in the jugular venous blood [12]. It is believed that brain tissue hypoxia in patients with post-anoxic coma may therefore be due not only to hypoperfusion (convective deficit) but also to reduced oxygen diffusion (diffusive deficit), probably caused by tissue edema [13].

20.2.3.1 Alterations of Cerebral Autoregulation

The cerebral circulation possesses autoregulation, which is the ability to maintain stable arterial flow independently of mean arterial pressure (MAP), within a certain range. In patients with acute brain injury, the autoregulation curve can be significantly altered. Specifically, in approximately 30–50% of comatose patients after cardiac arrest, the range of pressure in which CBF remains stable is narrower, and the cerebral autoregulation curve is shifted to the right [14]. The most important clinical consequence is that arterial hypotension after cardiac arrest can easily lead to cerebral hypoperfusion, worsening HIBI. Preventing this exacerbation of anoxic brain injury by optimizing MAP is one of the possible goals of post-resuscitation care, as will be discussed later.

20.2.4 Intracranial Hypertension

As in other forms of acute brain injury, comatose patients after cardiac arrest may develop intracranial hypertension [15]. The increase in intracranial pressure (*ICP*) likely results from cerebral edema and may be associated with a reduction in cerebral perfusion pressure (*CPP*), leading to secondary neurological injury and worsening prognosis. In a study of 84 comatose post-anoxic patients, more than a quarter exhibited increased cerebrospinal fluid pressure, measured by lumbar puncture, within the second day after ROSC, and in more than half, CPP dropped at least once below 50 mmHg [16]. In these patients, intracranial hypertension was significantly associated with unfavorable neurological outcome at 3 months.

20.3 Clinical Presentation

Many comatose patients after cardiac arrest exhibit severe neurological impairment. In a study of 585 patients included in the TTM trial on post-arrest body temperature, 228 (39%) had a decorticate or worse motor response (GCS motor ≤3) 4 days after ROSC [17]. Ocular reflexes (pupillary or corneal) were absent in 51/301 (17%) of the patients in whom they were assessed. The 2025 guidelines on post-resuscitation care published by the European Resuscitation Council (ERC) and the European Society of Intensive Care Medicine (ESICM) [18] recommend that in comatose post-anoxic patients, neurological examination be performed daily and be preceded by discontinuation of sedation. This examination should include the Glasgow Coma Scale score and assessment of ocular reflexes. Unlike the corneal reflex, the pupillary light reflex is not affected by the effects of neuromuscular blocking agents and can be quantitatively assessed using pupillometry (see below).

Clinically visible seizures are common, occurring in about one third of comatose post-anoxic patients [19] and may present as either generalized tonic-clonic or focal seizures, often in the same patient. As in other acute brain injury conditions, epilepsy may be nonconvulsive, that is, occurring in the absence of clinically evident muscle contractions, and detectable only by electroencephalogram (EEG). This also occurs because the administration of sedatives and neuromuscular blockers used to facilitate temperature control or mechanical ventilation suppresses the clinical manifestations of seizures.

A typical, though not exclusive, manifestation of anoxic brain injury is myoclonus. This consists of sudden, sometimes very intense, muscle contractions alternating with relaxation. Although post-anoxic myoclonus may sometimes be associated with epileptic activity, it is often entirely independent, suggesting a possible subcortical origin. A particular form of post-anoxic myoclonus, which must be recognized for its favorable prognostic significance, is Lance-Adams Syndrome (LAS) [20, 21]. In LAS, myoclonus typically appears during voluntary contractions of the facial or limb muscles. Although the presence of voluntary movements presupposes some degree of consciousness, this may be incomplete, and conversely, the myoclonus may be so intense as to mask it [22]. In patients with LAS, recovery of consciousness may therefore go unnoticed, and the intensity of muscle contractions may even lead caregivers to administer excessive sedation to suppress them. In such cases, EEG recording can help distinguish LAS from more malignant forms of myoclonus [23].

20.4 Management of Acute Post-anoxic Coma

Although various neuroprotective therapies have been tested, none have demonstrated proven efficacy in clinical trials [24]. Therefore, at present, the main goal of post-resuscitation care is to limit the risk of secondary brain injury by maintaining homeostasis and, in particular, ensuring stable oxygenation, blood pressure, ventilation, and body temperature within physiological limits.

20.4.1 Blood Pressure and Cerebral Perfusion

A 2015 post-hoc analysis of the TTM trial clearly demonstrated that an MAP below 65 mmHg is associated with a significantly higher risk of death after cardiac arrest [25]. However, it is not known whether MAP values above 65 mmHg improve prognosis in post-anoxic coma. The NEUROPROTECT trial [26] randomized 107 patients in post-anoxic coma to receive a hemodynamic optimization protocol targeting an MAP of 85–100 mmHg and a mixed venous oxygen saturation (SVO_2) of 65–75% versus maintenance of MAP at 65 mmHg alone. The trial showed no differences between the two groups in terms of anoxic brain injury as measured by neuroimaging, nor in long-term neurological outcomes among survivors. In 2022, the double-blind BOX trial [27] randomized 789 patients in post-anoxic coma to receive a protocol maintaining MAP at 63 mmHg versus 77 mmHg. The study found no differences in mortality or favorable neurological outcome at 3 months between the two groups, nor in the predefined subgroups included in the trial design.

In both of the above-mentioned trials, the same MAP target was maintained for all patients enrolled in each treatment arm. A more targeted intervention to optimize cerebral perfusion could involve maintaining MAP within the autoregulatory range of the individual patient. For this purpose, the cerebral oxygenation index (COx) has been studied, which is the correlation coefficient between regional cerebral oxygen saturation (rSO_2), measured by near-infrared spectroscopy (*NIRS*), and MAP. A change in COx with MAP suggests dysfunctional autoregulation, while a COx value close to zero or negative suggests intact autoregulation. Based on this model, the "optimal MAP" is the value at which COx variations are minimal, and autoregulation is preserved. Indeed, an observational study [14] showed that in patients with post-anoxic coma, the percentage of time spent below the optimal MAP was associated with worse neurological outcomes.

The single-center French GOODYEAR study evaluated the feasibility of optimizing cerebral blood flow based on transcranial Doppler (*TCD*). The results were modest, with only 20 includible patients out of 172 screened. Of these, three showed signs of cerebral hypoperfusion based on TCD. In two of these, an attempt was made to optimize MAP, but normalization of TCD parameters was not achieved [28]. The NEURO-INTACT trial (NEUROprotection Via optimizINg Cerebral Blood Flow afTer cArdiaC arresT; ClinicalTrials.gov NCT05679739), sponsored by the University Hospital of Singapore, is randomizing 90 patients to individualized MAP management during the first 72 h after ROSC aimed at optimizing cerebral blood flow versus standard MAP management according to current guidelines. In the intervention arm, optimal MAP is calculated using both NIRS and TCD.

At present, based on a recent individual patient data meta-analysis [29], the ERC-ESICM guidelines for post-resuscitation care recommend maintaining an MAP of at least 60–65 mmHg and targeting adequate urine output (>0.5 ml/kg/h) and normalization of blood lactate levels [18].

20.4.2 Ventilation

The partial pressure of carbon dioxide in arterial blood ($PaCO_2$) is one of the most important factors influencing CBF. An increase or decrease in $PaCO_2$ relative to normal values (35–45 mmHg) rapidly leads, respectively, to a decrease or increase in CBF [30]. In patients in post-anoxic coma after cardiac arrest, in whom cerebral edema is often present, cerebral vasodilation from hypercapnia could increase ICP and potentially be harmful. However, given the potential for cerebral hypoperfusion in the acute phase of HIBI, it has been hypothesized that a moderate increase in CBF resulting from moderate hypercapnia could be beneficial. Unfortunately, the multicenter randomized TAME trial [31], which enrolled 1700 patients to receive moderate hypercapnia (50–55 mmHg) versus normocapnia (35–45 mmHg) for 24 h after ROSC, did not show differences in rates of neurological recovery at 6 months.

The effect of moderate hypercapnia on cerebral blood flow in this trial remains unknown, as the study design did not include CBF assessment. The 2025 ERC-ESICM guidelines for post-resuscitation care [18] recommend maintaining post-anoxic coma patients with ventilation targeted to normocapnia.

20.4.3 Oxygenation

Oxygen is a substrate for the production of free radicals and, in patients with HIBI after ROSC, it may fuel cell damage following reperfusion. However, the results of major observational clinical studies have not consistently shown that hyperoxia is associated with worse prognosis after ROSC [32, 33]. The BOX trial [34] investigated the possible effects of maintaining two different levels of arterial partial pressure of oxygen (68–75 vs. 98–105 mmHg) in post-anoxic coma patients for 120 h after enrollment. The study found no differences in either three-month neurological outcomes or in concentrations of neuron-specific enolase (*NSE*), a biomarker of brain injury.

Recent evidence suggests that in the immediate phase following cardiac arrest, maintaining restrictive oxygen levels may be associated with a risk of hypoxia. The EXACT trial, conducted in the pre-hospital setting [35] randomized 428 patients to either restrictive (90–94%) arterial oxygen saturation (SaO_2) or liberal oxygen therapy (SaO_2 98–100%) from the time of ROSC until their arrival in intensive care. The study results showed that restrictive oxygen therapy was associated with a trend toward lower survival to hospital discharge (unadjusted odds ratio, [*OR*] 0.68 [95% CI, 0.46–1.00]; $p = 0.05$) and a significantly higher percentage risk of hypoxic episodes (OR 2.37 [95% CI, 1.49–3.79]; $p < 0.001$). The 2025 ERC-ESICM guidelines for post-resuscitation care recommend avoiding both hypoxia and hyperoxia, maintaining SaO_2 within a safe range of 94–98% [18]. In the immediate phase after ROSC, based on the EXACT trial, the use of 100% oxygen is recommended until accurate monitoring of PaO_2 or SaO_2 is possible. It is important to note that SaO_2 may overestimate the true value in individuals with dark skin tones.

20.4.4 Targeted Temperature Management

The induction of hypothermia prior to cardiac arrest has a protective effect against post-anoxic brain injury and is routinely used in cardiac surgery. Some animal studies have shown that hypothermia also has a neuroprotective effect when induced after the restoration of spontaneous circulation [36]. In 2025, the experimental trial Hypothermia After Cardiac Arrest in Large Animals (HACA-LA) randomized 33 pigs to receive immediate hypothermia at 33 °C, delayed hypothermia at 33 °C after 2 h, or normothermia for 30 h. The study demonstrated lower blood levels of neurofilament light chain (NfL), a marker of neurological injury, in animals with immediate hypothermia. However, there were no significant differences between groups in the primary outcome, the severity of histopathological brain injury, or in neurocognitive tests [37].

In 2002, two initial clinical trials in small populations with some important methodological limitations showed improved survival and neurological outcomes after hypothermia at 32–34 °C for 12–24 h in patients resuscitated from out-of-hospital cardiac arrest with a shockable rhythm [38, 39]. However, subsequent trials conducted with more rigorous methods and in larger populations did not confirm these results [40, 41]. Current consensus [18, 42] favors active prevention of fever in comatose patients after cardiac arrest, maintaining a core body temperature of ≤37.5 °C for at least 72 h. This can be achieved using either physical or pharmacological measures.

20.4.5 Antiepileptic Therapy

Epilepsy—both convulsive and non-convulsive—is common in post-anoxic coma and is associated with worse neurological prognosis, although its presence does not entirely preclude neurological recovery [43]. However, it is unclear whether the association between seizures and poor outcome is due to seizures causing further brain injury (for example, by increasing cerebral oxygen consumption) or if they are simply a marker of the severity of HIBI. To date, there is no direct evidence that antiepileptic treatment improves the outcome of HIBI. TELSTAR, the only randomized clinical trial conducted to date in this context, did not show benefit from incremental treatment with antiepileptic drugs up to deep sedation compared to no treatment [44]. It should be noted, however, that TELSTAR achieved suppression of epileptic activity in only 56% of patients after 48 h from the start of treatment, and that in the majority of patients, EEG epileptic activity consisted of periodic discharges rather than generalized convulsive seizures. For this latter subgroup, both a sub-analysis of the TELSTAR study and an observational study [45] suggest that aggressive antiepileptic treatment may instead lead to improved prognosis. In a recent multicenter study, aggressive pharmacological treatment was associated with better outcomes [46].

Current guidelines do not recommend seizure prophylaxis with antiepileptic drugs, but suggest treating seizures if they occur [18]. The sedative agents commonly used in intensive care have antiepileptic effects, and this should be taken into account since seizures often manifest upon discontinuation of sedation.

20.5 Monitoring in Post-anoxic Coma

In addition to monitoring basic cardiorespiratory parameters and temperature, patients in post-anoxic coma require continuous assessment of their neurological status.

20.5.1 EEG

Among instrumental neuromonitoring techniques, EEG is the most widely used and readily available [47]. In post-anoxic coma, EEG is useful both for detecting non-convulsive epilepsy and for prognostic purposes. In addition to the presence of epileptic activity, the amplitude and continuity of the EEG background rhythm are the most important pieces of information. Immediately after ROSC, EEG amplitude is often markedly depressed or discontinuous, but in patients who recover, there is a progressive improvement in the background rhythm, whereas persistent depression or discontinuity on EEG after the first 24–48 h is a very unfavorable prognostic sign. There is no unanimous consensus on whether continuous EEG monitoring should be used instead of standard 20–30-min EEG recordings in post-anoxic coma. Continuous EEG increases sensitivity for seizure detection [48], but is more expensive, and there is no evidence that it improves outcome prediction compared to routine EEG [49]. The 2025 ERC-ESICM guidelines on post-resuscitation care suggest early EEG recording in all comatose patients after cardiac arrest [18]. We suggest performing at least one routine EEG per day during the first 3 days in patients who remain unconscious after ROSC. EEG recording is particularly important in patients with myoclonus, both to exclude a state of consciousness masked by myoclonus and to provide prognostic information.

20.5.2 ICP and Transcranial Doppler

HIBI is frequently associated with cytotoxic and vasogenic cerebral edema, which can lead to increased ICP and reduced CPP. Invasive ICP monitoring in post-anoxic coma carries risks, as many cases of cardiac arrest are due to acute myocardial infarction requiring antiplatelet therapy, and is not recommended. Alternatively, TCD can provide an indirect estimate of intracranial hypertension based on measurement of increased arterial vascular resistance due to cerebral edema [50]. Vascular resistance on TCD is measured using the pulsatility index, calculated as the difference between systolic and diastolic CBF velocities (CBFV) divided by the mean CBFV. Pulsatility index values of 1.20 or higher indicate increased arterial resistance and suggest the presence of intracranial hypertension. In a study of 11 patients with HIBI, noninvasive ICP measured using the pulsatility index showed a linear correlation ($r = 0.30$) with invasive ICP measured using an intraparenchymal probe, and a good predictive value for the presence of intracranial hypertension (area under the ROC curve = 0.91; 95% CI = 0.83–1.00) [51] A larger study of 42 patients in post-anoxic coma showed that while mean CBFV values were within the normal range 6 h after ROSC in most patients, the pulsatility index was significantly increased (1.49 vs. 1.12; $p < 0.01$) in patients with unfavorable neurological outcomes, six of whom subsequently died of brain death [52].

The rationale for direct or indirect ICP monitoring after cardiac arrest is to treat intracranial hypertension resulting from HIBI-related cerebral edema. Although there are no prospective clinical studies on this topic, experimental evidence suggests that post-anoxic cerebral edema can be treated with hyperosmolar therapy [53]. In a retrospective clinical study of 65 patients in post-anoxic coma, treatment guided by invasive monitoring and aimed at maintaining ICP <25 mmHg and oxygenation parenchymal pressure >20 mmHg was associated with significantly higher rates of favorable neurological outcome at 6 months [54].

20.6 Prognosis of Post-anoxic Coma

20.6.1 Recovery of Consciousness

Most patients who survive with a favorable neurological outcome after cardiac arrest begin to regain consciousness within 48 h after discontinuation of continuous intravenous sedation. In a French study [55], the awakening rate at 48 h was 71%, and in two other studies [56, 57], it was 50%. In the French study [55], the latest recovery of consciousness occurred 12 days after ROSC, and in the other two studies, 22 and 25 days after, respectively [56, 57]. The presence of circulatory shock, renal failure, and advanced age [55] and the use of long-acting sedative agents [57, 58] are associated with longer times to regain consciousness. Delayed awakening (>4–5 days after ROSC) is associated with a higher risk of neurological disability [56, 57] or poorer quality of life [59]. The 2025 ERC-ESICM guidelines recommend the use of short-acting sedatives in patients with post-anoxic coma [18].

20.6.2 Causes of Death in Post-anoxic Coma

In the first 48–72 h after ROSC, the predominant causes of death in patients with post-anoxic coma are cardiocirculatory instability or multiorgan failure, while in the following days, neurological causes predominate. Overall, HIBI is responsible for about two-thirds of deaths in patients admitted to intensive care after cardiac arrest [3]. Most of these neurologically related deaths occur due to active limitation of treatments (*Withdrawal of Life-Sustaining Treatments, WLST*) based on a prediction of unfavorable neurological outcome [60, 61]. For this reason, accurate neurological prognostication is essential (see below). In a minority of cases, death occurs directly as a result of primary brain injury, and the diagnosis of death is made using neurological criteria (brain death). In 2016, a systematic review [62] including 23,388 patients from 26 studies reported that, on average, brain death was diagnosed in 5% of patients resuscitated with conventional CPR and in more than 20% of those resuscitated with ECPR, corresponding to 8% and 28% of all deaths, respectively. The mean time to brain death diagnosis was 3 days after ROSC, and the most common mechanism was massive cerebral edema. Recent studies on ECPR have confirmed these findings [63, 64]. It is important to perform daily clinical and instrumental neurological assessments in these patients to detect the onset of signs of brain death, both because it allows for the discontinuation of futile treatments and because CPR does not contraindicate potential organ donation in patients who die from brain death following HIBI. Observational studies in these patients have shown rates of successful donation to be comparable to those of donors without cardiac arrest and with brain death from primary neurological causes [62, 63, 65]. A systematic review published in 2025 confirmed these results [66].

20.6.3 Functional Recovery in Post-anoxic Coma

In those who survive cardiac arrest, functional outcome is measured in two main domains: neurological function and health-related quality of life (*HRQOL*).

20.6.3.1 Neurological Function

Neurological function in post-anoxic coma is most commonly assessed using the *Cerebral Performance Categories (CPC)* (Table 20.1) [67]. The CPC scale was adapted from the Glasgow Outcome Scale, developed for traumatic brain injury, and includes five categories, from 1 (no or mild disability) to 5 (death). CPC 1 and CPC 2 (moderate disability) are universally considered favorable neurological outcomes and correspond to patients who are independent in their activities of daily living. In contrast, CPC 3 corresponds to patients who are alert but severely disabled and dependent on others for daily activities, and is generally—though not universally—considered an unfavorable outcome. CPC 4 corresponds to a persistent vegetative state.

Despite its popularity, the CPC scale has limited ability to discriminate between mild and moderate disability, and current guidelines recommend using the modified Rankin Scale (mRS) [68] instead of the CPC. The mRS, originally developed for stroke, has seven scores, ranging from 0 to 6. A favorable outcome corresponds to categories from mRS 0 (no symptoms) to 3 (moderate disability), which can provide greater granularity compared to the two corresponding CPC categories. Patients with disability after cardiac arrest have locomotor issues less frequently than those

Table 20.1 Cerebral Performance Categories

Score	Description
1	Conscious: Alert, able to work and lead a normal life. May have mild psychological or neurological deficits (mild dysphasia, non-disabling hemiparesis, or minor cranial nerve abnormalities)
2	Conscious: Sufficient cerebral function for independent activities of daily living; able to work in a sheltered environment
3	Conscious but dependent on others for daily support due to impaired cerebral function. Can be managed in a long-term care facility or at home with considerable effort from the family Cognitive function is at least limited. Encompasses a wide range of cerebral abnormalities, from gait disturbances, severe memory impairment, or dementia precluding independent living, to paralysis or locked-in syndrome (patient able to communicate only with eye movements)
4	Unconscious, unaware of the surrounding environment. Absence of cognitive functions. No verbal or psychological interaction with the environment
5	Confirmed brain death or death by conventional criteria

with stroke. For this reason, in the mRS version recommended for use in post-anoxic coma (Table 20.2), the mRS 4 score considers dependence in meeting bodily needs separately from the ability to walk unaided (OR instead of AND).

Neither the CPC nor the mRS distinguishes between the two main causes of neurological death (i.e., brain death and death due to WLST) and, more importantly, they do not discriminate between neurological and non-neurological causes of death. As a result, resuscitated patients who die from extracerebral complications (e.g., a second arrest) after regaining consciousness are classified as CPC 5 or mRS 6, regardless of their neurological status at the time of death. In a European multicenter study [69], this "death after awakening" occurred in 4.2% of resuscitated patients. To address this issue, it is advisable to use the best neurological score, rather than the final score, achieved during the observation period.

The minimum recommended time for neurological function assessment in post-anoxic coma is at hospital discharge or 1 month after arrest [70]. However, the neurological outcome of resuscitated patients may further improve thereafter. In a longitudinal study of a large number of out-of-hospital cardiac arrests, the CPC recorded at hospital discharge improved in 80/550 (14.5%) survivors at 6 months [71]. Among the 58 patients with an initial CPC of 3 at discharge, 27 (53.4%) had a good neurological outcome 6 months later. The American Heart Association [70] recommends that—in addition to the minimum time of hospital discharge/1 month—neurological function be assessed at 3 and 6 months, and at 1 year, if resources allow.

Data from major studies on out-of-hospital cardiac arrest [41, 72] show that about 80% of resuscitated patients discharged alive from hospital have a good neurological outcome (CPC 1–2). However, this figure may be influenced by the high rate of early WLST in intensive care. In communities where WLST is not officially practiced, the percentage of good neurological outcomes may be less than 50%, while up to 39% of survivors were in a vegetative state at hospital discharge or at 1 month [73, 74].

At 6 months and 1 year after cardiac arrest, the rate of survival with good neurological outcome is about 90%, with most patients in CPC 1 and only about 1.5% of survivors in a persistent vegetative state [71, 72]. Although this result is partly

Table 20.2 Modified Rankin Scale (mRS)

Score	Description
0	No symptoms
1	No significant disability despite symptoms. Able to carry out all usual activities and duties
2	Slight disability. Unable to perform all previous activities, but able to manage daily affairs without assistance
3	Moderate disability. Requires some help, but able to walk unassisted
4	Moderately severe disability. Unable to walk or attend to personal needs without assistance
5	Severe disability. Bedridden, incontinent, and requiring constant nursing care and attention
6	Death

attributable to improvement over time in patients with CPC 2–3 [71, 74], an important cause is also the high mortality among patients discharged with neurological disability.

20.6.3.2 Quality of Life After Post-anoxic Coma

The ultimate goal of resuscitation is to achieve an adequate quality of life. However, this is a subjective measure for the patient and is not always well correlated with physician-assessed measures of neurological functional outcome. Since HRQOL can only be adequately assessed when the patient is given the opportunity to interact with their social environment, it should always be measured after hospital discharge and, in any case, not before 3 months after arrest. The Health Utilities Index (HUI) version 3, the Short-Form 36-Item Health Survey (SF-36), and the revised EuroQol EQ-5D-5L are the three tools recommended by experts to measure HRQOL after awakening from coma following cardiac arrest [75]. The abbreviated version, Short-Form 12-item Health Survey (SF-12), can also be used in place of the SF-36. Normative population data are available for all these measures.

Up to 55% of patients who awaken from post-anoxic coma report a decrease in HRQOL compared to pre-arrest levels [76, 77], very often due to limitations in work or other daily activities related to physical or emotional problems. Fatigue is very common. In one study [78], 52% of post-arrest patients had a higher fatigue severity score than the comparable population norm. About 50% of patients assessed for HRQOL at 6–12 months after ROSC were working at the time of cardiac arrest. Among these, the rates of return to work ranged between 62% and 75% [77–80]. In a study derived from the TTM trial [79], less than half of the patients who were employed at the time of arrest had returned to their previous level of work 6 months later. About one-third of these patients had shifted to part-time work.

The most common cognitive disorders after recovery from post-anoxic coma are memory deficits, followed by impairments in attention and executive functions [81]. These disorders can be subtle and often not directly visible, but they can significantly affect the patient's daily activities, participation in society, and quality of life [82].

20.7 How to Predict the Prognosis of Post-anoxic Coma?

About 80% of patients resuscitated from cardiac arrest are in a coma at the time of admission [83], and about two-thirds of them die or are discharged with severe neurological disability. Predicting the prognosis of post-anoxic coma is essential both to provide accurate information to *caregivers* and to avoid disproportionate care in patients with severe and irreversible injury who are destined for an unfavorable outcome.

Prognostic tests are widely used in intensive care. In post-anoxic coma, numerous predictors of neurological recovery exist [84], but only in 2025 were they integrated into the recommended prognostic strategy. Even today, prognostic tests are mainly used to identify severe brain injury. When the result of these unfavorable tests is positive (i.e., abnormal), the prognosis is poor. Ideally, the false-positive rate (*FPR*) of these tests should be zero to avoid erroneously predicting a poor prognosis in a patient who is destined to recover, which could lead to inappropriate WLST. However, the very fact that these tests are often used to make decisions about WLST creates a significant bias, known as a self-fulfilling prophecy. The most effective way to avoid or limit the risk of self-fulfilling prophecies is to study these tests in a blinded fashion, which has been successfully done for biomarkers [85], or to validate prognostic tests in countries or communities where WLST is not practised. Data from these studies have so far confirmed the accuracy of the unfavorable prognostic tests recommended by the guidelines [73, 86, 87].

Other important sources of confounding for prognostic tests include sedation and extracerebral causes of death. Sedatives alter the clinical examination and can depress the EEG. In particular, propofol can induce burst-suppression, which is an important EEG predictor of poor neurological outcome in post-anoxic coma; this occurs at higher doses than those generally used for sedation in the intensive care unit [88]. The N20 wave of short-latency somatosensory-evoked potentials is not abolished by deep sedation, but its amplitude may be reduced [89]. In contrast, biomarkers and imaging are not affected by sedatives, which is a significant advantage.

Extracerebral injury obviously influences the prognosis of patients in post-anoxic coma and must always be considered when making therapeutic decisions. Death from cardiocirculatory collapse or multiorgan failure is particularly frequent during the first 3 days after ROSC [3] but can also occur later in the clinical course after patients have regained consciousness [69]. In addition to extracerebral organ failure, when assessing the prognosis of a patient in post-anoxic coma, one must also consider the previous health status before the arrest and the precipitating cause of the arrest [18].

20.7.1 Clinical Examination

Clinical examination is crucial for predicting the prognosis of post-anoxic coma. Even before the definitive discontinuation of sedation, it is recommended to perform a daily clinical examination to detect signs of recovery of consciousness or deterioration, including brain death [90]. The absence of response to commands (motor score on the Glasgow Coma Scale <6) in a patient who appears unconscious is the entry point of the ERC-ESICM 2025 prognostic algorithm (see below).

The most widely used prognostic signs in the clinical examination are ocular reflexes and myoclonic status. Ocular reflexes are generated in the brainstem, which is relatively resistant to anoxic injury, so their persistent absence is a more specific sign of severe HIBI than alteration of the motor response. At 72 h or more after ROSC, the bilateral absence of pupillary and corneal reflexes predicts a poor neurological outcome with an FPR below 5% [91]. Unlike the corneal reflex, the pupillary light reflex (PLR) is not affected by muscle relaxants [92]. However, standard PLR (assessed visually) is operator-dependent, and its accuracy is reduced when the pupil diameter is less than 2 mm [93]. In contrast, quantitative automated pupillometry is accurate even when the pupil size is very small; moreover, it can predict prognosis as early as 24 h after ROSC. Finally, being quantitative, it is a reproducible and documentable measurement. The 2025 ERC-ESICM guidelines recommend the use of quantitative pupillometry over standard PLR to identify the absence of pupillary reflex.

Myoclonus is very often, but not always, associated with an unfavorable prognosis in post-anoxic coma. Certain features of myoclonus, such as early onset (<48 h), generalized rather than focal distribution, a synchronous and stereotyped pattern, and continuous myoclonus lasting more than 30 min (*status myoclonicus*), are associated with a worse outcome. The presence of a continuous and/or reactive EEG background during myoclonus is associated with more favorable outcomes compared to burst-suppression [23, 94]. Pharmacological treatment does not appear to improve the prognosis of post-anoxic myoclonus, but the evidence is limited [95]. As mentioned above, post-anoxic intention myoclonus, also known as Lance-Adams syndrome, generally has a favorable outcome, although the myoclonus may become chronic and cause some degree of disability.

20.7.2 Biomarkers

Biomarkers offer several advantages as prognostic tests in post-anoxic coma. First, they are easy for healthcare providers to obtain through a blood sample; in addition, they provide a quantitative and repeatable measure of the extent of post-anoxic brain injury. Finally, they are not affected by sedatives or muscle relaxants. However, for some biomarkers, there is a risk of confounding from extracerebral sources.

NSE (neuron-specific enolase) is the best-documented and most widely available marker of HIBI. In post-anoxic coma patients with a poor prognosis, blood levels of NSE increase within or shortly after 24 h and peak at 48–72 h after ROSC [91]. The currently recommended cut-off to predict a poor prognosis is 60 μgL^{-1} at 48–72 h. Rising NSE values within 72 h also suggest a poor prognosis. Conversely, NSE values within the normal range suggest a favorable prognosis [84]. When using NSE, it is particularly important to avoid hemolysis, as NSE is present in erythrocytes. This issue is especially relevant in patients resuscitated with ECPR [96]. Since the half-life of free hemoglobin (2–4 h) is considerably shorter than that of NSE (30 h), intravascular hemolysis occurring at the time of CPR may no longer be detectable when NSE is measured at 48–72 h [97, 98]. Neuroendocrine tumors are a less common but still important extracerebral source of NSE.

Neurofilament light chain (*NFL*) is a component of the cytoskeleton of large myelinated fibers in the central and peripheral nervous system and is an excellent predictor of both favorable and unfavorable prognosis in post-anoxic coma. Its overall accuracy has been shown to be superior to that of NSE and other biomarkers [85, 99]. The main limitations of NFL are its low blood concentrations, which require highly sensitive technologies for its measurement, and the wide variability in predictive thresholds reported in studies to date [91]. Its use as a prognostic test in post-anoxic coma is still limited. As of 2025, almost all clinical studies on NFL have been conducted with research-use assays not validated for clinical use. NFL is not currently recommended as a prognostic test after cardiac arrest by the 2025 ERC-ESICM guidelines [18].

20.7.3 Electrophysiology

20.7.3.1 Short-Latency Somatosensory-Evoked Potentials (SSEPs)

SSEPs (short-latency somatosensory evoked potentials) of the upper limb are elicited by stimulation of the median nerve at the wrist, and are recorded at the brachial plexus, posterior cervical level, and the sensory cortex contralateral to the stimulus. The negative wave recorded at about 20 ms on the scalp is called N20 and reflects activation of the primary sensory cortex. SSEPs are resistant to hypothermia and sedative drugs. In post-anoxic coma, bilateral absence of the cortical N20 wave almost invariably indicates a poor prognosis [91], although occasional false positive results have been reported [100]. In some of these cases, the N20 wave was not detected due to artifacts that prevented correct reading of the SSEP trace [101]. One of the main sources of artifacts is muscle activity, which can be eliminated by using muscle relaxants [102]. The ERC-ESICM 2025 guidelines recommend using muscle relaxants for recording SSEP for prognostication after cardiac arrest [18].

Unlike EEG, the bilateral absence of the N20 wave predicts a poor prognosis with 100% specificity as early as 12 h after ROSC [73, 103]. However, despite its high specificity, its sensitivity is low, often not exceeding 40%. Recent studies [103–105] suggest that even a low-voltage N20 wave predicts a poor prognosis with sufficient accuracy. Adding this criterion to the absence of the N20 wave may increase the sensitivity of SSEP-based prediction. Conversely, a high-voltage N20 wave, above 3.5 μV, suggests a favorable prognosis in post-anoxic coma [103, 105, 106].

20.7.3.2 EEG

EEG is the most widely used test to assess the severity of HIBI in clinical practice [47]. To limit subjectivity in its interpretation, in 2021 the American Clinical Neurophysiology Society (ACNS) proposed a standardized terminology for EEG in intensive care patients [107].

The two main aspects to consider when using EEG for prognosis in post-anoxic coma are (1) background activity and (2) the presence of reactivity to stimulation.

When the amplitude of the EEG record background rhythm does not exceed 10 μV, the term *suppression* is used. Although a suppressed EEG may still be compatible with neurological recovery if detected immediately after ROSC, the persistence of suppression after 24 h almost invariably predicts an unfavorable outcome [108, 109] .

An EEG background rhythm that is suppressed and alternates with bursts of electrical activity lasting <50% of the trace is defined as *burst-suppression* [107]. As with suppression, the accuracy of burst-suppression for predicting poor prognosis increases after 24 h from ROSC. The presence of repetitive bursts (*burst-suppression with identical bursts, BSIB*) predicts poor prognosis particularly accurately and early [110]. Suppression and burst-suppression have been defined in many studies as "highly malignant" EEG patterns [109, 111] in patients with post-anoxic coma. When standard ACNS definitions are used, there is good agreement among expert neurophysiologists in identifying these patterns [112].

EEG background reactivity consists of a measurable change in amplitude or frequency when a stimulus is applied. Methods for stimulation or assessment of reactivity vary widely, and only recently has an expert consensus proposed standardization of the type of stimulus, as well as its repetition and duration [113]. While the absence of EEG reactivity adds little prognostic value, its presence is a sign of good neurological outcome [84].

20.7.4 Imaging

The presence of cerebral edema on computed tomography (CT) after cardiac arrest indicates a poor prognosis with a high degree of accuracy. CT signs of post-anoxic edema include loss of gray-white matter differentiation, effacement of sulci, and reduction in the size of the cerebral ventricles. Another sign is pseudo-subarachnoid hemorrhage, caused by congestion of the cerebral venous sinuses [114, 115]. Recent prospective studies [116–118] have shown that the sensitivity of brain CT for identifying HIBI increases 3–4 days after ROSC. The ERC-ESICM 2025 guidelines suggest repeating cranial CT in comatose patients 3–4 days after ROSC if the initial CT is negative for signs of HIBI [18].

Cytotoxic edema on magnetic resonance imaging (MRI) appears as hyperintensity (brighter signal) on diffusion-weighted imaging (DWI) sequences. DWI assessment is usually visual, and therefore qualitative, but can be made quantitative by measuring apparent diffusion coefficient (ADC) values. Prognostic studies based on MRI have shown that a reduction in global cerebral ADC or the presence of a percentage of brain tissue with low ADC above a certain threshold [119–121] allow for the prediction of a poor prognosis with 100% specificity in post-anoxic coma. However, predictive thresholds vary between studies due to differences in measurement techniques, the brain region studied, and the interval between ROSC and MRI examination. Regarding timing, signs of altered diffusion are most evident in the basal ganglia during the first 3 days after ROSC, followed by the cortex and subcortical white matter [122].

Cerebral MRI provides a substantial amount of information, but summarizing it into a prognostic judgment is complex. Over the years, several scoring systems have been proposed to quantify the severity of HIBI on MRI [123, 124]. However, the criteria used are heterogeneous, and so far, none of these systems are recommended.

20.7.5 The ERC-ESICM 2025 Prognostic Algorithm

The 2025 ERC-ESICM guidelines on post-resuscitation care suggest a prognostic strategy for post-anoxic coma [18]. Its key elements are:

1. The neurological clinical examination is fundamental for prognosis; therefore, prognostic assessment can only be established after excluding potential confounding factors. Among these, residual effects of sedation or neuromuscular blocking agents are particularly important.
2. No predictor is 100% accurate; therefore, prognostic judgment cannot be based on a single predictor. Combining two or more tests for an unfavorable neurological outcome minimizes the risk of a falsely pessimistic prediction [125]. Since the 2021 guidelines, the principle of *concordance* between unfavorable test results has been introduced. To predict a poor prognosis, two or more concordant unfavorable test results are recommended, with no discordant result indicating a favorable prognosis.

The ERC-ESICM 2025 prognostic recommendations are summarized in the algorithm in Fig. 20.1. A patient who—after at least 72 h from ROSC and exclusion of confounding factors—is unconscious and does not follow commands (motor response 5 or less according to the Glasgow Coma Scale) enters the prognostic algorithm. The first step is to assess for a poor prognosis based on the presence of *two* concordant unfavorable prognostic signs among the following six: (1) absence of pupillary and corneal reflexes at ≥72 h after ROSC; (2) bilateral absence of the N20 wave on SSEP at ≥24 h after ROSC; (3) EEG background rhythm with suppression or burst-suppression at ≥24 h after ROSC; (4) blood NSE levels above 60 μg/L at 48 and/or 72 h after ROSC; (5) myoclonic status within 72 h after ROSC; or (6) severe and diffuse anoxic changes on brain CT or MRI.

If the criterion of ≥2 concordant unfavorable signs is not met, the next step is to assess for a potentially favorable prognosis. Signs indicating a potentially favorable outcome are: early return (within 24 h) of a favorable EEG background rhythm (continuous, reactive, and without epileptiform activity), blood NSE levels ≥17 μg/L within 72 h after ROSC, and absence of diffusion abnormalities on brain MRI. The likelihood of neurological recovery increases with the number of concordant favorable signs, while it is lower if there is a discordant unfavorable sign [126, 127].

If no favorable sign is present, the prognosis remains indeterminate and observation should be continued. In this patient population, the prognosis is mostly unfavorable, but neurological recovery can still occur in 20–30% of cases [126].

20.8 Conclusions

Post-anoxic brain injury, or HIBI, is the most important cause of disability and mortality after cardiac arrest and is due to a series of complex mechanisms triggered by both ischemia and reperfusion during and after resuscitation. In the absence of a

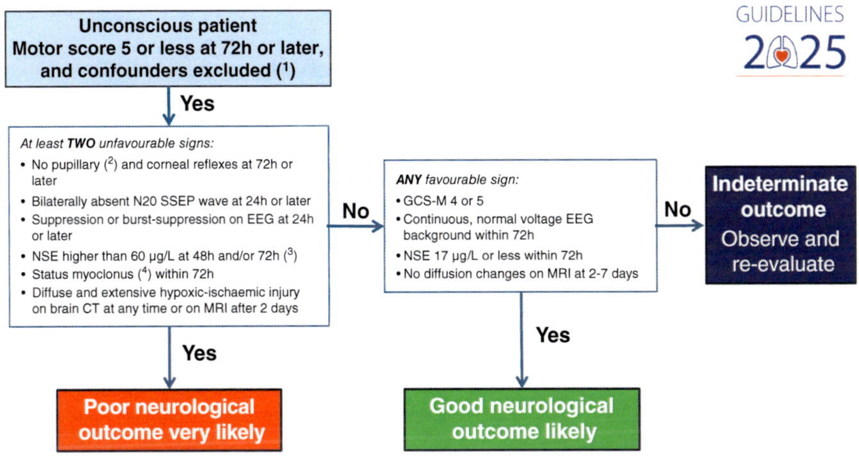

Fig. 20.1 ERC-ESICM 2025 prognostic algorithm. Redrawn from: Nolan J. P., et al. European Resuscitation Council and European Society of Intensive Care Medicine guidelines 2025: post-resuscitation care. Resuscitation 2025; 110,809, with permission of the European Resuscitation Council*Abbreviations: EEG* electroencephalogram, *NSE* neuron-specific enolase, *SSEP* short-latency somatosensory evoked potentials, *ROSC* return of spontaneous circulation*Notes*: (1) The main confounding factors are: sedation, neuromuscular blockade, hypothermia, severe hypotension, hypoglycemia, sepsis, and metabolic and respiratory disorders. (2) The use of an automated pupillometer is recommended, if available, to assess the pupillary light reflex. (3) An increase in blood NSE levels between 24 and 48 h or between 24/48 h and 72 h further supports a likely poor outcome. (4) Defined as continuous, generalized myoclonus persisting for 30 min or more.

direct neuroprotective treatment, secondary HIBI damage should be limited by maintaining blood pressure, oxygenation, ventilation, and temperature within physiological ranges. However, the optimal values for these parameters are currently unknown. In patients with post-anoxic coma, predicting neurological prognosis is essential to inform the patient's caregivers and ensure proportionate treatments. Prognostic assessment of post-anoxic coma is multimodal and should never rely on a single predictor. In case of uncertainty, it is recommended to prolong observation and ensure that confounding factors have been excluded.

References

1. Horsting MW, Franken MD, Meulenbelt J, van Klei WA, de Lange DW. The etiology and outcome of non-traumatic coma in critical care: a systematic review. BMC Anesthesiol. 2015;15:1–8.
2. Sandroni C, Cronberg T, Sekhon M. Brain injury after cardiac arrest: pathophysiology, treatment, and prognosis. Intensive Care Med. 2021;47:1393–414.
3. Lemiale V, Dumas F, Mongardon N, Giovanetti O, Charpentier J, Chiche JD, et al. Intensive care unit mortality after cardiac arrest: the relative contribution of shock and brain injury in a large cohort. Intensive Care Med. 2013;39:1972–80.

4. Sekhon MS, Ainslie PN, Griesdale DE. Clinical pathophysiology of hypoxic ischemic brain injury after cardiac arrest: a "two-hit" model. Crit Care. 2017;21:90.
5. Fischer M, Bockhorst K, Hoehn-Berlage M, Schmitz B, Hossmann KA. Imaging of the apparent diffusion coefficient for the evaluation of cerebral metabolic recovery after cardiac arrest. Magn Reson Imaging. 1995;13:781–90.
6. Buunk G, van der Hoeven JG, Meinders AE. Cerebral blood flow after cardiac arrest. Neth J Med. 2000;57:106–12.
7. Adrie C, Haouache H, Saleh M, Memain N, Laurent I, Thuong M, et al. An underrecognized source of organ donors: patients with brain death after successfully resuscitated cardiac arrest. Intensive Care Med. 2008;34:132–7.
8. Bhalala US, Koehler RC, Kannan S. Neuroinflammation and neuroimmune dysregulation after acute hypoxic-ischemic injury of developing brain. Front Pediatr. 2014;2:144.
9. Beckstead JE, Tweed WA, Lee J, MacKeen WL. Cerebral blood flow and metabolism in man following cardiac arrest. Stroke. 1978;9:569–73.
10. Hoedemaekers CW, Ainslie PN, Hinssen S, Aries MJ, Bisschops LL, Hofmeijer J, et al. Low cerebral blood flow after cardiac arrest is not associated with anaerobic cerebral metabolism. Resuscitation. 2017;120:45–50.
11. Hoiland RL, Ainslie PN, Wellington CL, Cooper J, Stukas S, Thiara S, et al. Brain hypoxia is associated with neuroglial injury in humans post-cardiac arrest. Circ Res. 2021;129:583–97.
12. Hoiland RL, Ainslie PN, Wellington CL, Cooper J, Stukas S, Thiara S, et al. Brain hypoxia is associated with Neuroglial injury in humans post-cardiac arrest. Circ Res. 2021;129:583.
13. Hoiland RL, Robba C, Menon DK, Citerio G, Sandroni C, Sekhon MS. Clinical targeting of the cerebral oxygen cascade to improve brain oxygenation in patients with hypoxic-ischemic brain injury after cardiac arrest. Intensive Care Med. 2023;49:1062–78.
14. Ameloot K, Genbrugge C, Meex I, Jans F, Boer W, Vander Laenen M, et al. An observational near-infrared spectroscopy study on cerebral autoregulation in post-cardiac arrest patients: time to drop 'one-size-fits-all' hemodynamic targets? Resuscitation. 2015;90:121–6.
15. Hayman EG, Patel AP, Kimberly WT, Sheth KN, Simard JM. Cerebral edema after cardiopulmonary resuscitation: a therapeutic target following cardiac arrest? Neurocrit Care. 2018;28:276–87.
16. You Y, Park J, Min J, Yoo I, Jeong W, Cho Y, et al. Relationship between time related serum albumin concentration, optic nerve sheath diameter, cerebrospinal fluid pressure, and neurological prognosis in cardiac arrest survivors. Resuscitation. 2018;131:42–7.
17. Moseby-Knappe M, Westhall E, Backman S, Mattsson-Carlgren N, Dragancea I, Lybeck A, et al. Performance of a guideline-recommended algorithm for prognostication of poor neurological outcome after cardiac arrest. Intensive Care Med. 2020;46:1852–62.
18. Nolan JP, Sandroni C, Cariou A, Cronberg T, D'Arrigo S, Haywood K, et al. European resuscitation council and European Society of Intensive Care Medicine Guidelines 2025 post-resuscitation care. Resuscitation. 2025;215(Suppl 1):110809.
19. Lybeck A, Friberg H, Aneman A, Hassager C, Horn J, Kjaergaard J, et al. Prognostic significance of clinical seizures after cardiac arrest and target temperature management. Resuscitation. 2017;114:146–51.
20. Lance JW, Adams RD. The syndrome of intention or action myoclonus as a sequel to hypoxic encephalopathy. Brain. 1963;86:111–36.
21. Aicua Rapun I, Novy J, Solari D, Oddo M, Rossetti AO. Early Lance-Adams syndrome after cardiac arrest: prevalence, time to return to awareness, and outcome in a large cohort. Resuscitation. 2017;115:169–72.
22. English WA, Giffin NJ, Nolan JP. Myoclonus after cardiac arrest: pitfalls in diagnosis and prognosis. Anaesthesia. 2009;64:908–11.
23. Elmer J, Rittenberger JC, Faro J, Molyneaux BJ, Popescu A, Callaway CW, et al. Clinically distinct electroencephalographic phenotypes of early myoclonus after cardiac arrest. Ann Neurol. 2016;80:175–84.
24. Marasini S, Jia X. Neuroprotective approaches for brain injury after cardiac arrest: current trends and prospective avenues. J Stroke. 2024;26:203–30.

25. Bro-Jeppesen J, Annborn M, Hassager C, Wise MP, Pelosi P, Nielsen N, et al. Hemodynamics and vasopressor support during targeted temperature management at 33°C versus 36°C after out-of-hospital cardiac arrest: a post hoc study of the target temperature management trial*. Crit Care Med. 2015;43:318–27.
26. Ameloot K, De Deyne C, Eertmans W, Ferdinande B, Dupont M, Palmers PJ, et al. Early goal-directed haemodynamic optimization of cerebral oxygenation in comatose survivors after cardiac arrest: the Neuroprotect post-cardiac arrest trial. Eur Heart J. 2019;40:1804–14.
27. Kjaergaard J, Møller JE, Schmidt H, Grand J, Mølstrøm S, Borregaard B, et al. Blood-pressure targets in comatose survivors of cardiac arrest. N Engl J Med. 2022;387:1456–66.
28. Meunier J, Engrand N, Saulnier P, Deye N, Landais M, Cariou A, et al. Transcranial Doppler goal-directed therapy after cardiac arrest (GOODYEAR): a feasibility study. Resusc Plus. 2025;25:101001.
29. Niemelä V, Siddiqui F, Ameloot K, Reinikainen M, Grand J, Hästbacka J, et al. Higher versus lower blood pressure targets after cardiac arrest: systematic review with individual patient data meta-analysis. Resuscitation. 2023;189:109862.
30. Willie CK, Tzeng YC, Fisher JA, Ainslie PN. Integrative regulation of human brain blood flow. J Physiol. 2014;592:841–59.
31. Eastwood G, Nichol AD, Hodgson C, Parke RL, McGuinness S, Nielsen N, et al. Mild hypercapnia or normocapnia after out-of-hospital cardiac arrest. N Engl J Med. 2023;389:45–57.
32. Kilgannon JH, Jones AE, Shapiro NI, Angelos MG, Milcarek B, Hunter K, et al. Association between arterial hyperoxia following resuscitation from cardiac arrest and in-hospital mortality. JAMA J Am Med Assoc. 2010;303:2165–71.
33. Bellomo R, Bailey M, Eastwood GM, Nichol A, Pilcher D, Hart GK, et al. Arterial hyperoxia and in-hospital mortality after resuscitation from cardiac arrest. Crit Care. 2011;15:R90.
34. Schmidt H, Kjaergaard J, Hassager C, Mølstrøm S, Grand J, Borregaard B, et al. Oxygen targets in comatose survivors of cardiac arrest. N Engl J Med. 2022;387:1467–76.
35. Bernard SA, Bray JE, Smith K, Stephenson M, Finn J, Grantham H, et al. Effect of lower vs higher oxygen saturation targets on survival to hospital discharge among patients resuscitated after out-of-hospital cardiac arrest: the EXACT randomized clinical trial. JAMA. 2022;328:1818–26.
36. Arrich J, Herkner H, Mullner D, Behringer W. Targeted temperature management after cardiac arrest. A systematic review and meta-analysis of animal studies. Resuscitation. 2021;162:47–55.
37. Persson O, Valerianova A, Tejkl L, Belohlavek J, Cronberg T, Nielsen N, et al. Hypothermia after cardiac arrest in large animals (HACA-LA): a randomized controlled experimental study. Intensive Care Med Exp. 2025;13:105.
38. Bernard SA, Gray TW, Buist MD, Jones BM, Silvester W, Gutteridge G, et al. Treatment of comatose survivors of out-of-hospital cardiac arrest with induced hypothermia. N Engl J Med. 2002;346:557–63.
39. HACA Study group. Mild therapeutic hypothermia to improve the neurologic outcome after cardiac arrest. N Engl J Med. 2002;346:549–56.
40. Dankiewicz J, Cronberg T, Lilja G, Jakobsen JC, Levin H, Ullen S, et al. Hypothermia versus normothermia after out-of-hospital cardiac arrest. N Engl J Med. 2021;384:2283–94.
41. Nielsen N, Wetterslev J, Cronberg T, Erlinge D, Gasche Y, Hassager C, et al. Targeted temperature management at 33 degrees C versus 36 degrees C after cardiac arrest. N Engl J Med. 2013;369:2197–206.
42. Sandroni C, Nolan JP, Andersen LW, Böttiger BW, Cariou A, Cronberg T, et al. ERC-ESICM guidelines on temperature control after cardiac arrest in adults. Intensive Care Med. 2022;48:261–9.
43. Backman S, Cronberg T, Friberg H, Ullen S, Horn J, Kjaergaard J, et al. Highly malignant routine EEG predicts poor prognosis after cardiac arrest in the Target Temperature Management trial. Resuscitation. 2018;131:24–8.

44. Ruijter BJ, Keijzer HM, Tjepkema-Cloostermans MC, Blans MJ, Beishuizen A, Tromp SC, et al. Treating rhythmic and periodic EEG patterns in comatose survivors of cardiac arrest. N Engl J Med. 2022;386:724–34.
45. Beretta S, Coppo A, Bianchi E, Zanchi C, Carone D, Stabile A, et al. Neurological outcome of postanoxic refractory status epilepticus after aggressive treatment. Epilepsy Behav. 2019;101:106374.
46. De Stefano P, Hofmeijer J, Quintard H, Damien C, Misirocchi F, Caroyer S, et al. Features, outcome, and treatment of postanoxic status epilepticus: pooled analysis of 3 cohorts. Neurology. 2025;105:e213913.
47. Friberg H, Cronberg T, Dunser MW, Duranteau J, Horn J, Oddo M. Survey on current practices for neurological prognostication after cardiac arrest. Resuscitation. 2015;90:158–62.
48. Elmer J, Coppler PJ, Solanki P, Westover MB, Struck AF, Baldwin ME, et al. Sensitivity of continuous electroencephalography to detect ictal activity after cardiac arrest. JAMA Netw Open. 2020;3:e203751.
49. Fatuzzo D, Beuchat I, Alvarez V, Novy J, Oddo M, Rossetti AO. Does continuous EEG influence prognosis in patients after cardiac arrest? Resuscitation. 2018;132:29–32.
50. Rasulo FA, Bertuetti R, Robba C, Lusenti F, Cantoni A, Bernini M, et al. The accuracy of transcranial Doppler in excluding intracranial hypertension following acute brain injury: a multicenter prospective pilot study. Crit Care. 2017;21:44.
51. Cardim D, Griesdale DE, Ainslie PN, Robba C, Calviello L, Czosnyka M, et al. A comparison of non-invasive versus invasive measures of intracranial pressure in hypoxic ischaemic brain injury after cardiac arrest. Resuscitation. 2019;137:221–8.
52. Rafi S, Tadie JM, Gacouin A, Leurent G, Bedossa M, Le Tulzo Y, et al. Doppler sonography of cerebral blood flow for early prognostication after out-of-hospital cardiac arrest: DOTAC study. Resuscitation. 2019;141:188–94.
53. Nakayama S, Migliati E, Amiry-Moghaddam M, Ottersen OP, Bhardwaj A. Osmotherapy with hypertonic saline attenuates global cerebral edema following experimental cardiac arrest via perivascular pool of Aquaporin-4. Crit Care Med. 2016;44:e702–10.
54. Fergusson NA, Hoiland RL, Thiara S, Foster D, Gooderham P, Rikhraj K, et al. Goal-directed care using invasive neuromonitoring versus standard of care after cardiac arrest: a matched cohort study. Crit Care Med. 2021;49:1333–46.
55. Paul M, Bougouin W, Geri G, Dumas F, Champigneulle B, Legriel S, et al. Delayed awakening after cardiac arrest: prevalence and risk factors in the Parisian registry. Intensive Care Med. 2016;42:1128–36.
56. Lybeck A, Cronberg T, Aneman A, Hassager C, Horn J, Hovdenes J, et al. Time to awakening after cardiac arrest and the association with target temperature management. Resuscitation. 2018;126:166–71.
57. Rey A, Rossetti AO, Miroz JP, Eckert P, Oddo M. Late awakening in survivors of postanoxic coma: early neurophysiologic predictors and association with ICU and long-term neurologic recovery. Crit Care Med. 2019;47:85–92.
58. Paul M, Bougouin W, Dumas F, Geri G, Champigneulle B, Guillemet L, et al. Comparison of two sedation regimens during targeted temperature management after cardiac arrest. Resuscitation. 2018;128:204–10.
59. Wimmer H, Lundqvist C, Saltyte Benth J, Stavem K, Andersen GO, Henriksen J, et al. Health-related quality of life after out-of-hospital cardiac arrest – a five-year follow-up study. Resuscitation. 2021;162:372–80.
60. Dragancea I, Rundgren M, Englund E, Friberg H, Cronberg T. The influence of induced hypothermia and delayed prognostication on the mode of death after cardiac arrest. Resuscitation. 2013;84:337–42.
61. Elmer J, Torres C, Aufderheide TP, Austin MA, Callaway CW, Golan E, et al. Association of early withdrawal of life-sustaining therapy for perceived neurological prognosis with mortality after cardiac arrest. Resuscitation. 2016;102:127–35.

62. Sandroni C, D'Arrigo S, Callaway CW, Cariou A, Dragancea I, Taccone FS, et al. The rate of brain death and organ donation in patients resuscitated from cardiac arrest: a systematic review and meta-analysis. Intensive Care Med. 2016;42:1661–71.
63. Bonizzoni MA, Scquizzato T, Pieri M, Delrio S, Nardelli P, Ortalda A, et al. Organ donation after extracorporeal cardiopulmonary resuscitation for refractory out-of-hospital cardiac arrest in a metropolitan cardiac arrest centre in Milan, Italy. Resuscitation. 2024;200:110214.
64. Smalcova J, Havranek S, Pokorna E, Franek O, Huptych M, Kavalkova P, et al. Extracorporeal cardiopulmonary resuscitation-based approach to refractory out-of-hospital cardiac arrest: a focus on organ donation, a secondary analysis of a Prague OHCA randomized study. Resuscitation. 2023;193:109993.
65. Morrison LJ, Sandroni C, Grunau B, Parr M, Macneil F, Perkins GD, et al. Organ donation after out-of-hospital cardiac arrest: a scientific statement from the international liaison committee on resuscitation. Circulation. 2023;148:e120–e46.
66. Sandroni C, Scquizzato T, Cacciola S, Bonizzoni MA, West S, D'Arrigo S, et al. Does cardiopulmonary resuscitation before donor death affect solid organ transplant function? A systematic review and meta-analysis. Resuscitation. 2025;213:110654.
67. Brain Resuscitation Clinical Trial I Study Group. A randomized clinical study of cardiopulmonary-cerebral resuscitation: design, methods, and patient characteristics. Brain resuscitation clinical trial I study group. Am J Emerg Med. 1986;4:72–86.
68. Rankin J. Cerebrovascular accidents in patients over the age of 60. II Prognosis. Scottish Med J. 1957;2:200–15.
69. Taccone FS, Horn J, Storm C, Cariou A, Sandroni C, Friberg H, et al. Death after awakening from post-anoxic coma: the "best CPC" project. Crit Care. 2019;23:107.
70. Geocadin RG, Callaway CW, Fink EL, Golan E, Greer DM, Ko NU, et al. Standards for studies of neurological prognostication in comatose survivors of cardiac arrest: a scientific statement from the American Heart Association. Circulation. 2019;140:e517–e42.
71. Arrich J, Zeiner A, Sterz F, Janata A, Uray T, Richling N, et al. Factors associated with a change in functional outcome between one month and six months after cardiac arrest: a retrospective cohort study. Resuscitation. 2009;80:876–80.
72. Phelps R, Dumas F, Maynard C, Silver J, Rea T. Cerebral performance category and long-term prognosis following out-of-hospital cardiac arrest. Crit Care Med. 2013;41:1252–7.
73. Scarpino M, Carrai R, Lolli F, Lanzo G, Spalletti M, Valzania F, et al. Neurophysiology for predicting good and poor neurological outcome at 12 and 72 h after cardiac arrest: the ProNeCA multicentre prospective study. Resuscitation. 2020;147:95–103.
74. Kim YJ, Ahn S, Sohn CH, Seo DW, Lee YS, Lee JH, et al. Long-term neurological outcomes in patients after out-of-hospital cardiac arrest. Resuscitation. 2016;101:1–5.
75. Haywood K, Whitehead L, Nadkarni VM, Achana F, Beesems S, Bottiger BW, et al. COSCA (Core Outcome Set for Cardiac Arrest) in adults: an advisory statement from the international liaison committee on resuscitation. Circulation. 2018;137:e783–801.
76. Bohm M, Lilja G, Finnbogadottir H, Cronberg T, Unden J, Friberg H, et al. Detailed analysis of health-related quality of life after out-of-hospital cardiac arrest. Resuscitation. 2019;135:197–204.
77. Smith K, Andrew E, Lijovic M, Nehme Z, Bernard S. Quality of life and functional outcomes 12 months after out-of-hospital cardiac arrest. Circulation. 2015;131:174–81.
78. Moulaert VRM, van Heugten CM, Gorgels TPM, Wade DT, Verbunt JA. Long-term outcome after survival of a cardiac arrest: a prospective longitudinal cohort study. Neurorehabil Neural Repair. 2017;31:530–9.
79. Cronberg T, Lilja G, Horn J, Kjaergaard J, Wise MP, Pellis T, et al. Neurologic function and health-related quality of life in patients following targeted temperature management at 33 degrees C vs 36 degrees C after out-of-hospital cardiac arrest: a randomized clinical trial. JAMA Neurol. 2015;72:634–41.
80. Kragholm K, Wissenberg M, Mortensen RN, Fonager K, Jensen SE, Rajan S, et al. Return to work in out-of-hospital cardiac arrest survivors: a Nationwide register-based follow-up study. Circulation. 2015;131:1682–90.

81. Cronberg T, Greer DM, Lilja G, Moulaert V, Swindell P, Rossetti AO. Brain injury after cardiac arrest: from prognostication of comatose patients to rehabilitation. Lancet Neurol. 2020;19:611–22.
82. Lilja G, Nielsen N, Bro-Jeppesen J, Dunford H, Friberg H, Hofgren C, et al. Return to work and participation in society after out-of-hospital cardiac arrest. Circ Cardiovasc Qual Outcomes. 2018;11:e003566.
83. Thomassen A, Wernberg M. Prevalence and prognostic significance of coma after cardiac arrest outside intensive care and coronary units. Acta Anaesthesiol Scand. 1979;23:143–8.
84. Sandroni C, D'Arrigo S, Cacciola S, Hoedemaekers CWE, Westhall E, Kamps MJA, et al. Prediction of good neurological outcome in comatose survivors of cardiac arrest: a systematic review. Intensive Care Med. 2022;48:389–413.
85. Moseby-Knappe M, Mattsson N, Nielsen N, Zetterberg H, Blennow K, Dankiewicz J, et al. Serum neurofilament light chain for prognosis of outcome after cardiac arrest. JAMA Neurol. 2019;76:64–71.
86. Park JS, In YN, You YH, Min JH, Ahn HJ, Yoo IS, et al. Ultra-early neurologic outcome prediction of out-of-hospital cardiac arrest survivors using combined diffusion-weighted imaging findings and quantitative analysis of apparent diffusion coefficient. Resuscitation. 2020;148:39–48.
87. Youn CS, Park KN, Kim SH, Lee BK, Cronberg T, Oh SH, et al. External validation of the 2020 ERC/ESICM prognostication strategy algorithm after cardiac arrest. Crit Care. 2022;26:95.
88. Huotari AM, Koskinen M, Suominen K, Alahuhta S, Remes R, Hartikainen KM, et al. Evoked EEG patterns during burst suppression with propofol. Br J Anaesth. 2004;92:18–24.
89. Sloan TB, Fugina ML, Toleikis JR. Effects of midazolam on median nerve somatosensory evoked potentials. Br J Anaesth. 1990;64:590–3.
90. Nolan JP, Sandroni C, Bottiger BW, Cariou A, Cronberg T, Friberg H, et al. European Resuscitation Council and European Society of Intensive Care Medicine guidelines 2021: post-resuscitation care. Intensive Care Med. 2021;47:369–421.
91. Sandroni C, D'Arrigo S, Cacciola S, Hoedemaekers CWE, Kamps MJA, Oddo M, et al. Prediction of poor neurological outcome in comatose survivors of cardiac arrest: a systematic review. Intensive Care Med. 2020;46:1803–51.
92. Gray AT, Krejci ST, Larson MD. Neuromuscular blocking drugs do not alter the pupillary light reflex of anesthetized humans. Arch Neurol. 1997;54:579–84.
93. Oddo M, Sandroni C, Citerio G, Miroz JP, Horn J, Rundgren M, et al. Quantitative versus standard pupillary light reflex for early prognostication in comatose cardiac arrest patients: an international prospective multicenter double-blinded study. Intensive Care Med. 2018;44:2102–11.
94. Seder DB, Sunde K, Rubertsson S, Mooney M, Stammet P, Riker RR, et al. Neurologic outcomes and postresuscitation care of patients with myoclonus following cardiac arrest. Crit Care Med. 2015;43:965–72.
95. Nutma S, Ruijter BJ, Beishuizen A, Tromp SC, Scholten E, Horn J, et al. Myoclonus in comatose patients with electrographic status epilepticus after cardiac arrest: corresponding EEG patterns, effects of treatment and outcomes. Resuscitation. 2023;186:109745.
96. Brodska H, Smalcova J, Kavalkova P, Lavage DR, Dusik M, Belohlavek J, et al. Biomarkers for neuroprognostication after standard versus extracorporeal cardiopulmonary resuscitation – a sub-analysis of Prague-OHCA study. Resuscitation. 2024;199:110219.
97. Rundgren M, Cronberg T, Friberg H, Isaksson A. Serum neuron specific enolase – impact of storage and measuring method. BMC Res Notes. 2014;7:726.
98. Czimmeck C, Kenda M, Aalberts N, Endisch C, Ploner CJ, Storm C, et al. Confounders for prognostic accuracy of neuron-specific enolase after cardiac arrest: a retrospective cohort study. Resuscitation. 2023;192:109964.
99. Pouplet C, Colin G, Guichard E, Reignier J, Le Gouge A, Martin S, et al. The accuracy of various neuro-prognostication algorithms and the added value of neurofilament light chain

dosage for patients resuscitated from shockable cardiac arrest: an ancillary analysis of the ISOCRATE study. Resuscitation. 2022;171:1–7.
100. Amorim E, Ghassemi MM, Lee JW, Greer DM, Kaplan PW, Cole AJ, et al. Estimating the false positive rate of absent somatosensory evoked potentials in cardiac arrest prognostication. Crit Care Med. 2018;46:e1213–e21.
101. Bouwes A, Binnekade JM, Verbaan BW, Zandbergen EG, Koelman JH, Weinstein HC, et al. Predictive value of neurological examination for early cortical responses to somatosensory evoked potentials in patients with postanoxic coma. J Neurol. 2012;259:537–41.
102. Hakimi K, Kinney G, Kraft G, Micklesen P, Robinson L. Reliability in interpretation of median somatosensory evoked potentials in the setting of coma: factors and implications. Neurocrit Care. 2009;11:353–61.
103. Scarpino M, Nencioni A, Bernardo P, Bonizzoli M, Nazerian P, Piccardi B, et al. Ultra-early short- and middle-latency SSEP accurately predict good and poor outcome after cardiac arrest. Resuscitation. 2025;216:110801.
104. Scarpino M, Lolli F, Lanzo G, Carrai R, Spalletti M, Valzania F, et al. SSEP amplitude accurately predicts both good and poor neurological outcome early after cardiac arrest; a post-hoc analysis of the ProNeCA multicentre study. Resuscitation. 2021;163:162–71.
105. Benghanem S, Nguyen LS, Gavaret M, Mira JP, Pène F, Charpentier J, et al. SSEP N20 and P25 amplitudes predict poor and good neurologic outcomes after cardiac arrest. Ann Intensive Care. 2022;12:25.
106. Gourd NM, Bigham C, Broomfield N, Nye L, Stapleton L, Stead E, et al. Enhanced analysis of somatosensory evoked potentials at 20-30 milliseconds can predict neurological outcome after cardiac arrest. Clin Neurophysiol. 2023;153:141–51.
107. Hirsch LJ, Fong MWK, Leitinger M, LaRoche SM, Beniczky S, Abend NS, et al. American clinical neurophysiology society's standardized critical care EEG terminology: 2021 version. J Clin Neurophysiol. 2021;38:1–29.
108. Cloostermans MC, van Meulen FB, Eertman CJ, Hom HW, van Putten MJ. Continuous electroencephalography monitoring for early prediction of neurological outcome in postanoxic patients after cardiac arrest: a prospective cohort study. Crit Care Med. 2012;40:2867–75.
109. Westhall E, Rossetti AO, van Rootselaar AF, Wesenberg Kjaer T, Horn J, Ullen S, et al. Standardized EEG interpretation accurately predicts prognosis after cardiac arrest. Neurology. 2016;86:1482–90.
110. Ruijter BJ, Tjepkema-Cloostermans MC, Tromp SC, van den Bergh WM, Foudraine NA, Kornips FHM, et al. Early electroencephalography for outcome prediction of postanoxic coma: a prospective cohort study. Ann Neurol. 2019;86:203–14.
111. Turella S, Dankiewicz J, Friberg H, Jakobsen JC, Leithner C, Levin H, et al. The predictive value of highly malignant EEG patterns after cardiac arrest: evaluation of the ERC-ESICM recommendations. Intensive Care Med. 2024;50:90–102.
112. Benarous L, Gavaret M, Soda Diop M, Tobarias J, de Ghaisne de Bourmont S, Allez C, et al. Sources of interrater variability and prognostic value of standardized EEG features in post-anoxic coma after resuscitated cardiac arrest. Clin Neurophysiol Practice. 2019;4:20–6.
113. Admiraal MM, van Rootselaar AF, Horn J. International consensus on EEG reactivity testing after cardiac arrest: towards standardization. Resuscitation. 2018;131:36–41.
114. Keijzer HM, Hoedemaekers CWE, Meijer FJA, Tonino BAR, Klijn CJM, Hofmeijer J. Brain imaging in comatose survivors of cardiac arrest: pathophysiological correlates and prognostic properties. Resuscitation. 2018;133:124–36.
115. Lang M, Kenda M, Scheel M, Martola J, Wheeler M, Owen S, et al. Radiological signs of hypoxic-ischemic encephalopathy on head computed tomography for prediction of poor functional outcome after cardiac arrest—a prospective observational cohort study. Resuscitation. 2025;214:110675.
116. Wang GN, Zhang ZM, Chen W, Xu XQ, Zhang JS. Timing of brain computed tomography for predicting neurological prognosis in comatose cardiac arrest survivors: a retrospective observational study. World J Emerg Med. 2022;13:349–54.

117. In YN, Lee IH, Park JS, Kim DM, You Y, Min JH, et al. Delayed head CT in out-of-hospital cardiac arrest survivors: does this improve predictive performance of neurological outcome? Resuscitation. 2022;172:1–8.
118. Case N, Coppler PJ, Mettenburg J, Ratay C, Tam J, Faiver L, et al. Time-dependent association of grey-white ratio on early brain CT predicting outcomes after cardiac arrest at hospital discharge. Resuscitation. 2025;206:110440.
119. Yoon JA, Kang C, Park JS, You Y, Min JH, In YN, et al. Quantitative analysis of apparent diffusion coefficients to predict neurological prognosis in cardiac arrest survivors: an observational derivation and internal-external validation study. Crit Care. 2024;28:138.
120. Kang C, Min JH, Park JS, You Y, Jeong W, Ahn HJ, et al. Association of ultra-early diffusion-weighted magnetic resonance imaging with neurological outcomes after out-of-hospital cardiac arrest. Crit Care. 2023;27:16.
121. Calabrese E, Gandhi S, Shih J, Otero M, Randazzo D, Hemphill C, et al. Parieto-occipital injury on diffusion MRI correlates with poor neurologic outcome following cardiac arrest. AJNR Am J Neuroradiol. 2023;44:254–60.
122. Greer D, Scripko P, Bartscher J, Sims J, Camargo E, Singhal A, et al. Serial MRI changes in comatose cardiac arrest patients. Neurocrit Care. 2011;14:61–7.
123. Iten M, Moser A, Wagner F, Haenggi M. Performance of the MRI lesion pattern score in predicting neurological outcome after out-of-hospital cardiac arrest: a retrospective cohort analysis. Crit Care. 2024;28:215.
124. Chan WP, Nguyen C, Kim N, Tripodis Y, Gilmore EJ, Greer DM, et al. A practical magnetic-resonance imaging score for outcome prediction in comatose cardiac arrest survivors. Resuscitation. 2024;202:110370.
125. Scarpino M, Lolli F, Lanzo G, Carrai R, Spalletti M, Valzania F, et al. Does a combination of >/=2 abnormal tests vs. the ERC-ESICM stepwise algorithm improve prediction of poor neurological outcome after cardiac arrest? A post-hoc analysis of the ProNeCA multicentre study. Resuscitation. 2021;160:158–67.
126. Lagebrant A, Sandroni C, Nolan JP, Bělohlávek J, Cariou A, Carrai R, et al. Prediction of good functional outcome decreases diagnostic uncertainty in unconscious survivors after out-of-hospital cardiac arrest. Resuscitation. 2025;214:110686.
127. Bougouin W, Lascarrou JB, Chelly J, Benghanem S, Geri G, Maizel J, et al. Performance of the ERC/ESICM-recommendations for neuroprognostication after cardiac arrest: insights from a prospective multicenter cohort. Resuscitation. 2024;202:110362.

Management of Adult Cardiac Arrest: Update 2025

21

Claudio Sandroni

21.1 Introduction

The aim of this chapter is to describe the main protocols for advanced cardiopulmonary resuscitation in adults (Advanced Life Support; ALS) as recommended by the 2025 guidelines of the European Resuscitation Council (ERC) [1]. In addition, where indicated, the major changes from the 2021 guidelines [2] are highlighted, ALS comprises the advanced interventions performed by healthcare professionals (physicians, registered nurses, or—where available—paramedics) in addition to, and as a continuation of, the basic life support (BLS) and the automated external defibrillation, which can be performed by lay rescuers. ALS includes the prevention and treatment of in-hospital cardiac arrest (IHCA) and out-of-hospital cardiac arrest (OHCA), the ALS algorithm, manual defibrillation, airway management during cardiopulmonary resuscitation (CPR), drugs, and their routes of administration. The protocols for the management of life-threatening arrhythmias are also commonly part of ALS, but will not be addressed in this chapter.

Figure 21.1 is a free adaptation of the ALS algorithm published by the European Resuscitation Council, which holds the copyright. Figures 21.2 and 21.3 are the work of the author.

C. Sandroni (✉)
Department of Intensive Care, Emergency Medicine and Anesthesiology, Fondazione Policlinico Universitario A. Gemelli-IRCCS – Università Cattolica del Sacro Cuore, Rome, Italy
e-mail: claudio.sandroni@unicatt.it

D. Chiumello, A. De Gasperi (eds.), *Practical Trends in Anesthesia and Intensive Care 2026*, https://doi.org/10.1007/978-3-032-25721-5_21

The ERC guidelines are based on the scientific consensus of the International Liaison Committee on Resuscitation (ILCOR), which brings together scientific societies involved in cardiopulmonary resuscitation worldwide. The ILCOR scientific consensus is based on a critical review of the literature, updated annually and conducted according to the GRADE methodology.

21.2 Prevention

21.2.1 Prevention of In-Hospital Cardiac Arrest

Several observational studies have shown that IHCA is preventable. In most cases, these arrests are not arrhythmic in origin, but are due to either the patient's acute illness that led to hospitalization or to its complications, and are preceded by a progressive deterioration of vital functions. If signs of deterioration are detected promptly, it is possible to prevent the final decline leading to cardiac arrest. This is particularly important in general wards, where patients are not monitored. To detect these signs and track possible deterioration over time in at-risk patients, Early Warning Scores (EWS) have been introduced into in-hospital clinical practice. These include, among others, the Modified Early Warning Score (MEWS) and the National Early Warning Score (NEWS) [3, 4]. EWS are used both in general wards and in emergency departments [3]. They work by assigning a score to the degree of abnormality in the patient's vital signs (e.g., respiratory rate, heart rate, blood pressure) and prescribing a proportionate response by the staff, such as increasing the frequency of assessments, initiating monitoring, or requesting evaluation by a physician or intensivist. Scores are recorded several times a day, and the frequency of measurement is increased if abnormalities in vital signs are detected, thereby allowing for the tracking of any deterioration in the patient's condition over time and enabling a timely response (track-and-trigger systems).

To increase the efficiency of the system, several hospitals are introducing in-hospital medical emergency teams (Medical Emergency Team: MET) composed of critical care personnel, not necessarily physicians, who respond to all requests for assessment of patients at risk of deterioration, even when their conditions are still relatively stable. These systems function optimally when staff are trained to use the detection system correctly and to call the MET promptly, even when there is a general clinical concern and not solely on vital sign scores [5].

In its 2025 guidelines, the European Resuscitation Council recommends that hospitals implement a track-and-trigger system and train staff in its use. Furthermore, hospitals must have a protocol for responding to warning signs, which may include activation of a MET or a similar resource [1].

21.2.2 Prevention of Out-of-Hospital Cardiac Arrest

Unlike IHCA, the main cause of out-of-hospital cardiac arrest (about 80% of cases) is coronary artery disease, and it is predominantly arrhythmic in origin, sometimes occurring without preceding symptoms. In younger individuals, although coronary artery disease cannot be excluded, the main causes of OHCA are inherited cardiomyopathies, congenital heart defects, myocarditis, and substance abuse.

In at least half of cases, OHCA occurs in individuals with undiagnosed heart disease, making prevention difficult. However, one-third of cardiac arrests due to acute coronary syndrome are preceded in the hours or days before the event by typical symptoms such as chest or epigastric pain, dyspnea, cold sweating, or syncope. Educating the general population to recognize these warning symptoms is obviously important for the prevention of OHCA. Notably, a British study of nearly 2000 patients with OHCA showed that in 9.4% of cases, the patient had already been assessed by ambulance personnel in the preceding 48 h [6].

In young people, the most important warning symptom of OHCA is syncope, mainly during intense physical activity. Among those who participate in sports, screening examinations, which at a minimum include an electrocardiogram and a physical examination, can help reduce the risk of sudden cardiac arrest. In a study conducted in the United Kingdom and published in 2018, cardiovascular screening identified conditions associated with sudden cardiac death in 42 out of over 11,000 athletes examined (0.4%) [7]. The athletes at highest risk are football and basketball players [8]. In an epidemiological study conducted in the USA between 2010 and 2023 on 29,311,597 marathon and half-marathon runners, 176 cardiac arrests were recorded, corresponding to an incidence of 0.56 events per 100,000 participants. The incidence remained unchanged during the observation period and was higher among men than among women, and among marathon runners compared to half-marathon runners [9].

21.3 Treatment of Cardiac Arrest

The treatment of cardiac arrest is summarized in the four interventions of the chain of survival: early recognition and call for help, early cardiopulmonary resuscitation, early defibrillation, and post-resuscitation care.

21.3.1 The Chain of Survival

Advanced resuscitation is simply a continuation, with more effective tools, of basic resuscitation, which must be initiated by the first witnesses of the event. Early activation of emergency services is essential to ensure that advanced help can be summoned timely. The presence of a witness and immediate bystander resuscitation are the most important factors increasing survival in cardiac arrest. Their importance outweighs that of advanced interventions such as drug administration or tracheal intubation. While awaiting the arrival of the ALS team, personnel from the Emergency Medical System (EMS) responding to emergency calls can assist rescuers in performing faster and more effective CPR by providing instructions over the phone (dispatch-assisted CPR). It has been shown that dispatch-assisted CPR improves both survival to hospital discharge and neurological outcomes in patients with out-of-hospital cardiac arrest [10]. Instructions are normally provided during the emergency call, but dispatch-assisted CPR can also be performed via smartphone video call [11]. Initial experiences suggest that video-assisted CPR yields better clinical outcomes than audio-only assisted CPR [12].

In the past two decades, automated external defibrillators (AEDs) have become increasingly available, allowing nonmedical rescuers who have received appropriate training to perform effective and safe defibrillation.

In hospitals, CPR and defibrillation are performed by ward staff while awaiting the arrival of the in-hospital ALS team, unless the arrest occurs in nonclinical areas. The organization of the emergency response may vary between hospitals, or within different clinical areas of the same hospital. Some clinical areas, such as intensive care units or cardiovascular departments, may have their own emergency team rather than relying on the centralized in-hospital emergency team. For activating the in-hospital emergency team, it has been recommended to implement the number 2222 in all European hospitals [13].

21.3.2 OHCA: Immediate Transport or On-Scene Resuscitation

In OHCA, the decision to prioritize transport to the hospital with ongoing ALS or to continue ALS treatment on scene depends on the available human and technical resources. The underlying principle remains to immediately perform on-site all interventions that can be carried out as effectively as in the hospital, and to transport the patient to the hospital for any interventions that cannot be effectively performed on-site. Systematic reviews [14] do not show that, in general, immediate transport improves survival from OHCA compared to on-scene treatment. However, the populations included in these studies were highly heterogeneous. A North American study of nearly 28,000 patients, whose characteristics were matched using a propensity score, showed that on-scene ALS was associated with double the survival rate compared to immediate transport [15].

The quality of care provided and the experience of EMS personnel influence the outcome of out-of-hospital cardiac arrest. For example, it has been shown that survival in OHCA patients increased with the number of cases attended by the rescuing personnel [16]. A recent systematic review of observational studies showed, albeit with low certainty, that when the majority of paramedics are trained in ALS, OHCA survival improves [17]. Recent studies have also explored the application of prehospital intensive care in selected patients, in addition to advanced resuscitation. The team consisted of physicians specialized in anesthesia or intensive care, or paramedics with specific training in critical care. A recent systematic review [18] showed that prehospital intensive care improves both survival and neurological outcomes in OHCA, and its use is recommended by the ERC 2025 guidelines, provided that resources and emergency system organization allow for it.

21.4 ALS Algorithm

One of the fundamental differences between a BLS provider and an ALS provider is that the latter bases interventions on electrocardiogram interpretation. The ECG underlying a cardiac arrest may show shockable rhythms (ventricular fibrillation [VF] or pulseless ventricular tachycardia [pVT]) or non-shockable rhythms (asystole and pulseless electrical activity [PEA]). The ALS algorithm (Fig. 21.1) therefore includes two parallel pathways for shockable and non-shockable rhythms, which differ in that defibrillation should be attempted in the former. Other interventions, such as CPR, airway management, intravenous or intraosseous access, drug administration, and emergency treatment of reversible causes, are common to both pathways. The ALS algorithm recommended in the 2025 guidelines remains essentially unchanged from the 2021 version, but includes minor modifications to better highlight the role of medications and the most appropriate timing for their administration.

Another important difference from basic resuscitation is that ALS is commonly performed by a team of several people, especially in hospitals and critical care settings. As a result, multiple interventions can be carried out simultaneously. ALS team interventions should be coordinated by a *team leader*, usually the most experienced provider. ALS training and certification courses help develop the skills needed to work effectively in a team and coordinate the team efficiently.

21.4.1 Defibrillation

ALS providers take over seamlessly from the basic responder, continuing CPR and, if not already done, connecting the patient to the defibrillator as soon as possible. If an AED has already been applied and defibrillation is indicated, ALS providers should follow its prompts, then switch to manual defibrillation as soon as possible. Both AEDs and manual defibrillators are equally effective in terminating VF/pVT, but manual defibrillation performed by a healthcare professional results in less CPR interruptions, as it does not require waiting for automated rhythm analysis.

Unlike the BLS provider who uses an AED, the ALS provider is able to interpret the ECG and must recognize shockable rhythms. Unlike previous editions, the 2025 ALS guidelines recommend defibrillating VF/pVT *of any amplitude*, including fine VF.

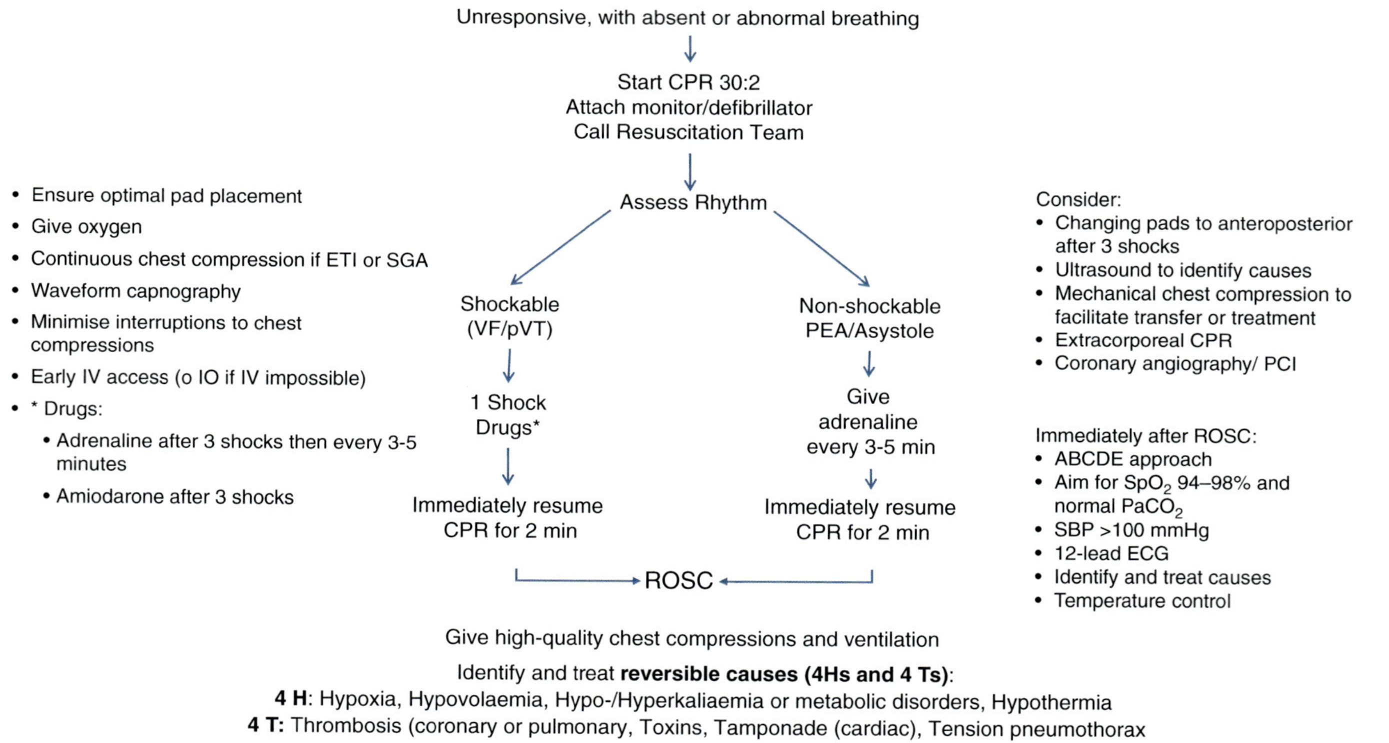

Fig. 21.1 ALS Algorithm (Redrawn from: Soar J et al. [1], with permission from the European Resuscitation Council). *Abbreviations*: CPR cardiopulmonary resuscitation, ETI endotracheal intubation, PCI percutaneous coronary intervention, PEA pulseless electrical activity, ROSC return of spontaneous circulation, SBP systolic blood pressure, SpO_2 peripheral oxygen saturation, measured by pulse oximetry, SGA supraglottic airway, VF/pVT ventricular fibrillation/pulseless ventricular tachycardia

21.4.1.1 Placement of Monitor-Defibrillator Electrodes/Pads

There are two options for ECG monitoring: the three standard leads (I, II, III) with electrodes, or adhesive pads on two leads. Adhesive pads allow both ECG monitoring and defibrillation, and are preferable. If electrodes are used, adhesive pads or manual defibrillation paddles will be required for defibrillation. The latter must be pressed by the rescuer onto the chest each time defibrillation is performed, after applying conductive gel. For this reason, they are less practical and potentially less safe than adhesive pads, which allow remote defibrillation.

In the standard configuration, the pads are positioned as follows (Fig. 21.2):

1. Anterior pad: below the right clavicle, to the right of the sternum.
2. Lateral pad: on the left mid-axillary line, below the armpit. In women, this pad should be positioned to avoid breast tissue.

The standard configuration is most convenient for a patient who is resuscitated in the supine position. Alternatively, an antero-posterior configuration is possible (Fig. 21.3):

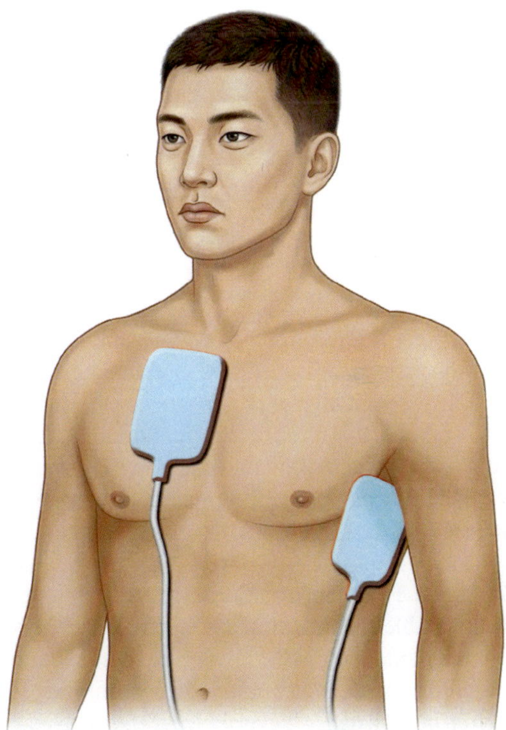

Fig. 21.2 Anterolateral pad placement for defibrillation. This configuration is ideal for minimizing interference with resuscitation efforts in a supine patient

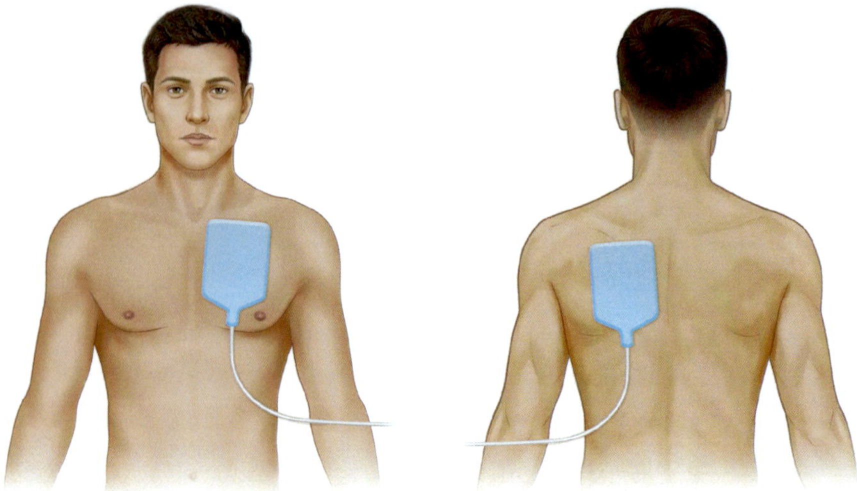

Fig. 21.3 Anteroposterior pad placement for defibrillation. This configuration is highly effective for optimizing current flow through the chest, but requires rotating the patient to position the posterior electrode

3. Anterior pad on the left side of the chest, between the midline and the nipple; in women, place the pad to the left of the lower half of the sternum, ensuring breast tissue is avoided.
4. Posterior pad to the left of the patient's spine, just below the left scapula.

A recent non-randomized study [19] showed that the anteroposterior configuration is associated with significantly higher rates of return of spontaneous circulation (ROSC) compared to the standard anterolateral configuration. However, it requires rotating the patient to access the subscapular region, resulting in greater difficulty and longer interruptions of resuscitation compared to the standard configuration. For this reason, in its 2025 ALS guidelines, the ERC suggests considering defibrillation vector change only in cases of persistent VF/pVT.

A particularly useful configuration for a resuscitated patient in the prone position (e.g., during ventilation of a patient with severe respiratory failure, or during certain surgical procedures) is the bi-axillary configuration. In this case, the two pads are placed under each armpit, on the lateral chest wall.

21.4.1.2 Precautions During Defibrillation

Implantable medical devices, such as pacemakers and cardioverter-defibrillators, can be damaged or deactivated by defibrillation shocks. These devices are commonly implanted subcutaneously in the left infraclavicular area, away from the defibrillation pads. Nevertheless, the pads should be placed at least 8 cm from the device.

During defibrillation, direct oxygen flow over the patient's chest should be avoided, such as from high-flow masks or nasal cannulas, due to the potential risk of fire. These devices should be kept at least 1 m away from the defibrillation pads. This precaution is not necessary if the patient is intubated and ventilated with a closed circuit.

21.4.1.3 Defibrillation Waveform and Energy Levels

Unlike the basic rescuer, the ALS provider independently selects the energy levels for defibrillation. These depend on the waveform used. Monophasic defibrillators have been almost completely abandoned in Western countries, and biphasic waveforms are now widely used. There are two main types of biphasic waveforms: truncated exponential biphasic and rectilinear biphasic. For these, the recommended energy for the first shock is 150 joules (J). A pulsed biphasic waveform is also available, for which the recommended defibrillation energy is 120–150 J. There is no evidence that one type of biphasic waveform is more effective than the others.

If the first defibrillation shock is ineffective, it is reasonable to increase the energy level for subsequent shocks. There are no recommendations for maximum energy levels, as they depend primarily on the defibrillator. Some defibrillators deliver shocks up to 200 J, while others reach 360 J.

There is no evidence that obese patients require higher defibrillation energies than patients of normal weight.

21.4.1.4 Refractory or Recurrent Ventricular Fibrillation

Refractory VF/pVT is defined as VF/pVT that persists after three consecutive shocks. This should be distinguished from *recurrent* ventricular fibrillation, which is the reappearance of VF/pVT after an initially successful defibrillation. More than half of the cases that appear refractory after the first defibrillation shock are actually recurrent fibrillations that reappear in the interval between the first effective shock and the subsequent assessment of cardiac rhythm [20]. The incidence of VF/pVT refractory to the first shock, initially estimated at around 20%, is more likely to be approximately 5% [21]. Patients with refractory VF/pVT have significantly lower survival rates compared to those who respond to standard resuscitation treatments. For the management of refractory or recurrent VF/pVT, the ALS algorithm recommends administering antiarrhythmic drugs (see below), but modifications to defibrillation technique may also be considered.

In addition to increasing defibrillation energy, as previously mentioned, in cases of VF/pVT truly refractory to shocks, it is essential to ensure that pad placement is appropriate and that optimal contact between the pads and the skin is achieved. Transthoracic impedance should be minimized by delivering shocks during the expiratory phase, and replacing the pads with a new set should also be considered. Finally, a change in pad orientation (*vector change*) should be considered.

21.4.1.5 Double Sequential Defibrillation

Double sequential defibrillation (DSD) has recently been investigated as a potential treatment for refractory VF/pVT. The technique involves the use of two defibrillators delivering either overlapping shocks or two shocks in rapid succession, one with the pads in the standard position and the other in the anteroposterior position. In 2022, the DOSE-VF [22] trial randomized 405 patients with refractory OHCA in VF/pVT to receive either DSD, anteroposterior *vector change* defibrillation, or conventional defibrillation. The results showed that both DSED and *vector change* were associated with higher survival, and—for DSED only—a higher rate of survival with good neurological outcome at discharge, compared to conventional defibrillation. Despite these positive results, the 2025 ERC guidelines do not recommend the routine use of DSD for refractory VF/pVT. There are several reasons for this decision. First, the DOSE-VF trial was stopped before reaching half of the planned sample size of 930 patients due to the COVID-19 pandemic. Second, this single trial contrasts with observational studies that did not show benefit. Finally, DSD is complex, as it requires repositioning the patient and the use of two defibrillators that must be discharged synchronously by two operators, since no defibrillators specifically designed for this technique currently exist. It should also be noted that many refractory VF/pVT cases are actually recurrent, and it remains uncertain whether DSD is more effective than conventional defibrillation in preventing recurrence of VF/pVT after successful defibrillation. The recommendation—already present in the 2021 guidelines—to consider *vector change* remains. Two European studies (STRAT-DEFI [NCT06781892] and Dual Defib [NCT06672159]) are currently underway and may provide further information on the potential use of this technique in the near future.

21.5 ALS Drugs

Drugs (vasopressors and antiarrhythmics) play a less important role than cardiopulmonary resuscitation in determining the prognosis of cardiac arrest. The only drugs currently indicated in advanced resuscitation are adrenaline, amiodarone, and lidocaine.

21.5.1 Adrenaline

The purpose of administering adrenaline during cardiac arrest is to increase vascular resistance, thereby improving perfusion of vital organs. Adrenaline is therefore used for its alpha (vasoconstrictive) effects and not for its beta (cardiac stimulatory) effects, which are potentially harmful as they increase myocardial oxygen consumption and the risk of fibrillation.

The main study supporting the use of adrenaline in cardiac arrest is the randomized, placebo-controlled clinical trial PARAMEDIC2, which enrolled 8104 patients with OHCA and demonstrated a significant increase in survival to hospital discharge with adrenaline compared to placebo (3.2% vs. 2.4%; $p = 0.02$). A subsequent follow-up study showed that this survival benefit persisted at 12 months [23]. Secondary analyses showed that the benefit is greater in non-shockable rhythms when adrenaline is administered early during cardiac arrest [24]. However, adrenaline has not been shown to improve long-term neurological outcomes.

As in the previous 2021 guidelines, the 2025 ERC ALS guidelines recommend giving adrenaline (1 mg IV every 3–5 min) as soon as possible in non-shockable rhythms, whereas in cases of cardiac arrest with initial VF/pVT, defibrillation should be attempted first (Fig. 21.1). In cases of initial refractory VF/pVT persisting after three consecutive shocks, the first dose of adrenaline should be administered after the third shock. Once the first dose of adrenaline has been administered, subsequent 1 mg boluses should be repeated every 3–5 min as per protocol, regardless of subsequent rhythms.

21.5.2 Amiodarone and Lidocaine

The evidence supporting the use of antiarrhythmics in cardiac arrest is weak and is mainly based on the randomized, placebo-controlled ALPS trial [25], which compared amiodarone, lidocaine, or placebo in OHCA with refractory VF/pVT. Compared to placebo, both amiodarone and lidocaine increased survival to hospital admission, but there was no difference between groups in survival to discharge or in survival with favorable neurological outcome at discharge. However, in the predefined subgroup of witnessed arrests, both amiodarone and lidocaine increased survival to discharge. An important limitation of the ALPS study is that it used a formulation of amiodarone hydrochloride (Nexterone®) instead of conventional amiodarone. This modification, intended to avoid the adverse hemodynamic effects of Polysorbate 80 contained in the conventional amiodarone preparation, limits the external validity of the study results.

As in the previous 2021 ALS guidelines, amiodarone is recommended in cases of persistent VF/pVT after three unsuccessful defibrillation attempts, *regardless* of whether these are consecutive shocks or interspersed with CPR cycles. The recommended dose of amiodarone is 300 mg IV bolus, which may be repeated once at half the dose (150 mg) after the fifth defibrillation attempt.

If amiodarone is not available, lidocaine may be used following the same protocol, at doses of 100 and 50 mg IV, respectively.

21.5.3 Fluids and Electrolytes

No randomized clinical trial has evaluated the routine administration of fluids versus no fluids as a treatment strategy for cardiac arrest. Rapid infusion of a large volume of fluids should be avoided unless there is evidence or suspicion that cardiac arrest is due to hypovolemia. Clinical assessment, history of events prior to cardiac arrest, and, when expertise is available, point-of-care emergency ultrasound may help identify hypovolemia as the cause of arrest.

There is no evidence supporting a specific type of fluid during cardiac arrest (e.g., isotonic saline vs. balanced crystalloids), and the benefit of hypertonic fluids has not yet been demonstrated [26].

21.5.3.1 Calcium

The 2025 guidelines have introduced new recommendations regarding calcium in ALS. A systematic review commissioned by ILCOR in 2023 examined three randomized trials and eight observational studies on calcium administration in adult cardiac arrest [27]. The largest and most recent trial included 391 patients with OHCA in a controlled manner and was stopped early because the *interim analysis* indicated potential harm from calcium compared to placebo [28]. Patients who received calcium had lower rates of favorable neurological outcome at 3 months and 1 year [27]. Based on these data, the 2025 ERC guidelines recommend against the routine administration of calcium during cardiac arrest. Calcium remains included in the 2025 guidelines for the treatment of cardiac arrest in special circumstances in cases of severe hyperkalemia ($K^+ \geq 6.5$ mmol/L) with ECG changes or arrhythmia, although there is no convincing evidence for or against its use [29].

21.5.3.2 Magnesium

Administration of magnesium during cardiac arrest due to refractory VF/pVT is not supported by sufficient evidence and is not recommended [1].

21.5.4 Vascular Access

The routine vascular access for administration of drugs or fluids during cardiac arrest is peripheral (IV) venous access, unless the patient already has a central venous line. However, observational studies show that in recent years the use of the intraosseous (IO) route as the first intravascular access in cardiac arrest has increased in an attempt to achieve more rapid drug administration [30].

In 2024, two open-label randomized clinical trials (IVIO, conducted in Denmark, and PARAMEDIC3, conducted in the United Kingdom) compared the IO-first strategy with the IV-first strategy in cardiac arrest [31, 32]. Neither of these studies showed that the IO-first strategy resulted in more rapid drug administration, although in both, the success rates for establishing vascular access were higher for the intraosseous route compared to the intravenous route. A meta-analysis of these studies commissioned by ILCOR [33] has shown that the IO-first strategy does not improve either survival or the rate of favorable neurological outcomes compared to an IV-first strategy. Given the lack of demonstrated benefit, the lower routine availability of the intraosseous route, its higher cost, and the need for additional training for its use, the ERC continues to recommend the intravenous route as the first-line vascular access, and suggests considering the intraosseous route only after two unsuccessful attempts to establish intravenous access.

21.6 Extracorporeal Cardiopulmonary Resuscitation (ECPR)

Extracorporeal CPR (ECPR) is a circulatory support technique achieved through an extracorporeal circuit combined with a veno-arterial membrane oxygenator (VA-ECMO) in a patient with cardiac arrest. Typically, ECPR is applied in patients in whom conventional CPR (c-CPR) fails. Between 2020 and 2023, three randomized clinical trials on ECPR were published, with significant differences in both design and randomization point, but all based on in-hospital ECPR performed on patients initially treated with c-CPR for OHCA. The first study chronologically (2019–2020) was the US ARREST trial, conducted in the USA on patients with an initial shockable rhythm, which showed higher survival to discharge after ECPR compared to c-CPR. However, this was a phase 2 study involving only 30 patients [34]. The Prague-ECPR study, conducted in the Czech Republic on 264 patients with refractory OHCA and any underlying rhythm, found improved survival with ECPR for favorable neurological outcome at 30 days, but not at 6 months, which was the primary outcome of the study [35]. INCEPTION, the third and most recent trial, and the only multicenter study, was conducted in the Netherlands on 134 adult patients with OHCA and an initial shockable rhythm who had received bystander CPR. The study found no significant difference between ECPR and c-CPR in the primary outcome, which was survival with favorable neurological outcome at 30 days [36]. A meta-analysis of these studies, which also included a pilot study, showed higher survival with favorable neurological outcome with ECPR compared to c-CPR [37]. Similar results were obtained for IHCA in a meta-analysis of observational studies [38]. In its 2025 guidelines, the ERC recommends considering ECPR as a rescue therapy for selected patients with IHCA or OHCA when conventional CPR fails to achieve ROSC, in settings where this can be implemented.

There are no universally accepted selection criteria for ECPR. In the clinical trials on ECPR described above, only a minority of patients were eligible for enrollment. A recent systematic review with meta-analysis found that younger age, an initial shockable rhythm, witnessed arrest, immediate CPR, ROSC, and a shorter duration of c-CPR before veno-arterial cannulation were associated with a higher likelihood of survival with favorable neurological outcome [39].

21.7 Airway Management and Ventilation

Unlike the basic rescuer, the ALS provider has access to an oxygen source. Although there are no randomized studies that have ventilated patients with different inspired oxygen fractions (FiO_2), ensuring adequate tissue oxygenation is one of the goals of CPR. During cardiac arrest, there are numerous causes of hypoxia, related both to the causes of the arrest itself (hypoxic arrest, pulmonary thromboembolism) and to complications of the arrest (massive pulmonary edema). For this reason, based on expert consensus, the ERC recommends ventilating the patient in cardiac arrest with the highest possible FiO_2. Observational studies show that a higher arterial partial pressure of oxygen (PaO_2) during resuscitation is associated with a greater likelihood of ROSC and survival [40, 41].

There is no evidence supporting the use of advanced airway devices during ALS. In 2018, a randomized trial conducted in the United Kingdom on over 9000 OHCA patients treated by paramedics compared initial insertion of a supraglottic airway (i-gel®) with tracheal intubation [42] and found no difference in the primary endpoint of survival with good functional outcome (6.4% vs. 6.8%; $p = 0.33$). A non-inferiority randomized trial involving over 2000 OHCA patients compared early tracheal intubation with bag-mask ventilation followed by tracheal intubation after ROSC. In this case, EMS personnel were physicians [43] Again, no difference was found in the primary endpoint of 28-day survival with favorable functional outcome (4.3% vs. 4.2%). The tracheal intubation success rate in this study was 98%. It is noteworthy that 146 patients in the bag-mask ventilation group underwent crossover to intubation due to difficulty with bag-mask ventilation or the presence of regurgitation.

Tracheal intubation allows for optimal airway management but requires interruption of chest compressions and may be associated with a high rate of failure or misplacement, especially in out-of-hospital systems where personnel have limited experience with the technique [44]. Based on this evidence, the ERC, reaffirming its previous 2021 recommendations, considers bag-mask ventilation and advanced airway management techniques to be equivalent.

Regarding the choice of advanced airway management techniques, efficacy data show substantial equivalence between the I-gel and tracheal intubation. The SAVE study, conducted in Taiwan, randomized 936 adult patients with nontraumatic OHCA to receive either tracheal intubation or I-gel by paramedics trained in both techniques, and found no difference in the primary outcome of sustained ROSC for at least 2 h.

The 2025 ERC ALS guidelines recommend the use of a supraglottic airway in systems where there is insufficient experience with tracheal intubation to ensure a high success rate. This is defined as correct placement in more than 95% of cases with no more than two attempts. Furthermore, interruption of CPR for intubation should not exceed 5 s. If available, videolaryngoscopy should be preferred over direct laryngoscopy. The 2025 ERC ALS guidelines suggest using the I-gel as the supraglottic airway device, rather than the laryngeal tube.

A potential advantage of advanced airways is that they allow for continuous chest compressions without pauses during ventilation. This advantage applies especially to tracheal intubation. Supraglottic airways provide a less effective seal; although they often allow for continuous chest compressions without excessive air leakage, in some cases intubation is required to continue effective asynchronous ventilation and compressions.

Another advantage of advanced airways is that they allow the patient to be connected to a mechanical ventilator. Continuous chest compressions interfere with ventilation. If mechanical ventilation is used during cardiopulmonary resuscitation, the 2025 ERC ALS guidelines recommend using volume-controlled mode, setting the peak pressure alarm at 60–70 cm H_2O, and disabling the flow trigger. Other recommended settings include a tidal volume of 6–8 ml/kg, or at least the minimum volume that produces a visible chest rise, an FiO_2 of 1, a respiratory rate of 10 breaths/min, an inspiratory time of 1–2 s, and a positive end-expiratory pressure (PEEP) of 0–5 cm H_2O. If mechanical ventilation is ineffective, manual ventilation should be used.

21.8 Physiologically Guided Resuscitation

The 2025 ERC ALS guidelines have introduced the principle of physiologically guided resuscitation to optimize CPR quality. This is only possible in highly monitored settings. Among the physiological parameters that can be used, the main ones are end-tidal CO_2 ($ETCO_2$) and invasive arterial pressure.

21.8.1 $ETCO_2$

CO_2 produced in perfused tissues by aerobic metabolism is transported by the venous circulation to the right side of the heart and propelled by the right ventricle into the pulmonary circulation, from which it is removed by alveolar ventilation. For this reason, $ETCO_2$ reflects cardiac output, tissue perfusion, pulmonary blood flow, and minute ventilation.

Monitoring $ETCO_2$ during resuscitation has three main objectives:

- Confirmation of correct tracheal tube placement; despite concerns that low CO_2 production and low cardiac output may reduce the sensitivity of CO_2 detection during CPR, $ETCO_2$ is considered the most reliable method for confirming endotracheal tube placement even during cardiac arrest, according to the PUMA (Project for Universal Management of Airways and International Airway Societies) guidelines [45].
- Detection of return of spontaneous circulation during resuscitation: when ROSC occurs, $ETCO_2$ may increase threefold. Capnography during CPR can therefore be useful to avoid unnecessary continuation of resuscitation efforts or the potentially harmful administration of adrenaline. However, no precise threshold for $ETCO_2$ increase has been reliably identified to diagnose ROSC. Moreover, the increase in $ETCO_2$ associated with ROSC is not immediate and may begin 10 min or more before a palpable pulse is detected [46–48].
- Prognosis during CPR. The lower the $ETCO_2$ during CPR, the lower the likelihood of ROSC. An unblinded observational study [49] suggested that failure to achieve an $ETCO_2$ value >10 mmHg was consistently associated with unsuccessful resuscitation, but subsequent studies have shown that this threshold should

not be interpreted as 100% accurate [50]. Conversely, an $ETCO_2$ greater than 10 mmHg does not guarantee survival, as it may be present in up to 88% of non-survivors [51]. A high $ETCO_2$ during cardiac arrest may also indicate hypoventilation rather than effective perfusion [52].

21.8.2 Arterial Pressure

Continuous arterial pressure monitoring is only possible in intensive care settings, and available data are limited. Based on expert consensus, the American Heart Association [53] has suggested that:

- If both an arterial line and a central venous catheter are in place during cardiac arrest, efforts should be made to achieve a coronary perfusion pressure (estimated as the difference between mean arterial pressure and central venous pressure) greater than 20 mmHg.
- If only an arterial line is in place during cardiac arrest, aim to maintain a diastolic arterial pressure above 25 mmHg.

Based on recent observational data [54], the ERC suggests targeting a diastolic arterial pressure of ≥30 mmHg when intra-arterial pressure monitoring is used during CPR.

21.9 Cardiac Arrest in Monitored Areas

Some in-hospital settings of special relevance for the anesthesiologist-intensivist, such as the operating room, intensive care unit, and cardiac surgery, require specific considerations.

In monitored areas such as the intensive care unit and operating rooms, invasive arterial pressure and $ETCO_2$ monitoring are generally available for the most unstable patients. In many of these patients, the objective elements on which the diagnosis of cardiac arrest is based, such as absence of consciousness and spontaneous breathing, may not be available due to clinical conditions or pharmacological sedation, and the diagnosis of cardiac arrest relies primarily on circulatory criteria. Since the circulatory criterion for initiating CPR is the loss of palpable central pulses, which usually occurs when systolic arterial pressure falls below 50 mmHg, a sudden drop in pressure below this level and lack of response to treatment of underlying causes are sufficient criteria to start chest compressions. A concomitant abrupt decrease in $ETCO_2$ provides further confirmation. In these patients, reduced adrenaline boluses of 50–100 μg IV, titrated as needed, should be considered instead of a 1 mg bolus, as the latter may induce tachyarrhythmias or severe hypertension [55]. If there is no response to incremental boluses, and after reaching a total dose of 1 mg, the standard dose should be used.

In the operating room, as well as in interventional radiology areas, the presence of the surgical field and equipment may hinder resuscitation maneuvers. When administering anesthesia to critically ill patients at high risk of cardiac arrest, it is advisable to place defibrillation pads before induction and keep the defibrillator connected and on standby. Both in the operating room and in the intensive care unit, it may be necessary to perform CPR in the prone position [56].

A specific condition in the operating room is cardiac arrest due to local anesthetic overdose. In addition to administration of 20% lipid emulsion infusions (1.5 ml/kg IV in 1 min + 0.25 ml/kg/min IV, which may be increased after 5 min) [29], it is recommended to administer adrenaline at a reduced dose of ≤1 mcg/kg IV, based on experimental data indicating that adrenaline may have arrhythmogenic effects and cause metabolic acidosis, hindering return of circulation [57].

Cardiac arrest in the post-cardiac surgery setting has a relatively high incidence (up to 2–5%) but a better prognosis than in-hospital cardiac arrest in general (survival 50% or higher), since it occurs in a highly monitored environment, with patients cared for by personnel experienced in cardiopulmonary resuscitation, and in most cases is due to reversible causes such as arrhythmias or surgical bleeding. The ALS protocol in this specific context is detailed in the 2025 Guidelines on arrest in special circumstances [29]. The main modifications compared to the general algorithm are as follows:

- In the case of VF/pVT, deliver three consecutive defibrillation shocks in less than1 min, without pauses between shocks for CPR.
- In the case of asystole or PEA with extreme bradycardia, apply pacing early.
- Consider early echocardiography, including transesophageal, to identify the causes of arrest.
- If there is no recovery within 5 min, perform emergency sternotomy.
- Consider mechanical circulatory support and ECPR.
- The administration of standard-dose adrenaline is controversial. The European Association of Cardio-Thoracic Surgery and the Society of Thoracic Surgeons advise against its use, due to concerns that the sudden hypertension induced by a 1 mg intravenous bolus of adrenaline may cause bleeding or rupture of surgical anastomoses after ROSC [58, 59]. The ERC 2025 guidelines suggest considering reduced doses (50–100 mcg bolus) in peri-arrest conditions, as recommended above in ALS in monitored settings.

21.10 CPR-Induced Consciousness

The 2025 guidelines have introduced a new chapter on CPR-induced consciousness. The occurrence of consciousness during CPR in the absence of ROSC, although rare (less than 1% of cases [60]), is being reported with increasing frequency [61]. The presence of consciousness is associated with a better prognosis [62] and should be considered when deciding whether to continue or terminate ALS. It is likely that resuscitation maneuvers may cause distress and pain in a conscious patient, and the presence of consciousness and patient reactivity may interfere with CPR itself. If ALS providers observe signs of consciousness during CPR, they may consider the use of sedative or analgesic drugs (or both) in small doses, but should avoid muscle relaxants, especially if used alone.

21.11 Immediate Treatment After ROSC

If resuscitation is successful and ROSC is achieved, post-resuscitation care should begin immediately. First, the patient should be rapidly reassessed, as in the initial approach, using the ABCDE checklist: Airway, Breathing, Circulation, Disability (neurological function), and Exposure (external physical examination for pathological signs). More than 80% of patients are unconscious after ROSC and require an advanced airway if one has not already been placed. Until peripheral oxygen saturation (SpO_2) can be measured, it is advisable to deliver an inspired oxygen fraction (FiO_2) of 100% to avoid the risk of hypoxia. As soon as SpO_2 can be reliably measured, FiO_2 and ventilatory parameters should be adjusted to achieve an SpO_2 of 94–98%. Immediately after ROSC, it is recommended to maintain a systolic blood pressure above 100 mmHg. It is often necessary to continue and complete the treatment of reversible causes initiated during ALS. To this end, it is important to obtain a 12-lead ECG, as acute coronary syndrome is the leading cause of OHCA.

21.12 When to Stop Resuscitation?

21.12.1 Out-of-Hospital Cardiac Arrest

Some EMS systems have developed Termination of Resuscitation (TOR) rules for out-of-hospital cardiac arrest. These rules are not the same in all systems, reflecting on the one hand differences in their organization, and on the other hand, the lack of high-certainty evidence supporting their use. ILCOR recommends implementing TOR rules only after verifying their accuracy in the context in which they are to be used. An important element of resuscitation termination criteria is specificity, that is, the ability to avoid false positives, which would lead to stopping resuscitation in a patient who may still have a chance of recovery. Since no rule is perfect, it is necessary to ensure that the risk of false positives is consistent with the expectations and local values of the context in which one operates.

21.12.2 In-Hospital Cardiac Arrest

Scientific evidence supporting the use of TOR rules for IHCA is relatively limited. A recent study enrolled patients with IHCA in Denmark, Sweden, and Norway, and developed and validated five TOR rules [63]. Of these, the most accurate rule includes four variables: unwitnessed and unmonitored arrest, asystole as the initial rhythm, and ineffective resuscitation for at least 10 min. This rule predicted 30-day non-survival with an error rate of 6 cases per 1000. Although this result is promising, external validation is required before the rule can be considered for practical use. Currently, the ERC recommends not using the TOR rules as the sole criterion for deciding to terminate resuscitation in IHCA. As with OHCA, TOR rules for IHCA should be validated in local, regional, or national cohorts before implementation, taking into account the local legal, organizational, and cultural context.

21.13 Organ Donation After CPR

Unfortunately, less than half of patients resuscitated with conventional CPR achieve ROSC [64]. In most cases, this leads to termination of resuscitation efforts, preferably using the TOR criteria described above. In selected patients, and where resources and organization allow, ECPR should be considered. This should be done as early as possible. Finally, in specific settings, the discontinuation of resuscitation and subsequent diagnosis of death based on circulatory criteria may be followed by uncontrolled donation after circulatory death (uDCD). uDCD donors are classified as Maastricht category I if the arrest was unwitnessed, and category II if the arrest was witnessed [65].

Uncontrolled donation after circulatory death requires significant resources and rapid decision-making, is complex, ethically sensitive, and therefore demands appropriate organization and a suitable legislative and social framework [66]. After discontinuation of CPR, rescuers observe a "no-touch" period to exclude the possibility of autoresuscitation, i.e., the occurrence of ROSC after resuscitation has been stopped [67]. In most countries where uDCD is practiced, the prescribed duration of this period is 5 min [68], but some countries, including Italy, require 20 min [69]. At the end of the "no-touch" period, organ preservation procedures are initiated and continue until consent for donation is confirmed.

Organs that can be donated from uDCD donors include kidneys, liver, pancreas, and lungs. In 2025, a systematic review promoted by ILCOR showed that in several studies, uDCD donation was associated with overall good outcomes, but with higher rates of early dysfunction for the kidney and both early and long-term dysfunction for the liver, not only compared to "standard" donors after brain death but also to donors after controlled circulatory death (cDCD) [70]. This may be at least partly due to the longer warm ischemia time in uDCD compared to other types of donors.

References

1. Soar J, Böttiger BW, Carli P, Jiménez FC, Cimpoesu D, Cole G, et al. European Resuscitation Council guidelines 2025 adult advanced life support. Resuscitation. 2025;215(Suppl 1):110769.
2. Soar J, Bottiger BW, Carli P, Couper K, Deakin CD, Djarv T, et al. European Resuscitation Council guidelines 2021: adult advanced life support. Resuscitation. 2021;161:115–51.

3. McGaughey J, Fergusson DA, Van Bogaert P, Rose L. Early warning systems and rapid response systems for the prevention of patient deterioration in acute adult hospital wards. Cochrane Database Syst Rev. 2021;11:Cd005529.
4. Covino M, Sandroni C, Della Polla D, De Matteis G, Piccioni A, De Vita A, et al. Predicting ICU admission and death in the Emergency Department: a comparison of six early warning scores. Resuscitation. 2023;190:109876.
5. Sandroni C, Cavallaro F. Failure of the afferent limb: a persistent problem in rapid response systems. Resuscitation. 2011;82:797–8.
6. Deakin CD, Morley P, Soar J, Drennan IR. Double (dual) sequential defibrillation for refractory ventricular fibrillation cardiac arrest: a systematic review. Resuscitation. 2020;155:24–31.
7. Malhotra A, Dhutia H, Finocchiaro G, Gati S, Beasley I, Clift P, et al. Outcomes of cardiac screening in adolescent soccer players. N Engl J Med. 2018;379:524–34.
8. Harmon KG, Drezner JA, Wilson MG, Sharma S. Incidence of sudden cardiac death in athletes: a state-of-the-art review. Heart. 2014;100:1227–34.
9. Kim JH, Rim AJ, Miller JT, Jackson M, Patel N, Rajesh S, et al. Cardiac arrest during Long-distance running races. JAMA. 2025;333:1699–707.
10. Nikolaou N, Dainty KN, Couper K, Morley P, Tijssen J, Vaillancourt C. A systematic review and meta-analysis of the effect of dispatcher-assisted CPR on outcomes from sudden cardiac arrest in adults and children. Resuscitation. 2019;138:82–105.
11. Dainty KN, Debaty G, Waddick J, Vaillancourt C, Malta Hansen C, Olasveengen T, et al. Interventions to optimize dispatcher-assisted CPR instructions: a scoping review. Resusc Plus. 2024;19:100715.
12. Lee SY, Song KJ, Shin SD, Hong KJ, Kim TH. Comparison of the effects of audio-instructed and video-instructed dispatcher-assisted cardiopulmonary resuscitation on resuscitation outcomes after out-of-hospital cardiac arrest. Resuscitation. 2020;147:12–20.
13. Whitaker DK, Nolan JP, Castrén M, Abela C, Goldik Z. Implementing a standard internal telephone number 2222 for cardiac arrest calls in all hospitals in Europe. Resuscitation. 2017;115:A14–a5.
14. Burns B, Hsu HR, Keech A, Huang Y, Tian DH, Coggins A, et al. Expedited transport versus continued on-scene resuscitation for refractory out-of-hospital cardiac arrest: a systematic review and meta-analysis. Resusc Plus. 2023;16:100482.
15. Grunau B, Kime N, Leroux B, Rea T, Van Belle G, Menegazzi JJ, et al. Association of intra-arrest transport vs continued on-scene resuscitation with survival to hospital discharge among patients with out-of-hospital cardiac arrest. JAMA. 2020;324:1058–67.
16. Dyson K, Bray JE, Smith K, Bernard S, Straney L, Finn J. Paramedic exposure to out-of-hospital cardiac arrest resuscitation is associated with patient survival. Circ Cardiovasc Qual Outcomes. 2016;9:154–60.
17. Wang SA, Lee HW, Ko YC, Sun JT, Matsuyama T, Lin CH, et al. Effect of crew ratio of advanced life support-trained personnel on patients with out-of-hospital cardiac arrest: a systematic review and meta-analysis. J Formos Med Assoc. 2024;123:561–70.
18. Boulton AJ, Edwards R, Gadie A, Clayton D, Leech C, Smyth MA, et al. Prehospital critical care beyond advanced life support for out-of-hospital cardiac arrest: a systematic review. Resusc Plus. 2025;21:100803.
19. Lupton JR, Newgard CD, Dennis D, Nuttall J, Sahni R, Jui J, et al. Initial defibrillator pad position and outcomes for shockable out-of-hospital cardiac arrest. JAMA Netw Open. 2024;7:e2431673.
20. Koster RW, Walker RG, Chapman FW. Recurrent ventricular fibrillation during advanced life support care of patients with prehospital cardiac arrest. Resuscitation. 2008;78:252–7.
21. Verkaik BJ, Walker RG, Taylor TG, Ekkel MM, Marx R, Stieglis R, et al. Defibrillation and refractory ventricular fibrillation. Eur Heart J. 2025;46:582–4.
22. Cheskes S, Verbeek PR, Drennan IR, McLeod SL, Turner L, Pinto R, et al. Defibrillation strategies for refractory ventricular fibrillation. N Engl J Med. 2022;387:1947–56.

23. Haywood KL, Ji C, Quinn T, Nolan JP, Deakin CD, Scomparin C, et al. Long term outcomes of participants in the PARAMEDIC2 randomised trial of adrenaline in out-of-hospital cardiac arrest. Resuscitation. 2021;160:84–93.
24. Perkins GD, Kenna C, Ji C, Deakin CD, Nolan JP, Quinn T, et al. The influence of time to adrenaline administration in the Paramedic 2 randomised controlled trial. Intensive Care Med. 2020;46:426–36.
25. Kudenchuk PJ, Brown SP, Daya M, Rea T, Nichol G, Morrison LJ, et al. Amiodarone, lidocaine, or placebo in out-of-hospital cardiac arrest. N Engl J Med. 2016;374:1711–22.
26. Jendoubi A, De Roux Q, Lê MP, Magnoni S, Ghaleh B, Tissier R, et al. Fluid therapy during and after cardiopulmonary resuscitation for nontraumatic cardiac arrest: a systematic review of evidence from preclinical and clinical studies. Shock. 2025;63:363–70.
27. Hsu CH, Couper K, Nix T, Drennan I, Reynolds J, Kleinman M, et al. Calcium during cardiac arrest: a systematic review. Resusc Plus. 2023;14:100379.
28. Vallentin MF, Granfeldt A, Meilandt C, Povlsen AL, Sindberg B, Holmberg MJ, et al. Effect of intravenous or intraosseous calcium vs saline on return of spontaneous circulation in adults with out-of-hospital cardiac arrest: a randomized clinical trial. JAMA. 2021;326:2268–76.
29. Lott C, Karageorgos V, Abelairas-Gomez C, Alfonzo A, Bierens J, Cantellow S, et al. European resuscitation council guidelines 2025 special circumstances in resuscitation. Resuscitation. 2025;215(Suppl 1):110753.
30. Vadeyar S, Buckle A, Hooper A, Booth S, Deakin CD, Fothergill R, et al. Trends in use of intraosseous and intravenous access in out-of-hospital cardiac arrest across English ambulance services: a registry-based, cohort study. Resuscitation. 2023;191:109951.
31. Couper K, Ji C, Deakin CD, Fothergill RT, Nolan JP, Long JB, et al. A randomized trial of drug route in out-of-hospital cardiac arrest. N Engl J Med. 2025;392:336–48.
32. Vallentin MF, Granfeldt A, Klitgaard TL, Mikkelsen S, Folke F, Christensen HC, et al. Intraosseous or intravenous vascular access for out-of-hospital cardiac arrest. N Engl J Med. 2025;392:349–60.
33. Couper K, Andersen LW, Drennan IR, Grunau BE, Kudenchuk PJ, Lall R, et al. Intraosseous and intravenous vascular access during adult cardiac arrest: a systematic review and meta-analysis. Resuscitation. 2025;207:110481.
34. Yannopoulos D, Bartos J, Raveendran G, Walser E, Connett J, Murray TA, et al. Advanced reperfusion strategies for patients with out-of-hospital cardiac arrest and refractory ventricular fibrillation (ARREST): a phase 2, single centre, open-label, randomised controlled trial. Lancet. 2020;396:1807–16.
35. Belohlavek J, Smalcova J, Rob D, Franek O, Smid O, Pokorna M, et al. Effect of intra-arrest transport, extracorporeal cardiopulmonary resuscitation, and immediate invasive assessment and treatment on functional neurologic outcome in refractory out-of-hospital cardiac arrest: a randomized clinical trial. JAMA. 2022;327:737–47.
36. Suverein MM, Delnoij TSR, Lorusso R, Brandon Bravo Bruinsma GJ, Otterspoor L, Elzo Kraemer CV, et al. Early extracorporeal CPR for refractory out-of-hospital cardiac arrest. N Engl J Med. 2023;388:299–309.
37. Scquizzato T, Bonaccorso A, Swol J, Gamberini L, Scandroglio AM, Landoni G, et al. Refractory out-of-hospital cardiac arrest and extracorporeal cardiopulmonary resuscitation: a meta-analysis of randomized trials. Artif Organs. 2023;47:806–16.
38. Low CJW, Ramanathan K, Ling RR, Ho MJC, Chen Y, Lorusso R, et al. Extracorporeal cardiopulmonary resuscitation versus conventional cardiopulmonary resuscitation in adults with cardiac arrest: a comparative meta-analysis and trial sequential analysis. Lancet Respir Med. 2023;11:883–93.
39. Tran A, Rochwerg B, Fan E, Belohlavek J, Suverein MM, Poll M, et al. Prognostic factors associated with favourable functional outcome among adult patients requiring extracorporeal cardiopulmonary resuscitation for out-of-hospital cardiac arrest: a systematic review and meta-analysis. Resuscitation. 2023;193:110004.

40. Spindelboeck W, Gemes G, Strasser C, Toescher K, Kores B, Metnitz P, et al. Arterial blood gases during and their dynamic changes after cardiopulmonary resuscitation: a prospective clinical study. Resuscitation. 2016;106:24–9.
41. Nelskylä A, Skrifvars MB, Ångerman S, Nurmi J. Incidence of hyperoxia and factors associated with cerebral oxygenation during cardiopulmonary resuscitation. Resuscitation. 2022;170:276–82.
42. Benger JR, Kirby K, Black S, Brett SJ, Clout M, Lazaroo MJ, et al. Effect of a strategy of a supraglottic airway device vs tracheal intubation during out-of-hospital cardiac arrest on functional outcome: the AIRWAYS-2 randomized clinical trial. JAMA. 2018;320:779–91.
43. Jabre P, Penaloza A, Pinero D, Duchateau FX, Borron SW, Javaudin F, et al. Effect of bag-mask ventilation vs endotracheal intubation during cardiopulmonary resuscitation on neurological outcome after out-of-hospital cardiorespiratory arrest: a randomized clinical trial. JAMA. 2018;319:779–87.
44. Wang HE, Schmicker RH, Daya MR, Stephens SW, Idris AH, Carlson JN, et al. Effect of a strategy of initial laryngeal tube insertion vs endotracheal intubation on 72-hour survival in adults with out-of-hospital cardiac arrest: a randomized clinical trial. JAMA. 2018;320:769–78.
45. Chrimes N, Higgs A, Hagberg CA, Baker PA, Cooper RM, Greif R, et al. Preventing unrecognised oesophageal intubation: a consensus guideline from the Project for Universal Management of Airways and international airway societies. Anaesthesia. 2022;77:1395–415.
46. Lui CT, Poon KM, Tsui KL. Abrupt rise of end tidal carbon dioxide level was a specific but non-sensitive marker of return of spontaneous circulation in patient with out-of-hospital cardiac arrest. Resuscitation. 2016;104:53–8.
47. Pokorná M, Necas E, Kratochvíl J, Skripský R, Andrlík M, Franek O. A sudden increase in partial pressure end-tidal carbon dioxide (P(ET)CO(2)) at the moment of return of spontaneous circulation. J Emerg Med. 2010;38:614–21.
48. Sandroni C, De Santis P, D'Arrigo S. Capnography during cardiac arrest. Resuscitation. 2018;132:73–7.
49. Levine RL, Wayne MA, Miller CC. End-tidal carbon dioxide and outcome of out-of-hospital cardiac arrest. N Engl J Med. 1997;337:301–6.
50. Smida T, Menegazzi JJ, Crowe RP, Salcido DD, Bardes J, Myers B. The association of prehospital end-tidal carbon dioxide with survival following out-of-hospital cardiac arrest. Prehosp Emerg Care. 2024;28:478–84.
51. Hambelton C, Wu L, Smith J, Thompson K, Neth MR, Daya MR, et al. Utility of end-tidal carbon dioxide to guide resuscitation termination in prolonged out-of-hospital cardiac arrest. Am J Emerg Med. 2024;77:77–80.
52. Heradstveit BE, Sunde K, Sunde GA, Wentzel-Larsen T, Heltne JK. Factors complicating interpretation of capnography during advanced life support in cardiac arrest—a clinical retrospective study in 575 patients. Resuscitation. 2012;83:813–8.
53. Meaney PA, Bobrow BJ, Mancini ME, Christenson J, de Caen AR, Bhanji F, et al. Cardiopulmonary resuscitation quality: [corrected] improving cardiac resuscitation outcomes both inside and outside the hospital: a consensus statement from the American Heart Association. Circulation. 2013;128:417–35.
54. Aziz S, Barratt J, Starr Z, Lachowycz K, Major R, Barnard EBG, et al. The association between intra-arrest arterial blood pressure and return of spontaneous circulation in out-of-hospital cardiac arrest. Resuscitation. 2024;205:110426.
55. Nolan JP, Armstrong RA, Kane AD, Kursumovic E, Davies MT, Moppett IK, et al. Advanced life support interventions during intra-operative cardiac arrest among adults as reported to the 7th National Audit Project of the Royal College of Anaesthetists. Anaesthesia. 2024;79:914–23.
56. Anez C, Becerra-Bolaños Á, Vives-Lopez A, Rodríguez-Pérez A. Cardiopulmonary resuscitation in the prone position in the operating room or in the intensive care unit: a systematic review. Anesth Analg. 2021;132:285–92.
57. Hiller David B, Gregorio Guido D, Ripper R, Kelly K, Massad M, Edelman L, et al. Epinephrine impairs lipid resuscitation from bupivacaine overdose: a threshold effect. Anesthesiology. 2009;111:498–505.

58. Dunning J, Fabbri A, Kolh PH, Levine A, Lockowandt U, Mackay J, et al. Guideline for resuscitation in cardiac arrest after cardiac surgery. Eur J Cardiothorac Surg. 2009;36:3–28.
59. Society of Thoracic Surgeons Task Force on Resuscitation After Cardiac Surgery. The Society of Thoracic Surgeons expert consensus for the resuscitation of patients who arrest after cardiac surgery. Ann Thorac Surg. 2017;103:1005–20.
60. Olaussen A, Nehme Z, Shepherd M, Jennings PA, Bernard S, Mitra B, et al. Consciousness induced during cardiopulmonary resuscitation: an observational study. Resuscitation. 2017;113:44–50.
61. Parnia S, Keshavarz Shirazi T, Patel J, Tran L, Sinha N, O'Neill C, et al. AWAreness during REsuscitation – II: a multi-center study of consciousness and awareness in cardiac arrest. Resuscitation. 2023;191:109903.
62. Talikowska M, Belcher J, Ball S, Majewski D, Finn J. CPR-induced consciousness in out-of-hospital cardiac arrest patients in Western Australia: case characteristics and CPR quality. Resuscitation. 2024;201:110278.
63. Holmberg MJ, Granfeldt A, Moskowitz A, Lauridsen KG, Bergum D, Christiansen CF, et al. Termination of resuscitation rules for in-hospital cardiac arrest. JAMA Intern Med. 2025;185:391–7.
64. Gräsner JT, Wnent J, Herlitz J, Perkins GD, Lefering R, Tjelmeland I, et al. Survival after out-of-hospital cardiac arrest in Europe – results of the EuReCa TWO study. Resuscitation. 2020;148:218–26.
65. Morrison LJ, Sandroni C, Grunau B, Parr M, Macneil F, Perkins GD, et al. Organ donation after out-of-hospital cardiac arrest: a scientific statement from the International Liaison Committee on Resuscitation. Circulation. 2023;148:e120–e46.
66. Lim WH, Dominguez-Gil B. Ethical issues related to donation and transplantation of donation after circulatory determination of death donors. Semin Nephrol. 2022;42:151269.
67. Kuisma M, Salo A, Puolakka J, Nurmi J, Kirves H, Väyrynen T, et al. Delayed return of spontaneous circulation (the Lazarus phenomenon) after cessation of out-of-hospital cardiopulmonary resuscitation. Resuscitation. 2017;118:107–11.
68. Zorko DJ, Shemie J, Hornby L, Singh G, Matheson S, Sandarage R, et al. Autoresuscitation after circulatory arrest: an updated systematic review. Can J Anaesth. 2023;70:699–712.
69. Campi R, Pecoraro A, Sessa F, Vignolini G, Caroti L, Lazzeri C, et al. Outcomes of kidney transplantation from uncontrolled donors after circulatory death vs. expanded-criteria or standard-criteria donors after brain death at an Italian Academic Center: a prospective observational study. Minerva Urol Nephrol. 2023;75:329–42.
70. Sandroni C, Scquizzato T, Cacciola S, Bonizzoni MA, West S, D'Arrigo S, et al. Does cardiopulmonary resuscitation before donor death affect solid organ transplant function? A systematic review and meta-analysis. Resuscitation. 2025;213:110654.

22 Cardiac Arrest in Children

Giovanna Chidini

The epidemiology, pathophysiology, and common causes of pediatric cardiac arrest differ from those in adults and neonates. In infants and children, cardiac arrest is generally not due to a primary cardiac problem, but rather represents the final stage of progressive respiratory deterioration or shock. In these patients, cardiac arrest is preceded by a period of worsening that leads to cardiopulmonary failure, bradycardia, and ultimately cardiac arrest. In children with congenital heart disease, cardiac arrest is often due to a primary cardiac cause, although the underlying causes differ from those in adults [1–4].

Outcomes for pediatric in-hospital cardiac arrest (IHCA) have improved over the past 20 years, in part due to early recognition, delivery of high-quality cardiopulmonary resuscitation (CPR), post-arrest care, and extracorporeal cardiopulmonary resuscitation (ECPR). In a recent analysis of the *Get With The Guidelines Resuscitation* registry, a large multicenter hospital-based cardiac arrest registry, survival to hospital discharge for pediatric cardiac arrest increased from 19% in 2000 to 38% in 2018. Survival improved by an average of 0.67% per year, although this increase plateaued after 2010. New directions in research and therapy may be needed to further improve cardiac arrest survival. Additionally, a greater number of cardiac arrests are now occurring in intensive care units (ICUs), suggesting that patients at risk of cardiac arrest are being identified earlier and transferred to a higher level of care.

Survival rates for pediatric out-of-hospital cardiac arrest (OHCA) remain less encouraging. In a recent analysis of the *Resuscitation Outcomes Consortium*

G. Chidini (✉)
Department of Emergency and Critical Care, Pediatric Intensive Care Unit – Fondazione IRCCS Cà Granda Ospedale Maggiore Policlinico, Milan, Italy
e-mail: Giovanna.chidini@policlinico.mi.it

D. Chiumello, A. De Gasperi (eds.), *Practical Trends in Anesthesia and Intensive Care 2026*, https://doi.org/10.1007/978-3-032-25721-5_22

Epidemiological Registry, a multicenter registry of out-of-hospital arrests, annual survival to hospital discharge between 2007 and 2012 ranged from 6.7% to 10.2%, depending on region and patient age. OHCA survival was higher in regions with more arrests witnessed by emergency medical services and higher rates of bystander CPR, underscoring the importance of early recognition and intervention [1–2].

In the same year, the incidence of pediatric in-hospital cardiac arrest (IHCA) was 12.66 events per 1000 pediatric and infant hospital admissions, with an overall survival to discharge rate of 41.1% [2–3]. Neurological outcomes remain difficult to assess across the entire pediatric population due to variability in reporting criteria and follow-up times among studies of OHCA and IHCA. However, it has been reported that up to 47% of survivors discharged from the hospital had a favorable neurological outcome. The International Liaison Committee on Resuscitation (ILCOR) Formula for Survival highlights three key components for achieving good resuscitation outcomes: guidelines based on robust scientific evidence, effective education for both laypersons and resuscitation professionals, and the implementation of a Chain of the well-coordinated Chain of Survival. In this review, we will refer to the AHA PALS guidelines for the management of pediatric patients in cardiac arrest. These guidelines provide recommendations for pediatric basic and advanced life support, excluding the neonatal period, and are based on the best available evidence in the field of resuscitation. The Chain of Survival, now expanded to include recovery from cardiac arrest, requires coordinated efforts among healthcare professionals from various disciplines and, in the case of OHCA, also among bystanders, emergency dispatchers, and first responders.

With increasing survival rates following pediatric cardiac arrest, greater attention has shifted toward the prevention of neurodevelopmental, physical, and emotional outcomes in survivors. Recent studies show that a quarter of patients with favorable outcomes exhibit global cognitive impairment, and that 85% of older children with favorable outcomes present with selective neuropsychological deficits.

The American Heart Association (AHA) Pediatric Advanced Life Support (PALS) guidelines are a key resource for lay rescuers and healthcare professionals. These guidelines provide a detailed framework for identifying and treating infants and children in all critical phases: pre-arrest, intra-arrest, and post-arrest. They are applicable in a variety of settings, including the community, prehospital environments, and hospital facilities, thus adapting to diverse and complex scenarios [4–5]. An integral part of the guidelines is Pediatric Basic Life Support Defibrillation (PBLSD), which details specific protocols for both single and two-rescuer scenarios, emphasizing the importance of coordination and efficiency during resuscitation maneuvers.

The aim of this review is to present the PALS-AHA guidelines, with a focus on the prevention of pediatric cardiac arrest, management during arrest, and the post-arrest phase. In addition, PBLSD protocols for one and two rescuers, as well as advanced PALS interventions, will be included to provide a comprehensive overview of the most up-to-date strategies for managing these critical emergencies in pediatric patients.

Regarding definitions, pediatric patients are defined as infants, children, and adolescents up to 18 years of age, excluding neonates. For basic life support (PBLSd), the guidelines apply as follows:

- The guidelines for infants apply to children under 1 year of age.
- The guidelines for children apply to those from about 1 year up to puberty. For educational purposes, puberty is defined as breast development in females and the appearance of axillary hair in males.
- For those showing signs of puberty or older, adult basic life support guidelines should be followed.

In collaboration with other societies, the American Heart Association (AHA) has provided interim guidance for basic and advanced life support in adults, children, and neonates with suspected or confirmed coronavirus disease 2019 (COVID-19). As evidence and guidelines are evolving alongside the COVID-19 situation, these interim recommendations are not included in the current guidelines.

The AHA working group reviewed all current and relevant American Heart Association (AHA) guidelines on Cardiopulmonary Resuscitation (CPR), along with the evidence and recommendations from the 2020 International Liaison Committee on Resuscitation (ILCOR) Consensus. The goal was to assess whether existing guidelines should be confirmed, revised, withdrawn, or if new recommendations were needed. The group then drafted, reviewed, and approved the recommendations, assigning each a Class of Recommendation (i.e., the strength of the recommendation) and a Level of Evidence (i.e., the quality and certainty of the evidence). The criteria for each COR and LOE are shown in Table 22.1 [6–7].

Traditionally, the management of cardiac arrest has focused primarily on treating the event itself, emphasizing the importance of high-quality cardiopulmonary resuscitation (CPR), early defibrillation, and effective teamwork. However, both pre-arrest and post-arrest interventions are also crucial for improving outcomes. With pediatric cardiac arrest survival rates having plateaued, prevention of cardiac arrest has become even more significant. In the out-of-hospital setting, prevention includes safety initiatives such as bicycle helmet laws, prevention of sudden infant death syndrome, training lay rescuers in CPR, and rapid access to emergency care. When cardiac arrest occurs, prompt resuscitation by bystanders is critical to improving outcomes. In the hospital setting, prevention of cardiac arrest relies on early recognition and treatment of at-risk patients, such as neonates undergoing cardiac surgery, patients with acute fulminant myocarditis, decompensated acute heart failure, or pulmonary hypertension.

Table 22.1 Classes of recommendation and levels of evidence

Classes of recommendation (strength of recommendation)
Class 1 (STRONG)—Benefit >>> risk
Class 2a (MODERATE)—Benefit >> risk
Class 2b (WEAK)—Benefit ≥ risk
Class 3 (NO BENEFIT)—Benefit = risk
Class 3 (HARM)—Risk > benefit
Levels of evidence (quality of evidence)
Level A: High-quality evidence from more than one RCT; high-quality meta-analyses of RCTs; one or more RCTs corroborated by high-quality studies
Level B-R (randomized): Moderate-quality evidence from one or more RCTs and/or meta-analyses of moderate-quality RCTs
Level B-NR (non-randomized): Moderate-quality evidence from one or more well-conducted non-randomized studies, observational studies, or studies of registry and/or meta-analysis of such studies
Level C-LD (limited data): Observational or registry studies, randomized/non-randomized, with design or execution limitations; meta-analyses of such studies
Level C-EO (expert opinion): Expert consensus based on clinical experience

After resuscitation, management of the post-arrest syndrome—which may include cerebral dysfunction, myocardial dysfunction with low cardiac output, and ischemia-reperfusion injury—is essential to prevent further damage, such as hypotension. Accurate neurological prognostication is vital to guide family discussions and decision-making. Finally, given the high risk of neurodevelopmental impairment in survivors of cardiac arrest, timely referral to rehabilitation programs for early assessment and intervention is important [8–10].

To highlight the various aspects of cardiac arrest management, the Pediatric Chain of Survival has been updated, as outlined in the 2020 AHA guidelines [6], and a separate version has been created for out-of-hospital cardiac arrest (OHCA), thus distinguishing it from in-hospital cardiac arrest (IHCA). In both chains, a sixth link has been added to emphasize the importance of recovery, focusing on the evaluation of short- and long-term treatments, as well as support for survivors and their families. In both versions of the chain of survival, activation of the emergency response is immediately followed by the initiation of high-quality CPR (cardiopulmonary resuscitation). If help is nearby or a mobile phone is available, emergency response activation and CPR initiation can occur almost simultaneously. However, in out-of-hospital settings, a lone rescuer without access to a mobile phone should begin CPR (compressions, airway, breathing) immediately on infants and children before calling for help, as respiratory arrest is often the primary cause of cardiac arrest and help may not be immediately available. In the case of a sudden, witnessed collapse, the rescuer should use an automated external defibrillator (AED) if available, as early defibrillation can be lifesaving even in pediatric cardiac arrest.

In the context of PALS (Pediatric Advanced Life Support), the concept of a "high-performance team" is crucial to ensure effective management of pediatric emergencies, especially during cardiac or respiratory arrest events. A high-performance team in PALS is characterized by its ability to work in a coordinated, efficient, and highly skilled manner, thereby improving the chances of survival for pediatric patients [11].

Below are some key aspects related to high-performance teams in PALS:

In PALS, each team member has a specific assigned role and must perform their task with precision.

Common roles include:

- Team leader: Directs activities, coordinates team members, assigns roles, and ensures everyone works together in synergy. The leader must make rapid, informed decisions based on the patient's condition and clinical responses, and coordinate consultations.
- CPR providers: These members perform chest compressions and ensure proper rate and depth, making sure there are no unnecessary interruptions between compressions.
- Airway manager: Responsible for maintaining airway patency (e.g., inserting ventilation devices) and ensuring adequate oxygenation.
- Medication administrator: Responsible for preparing and administering necessary medications, following the leader's instructions.
- Timer: Monitors the execution of CPR, tracks time intervals, and advises colleagues on the timing of adrenaline administration, defibrillation, and reassessment.
- CPR Coordinator: A role distinct from the team leader, responsible for verifying the correctness of ongoing procedures and politely correcting colleagues to optimize performance.

Communication within a high-performance team is clear and employs the "closed-loop communication" method, meaning that when a command is given, the recipient confirms receipt and executes it immediately. For example:

Leader: "Administer 0.01 mg/kg of epinephrine."
Team member: "Administering 0.01 mg/kg of epinephrine now."

This form of clear, circular communication helps prevent errors and ensures that all steps are followed accurately.

The quality of life support techniques is critical. In PALS, a high-performance team ensures that:

- Chest compressions are performed at a rate of 100–120 compressions per minute and to an appropriate depth.
- Interruptions in compressions are minimized to maintain a chest compression fraction (CCF) ideally above 80%, as also mentioned in the provided text.
- Airways are kept patent, and ventilation is adequate, with a rate of 1 breath every 6 s in intubated patients.

Team members must work in a coordinated manner, avoiding interference with each other and ensuring that every action is performed in a timely fashion. The leader is responsible for:

- Monitoring team performance and well-being.
- Reallocating resources as needed, for example, rotating personnel performing compressions when fatigue sets in.
- Verifying correct drug administration, monitoring vital signs, and ensuring adherence to PALS guidelines.

After an intervention, it is essential for the team to gather for a debriefing session. This allows the team to:

- Assess what went well and what could be improved.
- Receive constructive feedback to enhance future performance.
- Analyze collected data, such as the duration of uninterrupted compressions or the effectiveness of ventilation, using measurement and quality control tools (CQI—Continuous Quality Improvement).

The ability to remain calm and make rapid decisions in a highly stressful environment is a key quality for a high-performance team. Stress management techniques and regular simulation exercises help teams prepare both mentally and technically to handle critical situations.

A high-performance PALS team makes optimal use of technology. For example:

- Continuous monitoring of oxygen saturation and CO_2.
- Use of defibrillators with feedback on the quality of chest compressions.
- Advanced support devices, such as ventilators and multiparameter monitors, to ensure that actions are based on real-time data.

In PALS, a high-performance team does not limit itself to performing resuscitation maneuvers. Instead, it focuses on effective leadership, clear communication, optimal resuscitation techniques, resource management, and a holistic approach to continuous performance improvement. The ability to work synergistically and adapt quickly to the patient's condition is essential to achieve better outcomes and increase the survival chances of pediatric patients [12–13]. The team role configuration is consistent with the descriptions by Weiss et al. (2018) [3] and Berg et al. (2020) [4].

In the context of PALS, pediatric cardiac arrest is a condition that requires rapid, efficient, and coordinated intervention. Advanced resuscitation techniques, combined with optimal airway management, high-quality chest compressions, appropriate medications, and defibrillation when indicated, form the foundation for effective management. Prevention, early recognition, and high-performance teamwork are crucial to improving outcomes in children experiencing cardiac arrest.

One of the key aspects of PALS is the concept of preventing pediatric cardiac arrest through timely assessment and treatment of potentially life-threatening conditions before full arrest occurs.

This includes:

- Continuous monitoring of the child's vital signs (respiratory rate, oxygen saturation, heart rate, blood pressure) to identify signs of deterioration.
- Recognition of worsening respiratory or circulatory status, with the goal of intervening before cardiac arrest develops.
- Timely management of clinical deterioration, with the administration of fluids, oxygen, assisted ventilation, or appropriate medications.

The ranges of vital parameters considered physiological during childhood are reported in Table 22.2.

Cardiac arrest in children differs significantly from adults in both epidemiology and pathophysiology.

In children, primary cardiac arrest is rare; most arrests develop as a result of hypoxia or respiratory failure.

The most common causes include:

- Respiratory failure: May result from conditions such as severe asthma, pneumonia, aspiration syndrome, choking, or inhalation injuries.
- Shock: Septic, hemorrhagic, or cardiogenic shock can progress to circulatory failure and, ultimately, cardiac arrest.
- Congenital anomalies: Undiagnosed cardiac malformations or congenital defects.
- Trauma: Severe traumatic injuries, such as those resulting from accidents, can cause cardiac arrest.
- Choking or drowning: These events often lead to secondary arrests due to respiratory failure.

The AHA PALS guidelines propose a systematic approach to the critically ill pediatric patient based on the following key elements:

Table 22.2 Vital parameters in childhood

Heart rate (beats per minute)		
Age	Awake	Asleep
Newborn	100–205	90–160
Infant	100–180	90–160
Toddler	98–140	80–120
Preschool child	80–120	65–100
School-age child	75–118	58–90
Adolescent	60–100	50–90

Respiratory rate (breaths per minute)	
Age	Breaths
Infant	30–53
Toddler	22–37
Preschool child	20–28
School–age child	18–25
Adolescent	12–20

Blood pressure (mmHg)			
Age	Systolic pressure	Diastolic pressure	MAP (mean arterial pressure)
Birth (12 h, <1000 g)	39–59	16–36	45–60
Birth (12 h, 3 kg)	60–76	31–45	48–57
Newborn (96 h)	67–84	35–53	45–60
Infant	72–104	37–56	50–62
Toddler	86–106	42–63	49–62
Preschool child	89–112	46–72	58–69
School-age child	97–115	57–76	66–72
Adolescent	110–131	64–83	73–84

- Primary assessment (ABCDE).
- High-quality CPR.
- Early defibrillation.
- Pharmacotherapy.
- Post-ROSC care.

Primary Assessment ABCDE: The basic approach consists of assessing the airway (A), breathing (B), circulation (C), neurological status (D), and exposure (E), including temperature and blood glucose). This is a structured approach that helps identify and treat the underlying causes of arrest or conditions that may lead to arrest.

- A—Airway management: Ensure airway patency and, if necessary, proceed with intubation or the use of advanced airway devices.
- B—Ventilation: Hypoxia is a common cause of arrest in children. Adequate ventilation and oxygen administration are immediate priorities. Ventilations: In pediatric arrest, ventilations are essential, with a compression-to-ventilation ratio

of 30:2 during single-rescuer CPR; 15:2 for two-rescuer CPR, and delivering 20–30 breaths per minute during PALS with a protected airway in the intubated child.
- C—High-quality CPR: Pediatric cardiopulmonary resuscitation should be initiated immediately, with chest compressions at least one third the depth of the chest and at a rate of 100–120 compressions per minute. CPR effectiveness can be improved by minimizing interruptions between compressions and ensuring full chest recoil after each compression. Defibrillation: In children, cardiac arrest due to arrhythmias such as ventricular fibrillation (VF) or pulseless ventricular tachycardia (pVT) is less common than in adults, but can occur in some cases. Immediate defibrillation, when indicated, should be performed with a defibrillator that accounts for the child's weight and age, using an appropriately adjusted energy dose (e.g., 2–4 J/kg).
- Vascular/intraosseous access.
- D—Pharmacotherapy.
- E—Post-ROSC stabilization: After pulse and breathing have been restored, it is crucial to closely monitor the child to prevent further episodes of arrest. This includes management of hypoxia, hypothermia, blood glucose, and acidosis.

Rapid recognition of cardiac arrest, immediate initiation of effective chest compressions, and appropriate ventilation are essential to improve survival chances. Lay rescuers should not delay the initiation of CPR if a child shows no "signs of life." Healthcare providers may assess the pulse, provided this does not delay the initiation of CPR by more than 10 s. However, pulse palpation is not always reliable for determining cardiac arrest and the need for chest compressions. In infants and children, cardiac arrest due to respiratory failure is more common than primary cardiac events; therefore, ensuring effective ventilation during resuscitation is essential. Once CPR is initiated, the correct sequence to follow is compressions, airway, and breathing (CAB).

High-quality CPR generates blood flow to vital organs and increases the likelihood of return of spontaneous circulation (ROSC). The five main components of effective CPR are:

- Adequate depth of chest compressions.
- Optimal compression rate.
- Minimizing interruptions during CPR (i.e., maximizing chest compression fraction, the actual time compressions are performed during cardiac arrest).
- Allowing complete chest recoil between compressions.
- Avoiding excessive ventilation.

During pediatric resuscitation, inadequate compression depth and rate, incomplete chest recoil, and excessive ventilation frequency are common. [4, 14–15].

Table 22.3 presents the recommendations for performing high-quality CPR, with corresponding references [7–16].

Table 22.3 Recommendations for delivering components of high-quality CPR

Class of recommendation (COR)	Level of evidence (LOE)	Recommendations
1 B-NR	1 B-NR	1. CPR with chest compressions and rescue breaths should be performed on infants and children in cardiac arrest
1 B-NR	1 B-NR	2. For infants and children, if rescuers are unable or unwilling to provide rescue breaths, chest compressions alone are recommended
1 C-EO	1 C-EO	3. After each compression, rescuers should allow full chest recoil
2a C-LD	2a C-LD	4. It is reasonable to maintain a chest compression rate of about 100–120 per minute for infants and children
2a C-LD	2a C-LD	5. For infants and children, it is reasonable for rescuers to perform chest compressions to a depth of at least one-third of the anterior-posterior diameter of the chest, which is approximately 4 cm in infants and 5 cm in children. When children reach puberty, it is reasonable to use the adult compression depth, that is, at least 5 cm but not more than 6 cm
2a C-EO	2a C-EO	6. For healthcare providers, it is reasonable to perform a rhythm check, lasting no more than 10 s, approximately every 2 min
2a C-EO	2a C-EO	7. It is reasonable to ventilate with 100% oxygen during CPR
2a C-EO	2a C-EO	8. When performing CPR without an advanced airway, it is reasonable for a single rescuer to use a compression-to-ventilation ratio of 30:2 and for two rescuers to use a ratio of 15:2
2b C-LD	2b C-LD	9. When performing CPR on infants and children with an advanced airway, it may be reasonable to maintain a respiratory rate of 1 breath every 2–3 s (20–30 breaths per minute), taking into account age and clinical condition. Higher rates than these recommendations may compromise hemodynamics

Table 22.4 presents the PALS recommendations for high-quality early defibrillation.

Early defibrillation is an essential component in the management of pediatric cardiac arrest, especially in cases of ventricular fibrillation (VF) or pulseless ventricular tachycardia (pVT) [17–21]. The PALS guidelines emphasize the importance of a prompt response to significantly improve the chances of survival. Defibrillation works by interrupting potentially fatal arrhythmias, allowing the heart to restore a normal rhythm. The process involves the use of a defibrillator (manual or automated) to deliver an electric shock. According to updated recommendations, it is reasonable to start with an energy dose between 2 and 4 J/kg. If ventricular fibrillation persists despite the first defibrillation attempt, an increase to 4 J/kg is recommended for subsequent attempts. In particularly challenging situations, higher

Table 22.4 Defibrillation energy

COR	LOE	Recommendations
2a	C-LD	It is reasonable to use an initial dose of 2–4 J/kg of monophasic or biphasic energy for defibrillation, but for educational simplicity, an initial dose of 2 J/kg may be considered
2b	C-LD	For refractory ventricular fibrillation (VF), it may be reasonable to increase the defibrillation dose to 4 J/kg
2b	C-LD	For subsequent energy levels, a dose of 4 J/kg may be reasonable, and higher energy levels may be considered, but should not exceed 10 J/kg or the maximum adult dose

Table 22.5 Coordination between early defibrillation and the PALS sequence

COR	LOE	Recommendations
1	C-EO	Perform CPR until the device is ready to deliver a shock
1	C-EO	Deliver a single shock immediately followed by chest compressions for children with VF/pVT
1	C-EO	Minimize interruptions in chest compressions

energy levels may be considered, up to a maximum of 10 J/kg or the maximum adult dose, to avoid myocardial injury. Timeliness of intervention is crucial. The guidelines highlight that defibrillation should be performed as quickly as possible, ideally within a few minutes of arrest onset. Delays in treatment can significantly reduce the likelihood of a positive outcome. In addition to defibrillation, advanced life support includes high-quality chest compressions, airway management, and administration of appropriate medications. However, early defibrillation remains the treatment of choice for shockable arrhythmias. Finally, healthcare provider training and access to defibrillation devices are fundamental to ensuring effective treatment. The PALS guidelines promote the widespread availability of automated external defibrillators (AEDs) in public places, thereby increasing the likelihood of early intervention even outside the hospital setting [22–27].

Table 22.5 provides guidance on how to integrate early defibrillation into the PALS sequence.

- Perform CPR until the device is ready to deliver a shock.

It is recommended to continue chest compressions until the defibrillator is fully ready to deliver the shock.

- Deliver a single shock followed immediately by chest compressions:

For children with ventricular fibrillation (VF) or pulseless ventricular tachycardia (pVT), it is recommended to deliver a single shock and immediately resume chest compressions without checking the rhythm.

- Minimize interruptions in chest compressions:

It is essential to minimize pauses in compressions to ensure effective blood flow and improve the chances of survival.

Use of an Automated External Defibrillator (AED) with Pediatric Attenuator (COR 1, LOE C-LD):

When using an AED on infants and children under 8 years of age, the use of a pediatric attenuator is recommended.

Manual defibrillator (COR 1, LOE C-EO):

For infants under the care of a skilled healthcare provider, the use of a manual defibrillator is recommended when a shockable rhythm is identified.

Use of an AED without a pediatric attenuator (COR 2b, LOE C-EO):

If neither a manual defibrillator nor an AED with a pediatric attenuator is available, it is reasonable to use an AED without an attenuator [25–27].

BLS-D (Basic Life Support and Defibrillation) comprises a series of essential first aid interventions for anyone faced with managing cardiac arrest. This protocol, simple yet effective, enables rescuers to act quickly to increase the victim's chances of survival. The following are the main steps a rescuer should follow.

1. Ensure Safety

The first step for a rescuer is to ensure that the environment is safe, both for themselves and for the victim and anyone else present. It is important to check for hazards such as exposed electrical wires, traffic, or other threats that could endanger the rescuer or hinder the intervention.

2. Assess the Victim's Condition

Approach the victim and quickly assess the situation. Call out loudly to check for responsiveness, gently shaking the person to elicit a reaction. If the victim does not respond, check for breathing. Look for chest movement, listen for breath sounds, and feel for airflow near the nose and mouth. If the victim is not breathing or is gasping, consider the situation critical and proceed to action.

3. Activate Emergency Response

If the victim is unresponsive and not breathing normally, immediately call 112 (or the local emergency number). If you are alone, make the call before starting resuscitation maneuvers. If others are present, delegate someone to call for help and retrieve an automated external defibrillator (AED) while you begin resuscitation.

4. Start Cardiopulmonary Resuscitation (CPR)

Begin with chest compressions. Place the heel of one hand in the center of the victim's chest, on the sternum, and place your other hand on top. Keep your arms straight, and perform compressions forcefully, pressing down at least 5 cm (but not more than 6 cm) at a rate of 100–120 compressions per minute. After each compression, allow the chest to fully recoil.

If you are trained, alternate 30 compressions with 2 rescue breaths. For ventilation, tilt the victim's head back, pinch the nose, and blow into the mouth, ensuring a visible chest rise. If you are not trained or do not feel confident, continue with compressions only.

5. Use the Automated External Defibrillator (AED)

As soon as the AED is available, turn it on and follow the voice prompts. Place the pads on the victim's chest: one below the right clavicle and the other below the left armpit. The device will automatically analyze the victim's heart rhythm and indicate if a shock is needed. If so, ensure no one is touching the victim and press the button to deliver the shock. Immediately resume CPR without delay.

If the AED does not advise a shock, continue with compressions and ventilations. The device will periodically analyze the rhythm and guide you.

6. Continue until Help Arrives

Continue the cycle of compressions and ventilations until:

- Advanced rescuers arrive and take over the situation.
- The victim resumes normal breathing.
- You are too exhausted to continue.

For the detailed operational flow related to the PALS-AHA flow charts for single- and two-rescuer BLS-D, refer to the AHA PALS 2020 recommendations [6] and AHA educational materials (Hazinski et al., 2020).

In summary, the key steps can be outlined as follows:

1. Scene safety assessment.
2. Assessment of breathing and pulse:
   - If no pulse is detected within 10 s and there is no normal breathing or only gasping, start CPR immediately.
   - If a pulse is present but breathing is absent, provide rescue breaths.
3. CPR or rescue breaths:
   - If the heart rate (HR) is less than 60 beats per minute with signs of poor perfusion, start CPR.
   - If breathing is normal and a pulse is present, monitor until emergency personnel arrive.
4. If the arrest is witnessed, immediately activate the emergency response system and begin CPR.
5. Performing CPR: If you are a single rescuer, perform cycles of 30 compressions and 2 ventilations. If a second rescuer arrives, switch to cycles of 15 compressions and 2 ventilations.
6. Rhythm assessment: After 2 min, check the rhythm using an automated external defibrillator (AED) if available.
7. If the rhythm is shockable, deliver a shock with the AED and continue CPR.
8. If the rhythm is non-shockable, continue CPR until advanced help arrives or until the child begins to move.

The pediatric cardiac arrest algorithm is an essential tool to guide rescuers in managing cardiac arrest in children. Based on the updated guidelines of the American Heart Association (AHA), this tool is designed to optimize survival chances through a systematic and well-defined approach. It focuses on three main aspects: initiation of CPR, identification of cardiac rhythm, prompt execution of cardiopulmonary resuscitation (CPR), and the appropriate use of medications and defibrillation [28–31].

Management begins immediately with *high-quality CPR*, which is essential to ensure effective blood flow to vital organs. Chest compressions should be:

- Deep, reaching one-third of the chest diameter.
- Fast, at a rate of 100–120 compressions per minute.
- Interrupted as little as possible to preserve perfusion.

At the same time, provide bag-mask ventilation with oxygen and connect the monitor or defibrillator to analyze the cardiac rhythm.

After starting CPR, assess the rhythm to determine its nature:

- *Shockable Rhythm*: Ventricular fibrillation (VF) or pulseless ventricular tachycardia (pVT).
- *Non-shockable Rhythm*: Asystole or pulseless electrical activity (PEA).

The choice of therapeutic pathway depends on the type of rhythm identified.

1. Shockable Rhythm Pathway (VF/pVT)
   If the rhythm is shockable:
   (a) Deliver an electrical shock to interrupt the arrhythmia:
      - The first shock should be 2 J/kg.
      - The second shock should be 4 J/kg.
      - Subsequent shocks may be increased up to 10 J/kg, but should not exceed the maximum adult dose.

   (b) Perform CPR for 2 min immediately after the shock, without delay. During CPR:
      - Ensure intravenous (IV) or intraosseous (IO) access.
      - Administer epinephrine every 3–5 min.
      - Consider advanced airway management, such as intubation, with capnography monitoring.

   (c) If the rhythm persists, use medications such as amiodarone (5 mg/kg) or lidocaine (1 mg/kg) to treat persistent ventricular fibrillation.
2. Non-Shockable Rhythm Pathway (Asystole/PEA)
   If the rhythm is non-shockable:
   (a) Administer epinephrine as soon as possible (0.01 mg/kg IV/IO) and repeat every 3–5 min.
   (b) Continue CPR for 2 min, ensuring high-quality chest compressions.
   (c) Periodically assess the rhythm to detect any changes:
      - If it becomes shockable, switch to the appropriate pathway.
      - If it remains non-shockable, address reversible causes.

A crucial part of the protocol is to identify and correct reversible causes of cardiac arrest. These include:

- Hypoxia (lack of oxygen).
- Hypovolemia (loss of blood volume).
- Metabolic acidosis (accumulation of acids in the body).
- Hypothermia, cardiac tamponade, toxins, and thrombosis.

The quality of CPR is critical. Well-performed compressions with minimal interruptions can make a significant difference. It is important to switch rescuers every 2 min to prevent fatigue and ensure effectiveness.

Post-ROSC (Return of Spontaneous Circulation) management focuses not only on hemodynamic and respiratory stabilization but also on neuroprotection, as brain injury is one of the main complications after cardiac arrest. Neuroprotection protocols are designed to reduce ischemic injury and improve long-term neurological outcomes. The main neuroprotective interventions included in post-ROSC protocols are listed below.

1. Targeted Temperature Management (TTM)
   Temperature control is the cornerstone of post-arrest neuroprotection.
   - Goal: Reduce cerebral metabolism, limit reperfusion injury, and decrease neuronal inflammation.
   - Guidelines:
     - Maintain core body temperature between 32 and 36 °C for at least 24 h.
     - Avoid fever (temperature >37.5 °C), which is associated with worse neurological outcomes.
   - Application:
     - Use external cooling systems (e.g., cooling blankets) or endovascular devices.
     - Monitor core temperature with esophageal, bladder, or arterial probes.
2. Continuous Neurological Monitoring
   - Electroencephalogram (EEG):
     - Used to detect subclinical seizures, which are common after cardiac arrest.
     - Seizures should be treated immediately with antiepileptic drugs such as benzodiazepines, levetiracetam, or fosphenytoin.
   - Intracranial Pressure (ICP) Monitoring:
     - Indicated in patients with signs of cerebral edema.
     - Maintain intracranial pressure under control with mannitol, hypertonic saline, or deep sedation.
   - Capnography and Cerebral Oxygenation:
     - Monitor central venous oxygen saturation ($ScvO_2$) to avoid hypoxia or hyperoxia, both of which are associated with worsening neurological injury.
3. Oxygenation and Ventilation Management
   Oxygenation and ventilation must be carefully regulated to reduce ischemic and reperfusion injury:
   - Oxygenation:
     - Maintain oxygen saturation (SpO_2) between 94% and 98%.
     - Avoid prolonged hyperoxia (>100 mmHg PaO_2), which can cause oxidative stress.
   - Ventilation:
     - Maintain normal $PaCO_2$ (35–45 mmHg), avoiding hypocapnia (cerebral vasoconstriction), or hypercapnia (increased ICP).
     - Use capnography to monitor the effectiveness of ventilation.

4. Optimal Hemodynamic Management
   Stabilizing cerebral perfusion is crucial to prevent further injury:
   - Mean Arterial Pressure (MAP):
     – Target: Maintain MAP between 65 and 75 mmHg (adults) or above the fifth percentile for age (pediatric patients).
   - Fluid Therapy:
     – Use isotonic solutions (e.g., lactated Ringer's or normal saline).
     – Avoid fluid overload, which can worsen cerebral edema.
   - Inotropes/Vasopressors:
     – Use agents such as norepinephrine, epinephrine, or dopamine to maintain adequate perfusion.
5. Seizure Control
   - Post-arrest seizures, both clinical and subclinical, are common and associated with worse neurological outcomes.
   - Treatment:
     – First-line anticonvulsants: benzodiazepines (e.g., lorazepam).
     – Long-term treatment: levetiracetam or fosphenytoin.
   - Monitor EEG for at least 24–48 h in comatose patients.
6. Correction of Electrolytes and Glucose
   - Electrolytes:
     – Maintain sodium, potassium, calcium, and magnesium within normal limits to prevent arrhythmias.
   - Glucose:
     – Avoid hypoglycemia (<70 mg/dL), as well as prolonged hyperglycemia (>180 mg/dL), which is associated with worse neurological outcomes.
     – Target blood glucose: 140–180 mg/dL.
7. Sedation and Fever Control
   - Use sedatives such as midazolam or propofol to keep the comatose patient stable.
   - Prevent fever through the use of antipyretics (e.g., paracetamol) and physical cooling.

Post-ROSC neuroprotection protocols are complex but essential to improve neurological outcomes and quality of life for patients. They require a multidisciplinary approach that includes temperature management, oxygenation control, hemodynamic stabilization, and neurological monitoring. Each intervention must be tailored to the patient's condition, with the goal of optimizing both neurological and systemic prognosis (Table 22.6).

Table 22.6 Elements of post-ROSC management

Component	Description
Oxygenation and ventilation	Measure oxygenation and achieve normal oxygen levels (94–99%) or an appropriate saturation for the pediatric patient
	Adjust $PaCO_2$ to avoid severe hypercapnia or hypocapnia
Hemodynamic monitoring	Define hemodynamic targets and review them regularly
	Monitor cardiac telemetry
	Monitor blood pressure, serum lactate, urine output, and central venous oxygen saturation
	Use fluids, inotropes, or vasopressors to maintain adequate systolic blood pressure
Targeted temperature management (TTM)	Continuously monitor core temperature
	Prevent and treat fever during therapy
	Apply moderate TTM (32–34 °C) followed by normothermia (36–37.5 °C) or normothermia as the sole intervention
	Prevent shivering and treat hypotension during rewarming
Neuromonitoring	Perform continuous EEG monitoring, if indicated
	Treat seizures and consider prompt imaging for treatable causes
Electrolytes and glucose	Measure glucose to prevent hypoglycemia. Maintain electrolytes within normal limits
Sedation	Treat with sedatives or anxiolytics, if necessary
Prognosis	Assess prognosis by considering clinical factors, EEG, and imaging within the first 7 days

Cardiopulmonary resuscitation (CPR), according to Pediatric Advanced Life Support (PALS) guidelines, is not limited to the treatment of pediatric cardiac arrest, but emphasizes the importance of prevention through early identification of signs of clinical deterioration. Timely and appropriate interventions can often prevent a critical condition from progressing to cardiac arrest. Moreover, the success of resuscitation efforts depends not only on the advanced training of healthcare professionals but also on the education of laypersons, who are often the first to respond in an emergency. Promoting specific first aid courses for parents, teachers, and community members is crucial to reducing delays in intervention. Similarly, encouraging healthcare colleagues to participate in advanced simulation courses helps improve technical skills, communication, and teamwork in critical situations. Simulation, by recreating realistic scenarios, facilitates the acquisition of practical skills and the consolidation of standardized protocols, contributing to saving lives. Prevention and education therefore remain the cornerstones for improving outcomes in pediatric patients and ensuring rapid and effective interventions are effective in every situation.

References

1. Niles DE, Duval-Arnould J, Skellett S, Knight L, Su F, Raymond TT, Sweberg T, Sen AI, Atkins DL, Friess SH, de Caen AR, Kurosawa H, Sutton RM, Wolfe H, Berg RA, Silver A, Hunt EA, Nadkarni VM, pediatric Resuscitation Quality (pediRES-Q) Collaborative Investigators. Characterization of pediatric in-hospital cardiopulmonary resuscitation quality metrics across an international resuscitation collaborative. Pediatr Crit Care Med. 2018;19:421–32. https://doi.org/10.1097/PCC.0000000000001520.
2. Sutton RM, Niles D, Nysaether J, Abella BS, Arbogast KB, Nishisaki A, Maltese MR, Donoghue A, Bishnoi R, Helfaer MA, Myklebust H, Nadkarni V. Quantitative analysis of CPR quality during in-hospital resuscitation of older children and adolescents. Pediatrics. 2009;124:494–9. https://doi.org/10.1542/peds.2008-1930.
3. McInnes AD, Sutton RM, Orioles A, Nishisaki A, Niles D, Abella BS, Maltese MR, Berg RA, Nadkarni V. The first quantitative report of ventilation rate during in-hospital resuscitation of older children and adolescents. Resuscitation. 2011;82:1025–9. https://doi.org/10.1016/j.resuscitation.2011.03.020.
4. Sutton RM, Reeder RW, Landis WP, Meert KL, Yates AR, Morgan RW, Berger JT, Newth CJ, Carcillo JA, McQuillen PS, Harrison RE, Moler FW, Pollack MM, Carpenter TC, Notterman DA, Holubkov R, Dean JM, Nadkarni VM, Berg RA, Eunice Kennedy Shriver National Institute of Child Health and Human Development Collaborative Pediatric Critical Care Research Network (CPCCRN). Ventilation rates and pediatric in-hospital cardiac arrest survival outcomes. Crit Care Med. 2019;47:1627–36. https://doi.org/10.1097/CCM.0000000000003898.
5. Bahr J, Klingler H, Panzer W, Rode H, Kettler D. Skills of lay people in checking the carotid pulse. Resuscitation. 1997;35:23–6. https://doi.org/10.1016/s0300-9572(96)01092-1.
6. Magid DJ, Aziz K, Cheng A, Hazinski MF, Hoover AV, Mahgoub M, Panchal AR, Sasson C, Topjian AA, Rodriguez AJ, et al. Part 2: evidence evaluation and guidelines development: 2020 American Heart Association guidelines for cardiopulmonary resuscitation and emergency cardiovascular care. Circulation. 2020;142(suppl 2):S358–65. https://doi.org/10.1161/CIR.0000000000000898.
7. Levine GN, O'Gara PT, Beckman JA, Al-Khatib SM, Birtcher KK, Cigarroa JE, de Las FL, Deswal A, Fleisher LA, Gentile F, Goldberger ZD, Hlatky MA, Joglar JA, Piano MR, Wijeysundera DN. Recent innovations, modifications, and evolution of ACC/AHA clinical practice guidelines: an update for our constituencies: a report of the American College of Cardiology/American Heart Association Task Force on clinical practice guidelines. Circulation. 2019;139:e879–86. https://doi.org/10.1161/CIR.0000000000000651.
8. Dean JM, Moler FW. Neuropsychological outcomes of children 1 year after pediatric cardiac arrest: secondary analysis of 2 randomized clinical trials. JAMA Neurol. 2018;75:1502–10. https://doi.org/10.1001/jamaneurol.2018.2628.
9. Topjian AA, de Caen A, Wainwright MS, Abella BS, Abend NS, Atkins DL, Bembea MM, Fink EL, Guerguerian AM, Haskell SE, Kilgannon JH, Lasa JJ, Hazinski MF. Pediatric post-cardiac arrest care: a scientific statement from the American Heart Association. Circulation. 2019;140:e194–233. https://doi.org/10.1161/CIR.0000000000000697.
10. Laverriere EK, Polansky M, French B, Nadkarni VM, Berg RA, Topjian AA. Association of duration of hypotension with survival after pediatric cardiac arrest. Pediatr Crit Care Med. 2020;21:143–9. https://doi.org/10.1097/PCC.0000000000002119.
11. Rowland P, Lising D, Sinclair L, Baker GR. Team dynamics within quality improvement teams: a scoping review. Int J Qual Health Care. 2018;30(6):416–22. https://doi.org/10.1093/intqhc/mzy045.

12. Weiss SL, et al. The role of team dynamics in pediatric advanced life support: a systematic review. Pediatr Critic Care Med. 2018;19(2):117–23. https://doi.org/10.1097/PCC.0000000000001409.
13. Berg MD, Nadkarni VM, Berg RA. Cardiopulmonary resuscitation in children: teamwork and high-performance teams. Pediatr Clin N Am. 2020;64(5):1127–40.
14. Sutton RM, Niles D, Nysaether J, Abella BS, Arbogast KB, Nishisaki A, et al. Quantitative analysis of CPR quality during in-hospital resuscitation of older children and adolescents. Pediatrics. 2009;124:494–9.
15. McInnes AD, Sutton RM, Orioles A, Nishisaki A, Niles D, et al. The first quantitative report of ventilation rate during in-hospital resuscitation of older children and adolescents. Resuscitation. 2011;82:1025–9. https://doi.org/10.1016/j16-.
16. Kitamura T, Iwami T, Kawamura T, Nagao K, Tanaka H, Nadkarni VM, Berg RA, Hiraide A, Implementation Working Group for All-Japan Utstein Registry of the Fire and Disaster Management Agency. Conventional and chest-compression-only cardiopulmonary resuscitation by bystanders for children who have out-of-hospital cardiac arrests: a prospective, nationwide, population-based cohort study. Lancet. 2010;375:1347–54. https://doi.org/10.1016/S0140-6736(10)60064-5.
17. Mercier E, Laroche E, Beck B, Le Sage N, Cameron PA, Émond M, Berthelot S, Mitra B, Ouellet-Pelletier J. Defibrillation energy dose during pediatric cardiac arrest: systematic review of human and animal model studies. Resuscitation. 2019;139:241–52. https://doi.org/10.1016/j.resuscitation.2019.04.028.
18. Gutgesell HP, Tacker WA, Geddes LA, Davis S, Lie JT, McNamara DG. Energy dose for ventricular defibrillation of children. Pediatrics. 1976;58:898–901.
19. Berg MD, Samson RA, Meyer RJ, Clark LL, Valenzuela TD, Berg RA. Pediatric defibrillation doses often fail to terminate prolonged out-of-hospital ventricular fibrillation in children. Resuscitation. 2005;67:63–7. https://doi.org/10.1016/j.resuscitation.2005.04.018.
20. Meaney PA, Nadkarni VM, Atkins DL, Berg MD, Samson RA, Hazinski MF, Berg RA. American Heart Association National Registry of Cardiopulmonary Resuscitation Investigators. Effect of defibrillation energy dose during in-hospital pediatric cardiac arrest. Pediatrics. 2011;127:e16–23. https://doi.org/10.1542/peds.2010-1617.
21. Samson RA, Nadkarni VM, Meaney PA, Carey SM, Berg MD, Berg RA. American Heart Association National Registry of CPR Investigators. Outcomes of in-hospital ventricular fibrillation in children. N Engl J Med. 2006;354:2328–39. https://doi.org/10.1056/NEJMoa052917.
22. Cecchin F, Jorgenson DB, Berul CI, Perry JC, Zimmerman AA, Duncan BW, Lupinetti FM, Snyder D, Lyster TD, Rosenthal GL, Cross B, Atkins DL. Is arrhythmia detection by automatic external defibrillator accurate for children?: sensitivity and specificity of an automatic external defibrillator algorithm in 696 pediatric arrhythmias. Circulation. 2001;103:2483–8. https://doi.org/10.1161/01.cir.103.20.2483.
23. Atkinson E, Mikysa B, Conway JA, Parker M, Christian K, Deshpande J, Knilans TK, Smith J, Walker C, Stickney RE, Hampton DR, Hazinski MF. Specificity and sensitivity of automated external defibrillator rhythm analysis in infants and children. Ann Emerg Med. 2003;42:185–96. https://doi.org/10.1067/mem.2003.287.
24. Atkins DL, Scott WA, Blaufox AD, Law IH, Dick M II, Geheb F, Sobh J, Brewer JE. Sensitivity and specificity of an automated external defibrillator algorithm designed for pediatric patients. Resuscitation. 2008;76:168–74. https://doi.org/10.1016/j.resuscitation.2007.06.032.
25. Atkins DL, Jorgenson DB. Attenuated pediatric electrode pads for automated external defibrillator use in children. Resuscitation. 2005;66:31–7. https://doi.org/10.1016/j.resuscitation.2004.12.025.
26. Bar-Cohen Y, Walsh EP, Love BA, Cecchin F. First appropriate use of automated external defibrillator in an infant. Resuscitation. 2005;67:135–7. https://doi.org/10.1016/j.resuscitation.2005.05.003.

27. Hoyt WJ Jr, Fish FA, Kannankeril PJ. Automated external defibrillator use in a previously healthy 31-day-old infant with out-of-hospital cardiac arrest due to ventricular fibrillation. J Cardiovasc Electrophysiol. 2019;30:2599–602. https://doi.org/10.1111/jce.14125.
28. Lin YR, Wu MH, Chen TY, Syue YJ, Yang MC, Lee TH, Lin CM, Chou CC, Chang CF, Li CJ. Time to epinephrine treatment is associated with the risk of mortality in children who achieve sustained ROSC after traumatic out-of-hospital cardiac arrest. Crit Care. 2019;23:101. https://doi.org/10.1186/s13054-019-2391-.
29. Lin YR, Li CJ, Huang CC, Lee TH, Chen TY, Yang MC, Chou CC, Chang CF, Huang HW, Hsu HY, Chen WL. Early epinephrine improves the stabilization of initial post-resuscitation hemodynamics in children with nonshockable out-of-hospital cardiac arrest. Front Pediatr. 2019;7:220. https://doi.org/10.3389/fped.2019.00220.
30. Fukuda T, Kondo Y, Hayashida K, Sekiguchi H, Kukita I. Time to epinephrine and survival after paediatric out-of-hospital cardiac arrest. Eur Heart J Cardiovasc Pharmacother. 2018;4:144–51. https://doi.org/10.1093/ehjcvp/pv.
31. Hansen M, Schmicker RH, Newgard CD, Grunau B, Scheuermeyer F, Cheskes S, Vithalani V, Alnaji F, Rea T, Idris AH, Herren H, Hutchison J, Austin M, Egan D, Daya M, Resuscitation Outcomes Consortium Investigators. Time to epinephrine administration and survival from nonshockable out-of-hospital cardiac arrest among children and adults. Circulation. 2018;137:2032–40. https://doi.org/10.1161/CIRCULATIONAHA.117.033067.

Diuretics in Critically Ill Patients: An Update

23

Davide Chiumello and Alessandro Monte

23.1 Diuretics in the Critically Ill Patient

The administration of diuretics remains a cornerstone in the management of fluid overload in critically ill patients with heart failure, acute kidney injury, or following aggressive fluid resuscitation.

Retrospective data suggest that up to 70% of critically ill patients receive diuretics at least once during their ICU stay [1, 2], with furosemide being the most commonly prescribed agent (administered in 94% of cases), while combination therapy with different classes of diuretics is less common in intensive care [3, 4]. In the initial phase of critical illness, intravascular volume depletion due to capillary leak into the interstitium is common and requires aggressive fluid resuscitation with the ultimate goal of improving cardiac output and tissue perfusion [5–7]. After volume repletion, patients may develop fluid overload, either directly due to the infused

D. Chiumello (✉) · A. Monte
Department of Health Sciences, University of Milan, Milan, Italy

Department of Anesthesia and Intensive Care, ASST Santi Paolo e Carlo, San Paolo University Hospital, Milan, Italy
e-mail: davide.chiumello@unimi.it

D. Chiumello, A. De Gasperi (eds.), *Practical Trends in Anesthesia and Intensive Care 2026*, https://doi.org/10.1007/978-3-032-25721-5_23

fluids or secondarily as a result of acute kidney injury and oliguria, leading to further fluid retention and edema [1, 8–11]. Consequently, diuretics are generally used to counteract fluid overload by enhancing diuresis and promoting negative fluid balance [10, 12–16]. Several factors have been identified as associated with increased diuretic use, including mechanical ventilation, a history of chronic heart failure, recovery from septic shock, and acute kidney injury [4]. In addition, ICU patients typically present with several factors, such as reduced renal perfusion, acid-base disturbances, and hypoalbuminemia, which may reduce the effectiveness of diuretics and lead to resistance to this class of drugs.

23.2 Introduction and Renal Physiology

23.2.1 The Glomerulus

The average kidney contains about one million nephrons, each supplied by an afferent arteriole that, within Bowman's capsule, forms the glomerulus, a network of capillaries. The glomerulus is the kidney's filtration unit and is responsible for producing ultrafiltrate through Starling forces: in brief, the Starling equation defines filtration pressure as the difference between hydrostatic pressure and effective oncotic pressure. These forces drive the movement of water across the glomerular capillaries. The final ultrafiltrate is a fluid with a composition similar to that of the small molecules and ions present in the afferent arteriole. The fenestrated endothelium of the glomerular capillaries, the glomerular basement membrane, and the podocytes act as a semipermeable membrane, thanks to the presence of a negatively charged glycocalyx, which limits the filtration of proteins such as albumin. Under normal conditions, the kidneys can generate a glomerular filtration rate (GFR) of up to 125 mL min^{-1} of ultrafiltrate produced at the level of the Bowman's capsule.

However, most diuretics do not act at the glomerular level but rather at the tubular level: although no direct effect is observed on the glomerulus, diuretics can indirectly affect the glomerular filtration rate (GFR). This may be mediated through activation of the Renin-Angiotensin-Aldosterone System (RAAS) due to the reduction in circulating blood volume, which leads to vasoconstriction of the efferent arteriole. In addition to effects on glomerular hemodynamics, changes in electrolyte balance secondary to metabolic effects and to the acid–base balance alterations induced by diuretic administration can, in turn, influence the glomerular filtration rate.

23.2.2 The Proximal Convoluted Tubule (PCT)

Under physiological conditions, the proximal convoluted tubule (PCT) is the main site for the reabsorption of water and solutes after their loss through glomerular filtration. Approximately 65–70% of Na^+ and water are reabsorbed in the proximal convoluted tubule, resulting in a tubular fluid osmolarity similar to that of plasma. This remarkable reabsorptive capacity is achieved thanks to the presence of specific transporters on the apical membrane of the PCT (the Na^+/H^+ exchanger or NHE3 located on the luminal membrane). Na^+ reabsorption occurs in exchange for H^+ ions to maintain electroneutrality across the membrane. Subsequently, H^+ ions combine with filtered bicarbonate ions (HCO_3^-) to form carbonic acid (H_2CO_3) in the tubular lumen, which, through the action of carbonic anhydrase, generates H_2O and CO_2:

$$H^+ + HCO_3^- \leftrightarrows H_2CO_3 \leftrightarrows H_2O + CO_2$$

CO_2 freely diffuses back into the cells, and H_2O is reabsorbed through aquaporin-1 channels present in the tubular cells (aquaporin-1 is also present in the descending limb of the loop of Henle). H_2CO_3 is produced by the action of cellular carbonic anhydrase, which further catalyzes the reaction to form HCO_3^- and H^+ ions within the cells [17].

23.2.3 Loop of Henle

The loop of Henle is capable of establishing a hypertonic osmotic gradient in the renal medulla, with osmolarity increasing from about 300 mOsm/L in the cortex to 1400 mOsm/L in the medullary pyramid. This process is facilitated by passive water reabsorption in the descending (thin) limb and by reabsorption of Na^+ and Cl^- in the ascending (thick) limb of the loop (Thick Ascending Limb (TAL)), which is impermeable to water. This solute reabsorption occurs via an active transport mechanism with countercurrent blood flow, resulting in a net removal of sodium and chloride from the tubular fluid into the interstitium. Active solute transport across the TAL is mainly mediated by the sodium-potassium-chloride cotransporter 2 (NKCC2 or $Na^+/K^+/2Cl^-$) on the luminal surface of its cells, which reabsorbs about 25–30% of the Na^+ present in the tubular lumen [18, 19].

23.2.4 Macula Densa

At the distal end of the loop of Henle is the macula densa, a group of modified tubular epithelial cells that are part of the so-called "juxtaglomerular apparatus." This structure is located near the afferent arteriole and plays a key role in the autoregulation of renal blood flow and glomerular filtration rate. The macula densa senses sodium and chloride levels in the tubular fluid and, through granular cells—i.e., modified smooth muscle cells in the afferent arterioles—secretes renin [18].

In a state of circulating volume depletion (or in the case of reduced glomerular filtration rate), increased reabsorption of sodium and chloride in the TAL reduces the amount of sodium reaching the distal macula densa. This phenomenon leads to decreased vascular resistance in the afferent arterioles and increases renin release from juxtaglomerular cells, followed by the formation of angiotensin and vasoconstriction of the efferent arterioles. Both mechanisms just described lead to an increase in hydrostatic pressure at the glomerular level, resulting in an increased filtration rate; for this reason, this is referred to as the so-called tubuloglomerular feedback (TGF), of which both mechanisms are a part.

In the opposite situation, that is, in states of sodium overload and/or increased circulating volume, there is an increase in the concentration of sodium and chloride reaching the macula densa, due to elevated atrial pressure and the consequent release of natriuretic peptides. These peptides facilitate renal sodium excretion through direct tubular effects and by increasing the glomerular filtration rate. This results in suppression of the renin-angiotensin-aldosterone system, leading to systemic vasodilation and further promoting renal sodium excretion by reducing the tubular effects of angiotensin II and aldosterone (due to decreased renin release) [17].

23.2.5 Distal Convoluted Tubule

Approximately 5–10% of the filtered sodium load is reabsorbed in the distal convoluted tubule via the sodium-chloride co-transporter (NCC). In this segment of the nephron, about 10–15% of calcium (Ca^{2+}) is also reabsorbed through the TRPV5 receptor (Transient receptor potential cation channel subfamily V member 5 or vanilloid receptor 5), and 5–10% of magnesium (Mg^{2+}) is reabsorbed via the transient receptor potential melastatin 6 and 7 channels (TRPM6-7). This process is influenced by aldosterone-mediated stimulation of sodium reabsorption and potassium excretion, as well as by parathyroid hormone stimulation of Ca^{2+} reabsorption [20].

23.2.6 Cortical and Medullary Collecting Duct

The collecting duct reabsorbs about 0–2% of sodium and water. It is composed of two main cell types: principal cells, which facilitate sodium reabsorption and potassium excretion under the influence of aldosterone (while water reabsorption is mediated by antidiuretic hormone or ADH), and intercalated cells, which are responsible for hydrogen ion secretion (by alpha-intercalated cells) and bicarbonate ion secretion (by beta-intercalated cells) [17] (Table 23.1).

Table 23.1 The main roles and physiological mechanisms of the different segments of the nephron

Nephron segment	Main function	Physiological mechanisms
Glomerulus	Filtration of blood to form the ultrafiltrate.	Filtration is influenced by Starling forces, with hydrostatic pressure favoring the movement of water across a semipermeable membrane. The ultrafiltrate has a composition similar to that of small molecules and ions
Proximal convoluted tubule (PCT)	Massive reabsorption of water and solutes (Na^+, HCO_3^-) following glomerular filtration	Na^+ reabsorption occurs via the Na^+/H^+ exchanger (NHE3). H^+ ions combine with HCO_3^- to form H_2CO_3, which dissociates into H_2O and CO_2. CO_2 diffuses into the cells, and H_2O is reabsorbed via aquaporin-1
Loop of Henle	Creation of a hypertonic osmotic gradient in the renal medulla and reabsorption of Na^+ and Cl^-	The descending limb is permeable to water, while the ascending limb (TAL) is impermeable to water but actively reabsorbs Na^+ and Cl^- via the $Na^+/K^+/2Cl^-$ co-transporter (NKCC2), contributing to the osmotic gradient
Macula densa	Monitoring sodium and chloride levels in the tubular fluid and regulation of glomerular filtration rate (tubuloglomerular feedback)	If sodium is low in the tubular fluid, the macula densa stimulates renin release from the granular cells of the afferent arterioles, leading to vasoconstriction of the efferent arteriole and increased GFR. In cases of sodium overload, natriuretic peptide release is stimulated
Distal convoluted tubule (DCT)	Reabsorption of sodium (5–10%), calcium (10–15%), and magnesium (5–10%)	Sodium is reabsorbed via the Na^+/Cl^- cotransporter (NCC). Calcium is reabsorbed through the TRPV5 receptor and magnesium via the TRPM6-7 receptors. Aldosterone secretion promotes potassium excretion and sodium reabsorption
Collecting duct	Final reabsorption of sodium and water is regulated by aldosterone and ADH	Principal cells facilitate sodium reabsorption and potassium excretion under the influence of aldosterone, while water is reabsorbed under the effect of ADH. Intercalated cells secrete hydrogen ions (alpha) and bicarbonate (beta)

23.3 Mechanisms of Action of Different Classes of Diuretics

23.3.1 Loop Diuretics

Loop diuretics inhibit the majority of sodium reabsorption (about 25% of filtered sodium) and are the most potent drugs in terms of diuretic effect. They act at the tubular lumen after active secretion via the human organic anion transporter system (h-OAT) in the proximal tubule. From there, they are transported to the luminal NKCC2 or $Na^+/K^+/2Cl^-$ receptor (effector site) [21] (Fig. 23.1).

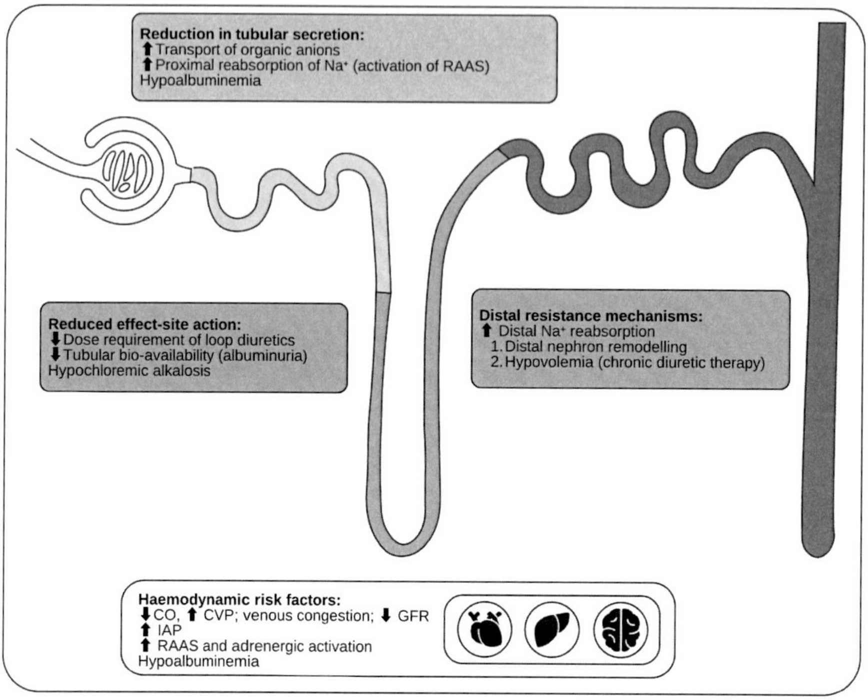

Fig. 23.1 The workflow of the diuretics

These molecules are all anionic in nature and bind to the chloride binding site of the transmembrane NKCC2 receptor located on the luminal membrane of the cells in the thick ascending limb of the loop of Henle (TAL) [18]. The binding of the loop diuretic to the chloride site of NKCC2 blocks the secondary active transport of solutes by NKCC2 out of the tubular lumen, thereby inhibiting the reabsorption of Na^+, K^+, and Cl^-, reducing the tonicity of the renal interstitium, and preventing the reabsorption of ultrafiltered water. The final effect of their administration is to induce natriuresis, accompanied by a greater loss of water than sodium. The macula densa cells also contain NKCC2 receptors, and binding of loop diuretics leads to inhibition of the tubuloglomerular feedback mechanism [22, 23].

From a pharmacokinetic perspective, absorption kinetics vary among different molecules, and it should be noted that loop diuretics are mostly bound to plasma proteins (>90%), thus their volume of distribution is limited. Comparing intravenous to oral administration, the former is twice as potent as the latter and has an onset of action of 5 minutes compared to 30–60 minutes after oral administration, with a half-life for furosemide of about 1.5 hours. In patients with preserved renal function, a steep dose-response curve is observed, reaching a plateau with doses commonly used in clinical practice, without further increase in diuretic effect with higher doses [24].

23.3.2 Thiazide and Thiazide-Like Diuretics

Examples of thiazide diuretics are benzothiadiazine derivatives: hydrochlorothiazide and chlorothiazide. Thiazide-like diuretics, which do not have the benzothiadiazine core structure characteristic of thiazide diuretics, include chlorthalidone, metolazone, and indapamide.

Regarding pharmacokinetics, with the exception of indapamide, these diuretics are bound to albumin, are not metabolized, and are excreted unchanged in urine and feces, with variable pharmacokinetic profiles, metabolism, bioavailability, and plasma half-life among drugs in this class. Most thiazides have an estimated duration of effect of about 12–18 hours, with a half-life of 2 to 5 hours for hydrochlorothiazide up to 14 hours for indapamide, two of the most commonly used thiazides [25].

From a pharmacodynamic standpoint, thiazide and thiazide-like diuretics act by blocking the Na-Cl cotransporter in the distal convoluted tubule (also known as the electroneutral NCC symporter), thereby inhibiting both sodium and chloride reabsorption. Both thiazide and thiazide-like diuretics competitively bind to the chloride binding site of the transmembrane domain of NCC and inhibit Na+ reabsorption, but since the distal convoluted tubule reabsorbs only about 5–10% of filtered sodium, the diuretic effect is relatively weak [22]. Also at the level of the distal convoluted tubule, thiazide diuretics are able to increase calcium reabsorption: by decreasing the intracellular sodium concentration in tubular epithelial cells, they increase the activity of the Na^+/Ca^{2+}—ATPase present on the basolateral membrane, resulting in an increase in active calcium reabsorption into the interstitium. The reduction of intracellular calcium in tubular cells promotes its entry from the tubular lumen through TRPV5 channels located on the apical side of the tubular cell [26, 27].

23.3.3 Carbonic Anhydrase Inhibitors

Carbonic anhydrase (CA) is a metalloenzyme belonging to the lyase class, containing zinc, and is present in red blood cells, the stomach, the central nervous system, and the kidney. At least 12 isoforms have been described, each with different biological roles; in the kidney, it is found in the proximal convoluted tubule either membrane-bound (CA isoform IV) or free in the cytoplasm (CA isoform II) [22]. Carbonic anhydrase plays a key role in bicarbonate ion reabsorption, reclaiming about 80% of filtered HCO_3^- and, together with hydrogen ion secretion, is crucial for the body's acid-base homeostasis. The only carbonic anhydrase inhibitor used as a diuretic in clinical practice is acetazolamide.

Acetazolamide is typically administered orally, with rapid absorption and peak plasma concentration reached about 2 hours after administration. It has a variable half-life of approximately 6–10 hours and a duration of effect of about 8–10 hours. It is highly bound to plasma albumin (over 90% is protein-bound), and about 90% is excreted unchanged in the urine via tubular secretion. Although it was previously thought not to undergo significant metabolism, possible acetazolamide metabolites have been identified, but their quantitative relationship to unmetabolized acetazolamide remains to be clarified by further studies.

Inhibition of carbonic anhydrase impairs the reabsorption of sodium, water, and bicarbonate ions, thereby promoting the excretion of sodium bicarbonate along with excess water in the urine. Another effect mediated by this enzyme is the facilitation of chloride excretion to maintain electroneutrality; thus, its inhibition leads to a reduction in luminal chloride. Associated with the urinary loss of bicarbonate ions, there is also an increase in the reabsorption of ammonia (NH_3). The net result is alkaline diuresis and, ultimately, metabolic acidosis (see dedicated section).

In summary, acetazolamide increases urinary sodium and bicarbonate ions and decreases urinary hydrogen and chloride ions (with the opposite effect observed in plasma). However, the diuretic effect of this drug is weak, but it can enhance the diuretic effect of loop diuretics by increasing sodium delivery to the thick ascending limb of the loop of Henle (TAL) [28].

23.3.4 Potassium-Sparing Diuretics

Potassium-sparing diuretics include those drugs capable of promoting diuresis while limiting urinary potassium loss. They can be divided into two subgroups:

- Mineralocorticoid receptor antagonists or aldosterone antagonists: spironolactone, eplerenone, canrenone, and finerenone (a more recent nonsteroidal mineralocorticoid antagonist)
- Epithelial sodium channel (ENaC) inhibitors: amiloride and triamterene

From a pharmacokinetic perspective, both spironolactone and eplerenone are metabolized in the liver and do not require secretion into the tubular lumen to exert their effect, whereas amiloride is excreted unchanged in the urine via tubular secretion and in the feces. The estimated onset of action is about 6 hours for amiloride and 24–48 hours for spironolactone, with half-lives of 21 hours and 15 hours for their active metabolites, respectively.

From a pharmacodynamic standpoint, all drugs in these two subgroups act on the distal part of the nephron, particularly on the cells of the distal convoluted tubule and the collecting duct. They inhibit sodium reabsorption either by binding to ENaC channels or by blocking aldosterone receptors, both of which, under physiological conditions, increase sodium and water reabsorption and promote urinary potassium loss. However, since they act distally, where sodium reabsorption accounts for less than 3%, these diuretics inhibit only about 3% of the filtered sodium load and therefore do not have a strong diuretic effect [17, 22].

23.3.5 Osmotic Diuretics

Osmotic diuretics act primarily by increasing the osmolarity of the tubular fluid in the proximal convoluted tubule and the thick ascending limb of the loop of Henle, thereby preventing the reabsorption of filtered water by osmotic gradient, without actively affecting the flow of electrolytes through the tubule. All are molecules that are filtered at the glomerulus and poorly reabsorbed at the tubular level (such as urea).

Mannitol, a non-metabolized sugar that is freely filtered through the glomerulus, is the most widely used. Due to its poor oral absorption, mannitol is administered only intravenously. intravenous and has 100% bioavailability with a half-life of 70–150 minutes. More than 90% of absorbed mannitol is excreted unchanged in the urine.

After being filtered into the tubular lumen, mannitol is minimally reabsorbed and remains in the tubular lumen, increasing the osmolarity of the luminal fluid and inhibiting the urine-concentrating function of the countercurrent mechanism, thereby promoting water transport in the collecting ducts and reducing the hyperosmolarity of the renal medulla; this results in marked diuresis. Its intravenous administration is acutely associated with plasma volume expansion, also leading to a reduction in renin release [17, 22] (Table 23.2).

Table 23.2 Main classes of diuretics used in clinical practice with site and mechanism of action

Class	Site of action	Mechanism of action	Examples	Half-life
Loop diuretics	Loop of Henle (TAL)	Inhibition of the Na^+/K^+/$2Cl^-$ co-transporter (NKCC2), blocks reabsorption of Na^+, K^+, and Cl^-, increases natriuresis	Furosemide	1.5–2 hours
Thiazide diuretics	Distal convoluted tubule	Inhibition of the Na^+/Cl^- co-transporter (NCC), prevents reabsorption of Na^+ and Cl^-	Hydro-chlorothiazide, Chlorthalidone	2–14 hours
Carbonic anhydrase inhibitors	Proximal tubule	Inhibition of carbonic anhydrase, reduces reabsorption of HCO_3^- and Na^+, increases reabsorption of H^+ and Cl^-	Acetazolamide	6–10 hours
Potassium-sparing diuretics	Distal convoluted tubule and collecting duct	Mineralocorticoid receptor antagonists (Spironolactone, Eplerenone): Inhibition of aldosterone ENaC inhibitors (Amiloride, Triamterene): Inhibition of the epithelial sodium channel (ENaC)	Spironolactone, Eplerenone, Amiloride	21 hours (spirono-lactone), 15 hours (active metabolites)
Osmotic diuretics	Proximal tubule, Loop of Henle, Collecting duct	Increases the osmolarity of tubular fluid, preventing water reabsorption by osmotic gradient	Mannitol	70–150 minutes

23.4 Clinical Use of Different Classes of Diuretics

23.4.1 Loop Diuretics

Loop diuretics are the most commonly administered class of diuretics in critically ill patients to treat volume overload, with furosemide remaining the most widely used. Other loop diuretics include bumetanide and torasemide, but their use in intensive care is less frequent. Although furosemide is the diuretic of choice in over 90% of cases of AKI (acute kidney injury) with associated fluid overload, a meta-analysis of 20 randomized controlled trials comparing the prevention or treatment of AKI with furosemide versus placebo showed that furosemide has no impact on mortality or the need for RRT (renal replacement therapy) [29]. Some studies have shown worsening of AKI and increased mortality in patients treated with loop diuretics, suggesting that such studies may have included a population with pre-renal failure [30]. Despite the lack of evidence suggesting that loop diuretics may improve mortality, it appears that these agents can improve renal insufficiency when used in the presence of fluid overload, thereby reducing renal congestion [31].

23.4.2 Methods of Administration of Loop Diuretics

Intermittent administration of diuretics, due to greater variability in drug concentration within the tubular lumen, is expected to provide a more predictable and controlled urinary response, whereas continuous administration of loop diuretics should theoretically maintain a constant luminal drug concentration and maximize urine output for as long as possible [32–36].

In critically ill patients, continuous infusion of furosemide has been associated with increased urine output and a more controlled diuretic response, using lower drug doses. A retrospective study conducted in a surgical patient population showed that continuous administration of 2 mg/h of furosemide, compared to a bolus of 10 or 20 mg per day, significantly improved diuresis with a more negative fluid balance, without a significant difference in ICU or hospital length of stay [37]. Similar results have been observed in the post-cardiac surgery setting: when comparing the diuretic effect of the same dose of furosemide administered as a bolus or continuous infusion, mean total urine volumes and sodium excretion were similar in the 12 hours following administration [38]. Notably, continuous infusion of furosemide resulted in less variation in urine output during treatment. The literature also reports evidence on higher doses of loop diuretics, comparing continuous infusion versus bolus administration of furosemide in a population of patients with acute heart failure [39]. The group treated with continuous infusion produced a greater volume of urine and showed a more pronounced trend toward reduction in natriuretic peptide levels, at the expense of worsening renal function during hospitalization [39–42].

Therefore, we can conclude that in patients admitted to intensive care, especially in the presence of AKI, continuous infusion of diuretics is safe and should be adopted to ensure a better diuretic response, although further studies are needed to assess the renal impact of high-dose loop diuretics and to define the most appropriate mode of administration.

23.4.3 Albumin and Furosemide

Loop diuretics, such as furosemide, bind reversibly to plasma proteins, with approximately 95–99% bound to circulating albumin; therefore, loop diuretics are not filtered by the glomerulus in their unbound form. The albumin–furosemide complex reaches the proximal tubular cells, interacts with the human organic anion transporter (h-OAT), leading to translocation of the diuretic molecule into the tubular lumen, where it acts on the thick ascending limb of the loop of Henle (TAL).

Hypoalbuminemia can lead to diuretic resistance (discussed in detail in the dedicated section) through several mechanisms:

1. It may reduce the amount of diuretic bound to albumin in plasma and the efficient transport of the drug to its site of action via the anion transporter system.
2. In hypoalbuminemic conditions, the volume of distribution of the diuretic increases, which may reduce drug availability at the site of action.
3. Hypoalbuminemia is often associated with conditions such as nephrotic syndrome or congestive heart failure, which lead to fluid retention and a further increase in the drug's volume of distribution and "dilution" at the plasma level, reducing its efficacy at the effector site.

Several authors have addressed this issue with conflicting results, for example:

- Mahmoodpoor et al. randomized 49 intensive care patients with normal renal function and moderate hypoalbuminemia to receive either furosemide alone or furosemide in combination with albumin, finding that furosemide excretion was initially higher in patients also treated with albumin, but without significant differences in urinary sodium or furosemide excretion at 4 and 8 hours after administration [43].
- Klinkmann et al. enrolled 50 intensive care patients treated with continuous furosemide infusion for at least 5 hours. Patients with an albumin binding capacity (ABiC: quantifies the residual binding capacity of one of the major binding sites of the albumin molecule) of at least 60% had a significantly lower proportion of free furosemide and a significantly greater amount of furosemide excreted renally compared to patients with a lower ABiC [44].
- Martin et al. conducted a randomized study in patients with acute lung injury (ALI), mechanically ventilated for more than 24 hours, with serum protein levels <6 g/dL, randomized to receive albumin followed by a loading dose of intravenous furosemide (20 mg) and a continuous infusion of furosemide at 4–10 g/h for 3 days, or an identical intravenous bolus and continuous furosemide infusion, with an equivalent volume of 0.9% saline solution. During the first 3 days, similar increases in serum albumin, daily urine output, and comparable changes in

body weight, cardiac index, and respiratory mechanics were observed, but with improved oxygenation at 24 hours [45].

- A meta-analysis that included a certainly more heterogeneous population, enrolling not only patients admitted to intensive care units but also patients with nephrotic syndrome or liver cirrhosis, found that the administration of furosemide in combination with albumin significantly increased diuresis in hypoalbuminemic patients (with baseline serum albumin levels below 2.5 g/dL) and in patients with creatinine levels above 1.2 mg/dL [46].

In conclusion, despite the pathophysiological rationale and pharmacological theory, the addition of albumin to furosemide administration in critically ill patients has not demonstrated a significant improvement in diuretic effect. However, considering the transient positive effect on diuresis and short-term natriuresis reported in the literature in populations treated with both diuretics and albumin, further large-scale randomized studies with more heterogeneous populations of critically ill patients are needed to define the role of this approach in the management of patients treated with loop diuretics, particularly in those with demonstrated drug resistance (see dedicated section).

23.4.4 Thiazides

Thiazide and thiazide-like diuretics are the most commonly used class of diuretics when loop diuretic resistance occurs in patients with fluid overload. This combination is recommended in patients with acute heart failure by the 2021 European Society of Cardiology Guidelines for Heart Failure [47], particularly when urine output remains inadequate despite appropriate doses of loop diuretics, in order to increase urine production and maximize negative fluid balance. A retrospective analysis of the "Medical Information Mart for Intensive Care III (MIMIC-III)" from Harvard University, conducted on a population of patients treated with high-dose loop diuretics, showed that in patients receiving more than 1 mg/kg/day of furosemide, co-administration of a second diuretic from another class (e.g., thiazides and carbonic anhydrase inhibitors) was associated with a moderate increase in 24-hour urine output [33].

23.4.5 Carbonic Anhydrase Inhibitors

Regarding CA inhibitors, acetazolamide appears to have a role in the treatment of metabolic alkalosis induced by loop diuretics, steroid therapy, and in patients with COPD undergoing mechanical ventilation. However, for the latter group, the first randomized study comparing acetazolamide to placebo did not find a reduction in the duration of invasive mechanical ventilation in patients with COPD [48].

Carbonic anhydrase inhibitors can also be used in combination with loop diuretics in patients with acute heart failure and fluid overload to enhance natriuresis. In a randomized study of patients with acute heart failure, when acetazolamide 250–500 mg per day plus bumetanide was compared to high-dose bumetanide monotherapy, the group receiving combination diuretic therapy increased the natriuresis. Additionally, in a study conducted on a large population of patients admitted to intensive care, the combination of acetazolamide and furosemide resulted in a greater 24-hour negative fluid balance compared to furosemide alone, although this result was not confirmed by a subsequent meta-analysis [33, 49–51].

In conclusion, in patients admitted to intensive care, acetazolamide can be used to increase diuresis and thus the 24-hour negative fluid balance in combination with diuretic therapy, to treat metabolic alkalosis induced by loop diuretics, and in patients with COPD undergoing mechanical ventilation.

23.4.6 Potassium-Sparing Diuretics

The clinical use of potassium-sparing diuretics in intensive care is mainly aimed at correcting hypokalemia induced by other diuretics and correcting hypomagnesemia; therefore, their use in intensive care is rather limited. Due to their limited diuretic effect, they should not be used to treat systemic congestion, but rather to manage persistent hypokalemia caused by other diuretic therapies (e.g., furosemide) [52].

23.4.7 Osmotic Diuretics

Mannitol has been recommended for the treatment/prevention of acute renal failure due to rhabdomyolysis, when a urine output of at least 300 mL/h is not achieved despite adequate volume resuscitation with crystalloids. However, it has not yet been demonstrated that mannitol therapy is superior to crystalloid alone fluid therapy/hydration. In addition to its diuretic effect, mannitol appears to have a beneficial role in preventing ischemia–reperfusion injury during kidney transplantation: a recent meta-analysis demonstrated that administration of mannitol during transplantation led to a reduction in the incidence of acute kidney injury and graft dysfunction, all without a significant increase in urine output from the transplanted kidney. This nephroprotective effect is likely based on the release of intrarenal vasodilatory prostaglandins and natriuretic peptides [53–55] (Table 23.3).

Table 23.3 Some of the main clinical indications for diuretics in intensive care

Class	Clinical indications
Loop diuretics	Management of volume overload in critically ill patients (e.g., acute heart failure, pulmonary edema, acute kidney injury) Treatment of AKI with fluid overload to reduce renal congestion, although this does not impact mortality or the need for RRT (renal replacement therapy)
Thiazides	Resistance to loop diuretics in patients with fluid overload Combination with furosemide when diuresis remains inadequate despite appropriate doses of furosemide in cases of acute heart failure
Carbonic anhydrase inhibitors	Used to enhance natriuresis in patients with acute heart failure and fluid overload Treatment of metabolic alkalosis in patients with COPD on mechanical ventilation Treatment of diuretic-induced metabolic alkalosis
Potassium-sparing diuretics	Correction of hypokalemia induced by other diuretic therapies, but with limited diuretic effect. Rarely used for congestion management
Osmotic diuretics	Treatment of AKI associated with rhabdomyolysis, when urine output does not reach at least 300 mL/h despite adequate volume resuscitation with fluids Protective effect against ischemia–reperfusion injury in kidney transplantation, reducing AKI and graft dysfunction without increasing urine output

23.4.8 Diuretic Resistance

Under conditions of normal renal function, increasing the dose of a (loop) diuretic results in a greater diuretic response and sodium excretion until a plateau is reached, where complete inhibition of the diuretic-sensitive channel occurs.

An adequate response to a diuretic can be defined as a urine output greater than 150 mL/h after 2 hours or a urinary sodium concentration greater than 50–70 mEq/L 2 hours after administration. Diuretic resistance is commonly defined as the failure to increase diuresis despite the use of maximal diuretic doses [56].

Diuretic resistance may occur through three main mechanisms [57]:

1. Reduced Drug Availability at the Site of Action

   Diuretics reach their site of action via tubular secretion at the proximal tubule, rather than by the normal process of glomerular filtration. Thus, most loop diuretics are secreted rather than ultrafiltered, also due to their high affinity for plasma proteins. A reduction in the concentration of these proteins (as in hypoalbuminemia) or a decrease in renal blood flow reduces the tubular secretion of loop diuretics. In addition, the accumulation of organic acids may compete with loop diuretics for secretion into the tubular lumen via anionic transporters, thereby reducing their efficacy at the effector site [57].
2. Increased Sodium Retention Due to Prolonged Therapy

   Prolonged use of loop diuretics can promote increased sodium reabsorption at both the proximal and distal sites of the tubule, counteracting the natriuretic and diuretic effects of these agents. This phenomenon may be caused by hypertrophy and hyperplasia of the distal tubules and collecting ducts, especially after chronic use, as well as by activation of the renin-angiotensin-aldosterone system (RAAS) and the release of vasopressin (ADH) after several days of diuretic administration, which together increase sodium reabsorption in the nephron [17, 57, 58].

3. Reduced Sodium/Chloride Sensing

   Sodium and chloride ions regulate the diuretic-sensitive sodium transporter; therefore, both hyponatremia and hypochloremia can reduce the effectiveness of loop diuretics by altering the ability to modulate sodium transport. Although there are no randomized controlled trials and thus the findings are not widely generalizable, the literature has suggested the simultaneous use of hypertonic saline and furosemide in patients with acute decompensated heart failure and fluid overload, resulting in increased daily diuresis, greater sodium excretion, and reduced hospital stay and mortality [59].

Possible solutions emerging from the literature include the use of combination strategies, such as combining furosemide with other agents like acetazolamide, thiazide diuretics, or spironolactone. Combination therapy has been shown to improve diuresis and achieve a more negative fluid balance [33, 49, 60–62].

In conclusion, to overcome diuretic resistance in intensive care patients with fluid overload, it has been suggested to increase the dose of the diuretic (furosemide) up to a maximum of 4 mg/kg/day to raise the drug concentration at the site of action. If this is insufficient, a second diuretic, such as a thiazide or acetazolamide, may be added to promote a more negative fluid balance [33–57].

23.5 Diuretic-Induced Acid-Base Disturbances

Diuretics can affect plasma and urinary acid-base balance by altering the ion concentrations in their respective compartments. According to the traditional approach using the Henderson-Hasselbalch equation, plasma pH depends on two variables: plasma bicarbonate concentration [HCO_3^-] and the amount of dissolved carbon dioxide in plasma. The former is regulated at the renal level, while the latter is controlled by alveolar ventilation [63].

Diuretics act at the renal level, influencing the reabsorption of electrolytes (sodium, potassium, and chloride), and by modulating volemia, they induce changes in plasma pH through various mechanisms.

The impact of diuretics on acid-base balance depends on their specific action and the site of the nephron activity. Effects can range from metabolic alkalosis (loop and thiazide diuretics) to metabolic acidosis (carbonic anhydrase inhibitors and potassium-sparing diuretics). The overall effect on pH also depends on the impact of their administration on volemia and on possible combined effects (between diuretics and between the drug and patient comorbidities). In fact, excessive use of diuretics can lead to depletion of circulating volume, reducing renal perfusion and glomerular

Table 23.4 Main acid-base disorders induced by diuretic administration and their pathophysiological mechanisms

Class	Mechanism of action	Cause of disorder	Effect
Loop diuretics	Inhibit the Na^+-K^+-$2Cl^-$ cotransporter in the loop of Henle	Chloride loss and activation of Na^+/H^+ exchange, with increased plasma bicarbonate	Hypochloremic metabolic alkalosis
Thiazide diuretics	Inhibit the Na^+-Cl^- co-transporter in the distal convoluted tubule	Similar to loop diuretics: chloride loss and activation of the Na^+/H^+ exchange	Hypochloremic metabolic alkalosis
Carbonic anhydrase inhibitors	Inhibit carbonic anhydrase in the proximal tubule	Decreased bicarbonate reabsorption, leading to accumulation of H^+ and Cl^- in plasma	Hyperchloremic metabolic acidosis
Potassium-sparing diuretics	Block Na^+ reabsorption and H^+ secretion in the collecting tubule	Reduced tubular secretion of H^+, resulting in decreased bicarbonate formation and a relative increase in Cl^-	Hyperchloremic metabolic acidosis

filtration rate (GFR). At the tubular level, this results in increased reabsorption of Na^+, HCO_3^-, and urea, thereby promoting greater secretion of hydrogen ions (H^+). Furthermore, depletion of intravascular volume can stimulate the release of renin and aldosterone, which in turn promote the loss of H^+ via the distal H^+/ATPase pump and the reabsorption of Na^+ in the collecting duct, resulting in metabolic alkalosis [59, 64, 65] (Table 23.4).

Mannitol also induces metabolic alkalosis through various mechanisms, such as increased renal bicarbonate production, tubular bicarbonate reabsorption, and H^+ secretion in the distal tubules, in addition to enhanced tubular bicarbonate reabsorption [66].

These effects on plasma pH can also be explained according to the Stewart approach (based on three independent variables: Strong Ion Difference, pCO_2, and weak acids) to acid-base balance [63]: the literature shows that, in mechanically ventilated patients, during continuous infusion of furosemide, a progressive increase in plasma Strong Ion Difference (SID) and pH has been observed, due to a reduction in plasma chloride levels (hypochloremic metabolic alkalosis) [67].

In conclusion, it should be remembered that metabolic alkalosis is the most common acid-base disorder in the Intensive Care Unit after the first few days of admission and has been associated with increased mortality. Metabolic alkalosis is rarely present as an isolated disorder and often coexists with respiratory disorders and metabolic acidosis [65]. Therefore, understanding the pathophysiological rationale of the impact that some of the most frequently administered therapies in the intensive care setting (e.g., furosemide) have on acid-base balance allows for broader management capabilities in critically ill patients.

23.6 Conclusions

Diuretics are among the most commonly prescribed drugs in Intensive Care. Nevertheless, there is a lack of information regarding outcomes and appropriate dosing. Furthermore, in the context of the use of different classes of diuretics and possible combination therapies, available data remain insufficient. The effects of diuretic therapy on acid-base balance are significant and should be an integral part of understanding the effects of these drugs, thus guiding their administration. Unfortunately, as is often the case in clinical practice, there is a lack of adequate evidence to support our therapeutic approaches, highlighting the need in this area as well to optimize medical therapy through further studies and clinical trials.

References

1. McCoy IE, Montez-Rath ME, Chertow GM, Chang TI. Estimated effects of early diuretic use in critical illness. Crit Care Explor. 2019;1:e0021.
2. Uchino S, Doig GS, Bellomo R, et al. Diuretics and mortality in acute renal failure*. Crit Care Med. 2004;32:1669–77.
3. Ostermann M, Alvarez G, Sharpe MD, Martin CM. Frusemide administration in critically ill patients by continuous compared to bolus therapy. Nephron Clin Pract. 2007;107:c70–6.
4. Jones SL, Mårtensson J, Glassford NJ, Eastwood GM, Bellomo R. Loop diuretic therapy in the critically ill: a survey. Crit Care Resusc. 2015;17:223–6.
5. Evans L, Rhodes A, Alhazzani W, et al. Surviving sepsis campaign: international guidelines for management of sepsis and septic shock 2021. Intensive Care Med. 2021;47:1181–247.
6. De Backer D, Aissaoui N, Cecconi M, et al. How can assessing hemodynamics help to assess volume status? Intensive Care Med. 2022;48:1482–94.
7. Nadeau-Fredette A-C, Bouchard J. Fluid management and use of diuretics in acute kidney injury. Adv Chronic Kidney Dis. 2013;20:45–55.
8. Ostermann M, Basu RK, Mehta RL. Acute kidney injury. Intensive Care Med. 2023;49:219–22.
9. Vignon P, Evrard B, Asfar P, et al. Fluid administration and monitoring in ARDS: which management? Intensive Care Med. 2020;46:2252–64.
10. Malbrain MLNG, Langer T, Annane D, et al. Intravenous fluid therapy in the perioperative and critical care setting: executive summary of the International Fluid Academy (IFA). Ann Intensive Care. 2020;10:64.
11. Chiumello D, Pozzi T, Fratti I, et al. Acid-base disorders in COVID-19 patients with acute respiratory distress syndrome. J Clin Med. 2022;11:2093.
12. Alaskar MA, Brown JD, Voils SA, Vouri SM. Loop diuretic use following fluid resuscitation in the critically ill. Am J Health Syst Pharm. 2022;79:165–72.
13. McCoy IE, Chertow GM, Chang TI-H. Patterns of diuretic use in the intensive care unit. PLoS One. 2019;14:e0217911.
14. Wichmann S, Barbateskovic M, Liang N, et al. Loop diuretics in adult intensive care patients with fluid overload: a systematic review of randomised clinical trials with meta-analysis and trial sequential analysis. Ann Intensive Care. 2022;12:52.
15. Wiedemann H, Wheeler A, Bernard G, Taylor Thompson B, Hayden D, deBoisblanc B. Comparison of two fluid-management strategies in acute lung injury. N Engl J Med. 2006;354:2564–75.
16. Bolgiaghi L, Umbrello M, Formenti P, et al. The furosemide stress test, electrolyte response and renal index in critically ill patients. Minerva Anestesiol. 2021;87:448.
17. Ronco C, Bellomo R, Ricci Z. Critical care nephrology. Elsevier; 2019.

18. Felker GM, Ellison DH, Mullens W, Cox ZL, Testani JM. Diuretic therapy for patients with heart failure. J Am Coll Cardiol. 2020;75:1178–95.
19. Ellison DH. Clinical pharmacology in diuretic use. Clin J Am Soc Nephrol. 2019;14:1248–57.
20. Hoover RS, Tomilin V, Hanson L, Pochynyuk O, Ko B. PTH modulation of NCC activity regulates TRPV5 Ca^{2+} reabsorption. Am J Physiol-Renal Physiol. 2016;310:F144–51.
21. Feig PU. Cellular mechanism of action of loop diuretics: implications for drug effectiveness and adverse effects. Am J Cardiol. 1986;57:A14–9.
22. Wile D. Diuretics: a review. Ann Clin Biochem: Int J Lab Med. 2012;49:419–31.
23. Peti-Peterdi J, Harris RC. Macula Densa sensing and signaling mechanisms of renin release. J Am Soc Nephrol. 2010;21:1093–6.
24. Ellison DH, Felker GM. Diuretic treatment in heart failure. N Engl J Med. 2017;377:1964–75.
25. Novak JE, Ellison DH. Diuretics in states of volume overload: core curriculum 2022. Am J Kidney Dis. 2022;80:264–76.
26. Ernst ME, Moser M. Use of diuretics in patients with hypertension. N Engl J Med. 2009;361:2153–64.
27. Carter BL, Ernst ME, Cohen JD. Hydrochlorothiazide versus chlorthalidone. Hypertension. 2004;43:4–9.
28. Tsikas D. Acetazolamide and human carbonic anhydrases: retrospect, review and discussion of an intimate relationship. J Enzyme Inhib Med Chem. 2024;39
29. Krzych ŁJ, Czempik PF. Impact of furosemide on mortality and the requirement for renal replacement therapy in acute kidney injury: a systematic review and meta-analysis of randomized trials. Ann Intensive Care. 2019;9:85.
30. Levi TM, Rocha MS, Almeida DN, et al. Furosemide is associated with acute kidney injury in critically ill patients. Braz J Med Biol Res. 2012;45:827–33.
31. Joannidis M, Druml W, Forni LG, et al. Prevention of acute kidney injury and protection of renal function in the intensive care unit: update 2017. Intensive Care Med. 2017;43:730–49.
32. Huang A, Luethi N, Mårtensson J, Bellomo R, Cioccari L. Pharmacodynamics of intravenous frusemide bolus in critically ill patients. Crit Care Resusc. 2017;19:142–9.
33. Côté J-M, Bouchard J, Murray PT, Beaubien-Souligny W. Diuretic strategies in patients with resistance to loop diuretics in the intensive care unit: a retrospective study from the MIMIC-III database. J Crit Care. 2021;65:282–91.
34. Ostermann M, Awdishu L, Legrand M. Using diuretic therapy in the critically ill patient. Intensive Care Med. 2024;50:1331–4.
35. Makhoul N, Riad T, Friedstrom S, Zvebil FR. Frusemide in pulmonary edema: continuous versus intermittent. Clin Intensive Care. 1997;8:273–6.
36. Ng KT, Yap JLL. Continuous infusion vs. intermittent bolus injection of furosemide in acute decompensated heart failure: systematic review and meta-analysis of randomized controlled trials. Anaesthesia. 2018;73:238–47.
37. Yeh DD, Van Der Wilden G, Cropano C, et al. Goal-directed diuresis: a case-control study of continuous furosemide infusion in critically ill trauma patients. J Emerg Trauma Shock. 2015;8:34.
38. Copeland JG, Campbell DW, Plachetka JR, Salomon NW, Larson DF. Diuresis with continuous infusion of furosemide after cardiac surgery. Am J Surg. 1983;146:796–9.
39. Palazzuoli A, Pellegrini M, Franci B, et al. Short- and long-term effects of continuous versus intermittent loop diuretic treatment in acute heart failure with renal dysfunction. Intern Emerg Med. 2015;10:41–9.
40. Caetano F, Mota P, Almeida I, Fernandes A, Botelho A, Leitão MA. Continuous infusion or bolus injection of loop diuretics for patients admitted for severe acute heart failure: is one strategy better than the other? Rev Port Cardiol. 2015;34:95–102.
41. Silbert BI, Ho KM, Lipman J, et al. Does furosemide increase oxidative stress in acute kidney injury? Antioxid Redox Signal. 2017;26:221–6.
42. Ter Maaten JM, Rao VS, Hanberg JS, et al. Renal tubular resistance is the primary driver for loop diuretic resistance in acute heart failure. Eur J Heart Fail. 2017;19:1014–22.

43. Mahmoodpoor A, Zahedi S, Pourakbar A, et al. Efficacy of furosemide-albumin compared with furosemide in critically ill hypoalbuminemic patients admitted to intensive care unit: a prospective randomized clinical trial. Daru. 2020;28:263–9.
44. Klinkmann G, Klammt S, Jäschke M, et al. Impact of albumin binding function on pharmacokinetics and pharmacodynamics of furosemide. Medicina (Kaunas). 2022;58:1780.
45. Martin GS, Moss M, Wheeler AP, Mealer M, Morris JA, Bernard GR. A randomized, controlled trial of furosemide with or without albumin in hypoproteinemic patients with acute lung injury*. Crit Care Med. 2005;33:1681–7.
46. Lee TH, Kuo G, Chang C-H, et al. Diuretic effect of co-administration of furosemide and albumin in comparison to furosemide therapy alone: an updated systematic review and meta-analysis. PLoS One. 2021;16:e0260312.
47. McDonagh TA, Metra M, Adamo M, et al. 2021 ESC guidelines for the diagnosis and treatment of acute and chronic heart failure. Eur Heart J. 2021;42:3599–726.
48. Verbrugge FH, Martens P, Ameloot K, et al. Acetazolamide to increase natriuresis in congestive heart failure at high risk for diuretic resistance. Eur J Heart Fail. 2019;21:1415–22.
49. Côté JM, Goulamhoussen N, McMahon BA, Murray PT. Diuretic combinations in critically ill patients with respiratory failure: a systematic review and meta-analysis. World J Crit Care Med. 2022;11:178–91.
50. Faisy C, Mokline A, Sanchez O, Tadié J-M, Fagon J-Y. Effectiveness of acetazolamide for reversal of metabolic alkalosis in weaning COPD patients from mechanical ventilation. Intensive Care Med. 2010;36:859–63.
51. Faisy C, Meziani F, Planquette B, et al. Effect of acetazolamide vs placebo on duration of invasive mechanical ventilation among patients with chronic obstructive pulmonary disease. JAMA. 2016;315:480.
52. Escudero VJ, Mercadal J, Molina-Andújar A, et al. New insights into diuretic use to treat congestion in the ICU: beyond furosemide. Front Nephrol. 2022:2.
53. Scharman EJ, Troutman WG. Prevention of kidney injury following rhabdomyolysis: a systematic review. Ann Pharmacother. 2013;47:90–105.
54. Somagutta MR, Pagad S, Sridharan S, et al. Role of bicarbonates and mannitol in rhabdomyolysis: a comprehensive review. Cureus. 2020;12:e9742.
55. van de Laar SC, Schouten GN, IJzermans JNM, Minnee RC. Effect of mannitol on kidney function after kidney transplantation: a systematic review and meta-analysis. Transplant Proc. 2021;53:2122–32.
56. Hoorn EJ, Ellison DH. Diuretic resistance. Am J Kidney Dis. 2017;69:136–42.
57. ter Maaten JM, Valente MAE, Damman K, Hillege HL, Navis G, Voors AA. Diuretic response in acute heart failure—pathophysiology, evaluation, and therapy. Nat Rev Cardiol. 2015;12:184–92.
58. Asare K. Management of loop diuretic resistance in the intensive care unit. Am J Health Syst Pharm. 2009;66:1635–40.
59. Liu FY, Cogan MG. Angiotensin II stimulates early proximal bicarbonate absorption in the rat by decreasing cyclic adenosine monophosphate. J Clin Invest. 1989;84:83–91.
60. Imiela T, Budaj A. Acetazolamide as add-on diuretic therapy in exacerbations of chronic heart failure: a pilot study. Clin Drug Investig. 2017;37:1175–81.
61. Bihari S, Holt AW, Prakash S, Bersten AD. Addition of indapamide to frusemide increases natriuresis and creatinine clearance, but not diuresis, in fluid overloaded ICU patients. J Crit Care. 2016;33:200–6.
62. Apte Y, Bellomo R, Warrillow S, Goldsmith D, Gillies M, McGain F. Pilot randomised double-blind controlled trial of high-dose spironolactone in critically ill patients receiving a frusemide infusion. Crit Care Resusc. 2008;10:306–11.
63. Kellum JA, Elbers PWG, editors. Stewart's textbook of acid-base. 2nd ed. Lulu Enterprises, UK Ltd; 2009.
64. Harrington JT, Hulter HN, Cohen JJ, Madias NE. Mineralocorticoid–stimulated renal acidification: the critical role of dietary sodium. Kidney Int. 1986;30:43–8.

65. Park M, et al. Metabolic alkalosis and mixed acid–base disturbance in anaesthesia and critical care. BJA Educ. 2023;4:128–35.
66. Kang KP, Lee S, Lee KH, Kang SK. Mannitol-induced metabolic alkalosis. Electrolyte Blood Press. 2006;4:61–5.
67. Zazzeron L, Ottolina D, Scotti E, et al. Real-time urinary electrolyte monitoring after furosemide administration in surgical ICU patients with normal renal function. Ann Intensive Care. 2016;6:72.

International Patient Safety Goals (IPSG) 24

Rita Cataldo, Rossana Alloni, and Sabrina Migliorelli

24.1 Introduction

The International Patient Safety Goals (IPSG) are a set of objectives established by the World Health Organization (WHO) to improve patient safety and the quality of healthcare worldwide. They were introduced into clinical practice by the Joint Commission International (JCI) starting in 2008 and have been progressively updated through 2023 [1]. The goals highlight key problem areas in healthcare delivery and describe expert consensus and *evidence-based* solutions, including guidelines and recommendations. The primary aim is to protect patients from preventable harm that may occur during medical treatment, to promote a culture of safety in healthcare, and to improve the quality of care provided to patients.

Patient safety should be understood as the prevention of errors associated with healthcare delivery [2] and the mitigation of their effects [3]. Safety is a right that ensures patients are free from accidental or preventable harm related to care [4]. Protecting this right requires the creation of systems that minimize the likelihood of

R. Cataldo (✉) · S. Migliorelli
Department of Anesthesia and Intensive Care, Fondazione Policlinico Universitario Campus BioMedico, Rome, Italy

Anesthesia and Intensive Care Research Unit, Department of Medicine and Surgery, Campus Bio-Medico University of Rome, Rome, Italy
e-mail: R.Cataldo@policlinicocampus.it; sabrina.migliorelli@policlinicocampus.it

R. Alloni
Fondazione Policlinico Universitario Campus Bio-Medico, Rome, Italy

General Surgery Research Unit, Department of Medicine and Surgery, Campus Bio-Medico University of Rome, Rome, Italy
e-mail: r.alloni@policlinicocampus.it

D. Chiumello, A. De Gasperi (eds.), *Practical Trends in Anesthesia and Intensive Care 2026*, https://doi.org/10.1007/978-3-032-25721-5_24

errors and maximize the ability to intercept them [5]. Although it is impossible to eliminate error entirely, harm and its impact on patients can certainly be limited. Patient safety is one of the three pillars of quality care, along with patient satisfaction and the provision of effective treatment [6]. Nevertheless, preventable patient harm remains a serious problem for health systems worldwide. The most striking indicator is the number of deaths attributable to preventable harm. In England, researchers attribute at least 3.6% of deaths in acute care hospitals to avoidable problems in care processes [7].

Below are the six International Patient Safety Goals (IPSG) currently recognized and accepted; each goal is developed through specific elements that make it applicable to the patient care process. Each goal must be implemented within individual healthcare facilities through specific guidelines and care processes that make it applicable to the patient, ultimately resulting in greater safety and quality. Implementing a virtuous pathway means developing proactive strategies aimed at reducing the risk of error by adopting best practices based on evidence and expert consensus.

To achieve this, it is first necessary to identify those risk factors, including local ones, that may lead to medical errors.

1. *Goal 1: Correct Patient Identification*
   - *IPSG.1* The hospital must develop and implement a process to improve the accuracy of patient identification.
2. *Goal 2: Improve the Effectiveness of Communication*
   - *IPSG.2* The hospital must develop and implement a process to improve the effectiveness of verbal and/or telephone communication among healthcare professionals.
   - *IPSG.2.1* The hospital must develop and implement a process for communicating critical results of diagnostic tests.
   - *IPSG.2.2* The hospital must develop and implement a process for communication during handover.
3. *Goal 3: Improve the Safety of High-Alert Medications*
   - *IPSG.3* The hospital must develop and implement a process to improve the safety of high-alert medications.
   - *IPSG.3.1* The hospital must develop and implement a process to improve the management of LASA (Look-Alike Sound-Alike) medications.
   - *IPSG.3.2* The hospital must develop and implement a process for the management and safe use of concentrated electrolytes.
4. *Goal 4: Ensure Surgical Safety*
   - *IPSG.4* The hospital must develop and implement a process for preoperative verification and for marking the site of the surgical/invasive procedure.
   - *IPSG.4.1* The hospital must develop and implement a process for conducting the *time-out* immediately before the start of the surgical/invasive procedure, and the *sign-out* at the end of the procedure.

5. *Goal 5: Reduce the Risk of Healthcare-Associated Infections*
   - *IPSG.5* The hospital must adopt and implement hand hygiene guidelines based on scientific evidence of effectiveness in order to reduce the risk of healthcare-associated infections.
   - *IPSG.5.1* Hospital leaders must identify care processes that can be improved and adopt and implement *evidence-based* interventions to improve patient health outcomes and reduce the risk of hospital-acquired infections.
6. *Goal 6: Reduce Harm Caused by Diagnostic Errors*
   - *IPSG.6* The hospital must implement processes to reduce harm caused by diagnostic errors.

24.2 Objective 1: Correctly Identify the Patient [1]

Errors in patient identification, such as performing a procedure on the wrong patient, unfortunately occur frequently in clinical practice; such errors can lead to serious consequences for the patient, including disability, prolonged hospitalization, and increased social costs. IPSG Goal 1 aims to prevent these errors by ensuring that any healthcare intervention (meal delivery, medication administration, blood transfusion, blood sampling, invasive procedure, etc.) is performed on the correct patient.

24.2.1 IPSG.1 Standard

The hospital must implement a process to improve the accuracy of patient identification [8].

24.2.2 Purpose of IPSG.1

Incorrect patient identification can result in procedural and treatment errors, medication administration errors, diagnostic errors, and more. All of these errors can cause harm to the patient.

24.2.3 Guidance for IPSG.1

Correct patient identification and matching with the intended treatment and services must be performed in all care settings [9]. The identification process used throughout the hospital must always involve two associated patient identifiers, chosen from: patient name, identification number, date of birth, a barcode wristband, and others; these must be checked in every circumstance preceding any intervention or even simple procedure on the patient [10]. Patients must be identified before administering medications or invasive treatments, performing procedures, or conducting any diagnostic maneuvers [11]. The patient's room or bed number, or their location within the hospital, must never be used for identification, not even as a secondary identifier [12]. Best practice also involves actively engaging the patient in the identification process whenever possible, by directly asking them to confirm their identifying information [13]. Procedures should be established for special circumstances where the identification process may require an alternative approach, such as for comatose or confused/disoriented patients without identification documents, or for newborns [14–17]; in addition, blood samples, biological material, histological specimens, meal trays, expressed breast milk, and all biological sample tubes should be labeled with dual identification.

24.3 Objective 2: Improve the Effectiveness of Communication [1]

Communication errors or delays at various levels, during handovers between colleagues, or in communicating laboratory or pathology results, are common and can lead to diagnostic and therapeutic errors. Oral or telephone communications/prescriptions are the leading cause of such communication errors and should, if possible, be avoided or at least regulated and standardized. The handover process, which is specifically intended for sharing and communicating patient data, is given particular emphasis. IPSG Goal 2 aims to ensure that the communication of clinical data regarding patients, especially those in critical condition, is smooth, rapid, and safe.

24.3.1 IPSG.2 Standard

The hospital must develop and implement a process to improve the effectiveness of verbal and/or telephone communication among healthcare providers.

24.3.2 IPSG.2.1 Standard

The hospital must develop and implement a process for reporting critical diagnostic test results.

24.3.3 IPSG.2.2 Standard

The hospital must develop and implement a process for communication during *handover* (shift change).

24.3.4 Guidance for IPSG.2, IPSG 2.1, and IPSG 2.2

Effective, timely, accurate, complete, and unambiguous communication that is correctly understood by the recipient reduces errors and improves patient safety [18].

Communication may occur verbally, electronically, or in writing on paper. Care situations that may be critically compromised by poor communication include verbal and telephone orders for patient care, verbal and telephone communication of critical diagnostic results, and communications during handover.

Clinical orders for patients that are given verbally or by telephone, where permitted by local regulations, are among the communications most prone to error. Dialects, inflections, different accents, a multicultural workforce, background noise, and similar factors can make it difficult for the recipient to correctly understand the order. For example, drug names and numbers that sound similar, such as erythromycin and azithromycin or six and seven, can compromise the accuracy of the order. The problem is often exacerbated by interruptions, distractions, and the use of unfamiliar terms or drug names. As soon as a verbal order is received, it must be transcribed into a written prescription, which adds complexity and risk to the prescribing process.

The communication of critical results from diagnostic tests also represents a challenge from the perspective of patient safety. A critical result is defined as a deviation from the normal reference range that indicates a pathophysiological state exposing the patient to a high risk or imminent life-threatening danger, requiring urgent or emergency intervention, and likely necessitating immediate medical action to preserve the patient's life or prevent a catastrophic event. A critical result differs from an abnormal or pathological result, which is defined as a result outside the expected reference range for the test type but does not pose a life threat. Critical results may concern both outpatients and inpatients, whether in critical care areas or standard wards.

Therefore, a formal reporting system must be implemented throughout the hospital to clearly define the procedures for communicating critical diagnostic test results to clinicians and for documenting this information. The goal is to communicate the critical result accurately and within a predetermined timeframe so that the responsible clinician can assess its significance in light of the patient's clinical condition and implement appropriate care strategies.

Clinical *handover* communications involve the exchange of up-to-date patient information and the transfer of responsibility or accountability for patient care [18]. *Handovers* within a hospital occur [19]:

- Between healthcare professionals (e.g., from physician to physician, physician to nurse, nurse to nurse, and so on)
- Between different levels of care within the same hospital (for example, when a patient is transferred from an intensive care unit to a general ward or from the emergency department to the operating room)
- From a ward to a diagnostic department or to a service for tests or treatments, such as radiology or physiotherapy
- Between healthcare professionals and patients/families/caregivers, for example, at discharge

A lack of clarity in communication during any *handover* can lead to adverse events. Interruptions and other distractions caused by unit activities can hinder the clear transmission of important patient information. Standardizing the critical content to be communicated among healthcare professionals, patients, families, and caregivers can significantly improve the outcomes of *handovers* [20].

Standardized forms, tools, or methods can support a consistent and comprehensive process for conducting *handovers* and should be provided [21]. The *handover* process may vary depending on the specific *needs and areas within the same hospital.* For example, the *handover* from the emergency department to a medical ward may require different procedures or content compared to that from the operating room to the intensive care unit; however, in all cases, *handovers* should be standardized within the various areas of healthcare facilities by selecting and implementing one of the established communication methods (SBAR, I-PASS, *Bedside nursing handover*, etc.).

Safe practices for effective communication require that hospital procedures define [22]:

- The restriction of verbal communication of diagnostic and therapeutic prescriptions to urgent situations in which it is not immediately possible to transmit information in writing or via electronic medical records. For example, verbal prescriptions are not permitted when the prescriber is present in the hospital, and the patient's medical record is available. Verbal prescriptions may be allowed in situations where it is difficult or impossible to transmit the prescription on paper or electronically, such as during a sterile procedure.
- Guidelines for requesting diagnostic tests in urgent or emergency situations and for receiving the results of such tests, for identifying and defining critical tests and critical values, and for recording to whom and by whom the reports of critical diagnostic results are communicated.
- That the person receiving telephone or verbal information writes down or enters into the computer the complete prescription or test result as dictated; once finished, reads back aloud the prescription or test result; waits for confirmation of the accuracy of what was written and read back from the other operator (*read back-repeat back*). Acceptable alternatives may be identified for cases in which the read-back process may not always be possible, such as in the operating room or in emergency situations in the emergency department or intensive care unit.
- The use of standardized methods, forms, or tools to facilitate complete and consistent *handovers.*

24.4 Objective 3: Improving the Safety of High-Alert Medications [1]

Errors in the medication "supply chain," from storage to administration, remain surprisingly frequent and are a cause of deaths and permanent harm. Some medications are particularly dangerous and are classified as "high-alert." The goal of ensuring the safety of the hospital medication process is fundamental in every hospital [23].

24.4.1 IPSG.3 Standard

The hospital must develop and implement a process to improve the safety of high-alert medications.

24.4.2 Purpose of IPSG.3

Errors involving high-risk medications can cause patient injury or death and may potentially generate additional costs related to the care of these patients [24].

24.4.3 Guidance for IPSG.3

The Institute for Safe Medication Practices (ISMP) defines high-risk medications as "…medications that bear a heightened risk of causing significant patient harm when used in error." [25] The most frequently cited examples of high-risk medications for adverse outcomes include insulin, opioids, chemotherapeutic agents, antithrombotic agents, anticoagulants, thrombolytics, drugs with a narrow therapeutic index (such as digitalis), neuromuscular blocking agents, and medications administered via epidural or intrathecal routes [26]. Examples of high-risk medication lists are readily available online from international organizations such as the *Institute for Safe Medication Practices* (ISMP) and the *World Health Organization* (WHO). For safe management, the hospital must develop its own list(s) of high-risk medications based on its specific patterns of medication use, internal data on near-misses, medication-related errors, sentinel events, and safety issues published in the scientific literature [27]. Information from the literature and/or the Ministry of Health may also be useful in identifying which medications should be included [28]. This list is updated at least annually, but may need to be revised more frequently in the event of additions or changes. Some high-risk medications or categories (such as neuromuscular blocking agents) have their own specific set of risks, in addition to those associated with being high-risk [29]. It is the hospital's responsibility to determine when a tailored strategy is needed in addition to standard measures. For example, neuromuscular blocking agents may be mistakenly confused when stored with other refrigerated medications. A strategy to reduce this risk is to store neuromuscular blocking agents separately from other medications, for example, in closed containers with prominent warning labels on both the container and the medications inside. Other examples include chemotherapeutic agents or insulin.

The overall process for managing high-risk medications must be standardized throughout the hospital, for example, through standardized labeling of high-risk medications and mandatory double-check procedures [30].

According to ISMP [26], examples of best practices include: standardizing processes related to storage, handling, preparation, and administration of medications; improving access to medication information; limiting staff access to high-risk medications; using additional labels and warnings; introducing redundancies in the medication management process such as double-check procedures, or reducing the available administration options (e.g., limiting the available concentrations of the same medication), and designating areas where the DO NOT DISTURB rule applies, allowing staff to avoid distractions during the handling and preparation of medications for administration.

24.4.4 IPSG.3.1 Standard

The hospital develops and implements a process to improve the safety of LASA (Look-Alike/Sound-Alike) medications.

24.4.5 Purpose of IPSG.3.1

Medications with similar packaging or names that sound alike can be easily confused by healthcare professionals and may lead to medication administration errors that can be potentially harmful and must therefore be properly managed.

24.4.6 Guidance for IPSG.3.1

Medications that look alike or sound alike (LASA) are very similar in their *packaging* or have names that can be confused with one another [31]. Similar medication packaging refers to vials or primary packaging that resemble those of another medication [32]. Examples of medications that sound or look similar to others [33] include, for instance, dopamine and dobutamine, or adrenaline and noradrenaline, which sound similar and whose printed names and packaging may also appear similar. LASA medications are a common cause of medication administration errors worldwide. Contributing factors to this confusion include: incomplete knowledge of drug names; newly marketed products and therefore new packaging as well; *packaging* or similar labeling, such as those from the same pharmaceutical company; similar clinical use; prescriptions written illegibly or misunderstandings during verbal orders [34].

Hospitals must determine which medications require safety measures to prevent LASA-related errors and must establish risk management strategies to improve patient safety [35]. Strategies should include, but are not limited to:

- Using both the brand name and the generic name on prescriptions and labels;
- Including the purpose of the medication on prescriptions
- Configuring safety features in computerized prescribing systems to require a minimum number of letters, for example, at least five letters, when healthcare professionals search for a medication by name
- Differentiating the appearance of similar drug names as much as possible, for example, by using so-called *TALLman lettering* on labels by inserting uppercase letters, such as DOBUTamine and DOPamine or oxyBUTynin and oxyCONTIN

The hospital should also stay up to date on emerging strategies, Good Clinical Practices, and national and international guidelines published to prevent LASA errors according to its available resources.

The risks of LASA-related errors are not limited to prescribing and dispensing. Other strategies to prevent LASA errors include avoiding the storage of these medications in close proximity, where a healthcare professional might accidentally select the wrong one for dispensing or administration. The hospital's process should also include a mechanism to reassess whether a LASA risk exists every time (frequently) the hospital needs to substitute medications to address shortages, for example, when replacing a drug with another brand that has similar packaging or a trade name similar to an existing one in the formulary. The hospital should implement a comprehensive approach to managing LASA medications, starting from pharmacy procurement, where decisions are made regarding brands (trade names, label appearance), and extending throughout the medication pathway to the staff who handle and administer them.

A separate section concerns concentrated electrolyte solutions.

24.4.7 IPSG.3.2 Standard

The hospital must develop and implement a process for the management and safe use of concentrated electrolytes.

24.4.8 Purpose of IPSG.3.2

Incorrect or unintentional administration of concentrated electrolytes can cause fatal errors, and the most effective way to reduce or eliminate such incidents is to implement a process for managing these medications.

24.4.9 Guidance for IPSG.3.2

Concentrated electrolytes are vials of concentrated electrolyte forms that require dilution or other preparation before intravenous administration. These include, but are not limited to: potassium chloride, potassium phosphate, magnesium sulfate, calcium chloride, and high-concentration sodium chloride.

Concentrated electrolytes should not be available or stored in *any* patient care unit (including the operating room/anesthesia department) whenever possible, considering the pharmacy's ability to provide immediate intervention. Where it is necessary to store concentrated electrolytes in intensive care units, they must be kept separate, labeled box by box and vial by vial, and must also display appropriate warnings (e.g., "CONCENTRATED ELECTROLYTE—Dilute before administration"). The dispensing or handling of concentrated electrolyte vials in patient care units (wards) should be prohibited by hospital policy.

The administration of electrolyte replacement therapy for hypokalemia, hyponatremia, and hypocalcemia is safer when standardized guidelines and/or shared internal protocols are used, and with pre-diluted electrolytes (such as 20 mEq of potassium chloride in 100 cc of normal saline).

24.5 Objective 4: Ensure Safety in Surgery [1]

Performing the correct procedure at the correct site, on the correct side, is another of the quality and safety principles of the IPSG; procedural errors and perhaps even more frequently errors in laterality of paired organs/limbs unfortunately still occur often. The Ministry of Health developed several years ago (2009) a "Manual for Safety in the Operating Room: Recommendations and Checklist" to which IPSG standards can be integrated [28].

24.5.1 IPSG.4 Standard

The hospital must implement a process for preoperative verification and for marking the surgical/invasive procedure site.

24.5.2 Purpose of IPSG.4

Errors regarding the patient, the surgical site, and the type of surgical procedure represent a safety risk, cause harm to the patient, and result in social costs [36].

24.5.3 Guidelines for IPSG.4

Errors involving the wrong patient, wrong site, and wrong procedure can result from ineffective or inadequate communication among members of the surgical team [37]. Common risk factors include:

- Lack of a standardized process for marking the procedural site
- Use of materials or methods that can be easily removed, such as adhesive tape or ink that may be washed off during sterile preparation of the surgical field
- Lack of active patient involvement in marking the site
- Inadequate preoperative patient assessment
- Insufficient review of the medical record
- Lack of clear communication among *team* members
- Issues related to illegible handwriting
- Use of unauthorized and non-standardized abbreviations

Surgical and invasive procedures in general include all procedures involving an incision or puncture, including but not limited to: open surgical procedures, percutaneous procedures, injections, biopsies, diagnostic or interventional cardiac and vascular procedures, laparoscopies, and endoscopies. For this reason, all areas within the hospital where surgical and invasive procedures are performed must be identified and protocolled, for example: operating rooms, cardiac catheterization labs, interventional radiology, endoscopy, and intensive care units [38].

The Joint Commission Universal Protocol "Universal Protocol for Preventing Wrong Site, Wrong Procedure, Wrong Person Surgery" [1] is based on the principle of using multimodal strategies to achieve the goal of always identifying the correct patient, the correct procedure, and the correct site. The essential elements of the Universal Protocol are the preoperative verification process (*Sign-in*), surgical site marking, and the *time-out* conducted immediately before the start of the procedure, as part of the perioperative checklist consisting of *Sign-in*, *Time-out*, and *Sign-out* [39, 40].

24.5.3.1 Preoperative Verification Process (*Sign-In*)

Preoperative verification is a continuous process of gathering and confirming information. The purpose of the preoperative verification process is to:

- Verify the correct patient, procedure, and site
- Ensure that all relevant documents, images, and investigations are available, properly labeled, and displayed
- Confirm that any required blood products and medical or surgical devices are present
- Assess specific risk factors such as anticipated difficult airway management

24.5.3.2 Surgical Site Marking

Surgical site marking can be performed in the preoperative waiting area, the day surgery unit (DSU), or patient units, before entering the operating/procedural room, by a physician who will participate in the entire procedure. In the case of surgical procedures, the responsible surgeon who will perform the operation usually marks the site. For nonsurgical invasive procedures, the operator is always responsible for identification. The hospital should specify and clarify who is authorized to perform surgical site marking in its policies, procedures, or medical staff documentation. According to international standards, there are circumstances in which a trainee physician or other designated authorized individual may perform site marking, specifically when the trainee will perform the entire procedure, requiring minimal or no supervision from the surgeon or responsible physician. In these cases, the trainee marks the surgical site. When a trainee acts as an assistant to the surgeon or responsible physician, unless otherwise specified in the procedure, only the latter may perform the site marking. University hospitals and hospitals hosting specialist trainees should explicitly regulate such cases in their internal procedures.

Surgical site marking can be performed at any time before the start of the surgical/invasive procedure, provided the patient is actively involved (i.e., awake and alert), and is done with a mark that is immediately recognizable, shared, and unambiguous. The mark must remain visible even after the patient has been prepared and the surgical site draped, so that it can be verified during the final *timeout*. Examples of situations where patient participation may not be possible include: patients who are not competent, children and patients requiring emergency surgery, and patients who have already received sedation prior to *sign-in*. Ideally, the "X" should not be used as a mark, as it could be interpreted as "not here" or "wrong side" and could potentially lead to errors in patient care. Other ambiguous marks, such as a line or a dot, should also be avoided. The mark must be distinctive, standardized, and therefore the same for all procedures performed within the hospital. The site should be marked in all cases involving laterality, multiple structures (fingers or toes, lesions), or multiple levels (spine).

24.5.4 IPSG.4.1 Standard

The hospital implements a process for the *time-out* to be performed immediately before the start of the surgical/invasive procedure, and a *sign-out* to be conducted after the procedure.

24.5.5 Purpose of IPSG.4.1

The *time-out* allows for the resolution of any preoperative uncertainties and provides a final opportunity to identify potential errors such as wrong-site surgery, wrong-patient surgery, or the wrong procedure on the correct patient. The *sign-out,* performed after surgery, allows for the identification of areas needing improvement and highlights any critical issues that arose during the procedure, enabling enhancements and optimization of surgical processes as a whole.

24.5.6 Guidelines for IPSG.4.1

The *time-out* applies to all surgical and non-surgical invasive procedures, both inside and outside the operating room, including, for example, endoscopy, hemodynamics, ICU, etc. Evidence indicates that procedures posing the greatest risk to patients are those involving general anesthesia or deep sedation.

24.5.6.1 Time-Out

The *time-out* is performed immediately before the start of the procedure with all team members present. The *team* agrees on the following components:

- Correct patient identity
- Correct procedure to be performed
- Correct site for the surgical/invasive procedure

The *time-out* is conducted at the location where the procedure will be performed, in the presence of the patient, and involves the active participation of the entire *team*. The patient is not required to participate in the *time-out*. Completion of the *time-out* is documented and includes the date and time it was completed.

24.5.6.2 Sign-Out

The WHO Surgical Safety Checklist [41] includes a *sign-out* process, which is conducted in the area where the procedure was performed. The following components of the *sign-out* are verbally confirmed by a member of the *team*, usually a nurse:

- Name of the surgical/invasive procedure that has been recorded/written
- Completion of instrument, sponge, and needle counts (if applicable)
- Labeling of specimens (when specimens are present during the *sign-out* process, labels are read aloud, including the patient's name)
- Any equipment issues (if applicable)
- Process-related critical issues, any problems encountered

24.6 Goal 5: Reduce the Risk of Healthcare-Associated Infections [1]

The global problem of the risks, mortality, morbidity, and healthcare costs associated with infections acquired in healthcare settings is well known and remains extremely serious [42]. Procedures that help contain this risk are sometimes remarkably simple, such as handwashing [43]. Following certain *evidence-based* recommendations can change patient *outcomes*.

24.6.1 IPSG.5 Standard

The hospital must adopt and implement evidence-based hand hygiene guidelines in order to reduce the risk of healthcare-associated infections.

24.6.2 IPSG.5.1 Standard

The hospital management identifies care processes that can be improved and adopts and implements evidence-based interventions to improve patient health outcomes and reduce the risk of hospital-acquired infections.

24.6.3 Purpose of IPSG.5 and IPSG.5.1

Proper hand hygiene is essential for containing infections associated with hospitalization and other healthcare-related infections.

24.6.4 Guidance for IPSG.5 and IPSG 5.1

Infection prevention and control present a range of challenges in most healthcare facilities, and the increasing rates of healthcare-associated infections are a major source of concern for both patients and healthcare professionals [44, 45]. The most frequent and common infections across all healthcare settings include urinary tract infections associated with bladder catheterization, bloodstream infections [46], and pneumonia (often associated with mechanical ventilation [47]).

A key factor in eliminating these and other infections is proper hand hygiene [48]. Evidence-based hand hygiene guidelines are available from the World Health Organization (WHO) [49], the US Centers for Disease Control and Prevention (CDC) [50], the Ministry of Health [28], and various other national and international organizations.

The hospital must therefore adopt and implement up-to-date evidence-based hand hygiene guidelines. These should be displayed using posters in appropriate areas, and staff must be trained in correct hand hygiene and washing procedures. Detergents, disinfectants, wipes, or other suitable means for washing and drying hands must be placed in areas where hand hygiene and washing procedures are required.

Certain treatments and healthcare procedures have been identified as major sources of hospital-acquired infections, such as surgical interventions, mechanical ventilation, and the placement of central venous or indwelling catheters. A hospital-acquired infection can severely and negatively affect a patient's clinical, emotional, and economic well-being, as it represents a significant source of complications that may result in further illnesses and even patient death [51]. Many of these infections are preventable: scientific studies suggest that implementing practices designed to prevent hospital-acquired infections can lead to a reduction of up to 70% [52].

In 2001, the Institute for Healthcare Improvement (IHI) [53] began developing and testing a concept to promote communication and teamwork within multidisciplinary teams to improve the clinical care provided to patients. This initiative led to the creation of so-called bundles of care. The IHI defines a bundle as "a set of evidence-based interventions, targeted at a specific patient population or care setting, which, when implemented together, result in significantly better outcomes than when implemented individually." [53] Examples of bundles include those for the prevention of central line-associated bloodstream infection (CLABSI) [54], prevention of ventilator-associated pneumonia (VAP) [55], prevention of catheter-associated urinary tract infection (CAUTI) [56], prevention of surgical site infection (SSI) [57–59], and prevention of severe sepsis [60].

The implementation of bundles has the greatest impact on patient outcomes when the hospital identifies gaps in the application of best practices or the persistence of negative outcomes in a particular care setting. Evidence-based bundles for infection prevention and control have been shown to have a greater impact on reducing infection risk than the implementation of individual improvement strategies. It is important for hospital management to declare, implement, and assess staff adherence to bundles, and to monitor improvements in outcomes, fostering teamwork and motivating healthcare professionals.

Perhaps the most direct way to achieve improvement in device-associated infections is to limit their use to the minimum necessary.

Maximize their use by structuring strategies (such as ERAS pathways) that drastically reduce the use of urinary catheters and central venous catheters, as well as by promoting a culture of appropriate antibiotic use and surgical site infection prevention (rules on hair removal, operating room dress code, quality of skin disinfectant, etc.); improving the prevention of cross-transmission of infections through routine and standardized identification of high-risk nosocomial isolates (MRSA, *K. pneumoniae* MDR, *C. difficile*, *P. aeruginosa*, etc.) can be another area of effective intervention.

24.7 Objective 6: Reduce Harm Caused by Diagnostic Errors [1]

Objective 6 has been updated compared to the 2021 IPSG version. Until then, the identified objective was to reduce the risk of patient harm resulting from falls in the hospital setting (inpatients and outpatients). In the 2023 version of the Joint Commission, the focus is instead on identifying and implementing strategies to reduce patient harm caused by diagnostic errors.

24.7.1 IPSG.6 Standard

The hospital must implement processes to reduce harm caused by diagnostic errors.

24.7.2 Intent of IPSG.6

Diagnostic errors are one of the leading causes of preventable harm in healthcare, and hospitals have a responsibility to minimize harm to their patients by identifying and addressing the causes of diagnostic errors [61, 62].

24.7.3 Guidelines for IPSG.6

"Diagnostic errors" refer to missed, incorrect, or delayed diagnoses, as evidenced by subsequent test results [63]. According to the Society of Diagnostic Medicine, a delayed diagnosis is one in which the diagnosis could and should have been made earlier than when the definitive diagnosis was actually established [64, 65]. Delayed diagnosis of oncological diseases is by far the most common entity in this category. An incorrect diagnosis occurs, for example, when a patient with a myocardial infarction is told that their pain is due to gastroesophageal reflux disease. The diagnosis is later found to be incorrect when the true cause is discovered after some time. Many patients with chronic fatigue or chronic pain are at risk of falling into this category, as are patients with more specific symptoms that are nonetheless not correctly diagnosed. According to a Harvard study, diagnostic errors account for 17% of preventable errors in patients [66]. Other studies [67] estimate diagnostic errors at 10%, while autopsy findings suggest an error rate ranging from 5% to 25% [68]. Another study from Johns Hopkins found that the most common diagnostic errors occur in cases of vascular events, neoplasms, and infections [69]. These are also, unsurprisingly, a major cause of medical malpractice claims.

The causes of diagnostic errors are complex and rarely attributable to the fault of a single clinician or staff member [70]. Factors leading to diagnostic errors range from diagnostic complexity, poor communication or care coordination [71], loss of certain diagnostic results, equipment malfunction, shortage of specialists, to cognitive errors or *bias* [72, 73]. The latter is particularly insidious because it is difficult to recognize and avoid: these are situations in which the clinician reaches a diagnosis by following habitual reasoning, uncritically, without considering alternative possible diagnoses. For example, a patient with acute neck pain and a history of chronic neck pain who presents to the emergency department with an exacerbation of neck pain may be "labeled" based on the known diagnosis of chronic pain, without considering that some features of the current pain differ from the history and should prompt consideration of acute myocardial infarction or meningeal irritation.

The impact of communication on diagnostic error can be significant; for this reason, some authors [74] refer to closed-loop communication as a safety factor: it ensures that the information transmitted has been correctly received and has led to an action consistent with the diagnosis [75]. In particular, communications given to caregivers or the patient after a diagnostic test, when the patient is no longer present in the facility, are at risk. If there is no well-defined process for conveying information to the patient or their caregiver, delays in further diagnostic workup and/or initiation of necessary therapy may occur for various reasons, resulting in harm of varying severity to the patient.

To improve communication of diagnostic test results, it is therefore advisable to:

- Identify at-risk workflows and processes and implement even redundant procedures to ensure that test results are received by someone responsible for the care of the patient concerned and that errors are more likely to be detected early. These procedures should also address the transfer of information between clinicians and handovers between different clinical settings.
- Establish standardized processes to ensure prompt communication of abnormal clinical investigation results to the physician responsible for patient care.
- Verbally notify patients of potentially risky test results and ensure that the patient has understood the information.
- Implement a process to ensure that, at the end of a shift, the responsibility to inform the patient of a potentially risky test result is handed over to the next colleague.

- Ensure that diagnostic test results are communicated promptly to another clinician if the ordering provider is unavailable, especially if the result exposes the patient to a high risk.
- Optimize information technology systems for communicating test results. Technology can be used to automate certain actions. However, IT systems should not be the sole method for communicating abnormal results to healthcare professionals and patients, as closing the follow-up *loop* can be affected by various nontechnical factors, including user behavior, the way electronic health records are used, institutional policies, training, organizational factors, and workflow.
- Improve patient portals to facilitate patient access to their diagnostic test results and medical history. Improvements may include ensuring the portal is accessible from both desktop and mobile devices, explaining the meaning of certain diagnostic results within the portal, providing patients with easy access to support services for treatment and follow-up, etc. The best form of communication of results to patients remains verbal communication: clinicians should not assume that patients necessarily use *online* portals. Some patients may feel uncomfortable or be unfamiliar with online portals and may prefer direct, verbal communication—consider, for example, elderly patients or those with visual or motor impairments.

Key areas to focus on for identifying and preventing diagnostic errors include: radiological screening, anatomical pathology, certain specific laboratory investigations such as microbiology tests, newborn disease screening—including metabolic disorders—and results indicative of pathological processes that may be asymptomatic, etc.

To implement this IPSG and foster a culture of error recognition in the diagnostic process to contain it, hospitals should analyze their own errors and risks and select at least one area of focus each year (radiology, anatomical pathology, or laboratory, etc.), and provide training and support to clinical staff on diagnostic errors, promoting a culture of "no blame" but rather of "learning" focused on diagnostic errors that have occurred [71].

24.8 Conclusions

Healthcare professionals should always keep in mind the principle of "primum non nocere" (Hippocrates (460–377 BC)), which is fundamental to ensuring high-quality care.

The goal of making healthcare safer involves management, professionals, and patients equally: safety is a key component of any quality improvement initiative.

The development and implementation of evidence-based risk containment and safety and quality improvement strategies in care could lead to significant improvements in clinical practice, also reducing overall healthcare costs.

References

1. Joint Commission International. International Patient Safety Goals. Jt. Comm. Int. – Accredited Organ. 2023 [Online]. Available: https://www.jointcommissioninternational.org/standards/international-patient-safety-goals/.
2. World Health Organization (WHO). Towards eliminating avoidable harm in health care-GLOBAL PATIENT SAFETY ACTION PLAN 2021–2030.
3. Emanuel L, et al. What exactly is patient safety? J Med Regul. 2008;95(1):13–24. https://doi.org/10.30770/2572-1852-95.1.13.
4. Chassin MR, Galvin RW, Donaldson MS. The urgent need to improve health care quality. Institute of Medicine National Roundtable on Health Care Quality. JAMA. 1998;280(11):1000–5. https://doi.org/10.1001/JAMA.280.11.1000.
5. Marinelarena M. Angood P, Colchamiro E, Lyzenga A. Meeting of the National Quality Forum Patient Safety Team. Washington, DC; 2009.
6. Maybin J, Thorlby R. Briefing: high quality care for all – Jo Maybin, Ruth Thorlby – The King's Fund, July 2008. 2008, Accessed: Feb. 14, 2024 [Online]. Available: www.kingsfund.org.uk.
7. H. Hogan, R. Zipfel, J. Neuburger, A. Hutchings, A. Darzi, and N. Black, "Avoidability of hospital deaths and association with hospital-wide mortality ratios: retrospective case record review and regression analysis," *BMJ*, vol. 351, Jul. 2015, doi:https://doi.org/10.1136/BMJ.H3239.
8. Sabatelli G, et al. Guidance document for the correct identification of the patient. Reg Lazio. 2020;
9. Solomon RP, et al. ECRI Institute. ECRI Institute PSO Deep Dive: Patient Identification: Executive Summary. 2016. Accessed: Feb. 11, 2024. [Online]. Available: https://www.ecri.org/resource-center/Pages/.
10. "People, processes, health IT and accurate patient identification – Quick Safety," 2018. https://www.jointcommission.org/-/media/tjc/newsletters/qs_hit_and_patient_id_9_25_18_finalpdf. Accessed 11 Feb 2024.
11. Riplinger L, Piera-Jiménez J, Dooling JP. Patient identification techniques-approaches, implications, and findings. 2020. https://doi.org/10.1055/s-0040-1701984.
12. ECRI Institute. Patient Identification Errors Policy Statement. 2016. Accessed: Feb. 11, 2024. [Online]. Available: http://www.ecri.org/patientid.
13. Hughes P, et al. Preventing patient identification errors – patient safety & quality healthcare." https://www.psqh.com/analysis/preventing-patient-identification-errors/. Accessed 11 Feb 2024.
14. Singh H, et al. IDENTIFY for making healthcare safer together PARTNERSHIP health IT patient safety health IT safe practices: toolkit for the safe use of health IT for patient identification. 2017.
15. Pereira A, et al. The importance of newborn identification to the delivery of safe patient care identification of the patient in neonatology for safe care identification of the patient in neonatology for safe care. 22:49501, 2017, https://doi.org/10.5380/ce.v22i3.49501.
16. Adelman JS, et al. Risk of wrong-patient orders among multiple vs singleton births in the neonatal intensive care units of 2 integrated health care systems. JAMA Pediatr. 2019;173(10):979. https://doi.org/10.1001/JAMAPEDIATRICS.2019.2733.
17. Härkänen M, Tiainen M, Haatainen K. Wrong-patient incidents during medication administrations. J Clin Nurs. 2018;27(3–4):715–24. https://doi.org/10.1111/JOCN.14021.
18. Buurman BM, et al. Improving handoff communication from hospital to home: the development, implementation and evaluation of a personalized patient discharge letter. Int J Qual Health Care J Int Soc Qual Health Care. 2016;28(3):384–90. https://doi.org/10.1093/INTQHC/MZW046.

19. Patton LJ, Tidwell JD, Falder-Saeed KL, Young VB, Lewis BD, Binder JF. Ensuring safe transfer of pediatric patients: a quality improvement project to standardize handoff communication. J Pediatr Nurs. 2017;34:44–52. https://doi.org/10.1016/j.pedn.2017.01.004.
20. The Joint Commission. Inadequate hand-off communication. Sentinel Event Alert. 2017. https://www.jointcommission.org/-/media/tjc/documents/resources/patient-safety-topics/sentinel-event/sea_58_hand_off_comms_9_6_17_final_(1).pdf. Accessed 11 Feb 2024.
21. Nasarwanji MF, Badir A, Gurses AP. Standardizing handoff communication: content analysis of 27 handoff mnemonics. J Nurs Care Qual. 2016;31(3):238–44. https://doi.org/10.1097/NCQ.0000000000000174.
22. Starmer AJ, et al. Effects of the I-PASS nursing handoff bundle on communication quality and workflow. BMJ Qual Saf. 2017;26(12):949–57. https://doi.org/10.1136/BMJQS-2016-006224.
23. Italian Society of Anesthesia, Analgesia, Resuscitation and Intensive Care – SIAARTI (2019). Good Clinical Practices. Safety in the management of drugs in the Operating Room, Intensive Care, Pain Therapy, and Emergency. 2019.
24. Ferracini FT, et al. Using positive deviance to reduce medication errors in a tertiary care hospital. BMC Pharmacol Toxicol. 2016;17(1):1–8. https://doi.org/10.1186/S40360-016-0082-9/TABLES/5.
25. Dispensing Sample Medications: Patient Safety Strategies | Institute For Safe Medication Practices. https://www.ismp.org/news/dispensing-sample-medications-patient-safety-strategies. Accessed 16 Feb 2024.
26. Institute for Safe Medication Practices. ISMP List of High-Alert Medications in Acute Care Settings. 2018. https://www.ismp.org/sites/default/files/attachments/2018-08/highAlert2018-Acute-Final.pdf. Accessed 11 Feb 2024.
27. Speth J. Guidelines in practice: medication safety. AORN J. 2023;118(6):380–9. https://doi.org/10.1002/AORN.14034.
28. Ministry of Health – Department of Quality. Quality and safety of care in the use of medicines. 2010, Accessed: Feb 14, 2024. [Online]. Available: http://www.salute.gov.it/qualita/qualita.jsp.
29. Tyynismaa L, Honkala A, Airaksinen M, Shermock K, Lehtonen L. Identifying high-alert medications in a university hospital by applying data from the medication error reporting system. J Patient Saf. 2021;17(6):417–24. https://doi.org/10.1097/PTS.0000000000000388.
30. Elliott RA, Camacho E, Jankovic D, Sculpher MJ, Faria R. Economic analysis of the prevalence and clinical and economic burden of medication error in England. BMJ Qual Saf. 2021;30(2):96–105. https://doi.org/10.1136/BMJQS-2019-010206.
31. Lizano-Díez I, Figueiredo-Escribá C, Piñero-López MÁ, Lastra CF, Mariño EL, Modamio P. Prevention strategies to identify LASA errors: building and sustaining a culture of patient safety. BMC Health Serv Res. 2020;20(1):1–5. https://doi.org/10.1186/S12913-020-4922-3/PEER-REVIEW.
32. Kondrak G, Dorr B. Automatic identification of confusable drug names. Artif Intell Med. 2006;36(1):29–42. https://doi.org/10.1016/J.ARTMED.2005.07.005.
33. Ostini R, Roughead EE, Kirkpatrick CMJ, Monteith GR, Tett SE. Quality use of medicines – medication safety issues in naming; look-alike, sound-alike medicine names. Int J Pharm Pract. 2012;20(6):349–57. https://doi.org/10.1111/j.2042-7174.2012.00210.x.
34. Naunton M, Gardiner HR, Kyle G. Look-alike, sound-alike medication errors: a novel case concerning a slow-Na, slow-K prescribing error. Int Med Case Rep J. 2015;8:51–3. https://doi.org/10.2147/IMCRJ.S78637.
35. Linden-Lahti C, Takala A, Holmström AR, Airaksinen M. What severe medication errors reported to health care supervisory authority tell about medication safety? J Patient Saf. 2021;17(8):e1179. https://doi.org/10.1097/PTS.0000000000000914.
36. Burssa D, et al. Safe surgery for all: early lessons from implementing a national government-driven surgical plan in Ethiopia. World J Surg. 2017;41(12):3038–45. https://doi.org/10.1007/S00268-017-4271-5.

37. Ragusa PS, Bitterman A, Auerbach B, Healy WA. Effectiveness of surgical safety checklists in improving patient safety. Orthopedics. 2016;39(2):e307–10. https://doi.org/10.3928/01477447-20160301-02.
38. Implementation manual WHO surgical safety checklist 2009. https://www.who.int/publications/i/item/9789241598590. Accessed 11 Feb 2024.
39. Cabral RA, Eggenberger T, Keller K, Gallison BS, Newman D. Use of a surgical safety checklist to improve team communication. AORN J. 2016;104(3):206–16. https://doi.org/10.1016/J.AORN.2016.06.019.
40. Jain D, Sharma R, Reddy S. WHO safe surgery checklist: barriers to universal acceptance. J Anaesthesiol Clin Pharmacol. 2018;34(1):7–10. https://doi.org/10.4103/JOACP.JOACP_307_16.
41. Schroeder SD. Surgical safety checklist. S D Med. 2009;62(5):209. https://doi.org/10.15448/1980-6108.2023.1.43223.
42. Sabatelli G, et al. Guidance document on best practices for the prevention and control of healthcare-associated infections (HAIs). Reg Lazio, 2022, [Online]. Available: https://www.regione.lazio.it/sites/default/files/2022-11/Documento-indirizzo-buone-pratiche-prevenzione-controllo-infezioni-correlate-assistenza-ICA.pdf.
43. Ales ME, et al. PPS-3 REPORT REGION-REGION LOMBARDY. Surveillance through point prevalence of HAIs and antimicrobial use in acute care hospitals.
44. Cassini A, et al. Burden of six healthcare-associated infections on European population health: estimating incidence-based disability-adjusted life years through a population prevalence-based modelling study. PLoS Med. 2016;13(10):e1002150. https://doi.org/10.1371/JOURNAL.PMED.1002150.
45. Magill SS, et al. Multistate point-prevalence survey of health care-associated infections. N Engl J Med. 2014;370(13):1198–208. https://doi.org/10.1056/NEJMOA1306801.
46. Blot K, Bergs J, Vogelaers D, Blot S, Vandijck D. Prevention of central line-associated bloodstream infections through quality improvement interventions: a systematic review and meta-analysis. 2014. https://doi.org/10.1093/cid/ciu239.
47. Jaffar A, Abed MS. Decreasing ventilator-associated pneumonia in adult intensive care units using the Institute for Healthcare Improvement bundle. Am J Infect Control. 2010;38(7):552–6. https://doi.org/10.1016/J.AJIC.2010.01.008.
48. Sickbert-Bennett EE, Dibiase LM, Schade Willis TM, Wolak ES, Weber DJ, Rutala WA. Reduction of healthcare-associated infections by exceeding high compliance with hand hygiene practices. Emerg Infect Dis. 2016;22(9):1628–30. https://doi.org/10.3201/EID2209.151440.
49. Clean care is safer care. https://www.who.int/news-room/events/detail/2005/10/13/default-calendar/clean-care-is-safer-care. Accessed 11 Feb 2024.
50. Healthcare-Associated Infections (HAIs) | HAI | CDC. https://www.cdc.gov/hai/index.html. Accessed 16 Feb 2024.
51. Allegranzi B, et al. Burden of endemic health-care-associated infection in developing countries: systematic review and meta-analysis. Lancet (London, England). 2011;377(9761):228–41. https://doi.org/10.1016/S0140-6736(10)61458-4.
52. Zingg W, et al. Hospital organisation, management, and structure for prevention of health-care-associated infection: a systematic review and expert consensus. Lancet Infect Dis. 2015;15(2):212–24. https://doi.org/10.1016/S1473-3099(14)70854-0.
53. White SV. Conference brief report: Institute for Healthcare Improvement National Forum on quality improvement in health care. J Healthc Qual. 2006;28(2):52–6. https://doi.org/10.1111/J.1945-1474.2006.TB00604.X.
54. Payne V, Hall M, Prieto J, Johnson M. Care bundles to reduce central line-associated bloodstream infections in the neonatal unit: a systematic review and meta-analysis. Arch Dis Child Fetal Neonatal Ed. 2018;103(5):F422–9. https://doi.org/10.1136/ARCHDISCHILD-2017-313362.

55. Martinez-Reviejo R, et al. Prevention of ventilator-associated pneumonia through care bundles: a systematic review and meta-analysis. J Intensive Med. 2023;3(4):352–64. https://doi.org/10.1016/J.JOINTM.2023.04.004.
56. Meddings J, Rogers MAM, Krein SL, Fakih MG, Olmsted RN, Saint S. Reducing unnecessary urinary catheter use and other strategies to prevent catheter-associated urinary tract infection: an integrative review. BMJ Qual Saf. 2014;23(4):277–89. https://doi.org/10.1136/BMJQS-2012-001774.
57. Wolfhagen N, Boldingh QJJ, Boermeester MA, De Jonge SW. Perioperative care bundles for the prevention of surgical-site infections: meta-analysis. Br J Surg. 2022;109(10):933–42. https://doi.org/10.1093/BJS/ZNAC196.
58. Pop-Vicas AE, Abad C, Baubie K, Osman F, Heise C, Safdar N. Colorectal bundles for surgical site infection prevention: a systematic review and meta-analysis. Infect Control Hosp Epidemiol. 2020;41(7):805–12. https://doi.org/10.1017/ICE.2020.112.
59. Martin EK, Beckmann MM, Barnsbee LN, Halton KA, Merollini KMD, Graves N. Best practice perioperative strategies and surgical techniques for preventing caesarean section surgical site infections: a systematic review of reviews and meta-analyses. BJOG. 2018;125(8):956–64. https://doi.org/10.1111/1471-0528.15125.
60. Levy MM, Evans LE, Rhodes A. The surviving sepsis campaign bundle: 2018 update. Intensive Care Med. 2018;44(6):925–8. https://doi.org/10.1007/S00134-018-5085-0.
61. Singh H, et al. Developing the safer dx checklist of ten safety recommendations for health care organizations to address diagnostic errors. Jt Comm J Qual Patient Saf. 2022;48(11):581–90. https://doi.org/10.1016/j.jcjq.2022.08.003.
62. Shen L, Levie A, Singh H, Murray K, Desai S. Harnessing event report data to identify diagnostic error during the COVID-19 pandemic. Jt Comm J Qual Patient Saf. 2022;48(2):71–80. https://doi.org/10.1016/J.JCJQ.2021.10.002.
63. Newman-Toker DE, et al. Diagnostic errors in the emergency department: a systematic review [Internet]. 2022. https://doi.org/10.23970/AHRQEPCCER258.
64. What is Diagnostic Error? – Society to Improve Diagnosis in Medicine. https://www.improvediagnosis.org/what-is-diagnostic-error/. Accessed 11 Feb 2024.
65. Diagnostic Errors | PSNet. https://psnet.ahrq.gov/primer/diagnostic-errors. Accessed 11 Feb 2024.
66. Brennan TA, et al. Incidence of adverse events and negligence in hospitalized patients-results of the Harvard medical practice study I. 2010;324(6):370–6. https://doi.org/10.1056/NEJM199102073240604.
67. Gunderson CG, et al. Prevalence of harmful diagnostic errors in hospitalized adults: a systematic review and meta-analysis. BMJ Qual Saf. 2020;29(12):1008–18. https://doi.org/10.1136/BMJQS-2019-010822.
68. Schwanda-Burger S, Moch H, Muntwyler J, Salomon F. Diagnostic errors in the new millennium: a follow-up autopsy study. Mod Pathol. 2012;25(6):777–83. https://doi.org/10.1038/MODPATHOL.2011.199.
69. Makary MA, Daniel M. Medical error—the third leading cause of death in the US. BMJ. 2016;353 https://doi.org/10.1136/BMJ.I2139.
70. Diagnostic errors – UpToDate. https://www.uptodate.com/contents/diagnostic-errors. Accessed 11 Feb 2024.
71. Auerbach AD, et al. Diagnostic errors in hospitalized adults who died or were transferred to intensive care. JAMA Intern Med. 2024;184(2) https://doi.org/10.1001/JAMAINTERNMED.2023.7347.
72. Quick Safety 28: Cognitive biases in health care | The Joint Commission. https://www.jointcommission.org/resources/news-and-multimedia/newsletters/newsletters/quick-safety/quick-safety-28/cognitive-biases-in-health-care/. Accessed 11 Feb 2024.
73. Hall KK, et al. Making healthcare safer III: a critical analysis of existing and emerging patient safety practices. Agency for Healthcare Research and Quality (US); 2020.

74. Quick Safety Issue 52: Advancing safety with closed-loop communication of test results | The Joint Commission. https://www.jointcommission.org/resources/news-and-multimedia/newsletters/newsletters/quick-safety/quick-safety-issue-52/. Accessed 11 Feb 2024.
75. Scicchitano E, Stark P, Koetter P, Michalak N, Zurca AD. Blindfolding improves communication in inexperienced residents undergoing ACLS training. J Grad Med Educ. 2021;13(1):123–7. https://doi.org/10.4300/JGME-D-20-00620.1.

Intensive Care Issues in Subarachnoid Hemorrhage (SAH)

25

Luciana Mascia, Rosanna D'Albo, and Irene Cavalli

25.1 Introduction

Globally, approximately 12.2 million people suffer a stroke each year; of these, 1.2 million are due to non-traumatic subarachnoid hemorrhage (SAH) [1]. Compared to the past, the global incidence of SAH has decreased from 10.2 (95% CI, 8.4–12.5) per 100,000 person-years in 1980 to 6.1 (95% CI, 4.9–7.5) per 100,000 person-years in 2010, with an annual decline of 1.7% [2], except in Japan, where there has been an annual increase of 1.6% (95% CI, 0.8–2.3) [2]. This downward trend can be partly explained by better control of risk factors for cerebral aneurysm rupture, such as improved management of blood pressure. Regarding sex-specific incidence, women remain more affected than men (57% vs 43%), while the average age at onset is ≥50 years [1, 2].

In 80% of cases, SAH is caused by rupture of a cerebral aneurysm [3, 4]; in 15% of SAH cases, the source of bleeding is not identified on neuroimaging; finally, other causes (arteriovenous malformations, vasculitis) account for the remaining 5% of cases [5]. SAH is associated with significant morbidity and mortality. Reported mortality rates in studies are around 20% [6] and do not include pre-hospital mortality, which is estimated to be about 25% [7]. Recent studies have shown a reduction in mortality over time [8–11], attributable to improvements in neurocritical care management as well as advances in surgical and endovascular techniques. However, about 20% of SAH survivors will have a disability with a

L. Mascia (✉)
Department of Experimental Medicine, University of Salento, Lecce, Italy
e-mail: luciana.mascia@unisalento.it

R. D'Albo · I. Cavalli
Department of Medical and Surgical Sciences, Alma Mater Studiorum, University of Bologna, Bologna, Italy
e-mail: rosanna.dalbo@studio.unibo.it; irene.cavalli@aosp.bo.it

D. Chiumello, A. De Gasperi (eds.), *Practical Trends in Anesthesia and Intensive Care 2026*, https://doi.org/10.1007/978-3-032-25721-5_25

permanent reduction in quality of life (at 5 years post-event, there is loss of work capacity and social independence, with compromised personal and family relationships) [11–13].

The aim of this chapter is to describe the main initial clinical manifestations, the diagnostic pathway, and the intensive care management of patients with aneurysmal SAH according to the recent guidelines of the American Heart Association/American Stroke Association (AHA/ASA) [7] and the Neurocritical Care Society (NCS) [14].

25.2 Clinical Manifestations

Most cerebral aneurysms remain undiagnosed during a person's lifetime or are found incidentally [4, 15]. The most common presentation of an aneurysm is SAH, which in 80% of cases typically manifests as a sudden, severe headache described by the patient as "the worst headache of my life," often accompanied by nausea, vomiting, photophobia, neck stiffness, and loss of consciousness [3, 16]. In 10–40% of patients, aneurysm rupture is preceded in the 2–8 weeks prior by a "sentinel headache," due to minor leaks from the aneurysm [17]. Occasionally, an aneurysm may present with focal neurological signs that vary depending on its location: bitemporal hemianopsia and bilateral lower limb weakness (anterior communicating artery), unilateral third cranial nerve palsy (posterior communicating artery), facial or orbital pain, epistaxis, progressive visual loss and/or ophthalmoplegia (intracavernous segment of the internal carotid artery), symptoms of brainstem dysfunction (posterior circulation) [3, 16]. Finally, Terson syndrome (vitreous hemorrhage associated with SAH) is present in up to 40% of patients with SAH [18, 19].

25.3 Diagnosis and Prognosis

A definitive diagnosis of SAH is based on a positive CT scan in the presence of suggestive clinical features. Imaging plays a crucial role in diagnosis, in identifying the site of bleeding, and in prognostic assessment [7, 20].

In the diagnostic algorithm, recent guidelines highlight the role of the "Ottawa SAH Rule" (Table 25.1) to exclude patients at low risk for SAH [7, 21]: patients over 15 years of age presenting with a new-onset, non-traumatic headache—even in the absence of altered consciousness or new neurological deficit—but with one or more of the "six rules" listed in Table 25.1 of the "Ottawa SAH Rule," require further diagnostic evaluation. The "Ottawa SAH Rule" is an excellent screening tool, with a sensitivity of 100%, albeit at the expense of low specificity, reported in various studies to range between 7% and 15%.

Table 25.1 Ottawa rules

Ottawa rules
Age ≥ 40 years old
Neck pain or stiffness
Witnessed loss of consciousness
Headache onset during exertion
"Thunderclap headache" (pain peaks instantly)
Limited neck flexion on examination

Cranial CT The initial diagnostic test most the most appropriate and sensitive test to identify patients with suspected SAH is a non-contrast head CT scan [7, 22]. According to a recent meta-analysis [23], the diagnostic accuracy of a head CT performed within 6 h of symptom onset in patients without neurological deficits shows a sensitivity and specificity of 98% and 99%, respectively. Thanks to technological advances, the sensitivity of CT remains high even after 48 h from symptom onset [22]: extravasated blood appears hyperdense and may be located in the basal subarachnoid cisterns, the sylvian and interhemispheric fissures, interpeduncular fossa, suprasellar, ambient, and quadrigeminal cisterns [24].

Lumbar Puncture In patients with a negative non-contrast head CT, symptom onset more than 6 h prior, and/or new neurological deficits, lumbar puncture is indicated [7]. Xanthochromic cerebrospinal fluid can be found in only 20% of patients starting from the sixth hour after symptom onset. The percentage of xanthochromic CSF rises to 90% of patients after 12 h [7, 25]. Cerebrospinal fluid should be collected in 4 consecutive tubes, and red blood cell counts should be performed in the first and fourth tubes. Elevated opening pressure, a high red blood cell count that does not significantly decrease in the fourth tube compared to the first, and especially xanthochromia of the CSF are findings that support the diagnosis of SAH [25–27]. Xanthochromia indicates intrathecal hemolysis and can be detected by visual inspection of the tube or by spectrophotometry [27].

Identification of the Source of Bleeding In the presence of a diagnostic head CT and/or lumbar puncture for SAH, the source of bleeding must be identified. According to the most recent guidelines, CT angiography of the head is the next imaging step after non-contrast head CT to identify the source of bleeding, mainly due to the wide availability of the technique [7]. CT angiography has the advantage of being readily available and can be performed during the same session as the head CT in cases of SAH diagnosis, with a sensitivity and specificity of 98% and 100%, respectively [28]. However, lower sensitivity and specificity have been attributed to technical factors such as the use of 16- or 64-slice scanners, image processing algorithms, aneurysm size (not visible on CT angiography when <3 mm), and operator experience [28–31]. The "gold standard" for identifying the source of bleeding remains digital subtraction cerebral angiography (DSA), which can be both diagnostic and therapeutic [7]. According to AHA/ASA guidelines [7], DSA is especially indicated in patients with a high suspicion of cerebral aneurysm but with negative or inconclusive CT angiography. The role of DSA remains important for identifying small aneurysms (<3 mm), in cases of SAH with positive head CT but negative CT angiography, or in cases of diffuse SAH [7, 32, 33]. In patients with a negative DSA, the exam should be repeated between 7 and 14 days after initial presentation, and if still negative, brain MRI angiography should be performed to detect possible cerebral, brainstem, or spinal vascular malformations [32, 34].

In about 15% of patients with SAH, imaging fails to demonstrate the source of bleeding. Of these, about 38% have a non-aneurysmal perimesencephalic SAH [35], which carries a lower risk of complications. Non-aneurysmal perimesencephalic SAH presents with negative CT angiography or DSA but with a characteristic head CT pattern [36]: the hemorrhage is located anterior to the midbrain, with or without extension of blood to the anterior part of the ambient cistern or the basal part of the sylvian fissures, and there is no intraventricular blood.

Prognosis The clinical and radiological severity of SAH at admission is the strongest predictor of poor outcome [7, 37]. In fact, the AHA/ASA guidelines [7] recommend the use of the following clinical scores to determine the severity and prognosis of patients with SAH: the WFNS (World Federation of Neurosurgical Surgeons) scale [38] and the modified Fisher scale [39]. The WFNS (Table 25.2) is a scoring system based on Glasgow Coma Scale (GCS) values and the presence of focal deficits at symptom onset: WFNS scores between 1 and 3 indicate a better prognosis, while a WFNS grade of 4–5 identifies a worse prognosis. The specific weight of focal deficits is relevant in cases with higher GCS, as prognosis depends primarily on the level of consciousness and then on focal neurological damage. The limitation of this assessment system is its dependence on the timing of clinical evaluation of SAH and the fact that it does not take into account cranial and extracranial complications [38, 40–42]. The modified Fisher scale (Table 25.3) classifies the amount and location of subarachnoid hemorrhage as a predictor of cerebral vasospasm, delayed cerebral ischemia (DCI), and patient outcome [39, 43]. Although other systems have been developed to assess the prognosis of patients affected by aSAH, such as the FRESH model [44] or the SAHIT model [45], the WFNS for clinical grading and the modified Fisher scale for radiological grading remain the most commonly used assessment scales due to their strong predictive power and ease of use.

Table 25.2 The World Federation of Neurosurgical Societies (WFNS) scale

The WFNS scale
Grade 1: GCS score of 15 without focal deficit
Grade 2: GCS score of 13 or 14 without focal deficit
Grade 3: GCS score of 13 or 14 with focal deficit
Grade 4: GCS score of 7–12
Grade 5: GCS score of 3–6

GCS Glasgow Coma Scale

Table 25.3 Modified fisher scale

Modified fisher scale
Grade 0: No SAH or IVH
Grade 1: Focal or diffuse, thin SAH, no IVH
Grade 2: Focal or diffuse, thin SAH, with IVH
Grade 3: Focal or diffuse, thick SAH, no IVH
Grade 4: Focal or diffuse, thick SAH, with IVH

Note: Thin SAH is <1 mm thick; thick SAH is >1 mm in depth
SAH subarachnoid hemorrhage, *IVH* intraventricular hemorrhage

25.3.1 Aneurysm Treatment

The two main approaches to the management of cerebral aneurysms are surgical clipping and endovascular coiling. Whenever possible, the goal of treatment is to achieve complete obliteration of the aneurysm and exclude it from the circulation. Clipping involves excluding the aneurysmal sac from the circulation by microsurgically placing a vascular clip at the aneurysm neck. Coiling is an endovascular technique in which a microcatheter is advanced into the aneurysmal sac, and extremely thin metal coils are deployed until the aneurysm is completely occluded [3]. The choice of treatment depends on several factors, including patient age, aneurysm location and morphology, and its relationship with adjacent vessels. For this reason, it is essential that the treatment decision is made by a multidisciplinary team comprising cerebrovascular neurosurgeons, interventional neuroradiologists, and neurointensivists [7, 46, 47]. The management of aSAH patients by a multidisciplinary team in high-volume centers plays a crucial role in improving patient outcomes, to the extent that it is now a strong recommendation in the latest guidelines [7].

To determine the best treatment for aneurysms, a randomized controlled clinical trial—the ISAT (International Subarachnoid Aneurysm Trial)—was published in 2002, including patients eligible for both endovascular coiling and surgical clipping [48, 49]. One year after treatment, patients assigned to the coiling group showed a significantly better outcome in terms of survival without disability, as assessed by the modified Rankin scale, and a lower risk of epilepsy compared to the clipping group. The risk of rebleeding was similar between the two treatments, although slightly higher in the coiling group. The major contribution of this study was the evaluation, in two subsequent prospective studies, of the 5- and 10-year outcomes of the ISAT trial cohort. At 5 years post-treatment [50], patients who underwent coiling had a lower risk of death compared to those who underwent clipping. However, the proportion of independent patients did not differ between the two groups, and the risk of rebleeding was higher in the coiling group. The 10-year follow-up [51] showed that patients treated with coiling had a higher probability of survival and independence compared to those treated with clipping. This finding holds true despite the higher risk of rebleeding in the endovascular group, which remains overall low and does not translate into worse clinical outcomes. Therefore, endovascular coiling should be preferred over surgical clipping whenever possible

[7]. Aneurysm closure, regardless of the approach, should be performed as soon as possible and preferably within 24 h of symptom onset [7]. Many aneurysms are not equally suitable for both clipping and coiling. Factors such as advanced age, poor clinical condition, presence of comorbidities, aneurysm location at the basilar artery apex, vertebrobasilar circulation, or the intracavernous segment of the internal carotid artery favor endovascular coiling. Conversely, giant or fusiform aneurysms, those with a wide neck-to-dome ratio (> 0.5), located at arterial bifurcations, aneurysms of the middle cerebral artery, or those associated with large parenchymal hematomas are better treated with surgical clipping. Young patients (< 40 years) benefit from surgical clipping as it provides better protection against recurrent aSAH[?]. The use of flow-diverting stents is reserved for cases where neither coiling nor clipping is feasible, generally for non-saccular aneurysms with a wide neck. At the end of the surgical or neuroradiological procedure, immediate cerebrovascular imaging is recommended to identify any residual or recurrent aneurysmal pathology that may require further treatment [7].

25.4 Intensive Care Management

As mentioned, the outcome of these patients depends on the initial clinical condition, the amount and distribution of blood on the first CT scan, and on cranial and extracranial complications that may occur during the intensive care unit stay [52–55].

Patients with aSAH are at increased risk of developing various neurological and systemic complications. Among the neurological complications, the most frequent are rebleeding, hydrocephalus, cerebral edema, delayed cerebral ischemia and vasospasm (delayed cerebral ischemia [DCI]), seizures, and neuroendocrine disturbances leading to impaired fluid and electrolyte balance. More than 75% of aSAH patients develop a systemic inflammatory response syndrome (SIRS), likely due to elevated levels of inflammatory cytokines, which may be associated with permanent neurocognitive dysfunction. In addition, increased circulating catecholamine levels are thought to underlie cardiac complications characterized by ECG changes, impaired contractility (Takotsubo cardiomyopathy), and elevated troponin levels plasma levels and myocardial necrosis. A similar pathophysiological mechanism is very likely also responsible for pulmonary complications such as neurogenic pulmonary edema or acute respiratory distress syndrome (ARDS).

25.4.1 Hemodynamic Management

In the past, the hemodynamic management of patients with SAH was based on triple-H therapy, namely "Hypertension, Hypervolemia, Hemodilution" [56], with the aim of preventing and treating vasospasm and DCI.

Hypervolemia This approach, which consists of maintaining a positive fluid balance, has been associated with an increased risk of hypoxemia and pulmonary complications, and has therefore been critically reconsidered [57–60]. In fact, in a retrospective study [59], a positive fluid balance during the first 7 days of hospitalization was associated with an unfavorable neurological outcome; in a randomized study [61], a hypervolemic fluid approach was not associated with improved cerebral blood flow or a reduction in vasospasm compared to normovolemic patients. Conversely, in a prospective observational study [58], a normovolemic fluid approach was associated with a reduction in hypoxemia episodes from day 3 to 7 of intensive care unit stay.

Based on this evidence, current AHA/ASA guidelines [7] state that induction of a hypervolemic state may be harmful, while NCS guidelines [14] suggest avoiding a liberal fluid approach due to the increased risk of pulmonary edema, and instead recommend a "goal-directed," i.e., individualized, approach [60]. The most recent methods for estimating volemic status proposed in the literature include transpulmonary thermodilution, volumetric monitoring of the global end-diastolic volume index (GEDVI), arterial waveform analysis, and echocardiography. Bergmans et al. [62] observed in a small cohort of SAH patients that fluid management based on transpulmonary thermodilution was able to reduce fluid overload while maintaining adequate diuresis and cardiac function. In a prospective observational study using *volumetric* monitoring, it was shown that a GEDVI value less than 822 mL/m [63] s1 was associated with a higher incidence of vasospasm, while a GEDVI value greater than 921 mL/m was associated with an increased risk of pulmonary edema. In a prospective observational study, arterial waveform analysis compared to transpulmonary thermodilution proved reliable, with an error of <20% in estimating cardiac output, although systems based on arterial waveform analysis require frequent recalibration to remain reliable.

Hypertension Blood pressure control plays a crucial role in the management of patients with SAH, as it must prevent rebleeding in the early phase, but also ensure adequate cerebral perfusion while minimizing the risk of DCI [64, 65]. Recent AHA/ASA [7] and NCS [14] guidelines recommend strict blood pressure control in the various phases: 1) systolic blood pressure values between 140 and 160 mmHg are suggested before securing the aneurysm, during anesthetic management, and during surgical or endovascular treatment of the aneurysm to avoid rebleeding; 2) controlled hypertension in the intensive management of SAH is suggested to prevent hypoperfusion injury (DCI) and to treat vasospasm [7, 66]. Although both recommendations only suggest a specific blood pressure target, controlling hypertension before securing the aneurysm on the one hand and avoiding hypotension and significant blood pressure fluctuations on the other hand remain reasonable indications to follow.

25.4.2 Management of Neurological Complications

Rebleeding Rebleeding is a major disabling complication of SAH, associated with high rates of mortality and morbidity. Between 4 and 15% of SAH patients experience rebleeding within the first 24 h. The highest risk is within the first 6 h after symptom onset, decreasing over the following 2 weeks [70]. The main associated risk factors include elevated systolic blood pressure (>160 mmHg), severe neurological clinical presentation, advanced age, ruptured aneurysms of the posterior circulation, and aneurysms larger than 10 mm in diameter. If anticoagulant therapy is present, early correction of coagulation status should be performed. The best therapeutic strategy to reduce the risk of rebleeding is early treatment of the aneurysm [71]. In cases where there is a delay in treatment (clipping or coiling), administration of antifibrinolytics was proposed to reduce the risk of rebleeding within 72 h [72]. However, in a recent randomized study [73], the ULTRA study (ultra-early tranexamic acid after subarachnoid hemorrhage), early administration of tranexamic acid in patients did not demonstrate an improvement of 6-month outcome. Therefore, the routine use of antifibrinolytics is not recommended by the AHA/ASA guidelines [7] and is discouraged by the NCS guidelines [14]. Blood pressure control, however, remains a crucial point in the prevention of rebleeding, both before and after aneurysm treatment. Nicardipine appears to provide better blood pressure control compared to labetalol and sodium nitroprusside, although no differences in clinical outcome have been demonstrated [74]. One working hypothesis concerns the use of V1a vasopressin receptor antagonists to treat systemic hypertension and prevent rebleeding [75]. However, patients with suspected rebleeding should be promptly evaluated, undergo a cranial CT and DSA, with immediate treatment if necessary.

ICP Control ICP monitoring is particularly useful in the perioperative management of patients who remain unconscious after the procedure [66]. In patients with SAH, this monitoring is preferably achieved by placing an external ventricular drain (EVD), which allows simultaneous measurement of ICP and therapeutic drainage of excess cerebrospinal fluid, especially in patients with aneurysmal SAH and acute symptomatic hydrocephalus [7, 67]. Management of elevated ICP involves a "stepwise" therapeutic approach, following the recommendations of the Brain Trauma Foundation for the treatment of traumatic brain injury. First, in comatose patients, treatment of elevated ICP and maintenance of normal CPP are essential to prevent further neurological damage. Initial medical management includes elevating the head of the bed to 30–45° in a neutral position, normocapnic ventilation, sedation with possible cerebrospinal fluid drainage, and osmotherapy with mannitol or hypertonic saline. The goal is to maintain ICP below approximately 20 mm Hg and CPP between 60 and 70 mm Hg [67, 68]. Regarding osmotherapy, there are no definitive data on the superiority of one solution over another, but the objective should remain to ensure adequate cerebral perfusion by reducing ICP and maintaining euvolemia; therefore, close monitoring of blood volume, blood pressure, serum sodium, and plasma osmolality is required.

In patients with SAH, it is important to maintain a PaCO2 level around 35–40 mmHg, but in cases of uncontrolled ICP, transient hyperventilation may be used, while avoiding the ischemic risk associated with hypocapnia [69]. Intracranial hypertension is a common complication during the first week in patients admitted to intensive care for SAH, and is associated with the severity of the initial brain injury and with high mortality.

In cases of refractory elevated ICP, both barbiturate coma induction and decompressive craniectomy (DC) may be considered as advanced therapies. Barbiturates help control ICP by reducing metabolism but are associated with multiple side effects, including hypotension and increased susceptibility to infections; therefore, this therapy should not be used prophylactically to prevent ICP elevation.

Decompressive craniectomy, considered an extreme therapy, may be used in the presence of cerebral edema and intractable intracranial hypertension. Removal of part of the cranial vault allows the brain parenchyma to expand, reduces compression and midline shift, and improves ICP, CPP, and thus cerebral blood flow. Unfortunately, the role of DC in SAH is not well established, and available data are limited and conflicting. Therefore, future randomized controlled trials are certainly desirable to identify the factors that should guide patient selection, timing, and indications for appropriate use of DC in SAH.

Hydrocephalus The risk of acute symptomatic hydrocephalus after SAH ranges from 15% to 87% [76]. Patients present with neurological impairment, reduced level of consciousness, and signs of increased ICP. Treatment of acute hydrocephalus involves placement of an external ventricular drain (EVD) [77], particularly in cases of obstructive hydrocephalus, or lumbar drainage, which can be used in cases of communicating hydrocephalus [78]. The AHA/ASA guidelines [7] recommend early placement of an EVD in cases of symptomatic hydrocephalus and the adoption of protocols for device management to reduce the complication rate (e.g., infections). About 60% of SAH patients treated with EVD will be successfully weaned, especially in the early phase [79], while the remaining patients will require placement of a permanent ventriculoperitoneal shunt. However, the guidelines do not provide recommendations on the best strategy for EVD weaning.

Seizures The exact frequency of post-SAH seizures is difficult to determine, and recent studies have shown a lower incidence (7–18%) [80] of this complication compared to the past (up to 26%), thanks to better and more appropriate continuous EEG monitoring. This is particularly indicated in patients at high risk, namely: middle cerebral artery aneurysms, presence of thick subarachnoid clots or intraparenchymal hematomas, rebleeding, cerebral infarction, history of hypertension, and clinical severity [81, 82]. The AHA/ASA guidelines [7] provide recommendations for the management of seizures and distinguish between the management of patients with SAH who present with seizures at onset and those who do not. In patients presenting with seizures at onset, treatment for a maximum of 7 days is appropriate, while there is insufficient evidence to justify longer therapy except in patients with a prior history of epilepsy [7, 82]. Conversely, in patients who do not present with seizures at onset, the guidelines recommend pharmacological seizure prophylaxis only in those at high risk. In this specific patient population, prophylaxis with phenytoin is associated with long-term cognitive impairment and is therefore now discouraged, whereas levetiracetam has been shown to have few side effects [83].

Delayed Cerebral Ischemia and Vasospasm Delayed cerebral ischemia (DCI) is the complication with the greatest impact on functional outcome [53]. It occurs in approximately 30% of patients with SAH, usually between days 4 and 14 after symptom onset. It is defined as any sign of neurological deterioration (focal or global, resulting in a loss of at least two points on the GCS) that persists for more than 1 h and cannot be explained by another neurological or systemic condition. The diagnosis of DCI involves a combination of neurological examination and imaging studies. A brain CT performed 24–48 h after aneurysm treatment that shows a new hypodense lesion not attributable to EVD placement or to an intraparenchymal hematoma should be considered a cerebral infarction caused by DCI. Expert consensus recommends that patients with SAH undergo routine neurological examination, continuous EEG monitoring if clinical assessment is not feasible, and transcranial Doppler (TCD) monitoring [89, 90]. Continuous EEG allows monitoring of large brain regions and noninvasive detection of epileptiform discharges [91]. It is particularly useful in patients with severe clinical conditions in whom neurological examination is significantly limited [92, 93]. DCI is therefore a diagnosis of exclusion: other confounding factors such as hydrocephalus, excessive sedation, hypoxemia, seizures, and electrolyte or metabolic disturbances must be absent. Multiple factors are implicated in its pathogenesis: proximal and/or microcirculatory vasospasm, microthrombosis, *cortical spreading depression,* disruption of the blood-brain barrier, cerebral edema, and impaired cerebral autoregulation [53, 84]. *Cortical spreading depression* in particular is defined as a wave of depolarization that propagates through the cerebral gray matter at a speed of 2–5 mm/min and suppresses both spontaneous and evoked EEG activity. The clustered spread of slow waves leads to severe vasoconstriction, disruption of cerebral ionic homeostasis, and ischemic tissue injury [86–88]. Microthrombosis results from activation of the coagulation cascade following the initial hemorrhage. Among these pathogenic factors, cerebral vasospasm plays a crucial role in the development of DCI, although these are two distinct entities, and the presence of vasospasm does not necessarily imply the development of DCI. Vasospasm occurs most frequently 7–10 days after aneurysm rupture and may resolve after 21 days. It involves both proximal and distal vessels; approximately *50%* of angiographically diagnosed vasospasm cases are associated with neurological symptoms. The risk of cerebral vasospasm is related to the density and location of subarachnoid blood and the severity of neurological impairment at onset. Monitoring of vasospasm with *transcranial Doppler (TCD)* is based on repeated assessment of blood flow velocity in the arterial circle of Willis over several days. TCD has high sensitivity and specificity for diagnosing vasospasm of the middle cerebral artery, but lower for the posterior circulation. The Lindegaard ratio (the ratio between the mean flow velocities of the middle cerebral artery and the extracranial internal carotid artery) is an index used to increase diagnostic accuracy [85]. The limitations of this method are related to operator experience and the presence of an adequate temporal acoustic window in the patient [94]. Transcranial Doppler was originally a technique that did not allow visualization of the brain parenchyma or cerebral vessels due to the intervening bone structure, and was therefore referred to as a "blind" technique; this aspect could make it difficult to correctly angle the probe relative to the monitored vessel. An important technological advancement was the addition of the "color" function to Doppler. In this way, the use of Transcranial Color Doppler (TCCD) allows direct visualization of the vessels. TCCD therefore optimizes the patient's acoustic window and the insonation angle of the vessel to explore [95, 96]. The reference threshold values for TCD in the diagnosis of vasospasm are as follows: mean flow velocity <120 cm/s excludes vasospasm; mean flow velocity >200 cm/s, Lindegaard ratio >6, and daily increases in mean flow velocity >50 cm/s are suggestive of vasospasm and warrant further investigation with more invasive diagnostic tests. CT angiography can be used instead of DSA with a high degree of specificity; in particular, a mean transit time greater than 6.4 s represents the threshold value suggestive of reduced cerebral perfusion and may predict DCI [97].

Invasive monitoring of intracranial pressure (and thus cerebral perfusion), brain tissue oxygen pressure (PtbO2), and microdialysis allows for the study of the relationship between flow, oxygen availability, and cerebral metabolism using three probes placed simultaneously. Approximately three-quarters of patients who develop intracranial hypertension show cerebral metabolic alterations with a shift from aerobic to anaerobic metabolism [101, 102]. Cerebral microdialysis offers the possibility of continuous, near real-time sampling of fluctuations in glucose, pyruvate, and lactate in the extracellular space. In ischemic conditions, the following can be detected: a) reduced extracellular glucose, reduced pyruvate, elevated lactate, and thus an increased lactate/pyruvate ratio [103]; b) increased extracellular glutamate concentration due to both increased neuronal release and reduced reuptake by the synaptic cleft, enhancing the neurotoxic effect of ischemia with consequent neuronal damage [104]. This technique can therefore assist not only in the early diagnosis of DCI, but also in evaluating the effect of treatments such as nimodipine and angioplasty, especially in patients with compromised clinical conditions [98–100].

Prophylaxis and Treatment Recent guidelines focus on the management of cerebral vasospasm and DCI after aSAH. In patients with aSAH, early enteral administration of nimodipine is recommended at a dose of 60 mg every 4 h, as it is beneficial in preventing the development of DCI and improving functional outcomes [7, 105, 106]. Nimodipine provides neuroprotection without reducing the frequency of angiographic vasospasm; however, the potential side effect of hypotension and consequent cerebral hypoperfusion must always be counteracted. Triple-H therapy (hypertension, hypervolemia, hemodilution) has been critically re-evaluated and replaced by the maintenance of euvolemia and induced hypertension when necessary [7].

The use of intra-arterial vasodilators or cerebral angioplasty is recommended only in cases of severe vasospasm. The neuroprotective role of statins, magnesium sulfate, and endothelin antagonists has also been studied, but there is no evidence that these agents improve outcomes or reduce the development of DCI [107–109].

25.4.3 Management of Non-neurological Complications

Cardiac Complications Cardiac complications are among the most common systemic complications of aSAH, and the risk of their development is particularly increased in the first 48 h following aSAH. These include ECG abnormalities (peaked T waves, T wave inversion, ST segment depression or elevation, and QT prolongation), arrhythmias of varying severity, and cardiac wall motion abnormalities detectable by echocardiography. Of these, only wall motion abnormalities have been identified as risk factors for outcome [110]. Sinus tachycardia is the most frequently observed arrhythmia [111]. ECG changes, together with elevated cardiac enzymes (troponin T and I, found in about 30% of patients) and left ventricular dysfunction, constitute the triad that defines neurogenic stunned myocardium syndrome or neurogenic stress cardiomyopathy (NSC), frequently described after acute brain injury. The pathogenesis appears to lie in an excessive catecholaminergic surge that mimics myocardial infarction [112]. In fact, plasma norepinephrine increases threefold compared to baseline within the first 48 h and remains elevated even after the first week [112, 113]. In more than 50% of NSC cases, imaging has shown a "spared apex" pattern, characterized by wall motion abnormalities of the basal and mid-ventricular segments of the left ventricle, without involvement of the apex (which is less innervated by the sympathetic nervous system). Takotsubo cardiomyopathy, on the other hand, is characterized by the typical ballooning of the ventricular apex visible on echocardiography and represents a manifestation of cardiac dysfunction in more severe patients, associated with an increased risk of DCI. Its incidence is less than 10%, and it is more common in postmenopausal women [114]. Echocardiography can help distinguish patients with diffuse cardiac dysfunction related to aSAH from those with underlying cardiac ischemia, by showing regional wall motion abnormalities corresponding to the respective coronary artery territories. From a clinical perspective, the cardiac dysfunction manifests as left ventricular failure, low cardiac output, hypotension, and consequent pulmonary edema. These cardiovascular dysfunctions can lead to severe cerebral hypoperfusion, further increasing damage to the already compromised brain parenchyma.

Respiratory Complications The most significant pulmonary complications include neurogenic pulmonary edema, the development of ARDS, and pneumonia. Neurogenic pulmonary edema, which is clinically difficult to distinguish from ARDS, has an incidence ranging from 2% to 43% of SAH cases and is associated with risk factors such as age, location of the vertebrobasilar aneurysm, and the severity of the hemorrhage [115]. As with NCS, neurogenic pulmonary edema (NPE) also appears to be explained by a significant sympathetic discharge caused by the sudden increase in intracranial pressure. The adrenergic surge is thought to be responsible for a volume shift from the systemic to the pulmonary compartment, which, together with possible left ventricular dysfunction, leads to the development of pulmonary edema [116]. In addition to this mechanism, another theory has been proposed suggesting impairment of the alveolar-capillary barrier with altered pulmonary endothelial permeability [117]. Recommendations for the management of pulmonary edema in patients with SAH include avoiding excessive fluid administration to maintain euvolemia and support cardiac function. Excluding the contribution of cardiac dysfunction, the same mechanisms underlying NPE are responsible for the development of ARDS, which is characterized by increased circulating pro-inflammatory cytokines. The likelihood of developing ARDS is correlated with the severity of SAH and is associated with poor outcomes [118]. Regarding treatment, protective mechanical ventilation is recommended, with particular attention to hypercapnia, which should be promptly managed to avoid further increases in ICP. Alveolar recruitment maneuvers and prone positioning for the treatment of refractory hypoxemia should be performed with caution and under close ICP monitoring [119, 120].

Pneumonia is a common complication in patients with SAH. The origin is most frequently bacterial, and the pathogenesis appears to involve immunosuppression that typically develops and persists for more than 3 days after the hemorrhage [121]. Identification of patients at risk (male, >65 years, with pulmonary hypertension and severe-grade SAH) aids in the prevention and management of these complications [122].

Fever Fever is the most common non-neurological complication of SAH, occurring in more than 70% of patients during their stay in the Intensive Care Unit [123]. It is more frequently observed in patients with severe neurological impairment and high Fisher scale scores. The pathogenesis is likely related in the early phase to a systemic inflammatory response syndrome (SIRS) rather than to an infectious event, and it appears to be associated with the risk of DCI [124]. Temperature control can be achieved through pharmacological agents or surface and endovascular cooling devices [125, 126]. In patients refractory to physical cooling methods, pharmacological temperature control is required, which may be associated with shivering and hypotension [127, 128].

Thromboembolic Prophylaxis In the prevention of thromboembolism, the benefits of antithrombotic therapy must be weighed against the risks of cerebral rebleeding. The risk of DVT is particularly high in the first 2 weeks after the event [129]: male sex, smoking, coagulation disorders, and the presence of heart failure appear to be associated with its development [130]. It is recommended to initiate DVT prophylaxis with unfractionated heparin within 24–48 h after stabilization of SAH, in agreement with neurosurgical colleagues. The use of elastic compression devices is recommended for all patients with SAH [7].

Glycemic Alterations and Nutrition Hyperglycemia is a common phenomenon following SAH, occurring in 70–90% of patients [131]. According to an observational study, it is associated with the development of vasospasm, DCI, and delayed neurological injury [132]. The methods, timing, and aggressiveness of glycemic control have not been well studied in SAH patients, but it is recommended to prevent hyperglycemia already during aneurysm surgery. On the other hand, any episode of hypoglycemia should be prevented and promptly treated, especially in unconscious patients; in fact, in general intensive care patients, the association between hypoglycemic episodes and worse outcomes has been well demonstrated. Early nutrition within 48 h of ICU admission is of fundamental importance for critically ill patients [133]. Poor caloric intake and a negative nitrogen balance are associated with worse outcomes in patients with SAH [134]. In this context, the NUTRIC score has proven effective in identifying patients who may benefit from artificial nutrition and in determining the optimal amount of required macronutrients [135].

Hyponatremia–Hypernatremia Disorders of sodium following SAH are very common: hyponatremia is the most frequent electrolyte disorder, occurring in approximately 30% of patients and is associated with the development of DCI [136, 137]. The main causes include cerebral salt wasting syndrome (CSWS) and syndrome of inappropriate antidiuretic hormone secretion (SIADH). CSWS is caused by excessive secretion of natriuretic peptides and leads to hyponatremia with associated hypovolemia due to excessive natriuresis, whereas SIADH results from abnormal vasopressin secretion, causing fluid retention and, ultimately, natriuresis. Determining the etiology of hyponatremia is therefore essential, as the therapeutic approach is opposite: CSWS requires fluid infusion, while SIADH is managed with fluid restriction. In both cases, the hemodynamic goal remains to maintain patient euvolemia and correct serum sodium levels [137]. Patients may be treated with continuous infusion of hypertonic saline solution (1.5–3%), which, in cases of severe SAH, appears to contribute to improved cerebral blood flow and oxygenation. In CSWS, if excessive natriuresis and volume depletion prevent maintenance of adequate fluid balance, fludrocortisone has proven effective, although without a significant impact on outcome [138]. Hypernatremia is less common and is due to excessive free water loss from diabetes insipidus, secondary to vasospasm of the hypothalamic region, resulting in the loss of very dilute urine. Treatment is based on volume replacement and, if necessary, administration of desmopressin [139]. Iatrogenic causes of hypernatremia, such as the use of mannitol or hypertonic saline, should always be excluded.

25.5 Conclusions

SAH is a neurological emergency associated with high morbidity and mortality. It is more common in women and ethnic minorities. Key elements in the management of a patient with SAH include: prompt assessment and diagnosis, transfer to a center with high-level expertise and multidisciplinary care, rapid aneurysm securing by surgical or endovascular means, and clinical management in a specialized intensive care unit in accordance with current guidelines. After patient discharge, it is reasonable to perform a follow-up neurological assessment, including cognitive, behavioral, and psychosocial status, to evaluate the impact of this condition on the patient's quality of life.

References

1. World Stroke Organization (WSO): Global Stroke Fact Sheet 2022. [Online]. Available: http://ghdx.healthdata.org/gbd-results-tool.
2. Etminan N, et al. Worldwide incidence of aneurysmal subarachnoid hemorrhage according to region, time period, blood pressure, and smoking prevalence in the population: a systematic review and meta-analysis. JAMA Neurol. 2019;76(5):588–97. https://doi.org/10.1001/jamaneurol.2019.0006.
3. Lawton MT, Vates GE. Subarachnoid hemorrhage. N Engl J Med. 2017;377(3):257–66. https://doi.org/10.1056/NEJMcp1605827.
4. Vlak MHM, et al. Prevalence of unruptured intracranial aneurysms, with emphasis on sex, age, comorbidity, country, and time period: a systematic review and meta-analysis. Articles Lancet Neurol. 2011;10:626–62. https://doi.org/10.1016/S1474.
5. Macdonald RL, Schweizer TA. Spontaneous subarachnoid haemorrhage. Lancet. 2017;389(10069):655–66. https://doi.org/10.1016/S0140-6736(16)30668-7.
6. Nguyen TN, et al. Global impact of the COVID-19 pandemic on subarachnoid haemorrhage hospitalisations, aneurysm treatment and in-hospital mortality: 1-year follow-up. J Neurol Neurosurg Psychiatry. 2022;93(10):1028–38. https://doi.org/10.1136/jnnp-2022-329200.
7. Hoh BL, et al. 2023 guideline for the management of patients with aneurysmal subarachnoid hemorrhage: a Guideline From the American Heart Association/American Stroke Association. Stroke. 2023;54(7) https://doi.org/10.1161/str.0000000000000436.
8. Lovelock CE, Rinkel FGJE, Rothwell PM. 'Time trends in outcome of subarachnoid hemorrhage: Population-based study and systematic review. 2010. Available at: www.neurology.org.
9. Chan V, Lindsay P, McQuiggan J, Zagorski B, Hill MD, O'Kelly C. Declining admission and mortality rates for subarachnoid hemorrhage in Canada between 2004 and 2015. Stroke. 2019;50(1):181–4. https://doi.org/10.1161/STROKEAHA.118.022332.
10. Mahlamaki K, Rautalin I, Korja M. Case fatality rates of subarachnoid hemorrhage are decreasing with substantial between-country variation: a systematic review of population-based studies between 1980 and 2020. Neuroepidemiology. 2023;56(6):402–12. https://doi.org/10.1159/000526983.
11. English SW. Long-term outcome and economic burden of aneurysmal subarachnoid hemorrhage: are we only seeing the tip of the iceberg? Neurocrit Care. 2020;33(1):37–8. https://doi.org/10.1007/s12028-020-00943-1.
12. Rinkel GJE, Algra A. Long-term outcomes of patients with aneurysmal subarachnoid haemorrhage. Lancet Neurol. 2011;10(4):349–56. https://doi.org/10.1016/S1474-4422(11)70017-5.
13. Tjahjadi M, et al. Health-related quality of life after spontaneous subarachnoid hemorrhage measured in a recent patient population. World Neurosurg. 2013;79(2):296–307. https://doi.org/10.1016/j.wneu.2012.10.009.
14. Treggiari MM, et al. Guidelines for the neurocritical care management of aneurysmal subarachnoid hemorrhage. Neurocrit Care. 2023;39(1):1–28. https://doi.org/10.1007/s12028-023-01713-5.
15. Johnsen LH, et al. Prevalence of unruptured intracranial aneurysms: impact of different definitions—the Tromsø study. J Neurol Neurosurg Psychiatry. 2022;93(8):902–7. https://doi.org/10.1136/jnnp-2022-329270.
16. D'Souza S. Aneurysmal Subarachnoid Hemorrhage. J Neurosurg Anesthesiol. 2015;27(3):222–40. https://doi.org/10.1097/ANA.0000000000000130.
17. Polmear A. Sentinel headaches in aneurysmal subarachnoid haemorrhage: what is the true incidence? A systematic review. Cephalalgia. 2003;23(10):935–41. https://doi.org/10.1046/j.1468-2982.2003.00596.x.
18. McCarron MO, Alberts MJ, McCarron P. A systematic review of Terson's syndrome: frequency and prognosis after subarachnoid haemorrhage. J Neurol Neurosurg Psychiatry. 2004;75(3):491–3. https://doi.org/10.1136/jnnp.2003.016816.

19. Hassan A, Lanzino G, Wijdicks EFM, Rabinstein AA, Flemming KD. Terson's syndrome. Neurocrit Care. 2011;15(3):554–8. https://doi.org/10.1007/s12028-011-9555-2.
20. Mittal AM, et al. Hunt-Hess score at 48 hours improves prognostication in grade 5 aneurysmal subarachnoid hemorrhage. World Neurosurg. 2023;171:e874–8. https://doi.org/10.1016/j.wneu.2023.01.018.
21. Perry JJ, et al. Clinical decision rules to rule out subarachnoid hemorrhage for acute headache. JAMA. 2013;310(12):1248–55. https://doi.org/10.1001/jama.2013.278018.
22. Vincent A, et al. Sensitivity of modern multislice CT for subarachnoid hemorrhage at incremental timepoints after headache onset: a 10-year analysis. Emerg Med J. 2022;39(11):810–7. https://doi.org/10.1136/emermed-2020-211068.
23. Dubosh NM, Bellolio MF, Rabinstein AA, Edlow JA. Sensitivity of early brain computed tomography to exclude aneurysmal subarachnoid hemorrhage: a systematic review and meta-analysis. Stroke. 2016;47(3):750–5. https://doi.org/10.1161/STROKEAHA.115.011386.
24. Marder CP, Narla V, Fink JR, Tozer Fink KR. Subarachnoid hemorrhage: beyond aneurysms. Am J Roentgenol. 2014;202(1):25–37. https://doi.org/10.2214/AJR.12.9749.
25. Cerebrospinal Fluid analysis.
26. Perry JJ. et al., Differentiation between traumatic tap and aneurysmal subarachnoid hemorrhage. 2015. https://doi.org/10.2307/26518312.
27. Perry JJ, et al. Should spectrophotometry be used to identify xanthochromia in the cerebrospinal fluid of alert patients suspected of having subarachnoid hemorrhage? Stroke. 2006;37(10):2467–72. https://doi.org/10.1161/01.STR.0000240689.15109.47.
28. Westerlaan HE, et al. Intracranial aneurysms in patients with subarachnoid hemorrhage: CT angiography as a primary examination tool for diagnosis—systematic review and meta-analysis. Radiology. 2011;258(1):134–45. https://doi.org/10.1148/radiol.10092373.
29. Yang ZL, et al. Small intracranial aneurysms: diagnostic accuracy of CT angiography. Radiology. 2017;285(3):941–52. https://doi.org/10.1148/radiol.2017162290.
30. Donmez H, Serifov E, Kahriman G, Mavili E, Durak AC, Menku A. Comparison of 16-row multislice CT angiography with conventional angiography for detection and evaluation of intracranial aneurysms. Eur J Radiol. 2011;80(2):455–61. https://doi.org/10.1016/j.ejrad.2010.07.012.
31. Mckinney AM, Palmer CS, Truwit CL, Karagulle A, Teksam M. Detection of aneurysms by 64-section multidetector CT angiography in patients acutely suspected of having an intracranial aneurysm and comparison with digital subtraction and 3D rotational angiography. Am J Neuroradiol. 2008;29(3):594–602. https://doi.org/10.3174/ajnr.A0848.
32. Catapano JS, et al. Digital subtraction cerebral angiography after negative computed tomography angiography findings in non-traumatic subarachnoid hemorrhage. J Neurointerv Surg. 2020;12(5):526–30. https://doi.org/10.1136/neurintsurg-2019-015375.
33. Rustemi O, et al. Detection of unruptured intracranial aneurysms on noninvasive imaging. Is there still a role for digital subtraction angiography? Surg Neurol Int. 2015;6(1) https://doi.org/10.4103/2152-7806.170029.
34. Dupont SA, Lanzino G, Wijdicks EFM, Rabinstein AA. The use of clinical and routine imaging data to differentiate between aneurysmal and nonaneurysmal subarachnoid hemorrhage prior to angiography: clinical article. J Neurosurg. 2010;113(4):790–4. https://doi.org/10.3171/2010.4.JNS091932.
35. Kapadia A, Schweizer TA, Spears J, Cusimano M, Macdonald RL. Nonaneurysmal perimesencephalic subarachnoid hemorrhage: diagnosis, pathophysiology, clinical characteristics, and long-term outcome. World Neurosurg. 2014;82(6):1131–43. https://doi.org/10.1016/j.wneu.2014.07.006.
36. Rinkel GJ, et al. Nonaneurysmal perimesencephalic subarachnoid hemorrhage: CT and MR patterns that differ from aneurysmal rupture. AJNR Am J Neuroradiol. 1991;12(5):829–34.
37. Jaja BNR, et al. Clinical prediction models for aneurysmal subarachnoid hemorrhage: a systematic review. Neurocrit Care. 2013;18(1):143–53. https://doi.org/10.1007/s12028-012-9792-z.

38. Van Heuven AW, Mees SMD, Algra A, Rinkel GJE. Validation of a prognostic subarachnoid hemorrhage grading scale derived directly from the Glasgow Coma Scale. Stroke. 2008;39(4):1347–8. https://doi.org/10.1161/STROKEAHA.107.498345.
39. Frontera JA, et al. Prediction of symptomatic vasospasm after subarachnoid hemorrhage: the modified Fisher scale. Neurosurgery. 2006;59(1):21–6. https://doi.org/10.1227/01.NEU.0000218821.34014.1B.
40. Fung C, et al. Reconsidering the logic of world Federation of Neurosurgical Societies grading in patients with severe subarachnoid hemorrhage. J Neurosurg. 2016;124(2):299–304. https://doi.org/10.3171/2015.2.JNS14614.
41. Van Donkelaar CE, et al. Timing of clinical assessment. J Neurosurg. 2017;126(1):52–9. https://doi.org/10.3171/2016.1.JNS152136.52.
42. Rosengart AJ, Schultheiss KE, Tolentino J, Macdonald RL. Prognostic factors for outcome in patients with aneurysmal subarachnoid hemorrhage. Stroke. 2007;38(8):2315–21. https://doi.org/10.1161/STROKEAHA.107.484360.
43. Nomura Y, et al. Retrospective analysis of predictors of cerebral vasospasm after ruptured cerebral aneurysm surgery: influence of the location of subarachnoid blood. J Anesth. 2010;24(1):1–6. https://doi.org/10.1007/s00540-009-0836-2.
44. Witsch J, et al. Prognostication of long-term outcomes after subarachnoid hemorrhage: the FRESH score. Ann Neurol. 2016;80(1):46–58. https://doi.org/10.1002/ana.24675.
45. Jaja BNR, et al. Development and validation of outcome prediction models for aneurysmal subarachnoid haemorrhage: the SAHIT multinational cohort study. BMJ. 2018;360(January):1–17. https://doi.org/10.1136/bmj.j5745.
46. Rabinstein AA, Lanzino G, Wijdicks EF. Multidisciplinary management and emerging therapeutic strategies in aneurysmal subarachnoid haemorrhage. Lancet Neurol. 2010;9(5):504–19. https://doi.org/10.1016/S1474-4422(10)70087-9.
47. Diringer MN, et al. Critical care management of patients following aneurysmal subarachnoid hemorrhage: Recommendations from the Neurocritical Care Society's multidisciplinary consensus conference. Neurocrit Care. 2011;15(2):211–40. https://doi.org/10.1007/s12028-011-9605-9.
48. Molyneux AJ, Kerr RSC, Yu L-M, Clarke M, Sneade M, Yamold JA. Articles Introduction International Subarachnoid Aneurysm Trial (ISAT) of neurosurgical clipping versus endovascular coiling in 2143 patients with ruptured intracranial aneurysms: a randomized comparison of effects on survival, dependency, seizures, rebleeding, subgroups, and aneurysm occlusion. 2005. Available: www.thelancet.com.
49. Molyneux A, et al. International Subarachnoid Aneurysm Trial (ISAT) of neurosurgical clipping versus endovascular coiling in 2143 patients with ruptured intracranial aneurysms: a randomized trial. Lancet. 2002;360(9342):1267–74. https://doi.org/10.1016/S0140-6736(02)11314-6.
50. Raper DMS, Allan R. International subarachnoid trial in the long run: critical evaluation of the long-term follow-up data from the ISAT trial of clipping vs coiling for ruptured intracranial aneurysms. Neurosurgery. 2010;66(6):1166–9; discussion 1169,. https://doi.org/10.1227/01.NEU.0000369613.44834.12.
51. Molyneux AJ, Birks J, Clarke A, Sneade M, Kerr RSC. The durability of endovascular coiling versus neurosurgical clipping of ruptured cerebral aneurysms: 18 year follow-up of the UK cohort of the International Subarachnoid Aneurysm Trial (ISAT). Lancet. 2015;385(9969):691–7. https://doi.org/10.1016/S0140-6736(14)60975-2.
52. Vergouwen MDI, Ilodigwe D, Macdonald RL. Cerebral infarction after subarachnoid hemorrhage contributes to poor outcome by vasospasm-dependent and -independent effects. Stroke. 2011;42(4):924–9. https://doi.org/10.1161/STROKEAHA.110.597914.
53. Macdonald RL. Delayed neurological deterioration after subarachnoid haemorrhage. Nat Rev Neurol. 2014;10(1):44–58. https://doi.org/10.1038/nrneurol.2013.246.
54. Etminan N, Macdonald RL. Medical complications after aneurysmal subarachnoid hemorrhage: an emerging contributor to poor outcome. World Neurosurg. 2015;83(3):303–4. https://doi.org/10.1016/j.wneu.2014.06.031.

55. Macdonald RL, Diringer MN, Citerio G. Understanding the disease: aneurysmal subarachnoid hemorrhage. Intensive Care Med. 2014;40(12):1940–3. https://doi.org/10.1007/s00134-014-3483-5.
56. Sen J, Belli A, Albon H, Morgan L, Petzold A, Kitchen N. Triple-H therapy in the management of aneurysmal subarachnoid haemorrhage. Lancet Neurol. 2003;2(10):614–21. https://doi.org/10.1016/s1474-4422(03)00531-3.
57. Anetsberger A, et al. Impact of goal-directed therapy on delayed ischemia after aneurysmal subarachnoid hemorrhage: randomized controlled trial. Stroke. 2020;51(8):2287–96. https://doi.org/10.1161/STROKEAHA.120.029279.
58. Drevet C-M, et al. Impact of restrictive fluid protocol on hypoxemia after aneurysmal subarachnoid hemorrhage. J Crit Care. 2017;42:152–6. https://doi.org/10.1016/j.jcrc.2017.07.031.
59. Sakr Y, et al. Poor outcome is associated with less negative fluid balance in patients with aneurysmal subarachnoid hemorrhage treated with prophylactic vasopressor-induced hypertension. Ann Intensive Care. 2016;6(1):25. https://doi.org/10.1186/s13613-016-0128-6.
60. Deem S, Diringer M, Livesay S, Treggiari MM. Hemodynamic Management in the Prevention and Treatment of delayed cerebral ischemia after aneurysmal subarachnoid hemorrhage. Neurocrit Care. 2023;39(1):81–90. https://doi.org/10.1007/s12028-023-01738-w.
61. Lennihan L, et al. Effect of hypervolemic therapy on cerebral blood flow after subarachnoid hemorrhage: a randomized controlled trial. Stroke. 2000;31(2):383–91. https://doi.org/10.1161/01.str.31.2.383.
62. Bergmans B, Egal M, Van Bommel J, Bakker J, Van der Jagt M. Effects of cardiac output-guided hemodynamic management on fluid administration after aneurysmal subarachnoid hemorrhage. Crit Care. 2014;18(Suppl 1):P455. https://doi.org/10.1186/cc13645.
63. Tagami T, et al. Optimal range of global end-diastolic volume for fluid management after aneurysmal subarachnoid hemorrhage. Crit Care Med. 2014;42(6):1348–56. https://doi.org/10.1097/CCM.0000000000000163.
64. Jaeger M, Soehle M, Schuhmann MU, Meixensberger J. Clinical significance of impaired cerebrovascular autoregulation after severe aneurysmal subarachnoid hemorrhage. Stroke. 2012;43(8):2097–101. https://doi.org/10.1161/STROKEAHA.112.659888.
65. Jaeger M, Schuhmann MU, Soehle M, Nagel C, Meixensberger J. Continuous monitoring of cerebrovascular autoregulation after subarachnoid hemorrhage by brain tissue oxygen pressure reactivity and its relation to delayed cerebral infarction. Stroke. 2007;38(3):981–6. https://doi.org/10.1161/01.STR.0000257964.65743.99.
66. Priebe H-J. Aneurysmal subarachnoid haemorrhage and the anaesthetist. Br J Anaesth. 2007;99(1):102–18. https://doi.org/10.1093/bja/aem119.
67. Addis A, Baggiani M, Citerio G. Intracranial pressure monitoring and management in aneurysmal subarachnoid hemorrhage. Neurocrit Care. 2023;39(1):59–69. https://doi.org/10.1007/s12028-023-01752-y.
68. Hawryluk GWJ, et al. A management algorithm for patients with intracranial pressure monitoring: the Seattle International Severe Traumatic Brain Injury Consensus Conference (SIBICC). Intensive Care Med. 2019;45(12):1783–94. https://doi.org/10.1007/s00134-019-05805-9.
69. Stocchetti N, Maas AIR, Chieregato A, van der Plas AA. Hyperventilation in head injury: a review. Chest. 2005;127(5):1812–27. https://doi.org/10.1378/chest.127.5.1812.
70. Kassell NF, Torner JC. Aneurysmal rebleeding: a preliminary report from the cooperative aneurysm study. Neurosurgery. 1983;13(5):479–81. https://doi.org/10.1227/00006123-198311000-00001.
71. Kassell NF, Torner JC, Haley EC, Jane JA, Adams HP, Kongable GL. The international cooperative study on the timing of aneurysm surgery. Part 1: overall management results. J Neurosurg. 1990;73(1):18–36. https://doi.org/10.3171/jns.1990.73.1.0018.
72. Starke RM, et al. Impact of a protocol for acute antifibrinolytic therapy on aneurysm rebleeding after subarachnoid hemorrhage. Stroke. 2008;39(9):2617–21. https://doi.org/10.1161/STROKEAHA.107.506097.

73. Post R, et al. Ultra-early tranexamic acid after subarachnoid haemorrhage (ULTRA): a randomised controlled trial. Lancet. 2021;397(10269):112–8. https://doi.org/10.1016/S0140-6736(20)32518-6.
74. Liu-Deryke X, Janisse J, Coplin WM, Parker D, Norris G, Rhoney DH. A comparison of nicardipine and labetalol for acute hypertension management following stroke. Neurocrit Care. 2008;9(2):167–76. https://doi.org/10.1007/s12028-008-9057-z.
75. Hockel K, Scholler K, Trabold R, Nussberger J, Plesnila N. Vasopressin V(1a) receptors mediate posthemorrhagic systemic hypertension thereby determining rebleeding rate and outcome after experimental subarachnoid hemorrhage. Stroke. 2012;43(1):227–32. https://doi.org/10.1161/STROKEAHA.111.626168.
76. Connolly ES, et al. Guidelines for the management of aneurysmal subarachnoid hemorrhage: a guideline for healthcare professionals from the American Heart Association/American Stroke Association. Stroke. 2012;43(6):1711–37. https://doi.org/10.1161/STR.0b013e3182587839.
77. Ransom ER, et al. External ventricular drainage response in poor grade aneurysmal subarachnoid hemorrhage: effect on preoperative grading and prognosis. Neurocrit Care. 2007;6(3):174–80. https://doi.org/10.1007/s12028-007-0019-7.
78. Hoekema D, Schmidt RH, Ross I. Lumbar drainage for subarachnoid hemorrhage: technical considerations and safety analysis. Neurocrit Care. 2007;7(1):3–9. https://doi.org/10.1007/s12028-007-0047-3.
79. Klopfenstein JD, et al. Comparison of rapid and gradual weaning from external ventricular drainage in patients with aneurysmal subarachnoid hemorrhage: a prospective randomized trial. J Neurosurg. 2004;100(2):225–9. https://doi.org/10.3171/jns.2004.100.2.0225.
80. Claassen J, et al. Predictors and clinical impact of epilepsy after subarachnoid hemorrhage. Neurology. 2003;60(2):208–14. https://doi.org/10.1212/01.wnl.0000038906.71394.de.
81. Ibrahim GM, Fallah A, Macdonald RL. Clinical, laboratory, and radiographic predictors of the occurrence of seizures following aneurysmal subarachnoid hemorrhage. J Neurosurg. 2013;119(2):347–52. https://doi.org/10.3171/2013.3.JNS122097.
82. Raper DMS, Starke RM, Komotar RJ, Allan R, Connolly ES. Seizures after aneurysmal subarachnoid hemorrhage: a systematic review of outcomes. World Neurosurg. 2013;79(5–6):682–90. https://doi.org/10.1016/j.wneu.2012.08.006.
83. Piani B, Andraos C, Mabry I, Siddiqi J. A comparison of seizure prophylaxis: phenytoin versus Levetiracetam. Cureus. 2021;13(5):e14956. https://doi.org/10.7759/cureus.14956.
84. de Rooij NK, Rinkel GJE, Dankbaar JW, Frijns CJM. Delayed cerebral ischemia after subarachnoid hemorrhage: a systematic review of clinical, laboratory, and radiological predictors. Stroke. 2013;44(1):43–54. https://doi.org/10.1161/STROKEAHA.112.674291.
85. Gonzalez NR, Boscardin WJ, Glenn T, Vinuela F, Martin NA. Vasospasm probability index: a combination of transcranial Doppler velocities, cerebral blood flow, and clinical risk factors to predict cerebral vasospasm after aneurysmal subarachnoid hemorrhage. J Neurosurg. 2007;107(6):1101–12. https://doi.org/10.3171/JNS-07/12/1101.
86. Lauritzen M, Dreier JP, Fabricius M, Hartings JA, Graf R, Strong AJ. Clinical relevance of cortical spreading depression in neurological disorders: migraine, malignant stroke, subarachnoid and intracranial hemorrhage, and traumatic brain injury. J Cereb Blood Flow Metab. 2011;31(1):17–35. https://doi.org/10.1038/jcbfm.2010.191.
87. Dreier JP, et al. Cortical spreading ischemia is a novel process involved in ischemic damage in patients with aneurysmal subarachnoid hemorrhage. Brain. 2009;132(Pt 7):1866–81. https://doi.org/10.1093/brain/awp102.
88. Woitzik J, et al. Delayed cerebral ischemia and spreading depolarization in the absence of angiographic vasospasm after subarachnoid hemorrhage. J Cereb Blood Flow Metab. 2012;32(2):203–12. https://doi.org/10.1038/jcbfm.2011.169.
89. Chen HY, et al. Combining transcranial Doppler and EEG data to predict delayed cerebral ischemia after subarachnoid hemorrhage. Neurology. 2022;98(5):e459–69. https://doi.org/10.1212/WNL.0000000000013126.
90. Kumar G, Shahripour RB, Harrigan MR. Vasospasm on transcranial Doppler is predictive of delayed cerebral ischemia in aneurysmal subarachnoid hemorrhage: a systematic review

and meta-analysis. J Neurosurg. 2016;124(5):1257–64. https://doi.org/10.3171/2015.4.JNS15428.
91. Kim JA, et al. High epileptiform discharge burden predicts delayed cerebral ischemia after subarachnoid hemorrhage. Clin Neurophysiol. 2022;141:139–46. https://doi.org/10.1016/j.clinph.2021.01.022.
92. Kondziella D, Friberg CK, Wellwood I, Reiffurth C, Fabricius M, Dreier JP. Continuous EEG monitoring in aneurysmal subarachnoid hemorrhage: a systematic review. Neurocrit Care. 2015;22(3):450–61. https://doi.org/10.1007/s12028-014-0068-7.
93. Claassen J, et al. Quantitative continuous EEG for detecting delayed cerebral ischemia in patients with poor-grade subarachnoid hemorrhage. Clin Neurophysiol. 2004;115(12):2699–710. https://doi.org/10.1016/j.clinph.2004.06.017.
94. Suarez JI, et al. Symptomatic vasospasm diagnosis after subarachnoid hemorrhage: evaluation of transcranial Doppler ultrasound and cerebral angiography as related to compromised vascular distribution. Crit Care Med. 2002;30(6):1348–55. https://doi.org/10.1097/00003246-200206000-00035.
95. Krejza J, Mariak Z, Melhem ER, Bert RJ. A guide to the identification of major cerebral arteries with transcranial color Doppler sonography. Am J Roentgenol. 2000;174(5):1297–303. https://doi.org/10.2214/ajr.174.5.1741297.
96. Robba C, Taccone FS. How I use transcranial Doppler. Crit Care. 2019;23(1) https://doi.org/10.1186/s13054-019-2700-6.
97. Wilson CD, Shankar JJS. Diagnosing vasospasm after subarachnoid hemorrhage: CTA and CTP. Can J Neurol Sci. 2014;41(3):314–9. https://doi.org/10.1017/s031716710001725x.
98. Veldeman M, et al. Invasive multimodal Neuromonitoring in aneurysmal subarachnoid hemorrhage: a systematic review. Stroke. 2021;52(11):3624–32. https://doi.org/10.1161/STROKEAHA.121.034633.
99. Tomé R, et al. Double hemispheric microdialysis study in poor-grade SAH patients. Sci Rep. 2020;10(1):7466. https://doi.org/10.1038/s41598-020-64543-x.
100. Craven CL, Sae-Huang M, Hoskote C, Watkins LD, Reddy U, Torna AK. Relationship between brain tissue oxygen tension and transcranial Doppler ultrasonography. World Neurosurg. 2021;149:e942–6. https://doi.org/10.1016/j.wneu.2021.01.070.
101. Nagel A, Graetz D, Vajkoczy P, Sarrafzadeh AS. Decompressive craniectomy in aneurysmal subarachnoid hemorrhage: relation to cerebral perfusion pressure and metabolism. Neurocrit Care. 2009;11(3):384–94. https://doi.org/10.1007/s12028-009-9269-x.
102. Patet C, et al. Bedside cerebral microdialysis monitoring of delayed cerebral hypoperfusion in comatose patients with poor grade aneurysmal subarachnoid haemorrhage. J Neurol Neurosurg Psychiatry. 2017;88(4):332–8. https://doi.org/10.1136/jnnp-2016-313766.
103. Rostami E, et al. Early low cerebral blood flow and high cerebral lactate: prediction of delayed cerebral ischemia in subarachnoid hemorrhage. J Neurosurg. 2018;128(6):1762–70. https://doi.org/10.3171/2016.11.JNS161140.
104. Bullock R, et al. Factors affecting excitatory amino acid release following severe human head injury. J Neurosurg. 1998;89(4):507–18. https://doi.org/10.3171/jns.1998.89.4.0507.
105. Dorhout Mees SM, et al. Calcium antagonists for aneurysmal subarachnoid haemorrhage. Cochrane Database Syst Rev. 2007;(3):CD000277. https://doi.org/10.1002/14651858.CD000277.pub3.
106. Allen GS, et al. Cerebral arterial spasm—a controlled trial of nimodipine in patients with subarachnoid hemorrhage. N Engl J Med. 1983;308(11):619–24. https://doi.org/10.1056/NEJM198303173081103.
107. Vergouwen MDI, de Haan RJ, Vermeulen M, Roos YBWEM. Effect of statin treatment on vasospasm, delayed cerebral ischemia, and functional outcome in patients with aneurysmal subarachnoid hemorrhage. Stroke. 2010;41(1) https://doi.org/10.1161/STROKEAHA.109.556332.
108. Shen J, et al. Effect of statin treatment on vasospasm-related morbidity and functional outcome in patients with aneurysmal subarachnoid hemorrhage: a systematic review and meta-analysis. J Neurosurg. 2017;127(2):291–301. https://doi.org/10.3171/2016.5.JNS152900.

109. Jeon JS, Sheen SH, Hwang G, Kang SH, Heo DH, Cho Y-J. Intravenous magnesium infusion for the prevention of symptomatic cerebral vasospasm after aneurysmal subarachnoid hemorrhage. J Korean Neurosurg Soc. 2012;52(2):75. https://doi.org/10.3340/jkns.2012.52.2.75.
110. van der Bilt I, et al. Cardiac dysfunction after aneurysmal subarachnoid hemorrhage: relationship with outcome. Neurology. 2014;82(4):351–8. https://doi.org/10.1212/WNL.0000000000000057.
111. Estafiol Vidal B, et al. Cardiac arrhythmias associated with subarachnoid hemorrhage: prospective study. Neurosurgery. 1979;5(6):675–80. https://doi.org/10.1227/00006123-197912000-00005.
112. Murthy SB, Shah S, Rao CPV, Bershad EM, Suarez JI. Neurogenic stunned myocardium following acute subarachnoid hemorrhage. J Intensive Care Med. 2015;30(6):318–25. https://doi.org/10.1177/0885066613511054.
113. Mazzeo AT, Micalizzi A, Mascia L, Scicolone A, Siracusano L. Brain-heart crosstalk: the many faces of stress-related cardiomyopathy syndromes in anaesthesia and intensive care. Br J Anaesth. 2014;112(5):803–15. https://doi.org/10.1093/bja/aeu046.
114. Wagner S, et al. Aneurysmal subarachnoid hemorrhage as a trigger for Takotsubo syndrome: a comprehensive review. Rev Cardiovasc Med. 2021;22(4):1241. https://doi.org/10.31083/j.rcm2204132.
115. Ochiai H, Yamakawa Y, Kubota E. Deformation of the ventrolateral medulla oblongata by subarachnoid hemorrhage from ruptured vertebral artery aneurysms causes neurogenic pulmonary edema. Neurol Med Chir (Tokyo). 2001;41(11):529–34; discussion 534-5,. https://doi.org/10.2176/nmc.41.529.
116. Vincent J-L, editor. Annual update in intensive care and emergency medicine 2012. Berlin/Heidelberg: Springer Berlin Heidelberg; 2012. https://doi.org/10.1007/978-3-642-25716-2.
117. Theodore J, Robin ED. Speculations on neurogenic pulmonary edema (NPE). Am Rev Respir Dis. 1976;113(4):405–11. https://doi.org/10.1164/arrd.1976.113.4.405.
118. Feldstein E, et al. Acute respiratory distress syndrome in patients with subarachnoid hemorrhage: incidence, predictive factors, and impact on mortality. Interv Neuroradiol. 2023;29(2):189–95. https://doi.org/10.1177/15910199221082457.
119. Roth C, et al. Does prone positioning increase intracranial pressure? A retrospective analysis of patients with acute brain injury and acute respiratory failure. Neurocrit Care. 2014;21(2):186–91. https://doi.org/10.1007/s12028-014-0004-x.
120. Dirnagl U, et al. Stroke-induced immunodepression: experimental evidence and clinical relevance. Stroke. 2007;38(2 Suppl):770–3. https://doi.org/10.1161/01.STR.0000251441.89665.bc.
121. Dasenbrock HH, et al. Hospital-acquired infections after aneurysmal subarachnoid hemorrhage: a Nationwide analysis. World Neurosurg. 2016;88:459–74. https://doi.org/10.1016/j.wneu.2015.10.054.
122. Scaravilli V, Tinchero G, Citerio G. Fever Management in SAH. Neurocrit Care. 2011;15(2):287–94. https://doi.org/10.1007/s12028-011-9588-6.
123. Suehiro E, et al. Importance of early postoperative body temperature management for treatment of subarachnoid hemorrhage. J Stroke Cerebrovasc Dis. 2016;25(6):1482–8. https://doi.org/10.1016/j.jstrokecerebrovasdis.2016.01.053.
124. Mayer SA, et al. Clinical trial of a novel surface cooling system for fever control in neurocritical care patients*. Crit Care Med. 2004;32(12):2508–15. https://doi.org/10.1097/O1.CCM.0000147441.39670.37.
125. Broessner G, et al. Prophylactic, Endovascularly based, long-term Normothermia in ICU patients with severe cerebrovascular disease. Stroke. 2009;40(12) https://doi.org/10.1161/STROKEAHA.109.557652.
126. Picetti E, et al. Early management of patients with aneurysmal subarachnoid hemorrhage in a hospital with neurosurgical/neuroendovascular facilities: a consensus and clinical recommendations of the Italian Society of Anesthesia and Intensive Care (SIAARTI) - part 2. J Anesth Analg Crit Care. 2022;2(1):21. https://doi.org/10.1186/s44158-022-00049-4.

127. Picetti E, et al. Intravenous paracetamol for fever control in acute brain injury patients: cerebral and hemodynamic effects. Acta Neurochir. 2014;156(10):1953–9; discussion 1959. https://doi.org/10.1007/s00701-014-2129-2.
128. Liang CW, Su K, Liu JJ, Dogan A, Hinson HE. Timing of deep vein thrombosis formation after aneurysmal subarachnoid hemorrhage. J Neurosurg. 2015;123(4):891–6. https://doi.org/10.3171/2014.12.JNS141288.
129. Kshettry VR, Rosenbaum BP, Seicean A, Kelly ML, Schiltz NK, Weil RJ. Incidence and risk factors associated with in-hospital venous thromboembolism after aneurysmal subarachnoid hemorrhage. J Clin Neurosci. 2014;21(2):282–6. https://doi.org/10.1016/j.jocn.2013.07.003.
130. Hall A, O'Kane R. The extracranial consequences of subarachnoid hemorrhage. World Neurosurg. 2018;109:381–92. https://doi.org/10.1016/j.wneu.2017.10.016.
131. Koyanna S, Panda NB, Mahajan S, Bharti N, Patel S, Singla N. The predictors of hyperglycemia and its effects on neurological outcome in the patients with aneurysmal subarachnoid hemorrhage undergoing surgical clipping: A prospective observational study. Surg Neurol Int. 2022;13:471. https://doi.org/10.25259/SNI_646_2022.
132. Badjatia N, et al. Relationship between hyperglycemia and symptomatic vasospasm after subarachnoid hemorrhage. Crit Care Med. 2005;33(7):1603–9; quiz 1623. https://doi.org/10.1097/01.ccm.0000168054.60538.2b.
133. Singer P, et al. ESPEN guideline on clinical nutrition in the intensive care unit. Clin Nutr. 2019;38(1):48–79. https://doi.org/10.1016/j.clnu.2018.08.037.
134. Badjatia N, et al. Inflammation, negative nitrogen balance, and outcome after aneurysmal subarachnoid hemorrhage. Neurology. 2015;84(7):680–7. https://doi.org/10.1212/WNL.0000000000001259.
135. Rahman A, Hasan RM, Agarwala R, Martin C, Day AG, Heyland DK. Identifying critically ill patients who will benefit most from nutritional therapy: further validation of the "modified NUTRIC" nutritional risk assessment tool. Clin Nutr. 2016;35(1):158–62. https://doi.org/10.1016/j.clnu.2015.01.015.
136. Hannon MJ, Finucane FM, Sherlock M, Agha A, Thompson CJ. Clinical review: disorders of water homeostasis in neurosurgical patients. J Clin Endocrinol Metab. 2012;97(5):1423–33. https://doi.org/10.1210/jc.2011-3201.
137. Suarez JI, Tarr RW, Selman WR. Aneurysmal subarachnoid hemorrhage. N Engl J Med. 2006;354(4):387–96. https://doi.org/10.1056/NEJMra052732.
138. Hasan D, et al. Effect of fludrocortisone acetate in patients with subarachnoid hemorrhage. Stroke. 1989;20(9):1156–61. https://doi.org/10.1161/01.str.20.9.1156.
139. Fisher LA, et al. Hypernatremia predicts adverse cardiovascular and neurological outcomes after SAH. Neurocrit Care. 2006;5(3):180–5. https://doi.org/10.1385/NCC:5:3:180.

26 Cardiorespiratory Monitoring in Patients with Acute Respiratory Distress Syndrome

Antonio Fioccola and Davide Chiumello

26.1 Introduction

Patients with acute respiratory distress syndrome (ARDS) develop inflammatory pulmonary edema caused by changes in endothelial permeability. Disease severity is classified according to the Berlin definition as mild, moderate, or severe (see Table 26.1). This definition was recently modified (Kigali) to broaden its application to patients not undergoing mechanical ventilation or in settings where blood gas analysis is unavailable, using the ratio of peripheral oxygen saturation to inspired oxygen fraction (SpO_2/FiO_2) as a surrogate for the P/F ratio (see Table 26.1) [1].

The application of different types of organ support is required depending on the severity of ARDS. Any hemodynamic compromise superimposed on pulmonary edema can complicate patient management and worsen prognosis. Therefore, a comprehensive assessment of patients with ARDS requires careful respiratory and hemodynamic monitoring, including both invasive and noninvasive technologies, as well as clinical and laboratory data. This approach is crucial for tailoring therapeutic strategies to individual patients and minimizing lung injury.

This chapter reviews strategies for respiratory and hemodynamic monitoring in patients with ARDS, highlighting their clinical utility and the most recent data in the literature.

A. Fioccola · D. Chiumello (✉)
Department of Health Sciences, University of Milan, Milan, Italy

Department of Anesthesia and Intensive Care, ASST Santi Paolo e Carlo, San Paolo University Hospital, Milan, Italy
e-mail: antonio.fioccola@unimi.it; davide.chiumello@unimi.it

D. Chiumello, A. De Gasperi (eds.), *Practical Trends in Anesthesia and Intensive Care 2026*, https://doi.org/10.1007/978-3-032-25721-5_26

Table 26.1 Berlin definition and Kigali modification for the diagnosis of ARDS

	Berlin criteria	Kigali modification
Symptom onset timing	Within one week of clinical insult	Within one week of clinical insult
Oxygenation	*Mild*: $200 < PaO_2/FiO_2 \leq 300$ *Moderate*: $100 < PaO_2/FiO_2 \leq 200$ *Severe*: $PaO_2/FiO_2 < 100$	*Mild*: $235 \leq SpO2/FiO2 \leq 315$ *Moderate*: $148 \leq SpO2/FiO2 \leq 235$ *Severe*: $SpO2/FiO2 \leq 148$
PEEP	Minimum of 5 cm H_2O	The application of PEEP is not required for diagnosis (in accordance with the AECC definition)
Imaging techniques	Bilateral opacities not fully explained by effusions, lobar collapse, or nodules on chest X-ray or CT	Bilateral opacities not fully explained by effusions, lobar collapse, or nodules on chest X-ray, CT, or by lung ultrasound
Origin of edema	Respiratory failure not fully explained by cardiac failure or fluid overload	Respiratory failure not fully explained by cardiac failure or fluid overload

Main updates introduced by the Kigali modification to the Berlin definition of ARDS are underlined
Legend: *PaO_2/FiO_2* ratio of arterial partial pressure of oxygen to inspired oxygen fraction, *SpO_2/FiO_2* ratio of peripheral oxygen saturation by pulse oximetry to inspired oxygen fraction, *PEEP* positive end-expiratory pressure, *cmH_2O* centimeters of water, *AECC* American European Consensus Conference, *CT* computed tomography

26.2 Respiratory Monitoring

Careful respiratory monitoring is essential in patients with ARDS. This approach allows for the application of appropriate treatment intensity and helps minimize lung injury caused by mechanical ventilation (*Ventilator-Induced Lung Injury* (VILI)).

26.2.1 Gas Exchange Efficiency

Gas exchange is directly affected by the pulmonary alterations induced by ARDS. It determines the classification of ARDS as mild, moderate, or severe according to the Berlin criteria. In this section, we examine the renewed role of pulse oximetry in patients with ARDS and new indices for monitoring dead space in patients undergoing mechanical ventilation.

26.2.1.1 Pulse Oximetry

Pulse oximetry is based on the principle of spectrophotometry to quantify the amount of oxygenated hemoglobin in the blood, allowing for continuous and non-invasive monitoring of arterial oxygen saturation [2]. The pulse oximeter is equipped with two diodes that emit light at two different wavelengths: red (660 nm) and infrared (940 nm). On the opposite side, a photocell measures the amount of light transmitted through the patient's skin. Oxygenated hemoglobin absorbs infrared light (940 nm) more effectively, while deoxygenated hemoglobin has a peak absorption at 660 nm. Consequently, detection of a lower amount of infrared light by the photocell indicates a higher presence of oxygenated hemoglobin, while detection of a lower amount of red light indicates a higher presence of deoxygenated hemoglobin. The pulse oximeter's photocell detects *pulsatile* variations in the amount of red and infrared light passing through the patient's skin, thereby determining the percentage of oxygenated hemoglobin only in arterial (pulsatile) blood, ignoring the signal from venous (nonpulsatile) blood (see Fig. 26.1).

The difference between oxygen saturation measured by arterial blood gas analysis (SaO_2) and oxygen saturation measured by pulse oximetry (SpO_2) is normally less than 3% [3]. However, as recently highlighted, the accuracy of pulse oximeters may be lower in patients with dark skin pigmentation, in whom saturation is overestimated. This phenomenon may increase the incidence of occult hypoxemia, defined as a situation in which SaO_2 is below 88% while SpO_2 is above 92% [4]. During the COVID-19 pandemic, it was shown that occult hypoxemia can lead to reduced intensity of treatment in Asian, Black, and Hispanic patients compared to White patients [5].

The ratio between arterial partial pressure of oxygen and FiO_2 (PaO_2/FiO_2, also known as the P/F ratio or Horowitz index) is used to monitor the adequacy of gas exchange and is the parameter by which ARDS severity is determined, as reported in the Berlin criteria (see Table 26.1). The SpO_2/FiO_2 ratio can be an acceptable surrogate for the P/F ratio, and its validity as a diagnostic and prognostic factor has been affirmed by the Kigali modifications to the Berlin definition. The use of SpO_2/FiO_2 has been described in both invasively and noninvasively ventilated patients

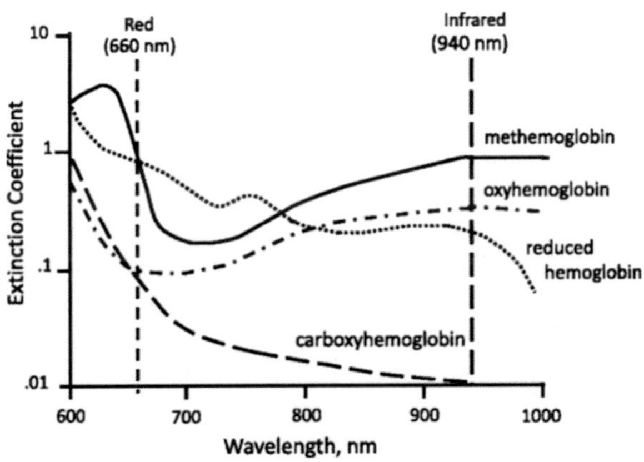

Fig. 26.1 Absorption peaks of red and infrared light in various types of hemoglobin. Note the absorption peak of reduced hemoglobin at red light (660 nm), while oxyhemoglobin has an absorption peak at 940 nm (infrared light). Legend: Extinction Coefficient = absorption coefficient; Red = red light; Infrared = infrared light; Wavelength = wavelength; nm = nanometers. (Adapted from Jubran et al. [2])

[6–9]. It appears to be a good prognostic index in both patients with coronavirus disease (COVID-19) and those with non-COVID-19 ARDS [10, 11]. In COVID-19 patients receiving oxygen therapy, the SpO_2/FiO_2 ratio at admission has shown good diagnostic accuracy, with an area under the curve (AUC, *Area Under the Curve*) of 85% for predicting the onset of ARDS [12]. Kim et al. demonstrated that the SpO_2/FiO_2 ratio can predict the need to escalate the level of care in patients receiving oxygen therapy with high-flow nasal cannula (HFNC, *High Flow Nasal Cannula*) [13]. Moreover, the SpO_2/FiO_2 ratio shows good correlation with PaO_2/FiO_2 in COVID-19 ARDS patients undergoing invasive ventilation and, when calculated on the second and third day of hospitalization, is a predictive index of mortality [12]. These data confirm the reliability of pulse oximetry for assessing gas exchange in ARDS patients and for monitoring its progression. SpO_2 is easy to measure, noninvasive, and particularly valuable in settings where blood gas analysis is not available.

The optimal SpO_2 target during the treatment of ARDS patients is still debated in the literature. In a recently conducted randomized controlled trial (RCT), Semler et al. showed that, in patients undergoing mechanical ventilation, the use of a lower SpO_2 target (90%, with a range from 88% to 92%), intermediate (94%, from 92% to 96%), or higher (98%, from 96% to 100%) does not affect either ventilator days or hospital outcomes [14].

26.2.2 Dead Space

Physiological dead space is the volume of inspired air that does not participate in gas exchange. It includes both anatomical dead space and alveolar dead space [15]. In patients undergoing mechanical ventilation, anatomical dead space remains relatively constant, whereas alveolar dead space can increase significantly depending on changes in the ventilation/perfusion (V/Q) ratio [16, 17].

In a highly relevant study, Nuckton et al. demonstrated that physiological dead space is significantly greater in non-ARDS survivors compared to survivors [18]. As in patients with ARDS, COVID-19 pneumonia is characterized by increased minute ventilation and a higher dead space fraction [19, 20]. Furthermore, in patients with COVID-19-related ARDS, there is a significant association between the amount of calculated dead space in the first 7 days and mortality [21]. According to a secondary analysis of the PRoVENT COVID-19 study, the dead space fraction is significantly higher in non-survivors and increases more during the first 4 days compared to survivors, suggesting that dynamic changes during the first week in the intensive care unit (ICU) are crucial prognostic factors [22]. These recent data highlight the important role of dead space and reinforce the rationale for its monitoring in patients with ARDS. Direct calculation of dead space is complex and requires measurement of the mean partial pressure of CO_2 in the exhaled air. Such measurement is possible using devices such as volumetric capnometry or indirect calorimetry, which are not always available in clinical practice.

Corrected minute ventilation (V_{Ecorr}), the *Ventilatory Ratio* (VR), and the ratio between end-tidal CO_2 and arterial CO_2 pressure ($P_{ET}CO_2/PaCO_2$) are three surrogate measures that can be used clinically to estimate dead space trends in patients undergoing mechanical ventilation, and are simpler to calculate than direct measurement of dead space.

26.2.2.1 Corrected Minute Ventilation

Corrected minute ventilation is a surrogate for dead space fraction that is easy to calculate, as it does not require measurement of exhaled carbon dioxide. V_{Ecorr} is calculated as the ventilation required to achieve a $PaCO_2$ value of 40 mmHg. In patients with COVID-19-related ARDS undergoing mechanical ventilation, Fusina et al. found a strong correlation between V_{Ecorr} and dead space fraction, with higher V_{Ecorr} values in non-survivors. In this study, the authors demonstrated that V_{Ecorr} is associated with mortality in patients with ARDS [23].

26.2.2.2 Ventilatory Ratio

In recent years, the *Ventilatory Ratio* (VR) has emerged as a useful surrogate for dead space in patients with ARDS, and is simple to calculate (see Eq. 26.1) [23]. VR is calculated as the product of minute ventilation and the partial pressure of arterial carbon dioxide, normalized to the patient's predicted body weight. In healthy individuals, this ratio is close to one, but it tends to increase progressively in patients with elevated dead space.

Ventilatory Ratio

$$VR = \frac{VM_{real} \times PaCO_{2\,real}}{VM_{ideal} \times PaCO_{2\,ideal}} = \frac{VM_{real} \times PaCO_{2\,real}}{PBW \times 100 \times 37.5} \tag{26.1}$$

Equation 26.1: Legend: VM_{real} = Minute ventilation (mL/min); $PaCO_{2real}$ = arterial CO_2 pressure measured at equilibrium; VM_{ideal} = ideal minute ventilation (mL/min); $PaCO_{2ideal}$ = arterial CO_2 pressure ideally obtained in a healthy subject with VM_{ideal}. PBW = predicted body weight; 100 = conversion factor to obtain ideal VM_{ideal} from predicted body weight; 37.5 = $PaCO_{2ideal}$.

In patients with ARDS, Sinha et al. reported a positive correlation between VR and alveolar dead space. VR is higher in patients with poor prognosis compared to survivors, being associated with an increased likelihood of in-hospital mortality with an *Odds Ratio* (OR) of 2.07 [23]. As recently demonstrated by Siegel et al., in combination with the APACHE III score at admission, VR has an AUC of 0.81 (95% CI 0.68–0.92) in predicting in-hospital mortality and outperforms the APACHE III score alone [24]. Changes in VR within the first 4 h after prone positioning in ARDS patients predict weaning from mechanical ventilation, with an AUC of 0.64 (95% CI 0.53–0.75) [25].

The reliability of VR may be affected by pulmonary shunt (Qva/Q, *venous admixture*) and the amount of CO_2 produced by the patient (VCO_2). These two factors can increase the difference between alveolar and arterial PCO_2, with the latter being used to calculate the Ventilatory Ratio. Maj et al. showed that the predictive value of VR decreases in patients with more severe ARDS, who are characterized by greater pulmonary shunt [26]. Another factor that may potentially reduce the predictive power of the Ventilatory Ratio is the body's production of CO_2 (VCO_2). To investigate this effect, Monteiro et al. performed a post-hoc analysis of the PETAL-ROSE study [27]. The authors showed that the presence of neuromuscular blockade, a factor that reduces muscular production of carbon dioxide, does not significantly affect the relationship between VR and mortality [29].

26.2.2.3 $EtCO_2/PaCO_2$ Ratio

An additional parameter for estimating gas exchange efficiency is the calculation of the ratio between end-tidal carbon dioxide pressure ($P_{ET}CO_2$) and $PaCO_2$ ($P_{ET}CO_2/PaCO_2$), which reflects the impact of pulmonary shunt and alveolar dead space on the efficiency of the pulmonary exchanger. Ideally, this ratio should be equal to one. Bonifazi et al. demonstrated that the $P_{ET}CO_2/PaCO_2$ ratio decreases significantly from mild to severe ARDS [28]. Moreover, the $P_{ET}CO_2/PaCO_2$ ratio is strongly correlated with the amount of non-aerated tissue measured by computed tomography (CT) and with respiratory compliance [28]. A subsequent study revealed a relationship between the $P_{ET}CO_2/PaCO_2$ ratio, alveolar ventilation, and in-hospital mortality [29]. For every 0.01 increase in the $P_{ET}CO_2/PaCO_2$ ratio, the risk of mortality decreases by 1%.

Currently, there are no well-defined criteria for weaning patients from veno-venous extracorporeal membrane oxygenation (VV-ECMO). In a recent multicenter study, Lazzari et al. demonstrated that the $P_{ET}CO_2/PaCO_2$ ratio, with a threshold of 0.83, is able to predict successful weaning [30].

In patients undergoing mechanical ventilation, dead space should be continuously assessed as an additional measure of reduction in gas exchange, together with the PaO_2/FiO_2 or SpO_2/FiO_2 ratio. The use of surrogate measures, which are easier to calculate, appears to be reliable and should encourage the use of such indices to predict patient outcomes.

Caution is warranted when calculating the ventilatory ratio in patients with moderate-to-severe ARDS, who have a higher pulmonary shunt and may therefore affect the assessment of the VR (greater difference between $PACO_2$ and $PaCO_2$), leading to an overestimation of dead space.

26.2.3 Ventilator-Induced and Patient Self-Inflicted Lung Injury

The respiratory system is continuously subjected to the application of energy, which can cause lung injury. Such injury may be induced by mechanical ventilation (VILI, *Ventilation-Induced Lung Injury*) or self-inflicted by the patient (PSILI, *Patient Self-Inflicted Lung Injury*). It is therefore important to quantify the energy transmitted to the airways, both in patients undergoing mechanical ventilation and in those breathing spontaneously. Mechanical Power (MP) is the summary variable used for this purpose. Recently, the concept of Mechanical Power Ratio (MP ratio) has been introduced in the literature, a variable that expresses the ratio between the mechanical energy delivered to the respiratory system in a mechanically ventilated patient and the mechanical energy to which the respiratory system is exposed during spontaneous breathin g under baseline conditions. Measurement of lung volumes, applied pressures, and respiratory rate is essential for calculating MP. In spontaneously breathing patients, measurement of esophageal pressure is necessary to quantify PSILI. Lung injury may be exacerbated by atelectrauma in non-recruited alveoli during expiration and by barotrauma in overdistended alveoli during inspiration. To optimize recruitment and reduce the occurrence of atelectrauma and barotrauma, the recruitment-to-inflation ratio (R/I) can be used clinically. Thoracic electrical impedance tomography (EIT) is gaining an increasingly important role in the literature for the assessment of lung recruitability.

26.2.3.1 Mechanical Power

Mechanical Power refers to the energy dissipated in the respiratory system as a specific volume is moved at a given PEEP. It is typically expressed in Joules per minute (J/min) [31]. The energy dissipated in the respiratory system plays a crucial role in promoting VILI. Mechanical Power is a unifying indicator calculated by considering the main ventilatory variables generated by the interaction between the patient and the ventilator. It can be calculated under passive conditions (controlled ventilation), and several algebraic formulas exist depending on the controlled ventilation mode used (pressure- or volume-controlled) [32]. The latest mechanical ventilators in intensive care offer the possibility of directly measuring Mechanical Power, with acceptable accuracy compared to traditional algebraic methods [33].

Recent studies have shown that Mechanical Power at admission is associated with hospital mortality in a heterogeneous patient population [34–36]. Urner et al. further explored the relationship between the intensity of Mechanical Power during ICU stay and mortality, revealing an increased risk of death in patients exposed to a Mechanical Power equal to or greater than 17 J/min [37]. Pozzi et al. analyzed the clinical course of respiratory variables in ARDS patients during the first 3 days of mechanical ventilation and identified Mechanical Power at admission as the only variable associated with ICU mortality [38]. By the third day, MP, alveolar dead space, and the PaO_2/FiO_2 ratio were associated with outcome. Therefore, it appears crucial to assess ventilatory variables in the early days of mechanical ventilation to predict outcomes in patients with ARDS.

Regarding the different components of Mechanical Power, Costa et al. showed that the dynamic components (i.e., respiratory rate and driving pressure) have a stronger association with mortality than the static components (tidal volume and PEEP) [39]. Finally, Coppola et al. demonstrated that adjusting MP at admission for respiratory system compliance and the amount of ventilated lung tissue calculated by CT scan may provide prognostic information in patients with ARDS [34].

26.2.3.2 Esophageal Pressure

Preserving spontaneous breathing offers several pathophysiological advantages [40, 41]. However, high inspiratory efforts in patients undergoing assisted ventilation modes are associated with significant negative swings in esophageal pressure (Pes).

The resulting transpulmonary pressure is the sum of the pressures applied within the airways (positive pressures delivered by the ventilator) and the negative pressures generated by the patient's spontaneous inspiratory effort (Eq. 26.2): this is the pressure applied across the alveolar membrane during the various phases of respiration. Transpulmonary pressure is the variable that integrates the effects of both mechanical and spontaneous components on the lung: the term VILI is used when the main component of transpulmonary pressure is the pressure within the airways, and PSILI when the main component of transpulmonary pressure consists of esophageal swings [42].

Transpulmonary Pressure

$$P_{\mathrm{L}(i)} = P_{\mathrm{aw}(i)} - P_{\mathrm{es}(i)} \tag{26.2}$$

Equation 26.2: Transpulmonary pressure, that is, the pressure applied across the alveolar-capillary membrane in a patient undergoing mechanical ventilation, is the sum of the (positive) pressure within the airways and the (negative) pressure measured by the esophageal catheter, which corresponds to pleural pressure. The latter becomes more negative as diaphragmatic contraction increases, that is, as the patient's spontaneous inspiratory effort increases. This pressure varies throughout the different phases of ventilation, moment by moment. Legend: $P_{L(i)}$ = instantaneous transpulmonary pressure; $P_{aw(i)}$ = instantaneous airway pressure; $P_{es(i)}$ = instantaneous esophageal (or pleural) pressure.

PSILI has been shown to be associated with organ dysfunction and increased mortality [43–45]. Monitoring esophageal pressure is essential in patients undergoing mechanical ventilation, as excessive inspiratory effort cannot be detected simply by monitoring airway pressure [46].

Calculating changes in esophageal pressure during inspiration (ΔP_{es}) as the difference between esophageal pressure at the start of inspiration and its lowest value is the simplest way to measure inspiratory effort. In patients with acute respiratory failure, several noninvasive respiratory support methods, such as high-flow nasal cannulae (HFNC), continuous positive airway pressure (CPAP), and noninvasive ventilation (NIV), should improve gas exchange and reduce inspiratory effort. Menga et al., in a study focused on noninvasive supports, showed that only helmet NIV is able to reduce ΔP_{es} [47]. In a large cohort of patients with COVID-19 ARDS receiving helmet CPAP, total stress, defined as the sum of transpulmonary pressure generated by the patient and airway pressure at end-expiration, is independently associated with unfavorable patient outcomes compared to other factors considered [48].

Measurements of transpulmonary pressure allow assessment of the effectiveness of lung recruitment. For this purpose, it may be useful to evaluate the effects of the prone position in awake patients, as during the COVID-19 pandemic. The prone position leads to a reduction in ventral alveolar overdistension and dorsal atelectasis, thereby promoting greater homogeneity of transpulmonary pressure across the airways and improving oxygenation indices. It has been shown that the prone position can significantly reduce mechanical power during ventilation [49].

The role of esophageal pressure in assessing inspiratory effort and preventing PSILI is increasingly recognized. Its measurement is strongly recommended for patients with ARDS undergoing controlled or assisted mechanical ventilation.

26.2.3.3 Lung Recruitment: The Recruitment/Overdistension Ratio and EIT

PEEP is an essential component in the management of patients with ARDS. The rationale for using PEEP is to keep alveoli open during all phases of mechanical ventilation, increasing the available alveolar-capillary membrane and improving gas exchange. Excessive application of PEEP in the absence of alveolar recruitment can lead to pulmonary overdistension, increased cardiac afterload, and worsening gas exchange. Therefore, selecting an appropriate PEEP level is essential in patients with pulmonary pathology, in whom oxygen delivery to the tissues (DO_2, oxygen delivery) is already compromised in itself. The recruitment to inflation ratio (R/I) has been proposed as a noninvasive method to calculate the potential for lung recruitment at different PEEP levels [50] and in patients with ARDS, both in the supine and prone positions [51]. It may serve as a valid alternative to computed tomography (CT), reducing the risks associated with patient transport and the use of human and material resources. The Recruitment to Inflation ratio can be calculated by measuring the compliance of the respiratory system under different recruitment conditions, that is, by measuring the changes in airway pressure resulting from the application of a given tidal volume at different PEEP levels. In principle, a higher R/I indicates that the respiratory system is overdistended, meaning that increasing PEEP is not beneficial. Conversely, a lower R/I is indicative of alveolar recruitment [50].

The available literature on the use of R/I confirms a high variability in lung recruitment among patients with ARDS, with different effects on gas exchange, respiratory mechanics, and hemodynamics. Zerbib et al. reported that an R/I ratio >0.62 predicts good lung recruitment following an increase in PEEP in patients with COVID-19-related ARDS [52]. Patients with high recruitability show improvement in both oxygenation and respiratory system compliance after the application of higher PEEP compared to baseline levels, whereas in patients with low recruitability, the application of higher PEEP is associated with a decrease in cardiac output. These data confirm that the Recruitment to Inflation ratio can be a valuable tool in selecting an appropriate PEEP level to improve respiratory mechanics, oxygenation, and optimize hemodynamics without resorting to imaging techniques.

New and interesting evidence is available regarding the role of thoracic electrical impedance (EIT, *Electrical Impedance Tomography*) in PEEP selection in patients with ARDS undergoing mechanical ventilation.

EIT is a bedside tool that allows continuous monitoring of thoracic impedance. Thanks to this property, it is possible to distinguish ventilated lung areas from non-ventilated areas that are either collapsed or overdistended. The device is capable of constructing a real-time two-dimensional map of ventilation distribution (Fig. 26.2). Analysis of collapsed and overdistended areas during mechanical ventilation at different PEEP levels enables the clinician to select the optimal PEEP, that is, the one

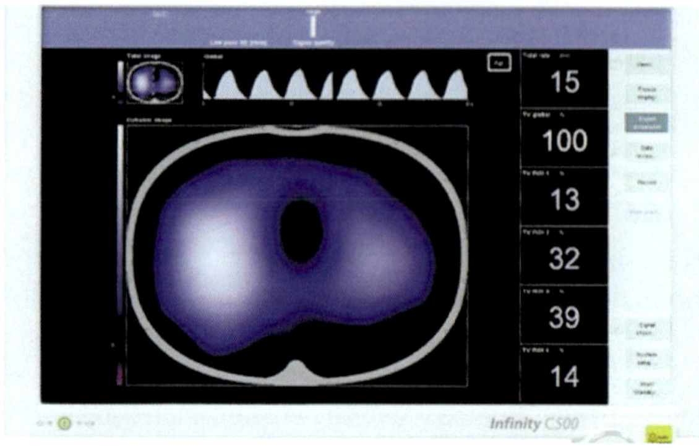

Fig. 26.2 Example of a real-time EIT panel showing regional distribution of mechanical ventilation

associated with the best compromise between atelectasis in dependent lung regions and overdistension in nondependent regions.

In a study conducted on 108 patients with COVID-19 ARDS, PEEP titration was performed with continuous monitoring using EIT, analyzing areas of collapse and overdistension through decremental PEEP maneuvers [53]. The authors identified the optimal PEEP as the point of intersection between the collapse and overdistension curves. Patients with higher lung recruitment indices had a crossing point corresponding to higher PEEP levels compared to patients with lower lung recruitment indices (*high* versus *low recruitability*).

The PEEP selected using EIT in the study by Jonkman et al. corresponded to the PEEP associated with the best lung compliance, demonstrating the reliability of the tool and its increasing potential applicability in clinical practice.

Further evidence of the reliability of EIT as an aid in PEEP setting was recently provided by Jimenez et al. [54]. In this study, the authors showed that EIT-guided PEEP selection allows for a reduction in mechanical power in patients undergoing mechanical ventilation and affected by ARDS.

26.3 Cardiovascular Monitoring

In patients with ARDS, hemodynamic instability and reduced cardiac output can decrease oxygen delivery to tissues, further worsening tissue hypoxia secondary to impairment of the pulmonary gas exchange system [55]. The main strategies to optimize cardiac output are fluid therapy and the use of vasoconstrictors and positive inotropic agents. Hemodynamic monitoring is therefore crucial in patients with ARDS to optimize fluid administration and cardiac output.

26.3.1 Dynamic Indicators of Fluid Responsiveness

As also emphasized by the recent Surviving Sepsis Campaign (SSC, 2021) guidelines on sepsis and septic shock, the first-line intravenous fluids to be administered in critically ill patients are balanced crystalloids [56]. The risks of a positive fluid balance in critically ill patients are well-documented in the literature. Among these, in patients with pulmonary disease, pulmonary edema is particularly noteworthy, as it further impairs gas exchange. The deliberate choice of a liberal versus a restrictive fluid therapy strategy does not show absolute benefits in terms of mortality reduction [57, 58]. These considerations highlight the importance of optimizing fluid administration in patients undergoing mechanical ventilation: appropriate fluid therapy should ensure adequate cardiac output, placing the patient on the flat portion of the Frank-Starling curve, without resulting in potentially harmful excess intravenous fluids (Fig. 26.3).

Pulse Pressure Variation (PPV) and *Stroke Volume Variation* (SVV) are two dynamic predictors of fluid responsiveness, whose clinical use is now strongly supported by the literature. PPV and SVV exploit the hemodynamic effects of heart-lung interactions in patients undergoing controlled mechanical ventilation to predict the response to a fluid bolus in terms of improvement in cardiac output. In the literature, these indices have been validated in patients ventilated with a tidal volume greater than 8 mL/kg. In fact, as also recognized by the LIMITS acronym (*Low*, low heart rate/respiratory rate ratio; *Irregular*, irregular heartbeats; *Mechanical*, low tidal volume mechanical ventilation; *Increase*, increased abdominal pressure; *Thorax*, open chest; *Spontaneous*, spontaneous breathing), low tidal volume mechanical ventilation can reduce the sensitivity of these tests [59]. This is a limitation for their application in patients ventilated with protective strategies, as

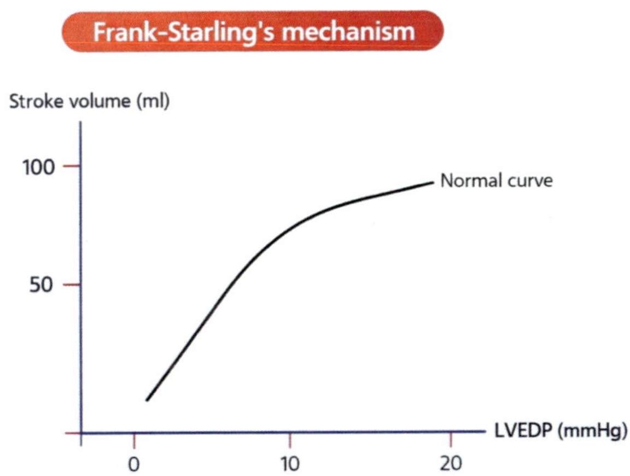

Fig. 26.3 Frank-Starling relationship. Frank-Starling relationship between preload and cardiac output in a subject without heart failure. Reductions in preload lead to a decrease in cardiac output. Hypervolemic states associated with excessive intravenous fluid administration result in increased preload on the flat portion of the curve: there is no substantial improvement in cardiac output, and the patient is exposed to the side effects of volume overload. Among these, pulmonary edema plays a key role in worsening the quality of gas exchange. Legend: Stroke volume = cardiac output; ml = milliliters; Normal curve = normal curve; LVEDP = left ventricular end-diastolic pressure, a surrogate for preload. (AI-generated image created with OpenAI, ChatGPT, version 5.2, 2026)

recommended by the guidelines for ventilation in ARDS patients and the evidence that led to the formulation of the "*baby lung*" concept [60].

Recently, Wang et al. [61] demonstrated that dynamic tests of fluid responsiveness can also have good sensitivity in patients ventilated with low tidal volumes. Similarly, as shown in Table 26.1, Taccheri et al. [62] showed that in patients ventilated with a low tidal volume (6 mL/kg), the application of a transient increase in tidal volume (*Tidal Volume Challenge*, TVc) can improve the diagnostic performance of dynamic indices of fluid responsiveness. In their interesting analysis, the authors demonstrated that an increase in PPV or SVV of 20% or by 1 point after the application of a TVc is a good predictor of fluid responsiveness in patients ventilated with protective ventilation (see Table 26.2).

Another important test for monitoring fluid responsiveness in patients ventilated with low tidal volumes was recently developed by Lai et al. [63] This is the

Table 26.2 Recent evidence on dynamic predictors of fluid responsiveness in patients undergoing mechanical ventilation

Predictor	Mechanical ventilation settings	Diagnostic cutoff	Recent evidences
PPV	Tidal volume >8 mL/kg of IBW	13% (*gray zone* between 9 and 13%)	In patients ventilated at low tidal volume (<8 mL/kg), a TVc increases PPV performance [73]
ΔSVV	Patients ventilated with low tidal volume and application of a TVc (from 6 to 8 mL/kg of IBW)	Increase of 20% or +1 point compared to the values before TVc	AUC of respectively 0.94 and 0.98 in predicting fluid responsivity from Taccheri et al. [62]
ΔPPV	Patients ventilated with low tidal volume and application of a TVc (from 6 to 8 mL/kg of IBW)	Increase of 20% or 1 point compared to the values before TVc	AUC of respectively 0.82 and 0.94 in predicting fluid responsivity from Taccheri et al. [62]
PLR	Independently from MV parameters	CO increase of 5% or $EtCO_2$ increase of 5%/2 mmHg or PPI increase of 9%	+4% of $\Delta ScvO_2$ after a PLR validated by Giraud et al. with an AUC of 0.92 [64]
ΔIVC	Patients ventilated at low tidal volume (6 mL/kg)	+4% of ΔIVC after a TVc or 24% after a PLR	AUC of 0.76 and 0.88 in prediction of fluid-responsivity as shown by Taccheri et al. [62]
PEEP test	PEEP decrease from 10 to 5 cmH_2O	CI increase of >8.6% when compared to initial values	AUC of 0.94 in prediction of fluid responsivity [63]

Recent evidence on predictors of fluid responsiveness in patients undergoing mechanical ventilation
Legend: *PPV* pulse pressure variation, *TVc* tidal volume challenge, *mL* milliliters, *kg* kilograms, *ΔSVV* relative changes in *stroke volume variation*, *ΔPPV* relative changes in *pulse pressure variation*, *AUC* area under the receiver operating characteristic curve, *PLR* passive leg raising, *MV* mechanical ventilation, *CO* cardiac output, $EtCO_2$ end-tidal carbon dioxide, *PPI* plethysmographic peripheral perfusion index, $\Delta ScvO_2$ relative changes in central venous oxygen saturation, *ΔIVC* relative changes in inferior vena cava diameter, *PEEP* positive end-expiratory pressure. (From Chiumello, Fioccola; Journal of Intensive Care, 2024)

PEEP-test: in patients undergoing mechanical ventilation with high PEEP (>10 cmH_2O), a reduction in positive end-expiratory pressure is a possible alternative to *Passive Leg Raising* (PLR) to demonstrate fluid responsiveness. The authors showed that an increase in cardiac output in the studied patients is evident both after a PLR and after reducing PEEP from 10 to 5 cm H_2O, with high sensitivity and specificity.

26.3.2 Central Venous Saturation

In patients monitored with a pulmonary artery catheter, mixed venous saturation (SvO_2) is a useful parameter for assessing the adequacy of oxygen delivery to the tissues (*oxygen delivery*, DO_2) relative to tissue oxygen consumption (*oxygen consumption*, VO_2). To date, only a minority of patients admitted to intensive care units are invasively monitored with a Swan-Ganz catheter, due to its invasiveness. In these cases, a good surrogate for SvO_2 can be central venous saturation ($ScvO_2$): it is a valuable indicator of the adequacy of DO_2 relative to VO_2, although it does not reflect whole-body oxygen consumption, but only that of the upper body (in particular, the brain). This latter characteristic may represent a diagnostic limitation for $ScvO_2$, especially in deeply sedated patients, where cerebral oxygen consumption is reduced due to the use of anesthetic agents. However, $ScvO_2$ can replace SvO_2 not so much in absolute terms as in relative terms, that is, in terms of improvement or deterioration over a given time interval.

In a recent prospective study [64], it was demonstrated that an increase in $ScvO_2$ ($\Delta ScvO_2$) after a PLR is a good predictor of fluid responsiveness, as it is associated with an increase in cardiac output following intravenous fluid administration. The authors also identified a threshold value (+4%) that is comparable to that found in a meta-analysis [65], which showed that $\Delta ScvO_2$ after a fluid bolus (*fluid challenge*, 500 mL of crystalloids) can adequately predict fluid responsiveness (see Table 26.1).

26.3.3 Echocardiography and Fluid Responsiveness

Echocardiography is considered the gold standard for measuring cardiac output, together with the thermodilution method, in patients monitored with a pulmonary artery catheter. In transthoracic echocardiography, one method for measuring cardiac output consists of measuring the diameter of the left ventricular outflow tract (LVOT) in the parasternal long-axis view, and the velocity time integral using continuous Doppler in the five-chamber view. The product of the LVOT cross-sectional area and the velocity time integral yields the amount of blood ejected with a single systole (see Eq. 26.3).

Measurement of Cardiac Output by Echocardiography

$$GC = \pi * \frac{\left(\text{LVOT diameter}\right)^2}{2} * \text{LVOT VTI} * \text{FC} \tag{26.3}$$

Equation 26.3: Measurement of cardiac output by echocardiography. In transthoracic echocardiography, the diameter of the left ventricular outflow tract can be measured in the parasternal long-axis view. The measurement of the velocity time integral in the outflow tract can be performed in the apical five-chamber view. To obtain cardiac output in milliliters, the outflow tract should be measured in cm^2 and the velocity time integral in centimeters.

The use of echocardiography allows for semicontinuous measurement of stroke volume (SV) and its variation over time (ΔSV) after a *fluid challenge* or *passive leg raising*. For this reason, echocardiography is considered a good method for estimating fluid responsiveness [66]. Recently, in a cohort of surgical patients, an excellent correlation was highlighted between LVOT-VTI as a single parameter and other indices of fluid responsiveness, such as PPV [67]. It should be kept in mind, however, that measurement of LVOT-VTI is not always straightforward and may be affected by operator-dependent variability [68]. Recently, the measurement of carotid systo-diastolic flow (CSD) has been proposed as a good surrogate for LVOT-VTI, being easier to measure and useful in patients with a poor cardiac ultrasound window [69]. However, further evidence is required for definitive validation of this technique for the assessment of fluid responsiveness.

Another potentially informative ultrasound measure of a patient's volemic status is the assessment of the vena cava. Generally, a vena cava diameter greater than 17 mm with inspiratory collapsibility less than 50% in mechanically ventilated patients is considered normal, indicating a patient with normal preload. Conversely, when inspiratory collapsibility exceeds 50% or the inferior vena cava diameter is reduced, the patient is considered hypovolemic. Changes in inferior vena cava diameter (ΔIVC, *changes of inferior vena cava diameter*) after maneuvers such as a *Tidal Volume challenge* or *passive leg raising* are easy to measure ultrasonographically, even by less experienced operators. However, it has been shown that its sensitivity is low in patients ventilated with low tidal volumes and in spontaneously breathing patients [62]. In their report, Taccheri et al. demonstrate that, similarly to PPV and SVV, ΔIVC is potentially applicable in patients ventilated with low tidal volumes, thus encouraging its use even in patients with ARDS. The authors report an AUC of 0.77 and 0.86 for ΔIVC in predicting fluid responsiveness after a TVc or PLR in patients ventilated with tidal volumes less than 6 mL/kg of ideal body weight [62].

26.3.4 Ratio of PCO_2 Arterial-Venous Deltas

Another possible indicator of fluid responsiveness and adequacy of cardiac output is the ratio between the venous-arterial difference in PCO_2 ($\Delta Pv\text{-}aCO_2$) and the arterial-venous difference in oxygen content ($\Delta Ca\text{-}vO_2$).

$\Delta Pv\text{-}aCO_2$ is identified in the literature as a good indicator of tissue perfusion: in patients with higher cardiac output, peripheral blood stagnation is reduced, and the blood has less time to accumulate carbon dioxide produced by the tissues. Conversely, in patients with lower cardiac output, $\Delta Pv\text{-}aCO_2$ is higher due to increased cardiovascular circulation time. $\Delta Pv\text{-}aCO_2$ also depends on tissue carbon dioxide production (VCO_2): higher VCO_2 corresponds to higher $\Delta Pv\text{-}aCO_2$. A cut-off of 6 mmHg for $\Delta Pv\text{-}aCO_2$ has been identified in the literature as an indicator of adequate cardiac output [70]. This index should be used with caution in patients with microcirculatory defects: in patients with septic shock, it has been shown that $\Delta Pv\text{-}aCO_2$ may be greater than 6 mmHg even in the presence of normal cardiac output. This effect results from the reduced capacity for CO_2 clearance in patients with decreased microcirculatory flow, despite adequate cardiac output [71].

$\Delta Ca\text{-}vO_2$ is an index of VO_2. Higher VO_2 corresponds to an increased $\Delta Ca\text{-}vO_2$.

The ratio of the two indices mentioned above ($\Delta Pv\text{-}aCO_2/\Delta Ca\text{-}vO_2$) contains two important pieces of information:

1. Adequacy of peripheral perfusion (cardiac output)
2. Ratio between VCO_2 and VO_2: in other words, the respiratory quotient (*respiratory quotient*, RQ). Under anaerobic conditions, when DO_2 is insufficient to meet tissue VO_2, the respiratory quotient increases: part of the carbon dioxide is produced as a consequence of anaerobic metabolism.

Based on this pathophysiological rationale, the ratio between these two indices has been proposed as a summary variable of peripheral perfusion. In a retrospective study, it was demonstrated that, in patients with ARDS secondary to COVID-19, a higher $\Delta Pv\text{-}aCO_2/\Delta Ca\text{-}vO_2$ was associated with a worse prognosis. The cutoff value identified by the authors is 2.1 mmHg/mL: above this threshold, a marked increase in in-hospital mortality was observed among the patients included in the analysis, with an Area Under the Curve (AUC) of 0.89 [72].

26.3.5 Capillary Refill Time

Capillary refill time (CRT) is a simple and noninvasive index for assessing peripheral tissue perfusion and microcirculation. It consists of compressing the nail bed of a patient's finger, which is then released. The time required for reperfusion of the nail bed is then measured. CRT is considered normal when the nail bed is reperfused in less than 2 s after release of digital compression. The test is considered positive if digital perfusion takes more than 2 s after release of digital compression. It has been shown that monitoring CRT in critically ill patients reduces multiorgan dysfunction and mortality compared to monitoring lactate levels alone [73]. In a prospective observational study, Raia et al. demonstrated a direct correlation between a decrease in CRT after a 500 mL fluid challenge and fluid responsiveness. In this study, CRT decreased only in patients who experienced an actual increase in cardiac output after a fluid bolus [74]. The authors also emphasized the importance of standardizing CRT measurement using digital timers to measure capillary reperfusion time. A low percentage (0.5%) of the variability in all measurements was due to measurement errors, thus allowing for high reliability. Another limitation of CRT in assessing fluid responsiveness in critically ill patients is the presence of distributive shock. Fage et al. demonstrated that, in septic patients, the correlation between a decrease in CRT after administration of fluids or vasoconstrictors is predictive of fluid responsiveness only when there are substantial increases in cardiac output (CO) or mean arterial pressure (MAP). Conversely, in patients with an increase in MAP and CO of less than 15% compared to baseline, CRT is poorly correlated with the response to fluids and vasoconstrictors, and thus loses sensitivity as a predictor of fluid responsiveness [75, 76]. These recent findings highlight that CRT is a mixed index, dependent both on perfusion (cardiac output) and on the distribution of perfusion (vasoconstriction/vasodilation), and has limited diagnostic power in patients with distributive shock. The close interdependence between CRT and microcirculation was recently highlighted in a study of 282 critically ill patients. The authors demonstrated a direct correlation between CRT and microcirculatory dysfunction, using the sidestream dark field imaging technique. CRT is independently correlated with the Microvascular Flow Index (MFI) [76]. Intensive care patients with higher CRT values have higher mortality. Similar results have been described in patients with COVID-19-related ARDS, in whom, despite hemodynamic stability and normal lactate levels, CRT and microcirculatory indices (such as MFI) are impaired, resulting in altered tissue perfusion. CRT is therefore among the useful and easily measurable parameters for assessing fluid responsiveness: given its completely non-invasive nature, its use should be encouraged, bearing in mind its diagnostic limitations in patients with distributive shock. In these cases, CRT monitoring to test fluid responsiveness may result in false negatives due to decreased test sensitivity. However, even when CRT loses its diagnostic power in terms of fluid responsiveness, it remains a useful parameter in critically ill patients, as it is correlated with patient prognosis.

26.4 Conclusions

In patients with ARDS, injurious mechanical ventilation combined with a positive fluid balance may amplify lung injury pulmonary. Therefore, careful respiratory and hemodynamic monitoring is crucial in these patients.

The SpO_2/FiO_2 ratio is a valid alternative to the PaO_2/FiO_2 ratio for assessing gas exchange. Corrected minute ventilation and the *Ventilatory Ratio* are two valuable

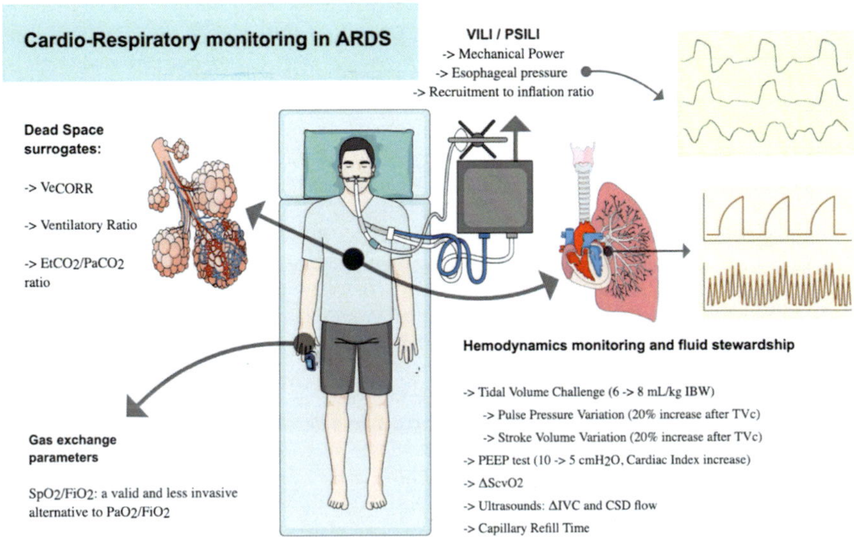

Fig. 26.4 Summary of cardio-respiratory monitoring indices in patients with ARDS. Recent evidence on respiratory and hemodynamic monitoring in patients undergoing mechanical ventilation. Legends: VeCORR corrected minute ventilation, $EtCO_2$ *end-tidal* carbon dioxide, SpO_2 peripheral oxygen saturation, FiO_2 fraction of inspired oxygen, PaO_2 arterial partial pressure of oxygen, mL milliliters, kg kilograms, IBW *ideal body weight,* TVc *tidal volume challenge,* PEEP positive end-expiratory pressure, $\Delta ScvO_2$ changes in $ScvO_2$, ΔIVC changes in inferior vena cava diameter

surrogates for estimating the dead space fraction, and their prognostic value is well recognized in patients with ARDS. Mechanical Power directly measures the energy dissipated in the airways during mechanical ventilation and is therefore able to predict VILI in patients undergoing invasive mechanical ventilation. The use of algorithms implemented directly in mechanical ventilators allows for continuous calculation of Mechanical Power. In patients receiving noninvasive mechanical ventilation, the role of esophageal pressure is crucial for estimating P-SILI.

In addition to monitoring respiratory variables, the management of intravenous fluids and fluid balance is also important to reduce the impact of VILI in patients with ARDS. Dynamic indices of fluid responsiveness have recently been validated even for patients undergoing lung-protective mechanical ventilation with low tidal volumes. There is increasing evidence supporting the validity of $\Delta ScvO_2$ and CRT after a PLR or a *fluid challenge*. The role of these parameters, which are easy to assess and noninvasive, may become increasingly important in patients with respiratory failure, especially in settings where advanced monitoring is not available.

Figure 26.4 summarizes the cardio-respiratory monitoring indices in patients with ARDS for which recent evidence is available in the literature.

References

1. Matthay MA, et al. A new global definition of acute respiratory distress syndrome. Am J Respir Crit Care Med. 2024;209:37–47.
2. Jubran A. Pulse oximetry. Crit Care. 2015;19:272.
3. Wick KD, Matthay MA, Ware LB. Pulse oximetry for the diagnosis and management of acute respiratory distress syndrome. Lancet Respir Med. 2022;10:1086–98.
4. Henry NR, et al. Disparities in hypoxemia detection by pulse oximetry across self-identified racial groups and associations with clinical outcomes. Crit Care Med. 2022;50:204–11.
5. Fawzy A, et al. Racial and ethnic discrepancy in pulse oximetry and delayed identification of treatment eligibility among patients with COVID-19. JAMA Intern Med. 2022;182:730–8.
6. Babu S, Abhilash KPP, Kandasamy S, Gowri M. Association between SpO2/FiO2 ratio and PaO2/FiO2 ratio in different modes of oxygen supplementation. Indian J Crit Care Med. 2021;25:1001–5.
7. Bashar FR, et al. Comparison of non-invasive to invasive oxygenation ratios for diagnosing acute respiratory distress syndrome following coronary artery bypass graft surgery: a prospective derivation-validation cohort study. J Cardiothorac Surg. 2018;13
8. Pisani L, et al. Risk stratification using SpO2/FiO2 and PEEP at initial ARDS diagnosis and after 24 h in patients with moderate or severe ARDS. Ann Intensive Care. 2017;7:108.
9. Rice TW, et al. Comparison of the SpO2/FIO2 ratio and the PaO2/FIO2 ratio in patients with acute lung injury or ARDS. Chest. 2007;132:410–7.
10. Fukuda Y, et al. Utility of the SpO2/FiO2 ratio for acute hypoxemic respiratory failure with bilateral opacities in the ICU. PLoS One. 2021;16
11. Roozeman JP, et al. Prognostication using SpO2/FiO2 in invasively ventilated ICU patients with ARDS due to COVID-19 – insights from the PRoVENT-COVID study. J Crit Care. 2022;68:31–7.
12. Choi KJ, Hong HL, Kim EJ. The association between mortality and oxygen saturation and fraction of inspired oxygen in patients requiring oxygen therapy due to COVID-19-associated pneumonia. Tuberc Respir Dis (Seoul). 2021;84:125–33.
13. Kim JH, et al. ROX index and SpO2/FiO2 ratio for predicting high-flow nasal cannula failure in hypoxemic COVID-19 patients: a multicenter retrospective study. PLoS One. 2022;17
14. Semler MW, et al. Oxygen-saturation targets for critically ill adults receiving mechanical ventilation. N Engl J Med. 2022;387:1759–69.
15. Andrew L. Nunn's applied respiratory physiology. Eur J Anaesthesiol. 2000;17(5):339–40.
16. Slobod D, Damia A, Leali M, Spinelli E, Mauri T. Pathophysiology and clinical significance of ventilation-perfusion mismatch in acute respiratory distress syndrome. Biology (Basel). 2022;12
17. Rossi A, et al. Effects of PEEP on VA/Q mismatch in ventilated patients with chronic airflow obstruction. Am J Respir Crit Care Med. 1994;149:1077–84.
18. Nuckton TJ, et al. Pulmonary dead-space fraction as a risk factor for death in acute respiratory distress syndrome. N Engl J Med. 2002;346:1281–6.
19. Farrow CE, et al. Increased intrapulmonary shunt and alveolar dead space post-COVID-19. J Appl Physiol (1985). 2023;135:1012.
20. Bertelli M, et al. COVID-19 ARDS is characterized by increased dead space ventilation compared with non-COVID ARDS. Respir Care. 2021;66:1406–15.
21. Mollura M, et al. Physiologic dead space is independently associated with mortality and discharge of mechanically ventilated patients with COVID-19 ARDS: a retrospective study. Sci Rep. 2023;13:5719.
22. Morales-Quinteros L, et al. Dead space estimates may not be independently associated with 28-day mortality in COVID-19 ARDS. Crit Care. 2021;25
23. Sinha P, Fauvel NJ, Singh S, Soni N. Ventilatory ratio: a simple bedside measure of ventilation. Br J Anaesth. 2009;102:692–7.

24. Siegel ER, et al. Ventilatory ratio is a valuable prognostic indicator in an observational cohort of patients with ARDS. Respir Care. 2022;67:1075–81.
25. Wang Z, et al. Early decrease of ventilatory ratio after prone position ventilation may predict successful weaning in patients with acute respiratory distress syndrome: a retrospective cohort study. Front Med (Lausanne). 2022;9
26. Maj R, et al. Ventilatory ratio, dead space, and venous admixture in patients with acute respiratory distress syndrome. Br J Anaesth. 2023;130:360–7.
27. Monteiro ACC, et al. The prognostic value of early measurements of the ventilatory ratio in the ARDS ROSE trial. Crit Care. 2022;26
28. Bonifazi M, et al. End-tidal to arterial PCO2 ratio: a bedside indicator of overall gas exchange performance. Intensive Care Med Exp. 2021;9
29. Kallet RH, Lipnick MS. End-tidal-to-arterial PCO2 ratio as a marker for physiologic dead-space ratio and oxygenation dysfunction in acute respiratory distress syndrome. Respir Care. 2021;66:263–8.
30. Lazzari S, et al. End-tidal to arterial PCO2 ratio as a guide to weaning from Venovenous extracorporeal membrane oxygenation. Am J Respir Crit Care Med. 2022;206:973–80.
31. Gattinoni L, et al. Ventilator-related causes of lung injury: mechanical power. Intensive Care Med. 2016;42:1567–75.
32. Chiumello D, et al. Bedside calculation of mechanical power during volume- and pressure-controlled mechanical ventilation. Crit Care. 2020;24:417.
33. Chiumello D, et al. A validation study of a continuous automatic measurement of mechanical power in ARDS patients. J Crit Care. 2022;67:21–5.
34. Coppola S, et al. Effect of mechanical power on intensive care mortality in ARDS patients. Crit Care. 2020;24:246.
35. Azizi BA, et al. Mechanical power and 30-day mortality in mechanically ventilated, critically ill patients with and without coronavirus Disease-2019: a hospital registry study. J Intensive Care. 2023;11:14.
36. Van Meenen DMP, et al. Effect of mechanical power on mortality in invasively ventilated ICU patients without acute respiratory distress syndrome: an analysis of three randomized clinical trials. Eur J Anaesthesiol. 2023;40:21–8.
37. Urner M, et al. Time-varying intensity of mechanical ventilation and mortality in patients with acute respiratory failure: a registry-based, prospective cohort study. Lancet Respir Med. 2020;8:905.
38. Pozzi T, et al. Early time-course of respiratory mechanics, mechanical power and gas exchange in ARDS patients. J Crit Care. 2024;79:154444.
39. Costa ELV, et al. Ventilatory variables and mechanical power in patients with acute respiratory distress syndrome. Am J Respir Crit Care Med. 2021;204:303–11.
40. Gattinoni L, et al. The future of mechanical ventilation: lessons from the present and the past. Crit Care. 2017;21:183.
41. Dreyfuss D, Soler P, Basset G, Saumon G. High inflation pressure pulmonary edema: respective effects of high airway pressure, high tidal volume, and positive end-expiratory pressure. 137:1159–1164 (2012). https://doi.org/10.1164/ajrccm/137.5.1159
42. Gattinoni L, et al. Targeting transpulmonary pressure to prevent ventilator-induced lung injury. Expert Rev Respir Med. 2019;13:737–46.
43. Brochard L, Slutsky A, Pesenti A. Mechanical ventilation to minimize progression of lung injury in acute respiratory failure. Am J Respir Crit Care Med. 2017;195:438–42.
44. Yoshida T, Grieco DL, Brochard L, Fujino Y. Patient self-inflicted lung injury and positive end-expiratory pressure for safe spontaneous breathing. Curr Opin Crit Care. 2020;26:59–65.
45. Goligher EC, et al. Lung- and diaphragm-protective ventilation. Am J Respir Crit Care Med. 2020;202:950–61.
46. Bellani G, et al. Driving pressure is associated with outcome during assisted ventilation in acute respiratory distress syndrome. Anesthesiology. 2019;131:594–604.

47. Menga LS, et al. Respective effects of helmet pressure support, continuous positive airway pressure, and nasal high-flow in hypoxemic respiratory failure: a randomized crossover clinical trial. Am J Respir Crit Care Med. 2023;207:1310–23.
48. Coppola S, et al. Role of total lung stress on the progression of early COVID-19 pneumonia. Intensive Care Med. 2021;47:1130–9.
49. Chiumello D, et al. Awake prone position reduces work of breathing in patients with COVID-19 ARDS supported by CPAP. Ann Intensive Care. 2021;11:179.
50. Chen L, et al. Potential for lung recruitment estimated by the recruitment-to-inflation ratio in acute respiratory distress syndrome. A clinical trial. Am J Respir Crit Care Med. 2020;201:178–87.
51. Del Sorbo L, et al. Association of lung recruitment and change in recruitment-to-inflation ratio from supine to prone position in acute respiratory distress syndrome. Crit Care. 2023;27
52. Zerbib Y, et al. Respiratory effects of lung recruitment maneuvers depend on the recruitment-to-inflation ratio in patients with COVID-19-related acute respiratory distress syndrome. Crit Care. 2022;26:12.
53. Jonkman AH, et al. Lung recruitment assessed by electrical impedance tomography (RECRUIT) a multicenter study of COVID-19 acute respiratory distress syndrome. Am J Respir Crit Care Med. 2023;208:25–38.
54. Jimenez JV, et al. Electric impedance tomography-guided PEEP titration reduces mechanical power in ARDS: a randomized crossover pilot trial. Crit Care. 2023;27:21.
55. Vignon P, et al. Fluid administration and monitoring in ARDS: which management? Intensive Care Med. 2020;46:2252–64.
56. Evans L, et al. Surviving sepsis campaign: international guidelines for management of sepsis and septic shock 2021. Intensive Care Med. 2021;47:1181–247.
57. Meyhoff TS, et al. Restriction of intravenous fluid in ICU patients with septic shock. N Engl J Med. 2022;386:2459–70.
58. Silversides JA, et al. Conservative fluid management or deresuscitation for patients with sepsis or acute respiratory distress syndrome following the resuscitation phase of critical illness: a systematic review and meta-analysis. Intensive Care Med. 2017;43:155–70.
59. Michard F, Chemla D, Teboul JL. Applicability of pulse pressure variation: how many shades of grey? Crit Care. 2015;19:144.
60. Brower RG, et al. Ventilation with lower tidal volumes as compared with traditional tidal volumes for acute lung injury and the acute respiratory distress syndrome. N Engl J Med. 2000;342:1301–8.
61. Wang X, Liu S, Gao J, Zhang Y, Huang T. Does tidal volume challenge improve the feasibility of pulse pressure variation in patients mechanically ventilated at low tidal volumes? A systematic review and meta-analysis. Crit Care. 2023;27:45.
62. Taccheri T, Gavelli F, Teboul JL, Shi R, Monnet X. Do changes in pulse pressure variation and inferior vena cava distensibility during passive leg raising and tidal volume challenge detect preload responsiveness in case of low tidal volume ventilation? Crit Care. 2021;25:110.
63. Lai C, et al. The increase in cardiac output induced by a decrease in positive end-expiratory pressure reliably detects volume responsiveness: the PEEP-test study. Crit Care. 2023;27:136.
64. Giraud R, Vujovic B, Assouline B, Neto Silva I, Bendjelid K. Do ScvO2 variations induced by passive leg raising predict fluid responsiveness? A prospective study. Physiol Rep. 2021;9
65. Pan J, Sun Y, Xu Z, Dong P, Zhou X. Variation in central venous oxygen saturation to evaluate fluid responsiveness: a systematic review and meta-analysis. Crit Care. 2023;27:203.
66. Lamia B, et al. Echocardiographic prediction of volume responsiveness in critically ill patients with spontaneously breathing activity. Intensive Care Med. 2007;33:1125–32.
67. Pérez-Manjarrez A, et al. Usefulness of the velocity-time integral of the left ventricular outflow tract variability index to predict fluid responsiveness in patients undergoing cardiac surgery. Echo Res Pract. 2023;10:9.
68. Shaikh F, et al. Measuring the accuracy of cardiac output using POCUS: the introduction of artificial intelligence into routine care. Ultrasound J. 2022;14

69. Cheong I, et al. Carotid flow as a surrogate of the left ventricular stroke volume. J Clin Monit Comput. 2023;37:661–7.
70. Dres M, Monnet X, Teboul JL. Hemodynamic management of cardiovascular failure by using PCO(2) venous-arterial difference. J Clin Monit Comput. 2012;26:367–74.
71. Ospina-Tascón GA, et al. Can venous-to-arterial carbon dioxide differences reflect microcirculatory alterations in patients with septic shock? Intensive Care Med. 2016;42:211–21.
72. Sánchez Díaz JS, et al. The ΔPv-aCO2/ΔCa-vO2 ratio as a predictor of mortality in patients with severe acute respiratory distress syndrome related to COVID-19. PLoS One. 2023;18:e0290272.
73. Hernández G, et al. Effect of a resuscitation strategy targeting peripheral perfusion status vs serum lactate levels on 28-day mortality among patients with septic shock: The ANDROMEDA-SHOCK Randomized Clinical Trial. JAMA. 2019;321:654–64.
74. Raia L, et al. Kinetics of capillary refill time after fluid challenge. Ann Intensive Care. 2022;12:74.
75. Fage N, et al. Effect on capillary refill time of volume expansion and increase of the norepinephrine dose in patients with septic shock. Crit Care. 2023;27:429.
76. Huang W, et al. Association of sublingual microcirculation parameters and capillary refill time in the early phase of ICU admission. Crit Care Med. 2023;51:913–23.

The Therapeutic Alliance and Healthcare Responsibility in the Care of Jehovah's Witness Patients

27

Davide Chiumello and Maria Chiara Lavorato

27.1 Introduction

The millenarian, theocratic, and Christian religious movement of Jehovah's Witnesses (JW) originated in 1870 in Pennsylvania (USA) and, among its precepts, includes the prohibition of both donating and receiving blood. This position is based on the interpretation of biblical texts, particularly certain passages of the Pentateuch, which define blood as a "sacred element"; both in Genesis (9:3, 4) and Leviticus (17:14, 15) it is stated that *"the life of every sort of flesh is its blood, and whoever eats it will be cut off."* [3]

Since 1979, the JW Governing Body, headquartered in Brooklyn, New York, has established numerous Hospital Liaison Committees (HLCs) worldwide; this has enabled the dissemination of the organization's position on blood transfusions and alternative treatments.

The prohibition of blood has had obvious repercussions on medical and surgical care, presenting healthcare professionals with the dilemma of how to manage the most critical hemorrhagic situations with a risk of death.

Meanwhile, medical science has advanced: the World Health Organization and the Ministry of Health recommend the adoption of Patient Blood Management (PBM) programs, that is, protocols designed to optimize the patient's own blood resources and to avoid, or at least reduce, blood transfusions during surgical procedures.

D. Chiumello (✉)
Department of Anesthesia and Intensive Care, ASST Santi Paolo e Carlo, San Paolo University Hospital, Milan, Italy

Department of Health Sciences, University of Milan, Milan, Italy

Coordinated Research Center on Respiratory Failure, University of Milan, Milan, Italy
e-mail: davide.chiumello@unimi.it

M. C. Lavorato
ASST Santi Paolo e Carlo. Complex Structure of Anesthesia and Intensive Care, San Paolo University Hospital Milan, Milan, Italy

D. Chiumello, A. De Gasperi (eds.), *Practical Trends in Anesthesia and Intensive Care 2026*, https://doi.org/10.1007/978-3-032-25721-5_27

At the same time, cultural and medicolegal developments have transformed the doctor-patient relationship. The predominance of the physician's opinion over the patient's wishes has been replaced by the "therapeutic alliance" [1] centered on the doctor-patient relationship, which is based on healthcare self-determination: it is the patient who decides whether and which therapies to undergo, including the possibility of making advance directives, even if only as a precaution. The therapeutic alliance thus becomes a "shared healthcare determination" [2]: the physician is obliged to inform the patient of their actual health status, to present the available treatment options, and to enable the patient to make the best possible choices, always leaving the final decision to the patient.

Greater clarity in the doctor–JW patient relationship was provided by the Court of Cassation in 2020, which provided reassuring elements regarding the hypotheses of healthcare liability.

27.2 The International Scenario: Elements of Cultural, Legal, and Bioethical Reasoning

The refusal of blood transfusions involves self-determination and advance healthcare directives, topics on which most countries have enacted ad hoc legislation.

In *Germany*, bioethics is influenced by two factors [4]: the history of the twentieth century, due to the involvement of many physicians in the Nazi program, and the Constitutional Law.

Articles 1 and 2 of the German legal system (*Grundgesetz*) state that "*human dignity is inviolable... respect for and protection of it is a duty of state authority*" and "*everyone has the right to freely express their personality, provided this does not infringe upon the freedom of others*."

The approach of the last century was characterized by authoritarianism and paternalism within the healthcare system, which delayed Germany's entry into the bioethical debate [5].

For Jehovah's Witnesses, autonomy plays a crucial role, and in Germany, the concept of autonomy is articulated in two fundamental ways: autonomy based on free choice and autonomy based on reason (according to Kantian thought). Autonomy is primarily associated with rationality and competence [6] rather than free choice. On June 18, 2009, the German *Bundestag* passed a law on advance healthcare directives regulating therapeutic self-determination[1]: any adult may provide written consent or refusal to undergo examinations, treatments, or medical interventions "in the event that they are unable to give consent."

In the *United Kingdom*, the issue of advance directives is addressed by the *Mental Capacity Act* of 2005. In fact, the right to refuse medical treatment had already been

[1] Prior to this date, even in the absence of specific regulations, the practice of the so-called *Patientenverfügung*, a specific form of advance directive, had become widespread.

discussed in the case of Anthony Bland[2]: the Court recognized the right—requested by his father—to withdraw care from the young man. This process closely resembles the Englaro case in Italy.

Regarding transfusions for Jehovah's Witnesses, the United Kingdom focuses on *decision-making* and *competence*, that is, the assessment of actual mental capacity in specific situations [7]. For patients under 16 years of age, assessment is based on the *Gillick* approach, which is widely used in healthcare decision-making.

The British emphasize that the position of Jehovah's Witnesses on blood transfusions has changed, shifting from an uncompromising refusal to a more accommodating stance: the Watchtower initially, in 1961, stated that receiving a blood transfusion meant "*must be cut-off from God's people by excommunication or disfellowship*"; later, in 2000, it clarified that "*fractions of all primary components are now permitted ... and when it comes to fractions of any of primary components, each Christian, after careful and prayerful meditation, must conscientiously decide for himself.*" Since April 2000, therefore, members are no longer "disassociated" for accepting certain blood components previously considered forbidden.

In *Belgium*, the law on patient rights (*Loi belge relative aux droits du patient*) dates back to 2002 and, in addition to allowing the refusal of artificial hydration and nutrition, decriminalizes the conduct of a physician who ends life upon request. Regarding Jehovah's Witnesses, in Belgium, there are particular concerns in cases of advance directives from adolescent patients [8]: especially in cases of unconsciousness, the physician informs the parents of the need for transfusions, and if consent is not obtained, informs a public judge who suspends parental authority and proceeds in the best interest of the minor.

In *Poland*, the Constitution of the Republic enshrines the principles of inviolable protection of personal rights and freedom of choice for all citizens; a physician who performs a therapeutic procedure without the patient's consent commits a criminal offense punishable under the penal code. An interesting 2023 study [9] used structured questionnaires to assess healthcare professionals' knowledge on the subject of blood and blood products.

In the study by Domaradzki et al., the questionnaires administered to healthcare professionals highlighted the urgent need to develop greater cultural [10] and technical competencies regarding so-called Bloodless Medicine, which should be an integral part of coordinated and personalized care, with particular attention to updating the information process for JW patients and their families.

We now turn to *India*, where healthcare professionals are calling on authorities for urgent laws and regulations on the matter, especially in the case of minors. Of interest is the *case report* published by a group of pediatric hemato-oncologists

[2]A young Liverpool supporter who, in 1989, suffered an accident at Hillsborough Stadium in Sheffield, resulting in severe injuries and an irreversible vegetative state. His father requested the withdrawal of treatment, the doctors refused, and the matter was brought before the House of Lords. The latter examined various scenarios regarding end-of-life issues and, after establishing several important principles, recognized the legitimacy of discontinuing treatment in this specific case.

from Kerala [11]: a 4-year-old child with Burkitt lymphoma, belonging to a JW family[3]. The authors emphasize that the majority of time was spent not so much on clinical decision-making, despite the complexity of an aggressive disease, but rather on engaging with the parents and attempting to overcome their refusal of transfusions, assembling a multidisciplinary team to strengthen the therapeutic relationship [12]. They ultimately highlight the need for clear regulation in Indian law as well, taking into account the broader range of tools used in Western countries [13].

In *Brazil*, by contrast, the scenario is radically different: in 2016, a multicenter group of anesthesiologists proposed a protocol for the "management" of JW patients who refuse transfusions [14]. After reviewing various legal rulings unfavorable to physicians, Brazilian doctors determined that refusal of a transfusion should not be accepted, especially in cases of emergency and necessity. The authors outline a protocol centered on the "intrinsic necessity" of transfusion and the primacy of their ethical and professional duty, whereby, when a transfusion is necessary, the physician is obliged to proceed and act, prioritizing saving life over the patient's freedom of choice.

Finally, in the *Russian Federation*, the government has at times stated that refusal of blood on religious grounds would lead to serious consequences, such as making it impossible for physicians to provide medical assistance. In one case, the Golovinskiy District Court in Russia[4] found that the JW community engaged in "*mind control*," subjecting members to mental subjugation, and that refusal of transfusions has a negative impact on health and life, equating refusal of transfusions to suicide. The European Court of Human Rights (ECHR) intervened on this point, commenting that the Russian government had not undertaken a proper balancing of public health concerns and personal autonomy.

The essence of the ECHR is founded on respect for human dignity and freedom, self-determination, and autonomy.

In *Europe*, the protection of rights and religious beliefs is provided by the European Convention for the Protection of Human Rights and Fundamental Freedoms (*European Convention of Human Rights, ECHR*)[5], as set forth in Articles 8, 9, and 10.

Article 8 ensures support for the manifestation of religious belief; Article 9 grants every person the right to freedom of thought, conscience, and religion, and includes the State's commitment to ensuring these rights; Article 10 concerns freedom of expression and offers protection to the religious sphere.

[3] The treatment plan preceded chemotherapy cytotoxic at high doses, myelosuppressive, requiring frequent blood transfusions. A prompt decision was urgently needed. The parents, after being informed about the rescue therapy program, initially did not consent; the physicians therefore initiated a series of meetings and discussions, involving a forensic physician and a senior pediatric expert, and at the third meeting, the parents gave their consent.

[4] Application no. 302/02—Case of Jehovah's Witnesses of Moscow and others vs. Russia.

[5] This is an international convention drafted and adopted within the framework of the Council of Europe. The 46 member states of the Council of Europe are contracting parties to the Convention. The Russian Federation, having been expelled from the Council of Europe as of March 16, 2022, ceased to be a party to the Convention as of September 16, 2022.

To what extent can the right to refuse a blood transfusion on religious grounds be asserted? The European Court has established that the will of a "competent" patient to determine aspects of their own treatment must be protected, even if such self-determination appears detrimental to their health and contrary to the common sense of sound medical decision-making, whether the decision is based on religious belief or otherwise. Religious belief, as the basis for refusal, is not the central issue in the discussion: the central issue is that the adult patient has made an autonomous decision, and physicians and courts must uphold that choice[6].

27.3 In Italy

In Italy, the principle of self-determination is enshrined in the Constitution (Art. 32: "*The Republic safeguards health as a fundamental right of the individual and as a collective interest, and guarantees free medical care to the indigent. No one may be compelled to undergo any particular health treatment except as provided by law*") and is expressed in the Code of Medical Ethics.

The key reference is Law 219 of 2017: "*Provisions on informed consent and advance directives.*" Of particular relevance, paragraph 5 of Article 1 states: "*Any person capable of acting has the right to refuse, in whole or in part, any diagnostic procedure or medical treatment proposed by the physician for their condition, or any individual act of treatment. They also have the right to revoke consent at any time, even if such revocation results in the discontinuation of treatment.*"

In this law, refusal of treatment is expressed as a reinforcement of the patient's right to self-determination and, in practice, results in "difficult decisions" for the physician: the real possibilities of the *ars* medica to provide benefit in the management of disease may come into conflict with the legitimate will of the patient to refuse such interventions. This can lead to feelings of frustration for the physician, an inner conflict in having to stop, in being unable to resolve a pathological condition despite having the tools and experience to aim for an improved *clinical outcome*, even in cases of potentially or partially reversible conditions [15].

The physician must also take into account that: "*if the patient expresses the intention to forgo or refuse medical treatments necessary for their survival, the physician must inform the patient and, with their consent, their family members, of the consequences of such a decision and possible alternatives, and must promote all forms of support, including the use of psychological assistance services.*" Therefore, when faced with a refusal, in whole or in part, of the proposed treatments, the physician must ensure supportive measures that allow the patient to face the deterioration of their health in the most tolerable way possible.

The physician's dilemma involves various factors, both ethical-deontological and medico-legal: on the one hand, inaction may lead to criminal charges of negligence or, in the event of the patient's death, manslaughter; intervention, on the other hand, could result in criminal charges of coercion or claims for damages for

[6] Op. cit. 1

violation of the right to self-determination. How should one proceed and protect oneself? The judiciary has also demonstrated its own cultural evolution.

Prior to 2017, the *Court of Cassation* [16] ruled in a case that a patient's written refusal of transfusions[7] could not be considered valid because it was expressed before the clinical condition worsened, in a different *setting,* and when the patient's life was not at risk. With the patient unconscious, the situation changed and rapidly deteriorated, and no fault could be attributed to the physician for administering the transfusion.

Also in the pre-Law 219 period, the *Court* upheld a similar position [17] in the case of a man, TG, who arrived unconscious at the Emergency Department in Pordenone, carrying a note stating "No Blood," and the physicians proceeded with a transfusion. The Court held that the physicians acted in accordance with the Hippocratic Oath and could not presume that the patient would still have refused in the face of imminent death. A note stating "No Blood" was not sufficient for the Court, as it lacked a detailed, precise, and unequivocal declaration of refusal of transfusion, even in the face of the risk of death.

In the following decade, the Supreme Court reversed its position, issuing rulings that affirm the right to refuse blood transfusions and the criminal liability of the physician who fails to comply, thus creating a progressive line of logical consistency that has come to align perfectly with the 2017 Law on Informed Consent and Advance Healthcare Directives [18, 19]. The final seal was set by the Supreme Court ruling in 2020 [20].

27.4 Supreme Court Ruling No. 29469/2020 [20]

The *Ruling No. 29469 of 2020* can be considered the most "up-to-date" and highlights that the case of refusal of transfusions by Jehovah's Witnesses is complex because it involves the "osmosis of two constitutional principles": self-determination in medical treatment and freedom of religion.

The principle established by the ruling states: "*the Jehovah's Witness who asserts the right to self-determination in healthcare, in order to protect the freedom to practice their religious faith, has the right to refuse a blood transfusion even after having consented to a different treatment that subsequently required a transfusion, including through a declaration made prior to the treatment itself, provided that the*

[7]A polytrauma patient was admitted to a hospital in Trento, fully competent, declared his refusal of blood transfusions, and requested transfer to another center equipped for bloodless medicine. In a short time, his condition worsened, he was taken to the operating room under general anesthesia and operated on; a large lesion of the subclavian was found. The team contacted the on-call magistrate by phone, who authorized the physicians to transfuse the patient. The patient awoke and claimed moral damages for being forced, against his explicit wishes, to receive blood. The Trento court rejected the claim. The patient appealed to the Court of Appeal, which also rejected the claim. The patient then appealed to the Supreme Court, with the same outcome and very interesting final reasoning.

declaration unequivocally expresses the will to prevent transfusion even in the event of life-threatening circumstances."

This was the case of a pregnant woman at term who was admitted for a scheduled cesarean section, fully conscious and carrying a detailed declaration refusing blood transfusions. During her hospitalization, the woman reiterated verbally to the physicians her refusal of transfusions, even in the face of life-threatening risk; she handed over her advance directives in which she specified that her choice was based on religious conviction. After the cesarean section, the woman suffered severe hemorrhage: the physicians proceeded with exploratory laparotomy and, despite the woman's explicit refusal in every possible way, subjected her—while conscious—to as many as seven blood transfusions. The woman filed a complaint against the physicians and the hospital, seeking damages for the forced transfusions, which she considered a violation of her right to self-determination and experienced as a true personal assault.

At first instance, the Milan Court rejected the woman's claims because: (a) by accepting the exploratory laparotomy, the woman had implicitly consented to all related procedures, including transfusions; (b) her refusal had been expressed without real awareness of the risk of death. The woman appealed, and the Milan Court of Appeal upheld the first instance decision.

The Supreme Court, however, with *ruling no. 29469 of 2020*, overturned the opinions of the lower courts and ruled in favor of the patient, with the following reasoning [20].

The Supreme Court held that consent to surgery is one thing, consent to transfusion is another: in this specific case, refusal of transfusion is not overridden by consent to surgery. The physician dealing with such cases must clearly understand that the strength of such a refusal is more akin to a "conscientious objection," rooted in religious grounds.

Furthermore, if the patient specifically refuses a medical treatment, it is irrelevant whether or not there is a risk to life; such refusal becomes insurmountable. According to the Supreme Court, a refusal made with full capacity does not lose its validity if the patient later becomes incapacitated or if a life-threatening situation arises [21]. Moreover, refusal of transfusion therapy for religious reasons actually suggests a stable and enduring will, stemming from unconditional adherence to religious precepts.

27.5 The Role of the Physician and Medical Liability

Let us begin with the pressing concern of possible civil and criminal liability. According to Law 219/2017, when the physician acts in accordance with the patient's autonomy and adverse consequences result from the patient's refusal, the physician is exempt from civil and criminal liability. In fact, to date, criminal jurisprudence has held physicians criminally liable for assault if they proceed with a transfusion against the patient's wishes: today, therefore, the physician is at greater risk of prosecution if they do not respect the refusal and perform the transfusion.

However, from a medicolegal perspective, some "risky" scenarios can be envisaged, in the sense of potential disputes, even when the refusal is respected:

1. The medical record contains inadequate information and consent/refusal forms, meaning it does not clearly show that the patient's choice was complete, informed, clear, explicit, unequivocal, and current.
2. It is not documented that the patient was provided with information regarding alternatives to transfusion.
3. It has not been verified that an adequate bloodless surgery support program is actually available and operational within the healthcare facility.
4. The information provided to the patient did not include a comprehensive explanation of all possible surgical complications, the incidence of bleeding, or the possibility of accidental vascular injuries that could suddenly alter the hemorrhagic risk profile.

This contribution aims to encourage the adoption of specific tools to ensure that information is "appropriate and safe." The medical record must contain written documentation of the information process, detailing all information provided to the TG patient, both regarding the type of surgical procedure proposed and the transfusions and feasible alternatives available within the healthcare facility. The information must include the statistical incidence of general risks, be dated, and signed by both the physician and the patient. Typically, there is a separate information form dedicated to transfusions, which must also be provided to the patient.

Subsequently, after allowing a reasonable period for the patient to review the information, the consent form (commonly referred to as "consent") should be presented: in the case of consent to the procedure and refusal of transfusions, consent to the surgery should first be obtained with a signature, after personalizing the form to include a detailed focus on hemorrhagic risk, the possibility of accidental vascular or visceral injuries which, depending on the anatomical site, could alter the hemorrhagic risk profile, with a concrete explanation of the irreversibility of anemia and the pathophysiology leading naturally to death. Then, on the transfusion-specific form, the patient will sign the refusal—which can be revoked at any time—and any real alternative measures for managing potential hemorrhage, if available, should be specified.

Advance Directives (DAT) deserve special mention. TGs have demonstrated prompt compliance with Law 219, and we expect that, in most cases, TG patients undergoing elective surgery will have DAT. Even in these cases, it is appropriate to submit the institutional information and consent forms, attaching the DAT to the medical record. Real concerns arise in the case of a patient without DAT:

- The patient is admitted for a scheduled procedure, is alert and conscious, has adequate mental *competence*, and refuses transfusions: after providing the information and consent forms, the refusal must be respected, even if the patient later becomes unconscious and experiences hemorrhage requiring transfusion.

- The patient arrives unconscious and anemic, requires urgent surgery, no proxy is present to provide DAT, but a family member reports the patient's religious beliefs and refusal of transfusions: the physician is required to use all available means, including transfusion. In this case, the will reported by third parties, the so-called surrogate will, is not sufficient.
- The patient is in a state of natural incapacity due to impaired consciousness and presents with stable anemia, with ongoing blood loss, and the possibility of a non-urgent procedure. Family members report religious beliefs or provide an unvalidated written statement: this is a case of a deferrable procedure, and especially in the presence of insistent family members, there is time to involve a Guardianship Judge in the decision, even though technically the situation is similar to the previous scenario: an invalid document does not preclude the use of all available means.

Finally, it is important to mention one last aspect provided for by Law 219: "*the patient cannot demand healthcare treatments that are contrary to the law, to professional ethics, or to good clinical practice; in response to such requests, the physician has no professional obligations*."

If a surgical procedure is planned in which hemorrhagic risk is "inherent" and virtually 100% predictable, the patient's refusal may entitle the physician to decline to perform the procedure, provided the patient has first been clearly informed—in writing—that this specific bloodless operation would be incompatible with life and there would be no hope of survival.

Conversely, in the presence of a low hemorrhagic risk, the patient must be given accurate and timely information, including the possibility of unpredictable or barely predictable and unpreventable events that could lead to death; if the patient signs the refusal, and hemorrhagic events and death subsequently occur, no blame can be attributed to the physician.

A very important element, in terms of medical liability, is to have a clear and appropriate pathway for the management of hemorrhagic emergencies, both in general and especially in TG patients. From a medicolegal perspective, an evaluative issue may arise if, during the procedure, the surgeon causes an accidental vascular injury resulting in a complication that becomes fatal because it cannot be treated with the most appropriate means.

The Supreme Court ruling discussed in the previous paragraph serves as a safeguard for both patients and healthcare professionals, who require certainty and guarantees, relieving them as much as possible from the feeling of working between a rock and a hard place when faced with the refusal of blood transfusions by Jehovah's Witnesses [22].

The dilemma: should one respect the patient's wishes and refrain from transfusing, with the fear that, in the event of an adverse outcome, civil and criminal actions may follow, or proceed with the transfusion despite the patient's refusal, thereby also risking civil and criminal actions from the patient? The evolution of case law and Law 219 appears to have clarified these doubts and concerns.

27.6 Strategies for the Healthcare Management of Jehovah's Witness Patients: Approaches to Ensure Appropriate Medical Care Without Blood Transfusions

While it is well known that Jehovah's Witnesses refuse allogeneic blood transfusions, many people, including healthcare professionals, are unaware of their openness to the use of blood products [23]. Jehovah's Witnesses refuse transfusions of whole blood (including preoperative autologous donations) and primary blood components such as red cells, white cells, platelets, and unfractionated plasma, as well as hemoglobin (both natural and recombinant). However, since 2000, they have been free, as a matter of "individual conscience," to use derivatives of primary blood components, hemoglobin-based blood substitutes, interferons, interleukins, albumin, globulins, cryoprecipitates, coagulation factor concentrates—including fibrinogen concentrates and immunoglobulins [24]. Generally, there are no objections to a number of medical procedures, such as blood donation, autologous blood transfusion (if maintained in a continuous circuit with the patient), organ transplantation (if the blood is drained), dialysis, intraoperative cell salvage, and acute normovolemic hemodilution, provided these are also maintained in a continuous circuit, as well as apheresis and cardiopulmonary bypass. The use of bloodless heart-lung machines is also permitted if extracorporeal circulation is uninterrupted. Recombinant products such as erythropoiesis-stimulating agents, granulocyte colony-stimulating factors, and pharmacological agents (intravenous iron or tranexamic acid) are also acceptable. While they refuse allogeneic blood, Jehovah's Witnesses often consent to blood management techniques and procedures that involve temporary diversion of autologous blood (e.g., autotransfusion); as previously mentioned, for healthcare professionals this represents both a clinical challenge and an ethical and medicolegal dilemma, specifically whether to accept or reject the Jehovah's Witness patient's refusal of a life-saving blood transfusion—a refusal that could result in death [25]. For many physicians, the refusal of transfusion by Jehovah's Witnesses is a significant challenge.

The international literature highlights the urgent need to develop greater cultural and technical competence in so-called Bloodless Medicine, which should be an integral part of coordinated and personalized care, with particular attention to keeping Jehovah's Witness patients and their families fully informed.

Medical and scientific knowledge regarding alternatives to transfusion must first be enhanced among healthcare professionals, and every healthcare facility should dedicate part of its training to deepening these aspects, with the aim of providing the best possible care not only to Jehovah's Witnesses. In essence, the alternatives that can be offered to patients must be carefully assessed, especially in terms of the facility's preparedness and the practical availability of a "bloodless" care pathway.

27.7 Conclusions

The patient's autonomy must be respected: this is the primary factor guiding every action. For this autonomy to be effective, the patient must be able to make choices consistent with their values, even when these may appear imprudent. The State, and therefore public healthcare professionals, cannot interfere with individual freedom in healthcare matters; at the same time, we as physicians must ensure that patients receive the most detailed information about proposed therapies and obtain from the patient a decision that, according to the Supreme Court, is "informed, clear, explicit, unequivocal, and current." What tools do we have to achieve a balance between these needs? The therapeutic relationship, knowledge symmetry, and a written record of all information provided, with the patient's consent being both informed and valid. Future developments in the field of healthcare liability and medical ethics will mainly concern the accuracy and preparedness in managing bloodless surgery, taking into account the alternatives to transfusion often accepted by Jehovah's Witness patients.

References

1. Law 2019/2017 "Provisions on informed consent and advance healthcare directives".
2. Consorti P. Freedom to choose therapy and medical violence. Brief considerations on the refusal of blood transfusions by Jehovah's Witnesses. State, Churches and Religious Pluralism; 2021.
3. Gianmatteo J, et al. Self-determination and healthcare responsibility: blood transfusions in Jehovah's witness patients. Medical Practice and Legal Aspects; 2017.
4. Rajtar M. Bioethics and religious bodies: refusal of blood transfusions in Germany. Soc Sci Med. 2013; 98:271-7.
5. Kottow MJ. Euthanasia after the holocaust—is it possible? A report from the Federal Republic of Germany. Bioethics. 1988;
6. Bock GL. Jehovah's witnesses and autonomy: honouring the refusal of blood transfusion. J Med Ethics. 2012;
7. O'Neill C. Jehovah's witnesses and blood transfusions: an analysis of the legal protections afforded to adults and children in European/English human rights contexts. Eur J Health Law. 2017;
8. Deneyer M, et al. Legislation and refusal of blood transfusion by a minor Jehovah's witness in Belgium. Acta Chir Belg. 2016;
9. Domaradzki J, et al. Between autonomy and paternalism: attitudes of nursing personnel towards Jehovah's witnesses' refusal of blood transfusion. Int J Public Health. 2023;
10. Zalewska-Puchaca J, et al. Attitudes of polish nurses towards representatives of certain religions. BMC Nurs. 2022;
11. Gopakumar KG, et al. Jehovah's Witness and consent for blood transfusion in a child: the Indian scenario. Asian J Transfus Sci. 2017;
12. Marsh JC, et al. Hematological care of the Jehovah's witness patient. Br J Hematol. 2002;
13. Petrini C. Ethical and legal aspects of refusal of blood transfusions by Jehovah's witnesses, with particular reference to Italy. Blood Transfus. 2014;
14. Takashima AKK, et al. Ethical and legal duty of anesthesiologist regarding Jehovah's witness patient: care protocol. Revista Brasilera de Anestesiologia. 2016;
15. Chiumello D, Lavorato MC, Faraone C. Between emergency, end of life, and the right to knowledge: informed consent in anesthesia and intensive care. ATI; 2023.
16. Supreme Court, judgment of February 23, 2007.

17. Supreme Court, judgment no. 23676 of September 2008.
18. Supreme Court, judgment of June 7, 2017 no. 14158.
19. Supreme Court, judgment of May 15, 2019 no. 12998.
20. Supreme Court, judgment of January 15, 2020 no. 515.
21. Papini et al. Commentary on Supreme Court Judgment no. 29469/2020, Biodiritto, 2021.
22. Op. sub. cit. 20.
23. Knapp van Bogaer D, et al. Ethics and medicine: Jehovah's witnesses and the new blood transfusion rules. S Afr Fam Pract. 2013;
24. Bodnaruk ZM, et al. Meeting the clinical challenge of care for Jehovah's witnesses. Transfus Med Rev. 2004;18(2):105–16.
25. West JM. Ethical issues inherent to Jehovah's witnesses. Curr Opin Anaesth. 2014;

Kolibri 360 GmbH
Ferdinand-Jühlke-Straße 7
99095 Erfurt, Deutschland
produktsicherheit@kolibri360.de